CONDENSE WISDOM
and
CONQUER CANCER
for the
BENEFIT OF MANKIND

HOW TO CONQUER CANCER? HOW TO TREAT CANCER?

Part II

Xu Ze; Xu Jie; Bin Wu

authorHOUSE

AuthorHouse™
1663 Liberty Drive
Bloomington, IN 47403
www.authorhouse.com
Phone: 1 (800) 839-8640

Published by AuthorHouse 02/13/2018

ISBN: 978-1-5462-1971-2 (sc)
ISBN: 978-1-5462-1970-5 (e)

Library of Congress Control Number: 2017917861

Print information available on the last page.

Table of Contents

A Brief Introduction to the First Author

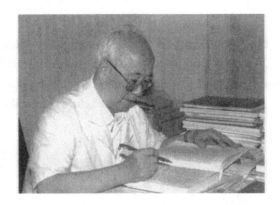

Xu Ze, male, born in Leping County of Jiangxi Province in Oct. 1933, gradated from Tongji Medical University in 1956, successively held the post of director of department of surgery of Affiliated Hospital of Hubei College of Traditional Chinese Medicine, professor, chief physician, tutor of postgraduate and doctoral student, President of Experimental Surgery Restitute Institute of Hubei College of Traditional Chinese Medicine, Director of Abdominal Tumor Surgery Research Room and Director of Anti Carcinomatous Metastasis and Reoccurrence Research Room. in addition, he held concurrent posts of Standing Director of China Medical Association Wuhan Branch, Vice President of Wuhan Micro-circulation Academy, Academic Member of International Liver Disease Research, Cooperation and Exchange Center, Member of International Surgeon Union, Standing Member of 1st, 2nd, 3rd and 4th Editorial Board of China Experimental Surgery Journal, Standing Member of 1st, 2dn and 3rd Editorial Board of Abdominal Surgery Journal. Enjoying Special Allowance of State Council.

He has been engaged in surgery work for 49 years and accumulated rich experience in radical operation of lung cancer, esophageal carcinoma, liver cancer, carcinoma of gallbladder, adenocarcinoma of pancreas, gastric carcinoma and intestinal cancer as well as in clinical therapy with Chinese Traditional Medicine combined with Western Medicine of prevention of reoccurrence and metastasis after operation.

He has been engaged in scientific research of surgery for 15 years and obtained many fruits, among which the task of Experimental Study and Clinical Application of Self-made Type Z-C1 Abdominal Cavity---Vein Flow Turning Unit in Therapy of Chronic Ascites of Hepatic Cirrhosis issued by Science Commission of Hubei Province was awarded Second Prize of Scientific Fruit by People's Government of Hubei Province and was popularized and applied in 38 hospitals in 12 provinces all over the country in 1982. The task "Experimental Study on Physiological Mechanism and Pathogenesis of

Schistosome with Method of Experimental Surgery", issued by National Natural Fund Commission was awarded Second Prize of Scientific Fruit by People's Government of Hubei Province in 1986.

He began to study the tumor experience, established the tumor animal model and metastasis and reoccurrence animal model and probed into the mechanism and rules of carcinomatous metastasis and reoccurrence to find out the method to inhibit the metastasis. 48 kinds of Chinese traditional herbs that could counteract the intrusion, metastasis and reoccurrence were found and selected from a large number of natural herbs. Based on this, he invented and developed China Xu Ze (Z-C) Medicine Treating Malignancy, which had remarkable curative effects through over 10 years' clinical validation of many cases.

He has been engaged in teaching for 40 years and has cultivated many young doctors, 10 masters and 2 doctors. He has released 126 papers, published New Understanding and New Mode of Therapy of Cancer as the editor in charge, participate in writing 8 medical exclusive books including Therapeutics of Liver Disease, Surgery of Liver, Gallbladder and Pancreas and Surgical Operation of Abdomen.

A Brief Introduction to the Second Author

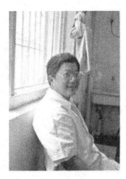

Xu Jie, male, graduated from Hubei College of Traditional Chinese Medicine in 1992, graduated from Hubei Medical University in 1996, Department of Clinical Medicine. Now He is chief physician in Hubei University of Traditional Chinese Medicine Hospital and Hubei Provincial Hospital of Surgery, engaged in experimental surgical tumor research and general surgery, urology clinical work.

Since 1992, he has been involved in the experimental tumor research of the Institute of Experimental Surgery of Hubei College of Traditional Chinese Medicine. He has carried out cancer cell transplantation and established a tumor animal model. He has carried out a series of experimental tumor research: exploring the mechanism of recurrence and metastasis of cancer and in vivo screening experiment of more than 200 kinds of Chinese herbal medicine in vivo tumor model of tumor inhibition s from a large number of natural medicine to find out, screening out of 48 kinds of anti-cancer invasion, metastasis, relapse traditional Chinese medicine

He participates in clinical validation and followed up for XZ - C immunoregulatory Chinese herbal medicine and completes the experimental research and clinical verification, data collection, collection and summary of this book.

A Brief Introduction to the Third Author and the main Translator and one of the Editors

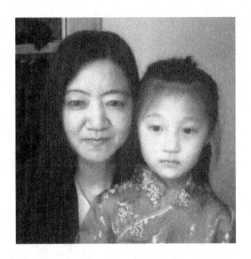

Bin Wu, MD, Ph.D., graduated from College of Yunyang of Tongji University of Medical Sciences for her MD degree; Studied her Master degree and her Ph. D degree in Sun Yat-Sen University of Medical Sciences. After she received her Ph.D., she worked as a Post-doctoral Follews in the Johns Hopkins Medical School and University of Maryland Medical School. She passed her USMLE tests and is going to do her residency training in America. She dedicated herself to oncology clinical and research. Her goal is to conquer cancer, which she believes this great contribution to our health. She has a daughter, named Lily Xu who drew all of the pictures in this book.

A Brief introduction to the Illustrator and the Advisor

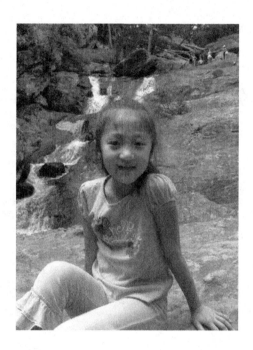

Lily Xu was born on November 17th 2006 and had an art presented in the Walter Art Museum in Baltimore at the age of 6; she got the fourth place trophy in the ES Double Digits or 24 and 24 games in the Baltimore County in Maryland; she got the first trophy in the BCPS STEM FAIR PHYSICS in Baltimore County; when she was in the sixth grade, she passed the advanced Math for 7th grade(which means the 8th grade math) test and moved the 8th grade math class; she loves the reading and the writing and she finished many seires of books. She got $3000 scholarship award for the Peabody music program in the Johns Hopkins University. She edits all of my books for the publication. She is a very smart advisor on the computer and on some medical-related topics.

Science is endless

XU ZE think of conquering cancer, where is the road? The road is in the scientific research – the road is on the prevention and treatment of cancer scientific research and the road is the study under the guidance of the concept of the scientific development.

Science is an endless frontier, our scientific work has followed the scientific concept of development, based on the known medical, future-oriented medicine, the new disciplines,interdisciplinary, cross-disciplinary,basedon the known material science, to explore the future of science and unknown knowledge, look forward, through the static mind, a long-term hard work and practice the scientific concept of development , in scientific, difficult journey , a scientific step by step and step, to the forefront of science, for innovative and forward, to overcome cancer research hall brick by Tim watts.

Preface

This book is to help with conquering cancer and with launching a total attack and with building the scientific city of conquering cancer.

The overall design and the planning and the blueprint of XZ-C 's conquering cancer are the scientific thinking and the theoretical innovation and the experimental basis of conquering cancer are the reform and development of the overall strategy of cancer treatment and the crystallization of my 60 years of experience in medical work and 30 years of the scientific research results and achievement and the scientific and technological innovation and the scientific thinking and the scientific research wisdom which the direction of the research is to conquering cancer. It is proposed that to set up a test area sitting in Wuhan City, Huang Jiahu University City; the implementation of this research program will be done by my research team experts, professors ... ... and so.

The scientific research plan of conquering cancer is put into the focused on scientific research in the international and is the forefront of science.

In January 12th, 2016 the US President Barack Obama in the State of the Union addressed the national cancer program of "to conquer cancer" and named the new moon plan (Cancer moon shot) which is responsible by the vice president Joe Biden for the implementation which its specific plan is unknown.

Cancer is a disaster of the mankind. It must struggle with cancer all over the world and people of the world struggle together and gather wisdom and move forward together to overcome cancer.

Cancer disaster is covered by the world. The people worldwide are eager to overcome the cancer one day. It is the urgent hope that the states and the governments and the experts and the scholars and the scientists can find anti-cancer measures to keep people from cancer.

Acknowledgements

This book is for all of people who concern human being health. We are deep grateful to all of people who like our new ways to improve our human being health.

My daughter Lily Xu gives me many smart and creative ideas while we were finishing this book. Lily Xu drew all of the pictures such as the Thymus etc.

I would like to express our sincere gratitude to the following:

1. All of Authorhouse staffs
2. Dr. Xu Ze's family and Dr. Xu Jie's family
3. Mrs. Bo Wu's family and Mrs. Tao Wu's famly: espeicaly their daughters Chongshu Luo and Xunyue Wang
4. Medchi CEO: Gene Ransom III gives us great help

Bin Wu, M.D., Ph.D

In October, 2017 in Baltimore , Maryland in USA

The Guidance Information

Condense Wisdom and Conquer Cancer
------ for the benefit of mankind

How to conquer cancer? how to prevent cancer by my opinions?how to treat cancer by my opinions

Table of Contents

1, the guidance to read

2, the guidance words

3, the guidance to act

I, the guidance to read

1), In this medical monograph the book is divided into the next two parts, a total of 10 volumes, which wisdom are condensed to be used to conquer cancer?

Part I (Volume 1-4) condense how to conquer cancer and how to prevent cancer by my opinions

Part II (5-10 volumes) condense how to conquer cancer and how to treat cancer by my opinions?

Prevention cancer and anti-cancer, and the prevention is as the main are the health work policy, especially the prevention cancer for the top priority so that people can be away from cancer to reduce cancer incidence.

This is a medical monograph with the more complete and more systematic and more comprehensive design and more specific planning of how to conquer cancer which can be used as the reference for the various countries and the provinces and the states to carry out the implementation of how to overcome cancer? How to prevent cancer? How to control cancer? How to treat cancer?

2), the agglutination of the following wisdom which can be used to overcome cancer:

PART ONE

CONDENSE HOW TO CONQUER CANCER? HOW TO PREVENT CANCER I SEE.

VOLUME I

(A), How to overcome cancer? XZ-C proposed three targets

After analysis: XZ-C proposed that the target or the goal of conquering cancer should be:

A. target: it should be directed against the gene mutations and the abnormal expression or the deletion.
B. target: it should be for environmental factors:
    The external environment ----- air, water, soil, physical, chemical, biological factors, clothing, food, shelter.
    The internal environment -------immune, endocrine, neurohumoral
    It should create "the environmental protection research institute" and carry out   the prevention cancer system engineering research.
C. target: it should be to adjust the normal immune system and to restore the immune system to identify cancer cells, thereby remove tumor cells, and conduct the immunotherapy and the immunoprophylaxis.

(B), how to overcome cancer? XZ-C presents: two wheels

The details of the situation analysis (a), (b), (c), (d)
The basic situation is:
The United States:

life sciences, biomedicine, genetic engineering, targeted therapy, drugs, minimally invasive techniques, instruments , and precision medicine are far ahead.

China:

It has the rich resources of the immune regulation and control traditional Chinese medication and the immune regulation traditional Chinese medications, the traditional Chinese medications with activating blood and removing stasis and anti-microvascular thrombosis and anti-micrometastasis as well as the traditional Chinese medication which controls precancerous nodules by soften the firm and scatter the knot.

It should cooperate complement each other and move forward together.

(C). Why is the cooperation between China and the United States?

Because:

    (1) in 1971 the US Congress passed a "national cancer regulations", and President Nixon issued "anti-cancer declaration" in order to overcome cancer in one fell swoop.

    (2) In January 12, 2016 US President Barack Obama announced **" the national plan to conquer cancer"** and the plan is responsible by Vice President Joe Biden.

The Plan name: **"Cancer moon shot"**

The Goal: to overcome cancer

    (3) In 2011 Chinese doctor Xu Ze put forward in his published monographs: " the strategic thinking and suggestions of conquering cancer."

In August 2013 at the International Cancer Conference it was put forward " the XZ-C research program of conquering cancer and launch a total attack "

In July 2015 it proposed" the dawn of the C-type plan of conquering cancer and launch a total attack "

In December 2016 in the English version of the monograph it was put forward " the initiative of conquering cancer and launch the general attack."

Therefore: China and the United States both are conducting the scientific research of conquering cancer and it should be co-operation and move forward toward the scientific hall of conquering cancer.

(VOLUME II)

What wisdom is condensed which can be used to overcome cancer?

Its focus is:

- How to prevent cancer I see and how to carry out conquering cancer and launching a total attack?
- How to create the scientific research bases and the Science city with a multidisciplinary and cancer research group?
- it must create an "Innovative Oncology School" and a graduate school in order to o overcome cancer.
- it must set up To overcome the cancer, it must create " the prevention and treatment hospital with innovative tumor integrated traditional Chinese and Western medications during tumor whole process and the prevention, control and treatment of cancer are at the same attention in order to conquer cancer.
- it must create an "Innovative Molecular Cancer Institute" in order to overcome cancer.
- it must create "Innovative Environmental Protection Cancer Research Institute" and prevention cancer system engineering.

VOLUME III

What wisdom is condensed which can be used to conquer cancer?

Its focus is:

How to prevent cancer I see: how to prevent cancer from the big environment and the small environment?

- How to prevent cancer from clothing, food, shelter, and walking?
- it should be carried out prevention cancer from improving carcinogenic factors in external causes (external environment) and internal causes (internal environment).
- Environmental and cancer research groups should be set up to study the relationship between environment and cancer.
- To study what the carcinogenic factors are in the environment and how should they be prevented?
- XZ-C proposes to create the "Innovative Environmental Protection Institute" and the prevention cancer system project
- How can we prevent cancer from "two types of society"?
- The catastrophe of cancer is the global and the people of the world must struggle with it and struggle together.

VOLUME IV

What wisdom is condensed which can be used to conquer cancer?

Its focus is:

- the proposals was put forward «cancer treatment reform, innovation and development.»
- XZ-C proposes a plan to tackle the total attack on cancer.
- it was put forward the necessity and feasibility of proposing a total attack on cancer.
- it was proposed "the general design and imagine of conquer cancer and the basic design of the Science City" and the feasibility report.
- it was put forward the suggestions that at the same time when a well-off society is constructed, the ride research is built and the scientific research on prevention cancer and anti-cancer is conducted.

PART II

THE AGGLOMERATION OF HOW TO OVERCOME CANCER? EACH OPINION I SEE OF HOW TO TREAT CANCER IS THIS PART.

VOLUME V

What wisdom is condensed which can be used to conquer cancer?

Its focus is: "walked out of a new way to overcome cancer"

- From the experimental results it was found that: the thymus has the acute progressive atrophy in the host with inoculated cancer cells and the cell proliferation was blocked and the volume was significantly reduced.
- From the above experimental study it was found that thymic atrophy and the immune dysfunction may be one of the etiology and pathogenesis of the tumor, it must try to prevent from the thymic atrophy and to promote thymocyte proliferation and to increase immune function.
- In order to try to prevent thymic atrophy and to promote thymocyte hyperplasia and to increase immune function, it was to find from both the traditional Chinese medication and Western medication. In western medication there is rare medication which can improve immunity and promote the proliferation of thymocytes so that it was changed from the Chinese medication to find because in the traditional Chinese medication the increasing tonic drugs generally have immune regulation.
- After 7 years of laboratory scientific research, XZ-C1-10 immune regulation and control anti-cancer and anti-transfer medications were screened out from the natural and traditional Chinese medication and composed of which can protect the thymus and the hematopiene in bone marrow . On the basis of the success of the animal experiment The clinical validation work was performed, after 20 years of more than 12,000 cases of cancer specialist clinical application it achieved good results.
- After the experimental study and the anti-cancer research of Chinese medicine immunopharmacology and the combination of Chinese and Western medications on the molecular level, it walked out of a new path of conquering cancer with XZ-C immune regulation and control which regulates immune activity, prevents thymus atrophy, promotes thymocyte proliferation, protects bone marrow hematopoietic function, improves immune surveillance and with the Combination of Chinese and Western medication----the "Chinese - style anti - cancer" new road.

VOLUME VI

What wisdom is condensed which can be used to conquer cancer?

Its focus is:

- During more than 20 years it has been walked out of a new path to overcome the cancer and has formed the theoretical system of XZ-C immune regulation and control and has undergone the clinical application, observation and verification.
- The new model that it is considered cancer treatment is that **healing should be done through immunoregulation rather than a single killer**, and the last step in curing cancer is to regain the control of the host's immune regulation and control function rather than destroy the last cancer cells.
- From the experimental results to analyze thinking, the new revelation is that : thymus atrophy are immune dysfunction are one of the factors of the cause and pathogenesis of cancer so that in the international academic conference Xu Ze Professor proposed that one of the cause and the pathogenesis of cancer may be thymus atrophy, central immune organ motility damage, immune dysfunction, immune surveillance capacity decline and immune escape.
- Based on the findings of the laboratory above experimental results, the treatment principle must be to prevent thymus atrophy, promote thymic hyperplasia, protect bone marrow hematopoietic function, improve immune surveillance, control malignant cells immune escape.
- XZ-C (XU-ZE-China) immunoregulation therapy was first presented by Professor Xu Ze in his book "New Concepts and Methods for Cancer Transfer Treatment" in 2006, and he believes **that under the normal circumstances, both cancer and body defense are in a dynamic balance ; the occurrence of cancer is caused by this dynamic imbalance. If the state has been adjusted to the normal level, you can control the growth of cancer and make it subside.**
- **It is well known that the occurrence, progression and prognosis of cancer is determined by a combination of two factors, namely, the biological characteristics of cancer cells and the host body itself; if the balance between the two can be controlled, the cancer cells can be controlled; if the two are imbalance, the cancer will occur and develop.**
- Cancer treatment should be changed to observe and establish **a comprehensive treatment concept.**

The goal of treatment only kill cancer cells which is only one aspect and it is one-sided treatment concept and it can not overcome cancer. **The goal of treatment should be in both the areas of the host and cancer cells and not only kill cancer cells , but also protect the host, enhance immune function and protect thymus and increase immune functions and protect the hematopiene of the bone marrow and enhance the host anti-cancer ability; this is a comprehensive treatment concept, it is possible to overcome cancer.**

Therefore, the principle of cancer treatment should change the concept and it should establish a comprehensive treatment concept.

VOLUME VII

What wisdom is condensed which can be used to conquer cancer?

To challenge the status quo of cancer treatment and to reform can develop.

Its focus is:

- the review and the analysis and the questioning of the three major treatments for cancer

Through the review and the analysis and the reflection it is found the traditional problems and shortcomings of traditional therapy.

- The analysis and the evaluation and the questioning of systemic intravenous chemotherapy for solid tumors:

The analysis and questioning of whether the method and the route of the systemic intravenous administration for the solid tumors are scientific and reasonable or not?

The analysis and questioning of whether the method of calculating the dose of the systemic intravenous chemotherapy for the solid tumors is reasonable or not?

The analysis and query on the evaluation standard of Intravenous Chemotherapy and Curative Effect of Solid Tumor.

- the century review, analysis and comment of the three major treatments for cancer.

Respectively, the problems existing in the surgery and the radiotherapy and the chemotherapy are analyzed and commented:

The Surgical treatment:

Comments:

It is the main technology and the main treatment method in the future of conquering cancer. The surgical treatment of cancer is the exact and effective method.

The Radiation Therapy:

Comments:

The radiotherapy is for local treatment and the transfer is the entire body and the systemic problems which is a major contradiction. The reason for its failure is not for the transfer and is not for controlling the transfer because the main problem of cancer treatment is to anti-transfer and how to play its role during anti-transfer therapy which must be carefully considered and in-depth study.

The Chemotherapy:

Comment 1:

Comment on the route of administration of systemic intravenous chemotherapy

This route of administration is not the real point of targeted administration, but through the heart pump to the blood spray to the body and has the whole body cytotoxic distribution and the whole body target so that the whole body organs obtain the cytotoxic. It is very unreasonable and is very unscientific . The result is:

① very few foci cancer, only about 0.4%, the effect is minimal (because the foci accounts for a small body surface area and is very small proportion).

② 99.6% of the cytotoxic kill to the body of normal cells, causing the adverse reaction to the brain, heart, liver, lung, kidney, gastrointestinal system, hematopoietic system, the immune system, endocrine system.

The toxic side effects of these chemotherapy is irrational route of administration, which should be avoided.

Therefore, this route of intravenous chemotherapy is unreasonable, unscientific, easily lead to iatrogenic toxic side effects.

How to do? Should it be reformed? should it be changed the route of administration into target organ intravascular chemotherapy pathways? the drug can directly go the "target" organs so that the dose is very small, effective, no side effects, and is conducive to patients.

Comment 2:

The assessment of the dose calculation of the solid body tumor intravenous chemotherapy is applied according to the experience and methods of leukemia treatment; the guiding ideology is calculated by the body surface area, which is unwise, unreasonable, easy to lead Iatrogenic toxic side effects.

Why?

It is because solid tumors are confined to an organ, it should not be calculated with whole body surface area, which is unreasonable and unscientific.

Comment 3:

The evaluation of the efficacy evaluation criteria for the solid tumor systemic intravenous chemotherapy:

The current assessment criteria for the efficacy of solid tumors are:

a, the size of the tumor; b, remission periods, remission (CR, PR) - as the name suggests, to be ease is not cured and it is only the improvement in a few short weeks; after this short-term improvement, it will progress, increase, transfer, so that to be ease is not the purpose of treatment, it can not be cured and it can only alleviate and it is only the short-term relief, so that this is not the desired purpose of the patients and should not be the goal of treatment.

Comment 4:

Why did the abdomen solid tumor after adjuvant chemotherapy fail to prevent the recurrence and metastasis of cancer ? In the abdominal solid tumor (gastric cancer, cardiac cancer, colorectal cancer, liver cancer, gallbladder cancer, pancreatic cancer, abdominal tumor) the postoperative adjuvant chemotherapy is the systemic intravenous chemotherapy, this way from the vena cava can not directly reach the portal vein.

Abdominal solid tumor cancer cells are mainly in the portal vein system; the vena cava system and the portal vein system is generally not connected; the medications administered by the superior vena cava can not reach the portal vein so that this route of administration is unreasonable, does not meet the anatomy ,not scientific.

Comment 5:

There are some important errors and shortcomings in current chemotherapy.

Chemotherapy can suppress immune function and inhibit the bone marrow hematopoietic function so that the overall immune function decreased. In cancer patients thymus is inhibited and chemotherapy can inhibit bone marrow, as "snow adds frog or worse" so that the entire central immune organs are damaged and it promotes the further decline in immune surveillance and it may cause that while chemotherapy , cancer metastasis ; the more treatment , the more chemotherapy.

VOLUME VIII

What wisdom is condensed which can be used to conquer cancer?

The Study on Anti - cancer Traditional Chinese Medication of XZ - C Immunomodulation

Its focus is:

(1) In our laboratory the experimental study of finding and screening anti-cancer and anti-transfer medications was conducted from the Chinese medications:

    1.) **The in vitro culture method of cancer cells was used to study the anti-tumor rate of Chinese herbal medication.**

        a, in vitro screening test: the cancer cells were used in vitro culture to observe the direct damage to cancer cells.

        b, the test in the tube screening test: in the tubes which the cancer cells were cultured, the biological crude products (500ug / m) were placed to observe whether it could inhibit the cancer cells.

    2.) To make the animal models and to do the experimental study on the tumor inhibition rate of Chinese herbal medications:

Each group of mice were divided into 8 groups, each group of 30, the group 7 for the blank control group, the group 8 with 5-F or CTX as the control group. The whole mice groups were inoculated with EAC or S180 or H22 cancer cells. After 24 hours of inoculation, each mouse was orally fed with the crude drug powder, and then the selected Chinese herbal medication was fed for a long period of time. The survival time and the medication toxicity and side effects were observed, and the survival rate was calculated and the tumor inhibition rate was calculated.

In this way, we conducted four consecutive years of experimental study, each year with more than 1,000 animals models, during 4 years there were the total of nearly 6000 cancer-bearing animal models; after each mouse died the pathological sections and the slides were made for the liver, spleen, kidney, lung , thymus, which a total has more than 20,000 slices.

The experimental results:

In our laboratory 200 kinds of Chinese herbal medications were screened through animal experiments and then screened out 48 kinds with the certain, even excellent tumor inhibition rate which is 75% -90% or more. During the experimental screening tests 152 kinds of Chinese herbal medication with no obvious anti-cancer effects were gotten rid of .

(2) The clinical validation:

On the basis of the success of the animal experiments the clinical validation was conducted and it was established the cancer specialist outpatient and it was retained outpatient medical records and each outpatient record was recorded. It established the regular follow-up observation system to observe long-term efficacy. The standard of the Observation of the efficacy of the standard is: the patients have the long survival time and the good quality of life.

After 30 years of the clinical application and verification in the cancer specialist outpatient service in more than 12000 cases of advanced patients XZ-C immunoregulation anti-cancer traditional Chinese medication preparation has achieved significant effect. XZ-C immunomodulatory medications can improve the quality of life of patients with advanced cancer and enhance immune function and increase the body's anti-cancer ability and enhance appetite and significantly extend the survival period.

VOLUME IX

What wisdom is condensed which can be used to conquer cancer?

The focus is:

(1) **how to carry out clinical research data summary and collation and expression?**

    ① China is a large country with 1.3 billion population and thus it is a large resource for cancer cases. China has a large number of cancer cases for the clinical observation and the analysis.

    In the daily clinical work the clinicians conduct the subtle observation of cancer and the careful thinking and the analysis and the actively exploring study. After the long-term accumulation of the practice medical experience it will also have some discovery and the development and the continuous progress; the medical research is to improve clinical diagnosis and treatment work. The medical research is to Improve the quality of medical care and medical level so that the clinical research work is also an important part of clinical work.

    ② **it creates a table form to explain the scientific research materials which can be achieve to be both concise and comprehensive and to be easy to read and easy to understand.** Through a few decades of the bitter and meticulous clinical research work it received a lot of scientific research data and experimental data and the summary and the collation and the collection. Through the table form for the narrative expression it is concise and structured and the readers can understand their core content in ten minutes.

    ③ to retain the outpatient medical records and the information accumulation about the outpatient visits, treatment, rehabilitation and follow-up; to fill in a complete detailed table outpatient medical records so as to obtain clinical validation of complete information and it is easy analysis, statistics and in order to facilitate follow-up treatment of patients.

If there is no preservation of the outpatient medical records, the analysis and the statistics of the outpatient efficacy of scientific research work can not be carried out.

    ④ to stay outpatient medical records is to observe the long-term efficacy, is conducive to clinical research outpatient to improve the quality of medical care.

VOLUME X

What wisdom is condensed which can be used to conquer cancer?

Its focus is:

- How to overcome the cancer ? I see one: the road to scientific research is the experimental basic research to explore the cause of cancer, pathogenesis, pathophysiology.

- **the experimental surgery is extremely important in the development of medication. It is a key to open the medical closed area, many diseases prevention and control methods were applied to the clinical practice after many animal experimental research to achieve a stable effect and promote the development of medical career.**

- We conducted a series of animal experiments to explore the etiology, pathogenesis and pathophysiology of cancer. We have obtained new findings from the experimental results. The new findings: thymus atrophy and the immune dysfunction are one of the the cause and pathogenesis of cancer.

- As a result of our laboratory study, we found that thymus has atrophy, and the central immune sensory has dysfunction, and the immune function decreases, and the immune surveillance decreases in the cancer-bearing mice. Therefore, the principle of treatment must be to prevent thymic atrophy and promote thymus Cell proliferation and protect bone marrow hematopoietic function and improve immune servillence . For the immune regulation of cancer, it provides a theoretical basis and experimental basis.

- **XZ-C believes that under normal circumstances the cancer and the body defense are in a dynamic balance . The occurrence of cancer is caused by dynamic imbalance. If the state has been adjusted to the normal level, you can control the growth of cancer and may make it subside.**

- **No matter how complex the mechanism behind cancer, immunosuppression is the key to cancer progression**. Removal of immunosuppressive factors and restoring the immune system to cancer cell recognition can effectively inhibit cancer. More and more evidence shows that by regulating the body's immune system, it is possible to achieve the purpose of cancer control. Through the activation of the body's anti-tumor immune system to treat tumors is currently the majority of researchers excited areas.

Second, the guidance words

1, It outlined the research process of anti-cancer research:

(A) a brief description of the research process of anti-cancer research

In 1985 I have done the petition for more than 3,000 cases of thoracic and abdominal cancer patients whose surgeries were operated by my own. The results were found that most patients had the recurrence and the metastasis and died within 2-3 years, and some were even after a few months, or 1 year. So that I realized that surgery was successful and the long-term efficacy was not satisfied and the postoperative recurrence and metastasis are a key factor affecting the long-term efficacy of surgery. And therefore it also raised a question: to study the prevention and treatment of postoperative recurrence and metastasis is the key to improve the survival. Therefore, it is the need for clinical basic research. If there is no breakthrough in basic research, the clinical efficacy is difficult to improve.

So we established the Institute of Experimental Surgery, from the following three aspects it took 30years to carry out a series of experimental research and clinical validation work:

(1) The experimental study of exploring the pathogenesis of cancer, invasion mechanism and recurrence and metastasis mechanism and of finding the effective control of invasion and the effective methods of cancer recurrence and metastasis.

I and my colleagues in our laboratory did the experimental tumor research work for a full four years; the research project topics are from the clinical problems and it attempted to explain or to solve some clinical problems through the experimental stud. All of them are the clinical basic research.

(2) The new drug experimental study of finding the new anti-cancer, anti-metastasis ad anti-recurrence from the natural herbal medication.

The existing anti-cancer drugs are that kill both cancer cells and the normal cells and have the toxic side effects . In our laboratory through the tumor-bearing mice in vivo tumor inhibition test, it was to find the new drugs that it only inhibited cancer cells without affecting the normal cells from the natural Chinese medication. We spent a total of three years in the laboratory testing 200 kinds of Chinese herbal medications which were the traditional commonly used anti-cancer prescription and reported anti-cancer prescriptions in the cancer-bearing animals in vivo tumor inhibition experiments to find the new drugs which only inhibit cancer cells without affecting the normal cells. The results: 48 kinds of Chinese medication with good tumor inhibition rate were screened out and at the same time with the better effect of increasing immune function and it was also found the traditional Chinese medication TG which could inhibit neovascularization.

(3) the clinical validation work: through the above four years of the basic experimental study to explore the recurrence and metastasis mechanism, and after three years of the basic experimental study screening the natural herbal medication it was found a group of XZ-C1-10 anti-cancer immune regulation traditional Chinese medications, and then through 30 years of clinical validation in

more than 12,000 cases of patients with advanced or postoperative metastatic cancer the application of XZ-C immunomodulation of traditional Chinese medication had achieved the good results, improved the quality of life, improved the symptoms and significantly prolonged survival period.

After the review, analysis, reflection of nearly 60 years of clinical practice cases and their own experience and more than 30 years of experimental results and discovery in the animal experiments, from the experimental to clinical, also from the clinical to the experiments and the data sorting and ummary of the collection from the experimental researches and clinical validation, it was published three monographs:1).In 67-year-old sixtieth year it was published the first monograph "new understanding and new model of cancer treatment " by Hubei Science and Technology Press in January 2001; 2).In 73 years old seventy years it was published the second monograph " new concepts and new methods of cancer metastasis treatment " by Beijing People's Medical Publishing House in January 2006;In April 2007 the People's Republic of China Publishing House issued a "three hundred" original book certificate.3).In 78 years old seventy years it was published the third monograph "new concept and new methods of cancer treatment " by Beijing People's Medical Publishing House in October 2011; followed by American medical doctor Dr. Bin Wu who translated it into English, the English version on March 26, 2013 was published in Washington, the international distribution; 4).The New Concept and the New Way Of Treatment of Cancer, published in Washington, DC in March 2013, in English, the international distribution of the third edition. 5).In 82-year-old it was published the fifth monograph "On Innovation of Treatment of Cancer" - "cancer treatment innovation" published in full English, worldwide in December 2015 in Washington, 6). At the age of 83 it was published the sixth monograph "New Concept and New Way of Treatment of Cancer Metastais" in August 2016 in Washington in the full English version, the global release;7).In 83 years old the seventh monograph "The Road To Over come Cancer" - to overcome the road of cancer in December 2016 in Washington, published in full English, the global release.

(B). The Cognition and Scientific Thinking of Our Scientific Research journey

Our 30 years of cancer research work research journey of ideological awareness and scientific research thinking can be divided into four stages :

(A) The first phase of 1985-- 1999

- Find problems from follow-up results → Ask questions → Research questions;
- From the review, analysis, reflection to find the questions existing in the current cancer traditional therapies and it needs to be further studied and improved;
- Recognize the existence of problems and it should change thinking and change ideas;
- summarized and organized and collected the information, it was publish the first monograph "new understanding and new model of cancer treatment " in January 2001 by Hubei Science and Technology Publishing House.

(B) The second phase after 2001 –

- The "target" and key of cancer research and treatment is anti-metastatic cancer therapy;

- Conducted a series of basic and clinical validation studies of anti-cancer metastasis, recurrence and rised to the theory of innovation, put forward new ideas, new methods of anti-metastasis;
- Summarized information, sorted into collection, published "new concepts and new methods of cancer metastasis treatment" second monograph January 2006 by People's Medical Publishing House, Xinhua Bookstore issued in April 2007 won the People's Republic of China and Publication issued by the department "Three hundred" original book award.

(C) The third phase after 2006 -

A. Study the whole process of development of cancer prevention and treatment;
B. Reform and innovation of cancer research and development ;
C. "three early" is the strategies of cancer prevention and treatment
D. I have been 60 years in the tumor surgery, more and more patients, the incidence of cancer is also on the rise, the mortality rate remains high, so I deeply appreciate, not only pay attention to the treatment of cancer, but also to focus on prevention from cancer source. There is a series of related studies, summary data, sorting and collection which was published in the third of my monograph "The new concept and a new approach to cancer treatment," in October 2011 by People's Medical Publishing House, Xinhua Bookstore. Later it was published in English on March 26, 2013 in Washington publication, international distribution.

(4) the fourth stage after 2011 -

- It is now the fourth stage of our research work, which is being carried out and developed ; the research work is conducted with step by step; the research goal or "target" is positioned to reduce the incidence of cancer, to improve the cure rate and to prolong the survival period.
- Our 30 years of cancer research work: the first three stages of experimental research and clinical research work were mainly in the treatment to study the new drugs, new methods of diagnosis, new technologies, new concepts of treatment, new methods.

But today in the 21ˢᵗ century, the second 10 years cancer is still rampant, the more treatment and the more patients, the incidence of cancer continues to rise, it has the high mortality rate so that I deeply appreciate that the cancer is not only to pay attention to treatment, but also to pay attention to prevention in order to stop at the source.

The current tumor hospital or oncology mode to go all out is to focus on treatment and aimed for patients with advanced disease and it had poor efficacy and it exhausted human and financial resources, and failed to achieve lower morbidity, the more treatment and the more patients. The status quo is: through a century the road which was walked on was to focus on treatment and ignore the prevention , or only treatment. Over the years we have just been working on cancer. But the prevention of cancer was done very little, almost did not do so that the incidence of cancer continues to rise.

The Review, reflection, cliché anti-cancer of the prevention of cancer and anti-cancer work: for a century, what have we done in the prevention of cancer research or work? What has it been done?

Medical school textbooks teaching content does not attach importance to the knowledge of the prevention of cancer ;

Hospital hospital mode does not attach importance to the prevention of cancer science setting up work;

Medical school or hospital research projects do not attach importance to the prevention of cancer research projects;

Journal of Cancer Medical Science does not attach importance to the cancer prevention work papers .

In short, the cancer prevention is not attached importance and the prevention is not paid attention. Cliché the cancer prevention is as the main and was not paid attention to and is not implemented.

How to do? How to reduce the incidence of cancer? How to improve cancer cure rate? How to reduce cancer mortality? How to extend life? How to improve the quality of life?

It should be launched the total attack to conquer cancer and the prevention and treatment are at the same attention and the level.

The goal of conquering cancer should be: reduce morbidity, improve the cure rate, reduce mortality, prolong survival, improve quality of life, reduce complications.

The current global hospitals and the hospitals in China are going all out to engage in treatment and focus on treatment and ignore the defense, or only treatment .

XZ-C thinks of that this hospital model or cancer treatment model can not overcome the cancer, can not reduce the incidence. Global hospitals and the hospitals in China must change the overall strategy of cancer treatment from focusing on treatment into focusing on prevention and treatment.

Therefore, we propose the general idea and design of launching the attack to conquer cancer and XZ-C (Xu Ze-China) proposed to launch the general attack, that is, the prevention of cancer and cancer control and the treatment of cancer three-phase work are carried out simultaneously .

It is put forward the " the necessity and feasibility report of conquering cancer to start the general attack . "

It is put forward " the XZ-C research program to conquer cancer and launch a total attack "

(C) why do I study cancer and propose to launch a total attack and to build "the science city to overcome cancer"? it is because:

① In 1985, I have done the petition for more than 3,000 cases of thoracic and abdominal cancer patients whose surgeries were operated by my own, the results were found that within 2-3 years most patients had the recurrence or metastasis. Therefore, we must study the prevention methods of the postoperative recurrence and metastasis to improve postoperative long-term efficacy.

② I suddenly had acute myocardial infarction in 1991. After treatment it was mproved; after recovery I should not be on the operating table and I was to calm down and to hide in the small building to concentrate on scientific research.

③ through experimental studies it was found that thymus atrophy and immune dysfunction are one of the etiology and pathogenesis of cancer and it should be to be expanded in-depth study.

④ through experimental research and clinical validation, after 30 years of more than 12,000 cases of clinical validation observation, I found the new path of the combination of chinese medication and western medication in the molecular level with the modernization of this «Chinese-style anti-cancer» and walked out this innovation new path of Chinese medicine immunoregulation which prevent thymus atrophy, promote thymic hyperplasia, protect bone marrow hematopoietic function, improve immune surveillance, at the molecular level of the combination of chinese medication and Western medication to overcome cancer, so that it is to be perseverance and persistence to stuy. Therefore, it is proposed to overcome the cancer and launch the total attack, to build the "Science City" of conquering cancer in an attempt to achieve: reduce the incidence of cancer; improve cancer cure rate; extend cancer survival; to be "three early" (early detection, early diagnosis, early Treatment), early can be cured; to achieve cancer prevention and treatment at the same attention and level; Both of prevention and treatment at the same attention and level can overcome the cancer, reduce the incidence of cancer.

All basic research must be for clinical to improve patient efficacy so that patients benefit. The evaluation criteria for the efficacy of cancer patients should be: prolong survival, good quality of life, less complications.

In 1951 I come to Wuhan and attended the Zhongnan Tongji Medical College, in 1956 graduated from Tongji Medical College, assigned to the Hubei College of Traditional Chinese Medicine Hospital, has served as director of surgery, Professor, Hubei College of Experimental Surgery, director of the Institute.

In 1991 due to sudden acute myocardial infarction, I was to have emergency rescue and rehabilitation after six months hospitalization . It was because I can not go to power surgery, I was quiet to hide into the small building to do the basis of cancer and clinical research. As a result of that my experimental laboratory equipment conditions were better, it made a large number of the experimental research about the cancer etiology, pathology, pathogenesis, cancer metastasis mechanism and the experimental screening study for anti-cancer Chinese herbal medicine suppression rate in cancer-bearing animal model mice.

I was 63 years old in 1996 and applied for retirement. After the retirement I was to continue to do the scientific research; the science (science) journey is non-stop. (No one to ask, no one support), go it alone, self-reliance, from the years over sixty, to the seventy years of the year , to more than eighty ripe old age, it still perseveres and is to be perseverance, continues to carry out a series of experimental research and clinical validation observation. And it finally made a series of scientific research and scientific and technological innovation series. All of these experimental and clinical data, data conclusions, summary collection were written into more than 100 research papers, published by the new book monographs. It was to be published a series of monographs about these cancer study, of which 3 for the Chinese version, 4 for the English version. The English version is published in Washington, USA. **In the books it was put forward a series of new concepts and new methods to overcome cancer, put forward the theory of cancer treatment innovation, put forward the road to overcome the cancer and it formed the theoretical system of the immune regulation and control which is the experimental basis of cancer immunotherapy and the observation and verification of clinical application; it walked out of a new way to overcome cancer. Why is the English version? It is because cancer is a disaster of all mankind, the people of the world must work together. I contribute the scientific thinking, scientific research, experience, lessons, wisdom of my 60 years of clinical work and 30 years engaging in cancer research experimental research and clinical validation to the people for the benefit of mankind.**

I am 83 years old this year, I was the total designer of XZ-C research program "to capture the cancer and to attack the total attack and to build the cancer research base science city" , I will participate in this practice of the preparation of "the science city to overcome the Cancer " with my academic, knowledge, wisdom and strength , to build "global demonstration of cancer prevention and treatment hospital", the cancer prevention and treatment and control of cancer at the same attention to build a good laboratory and multidisciplinary and cancer research group.

Change the mode of hospital from the focusing treatment with light defense into prevention and control and treatment of cancer at the same level! Change the treatment mode from the treatment of serious illness in the late stage to focus on the "three early" (early detection, early diagnosis, early treatment) precancerous lesions and early in situ cancer! This will benefit the human race and will open up a new era of anti-cancer research so that our prevention and treatment of cancer medical care go into the forefront of the world.

(D) I experienced 30 years to overcome the cancer as the direction of cancer research and clinical research, deeply appreciate: to achieve the purpose of cancer prevention and control:

①　It must start the total attack. The prevention of cancer and cancer control and cancer treatment three stages of work should be the same attention; three carriages go hand in hand in order to achieve lower incidence of cancer, improve cancer cure rate, reduce cancer mortality and prolong cancer survival. If it is only treatment , or the focusing treatment with light defense, it will never be able to overcome the cancer, because it can not reduce the incidence, the more treatment and the more patients.

How to launch a total attack and to implement the cancer prevention + control cancer + cancer treatment ? It is necessary to establish the hospital with the prevention and treatment of cancer during the whole process of the occurrence and the development of cancer and to change the current only treatment mode. Change the current treatment model for the middle and advanced cancer patients.

② It must be the government-led, the masses to participate, the mobilization of all the people, the work of thousands of households involved in order to conquering cancer ; in preset our country is building the new country, which it is the government-led, the masses involved; Time is good; if it can do the medical science research of cancer prevention and treatment and cancer control, it will be able to improve the awareness of the whole people prevent cancer to achieve the effects of the prevention cancer and control cancer to significantly reduce the incidence of cancer in our city and province and country.

③ **Why should it launch the total attack? It is because the status quo is:**

a, the current hospital mode is to pay attention to treatment with light defense, or only treatment , the more treatment the more patients.

b, the current treatment model is mainly cancer patients in the middle and late stage and late transfer, the effect is very poor.

c, the current radiotherapy and chemotherapy can not be cured, can only alleviate, slow interval of 4 weeks which can still progress, the effect is very poor, there are still problems and drawbacks.

It must emphasize early diagnosis, early treatment, early rehabilitation and adhere to the main prevention:

a, To change the hospital mode for the prevention, control, treatment at the same attention.

b, To change the treatment model for the "three early", precancerous lesions.

c, the anti-cancer way-out is the prevention and the research and the cancer prevention research.

(5) I have been working on experimental research and clinical validation for the study of cancer for 30 years both in the laboratory and in the hospital. Why now is it to apply for government support?

It is because 90% of the cancer is related to the environment. The occurrence of cancer is closely related people's clothing, food, shelter, line and living habits so that I think deeply about prevention cancer and cancer control work are not just to rely on medical staff, experts, scholars to do it. It must rely on the government's major policy ; the current serious environmental pollution and ecosystem degradation may be closely related to the rising incidence of cancer.

Cancer treatment is dependent on medical staff and researchers to study new drugs, new treatment techniques.

However, the prevention and control of cancer, how to reduce the incidence of cancer and the cancer prevention work must rely on the government's major policy and rely on government-led and leadership, experts, scholars efforts to participate in the masses to make true.

The current status quo is:

1, the more treatment and the more patients ; the incidence is on the rise, which 90% are related to the environment. **We deeply appreciate not only to pay attention to cancer treatment, but also to pay attention to prevention; in order to stop at the source** , it must be prevention and treatment at the same attention and level.

2, the current diagnostic methods, B ultrasound, CT, MRI are currently the most advanced diagnostic methods, but once diagnosed, it mostly in in the late, the effect is very poor. **We must try to do the research and find new methods, new reagents and new technologies that can be diagnosed early.** If the early and precancerous lesions can be diagnosed, the early cancer can be cured. Therefore, the way out of cancer treatment is the "three early". (Early detection, early diagnosis, early treatment).

What should I do next? Now it is proposed to overcome cancer and to launch a total attack. Hope to get leadership support at all levels. I know that to achieve the purpose of cancer prevention and control cancer and treatment of cancer must be government leadership, government-led, experts, scholars efforts, the masses involved, thousands of households to participate in order to do.

In China daily about 8550 people were diagnosed with cancer, 6 people per minute was diagnosed with cancer. Therefore, the study of launching a total offensive research work can not walk slowly and it should run forward, save the dying.

We should avoid empty talking about and conduct the hard work and start to go. No matter how far the way to overcome cancer it is , it should always start to go.

(6) In 2013 → 2014 → 2015, I have been studying and formulating the basic idea and design of how to overcome cancer; formulate the theoretical basis and experimental basis for how to overcome cancer; formulate the planning and blueprint and guideline and method of how to overcome cancer.

It came up with:

① « the XZ-C research program of capturing the cancer and launch a total attack «

② « the necessity report to build a comprehensive cancer prevention and treatment of hospital necessity report»

③ « the the necessity and feasibility report of the proposed» ride research in building a moderately society at the same time « ----- conducting the medical science research of cancer prevention and cancer control and cancer prevention and treatment work.»

④ «The planning and the total design to build a science city of conquering cancer and launching the total attack.»

These four research projects were put forward in the international community for the first time, opened up a new field of anti-cancer research. Professor Xu Ze proposed to capture the total attack of cancer, which is unprecedented work. To July 2015, it was developed as "dawn of the C-type plan." That dawn is the morning sun and the sunrise, C type = China, the "Chinese model" to overcome the cancer plan. This "4" reports " is "tackling cancer and launching a total attack" and "establishing a science city to overcome cancer".

How to implement the specific plan to overcome the cancer? I detailed the overall design, the overall planning, the specific program research team talent ... ... and other planning, blueprint.

It was put forward the " the total blueprint and design of the science city of launching the total attack of cancer "

The total design and preparation work of the Science City; to establish a pilot area for cancer prevention work (station)

To set up the following :

1, the Cancer Academic Committee of overcoming cancer

2, the working group to build Science City (of the medical, teaching, research, science schoo to attack the cancer and launch a total attack)

(7) This work is ongoing, we have taken three to four years in the cancer research, but step by step to move slowly forward.

In January 12, 2016 US President Barack Obama in the State of the Union made a national cancer plan: to overcome cancer.

The program name: "Cancer moon shot"

Goal: to overcome cancer

Nature: A national plan to overcome cancer

The program leader: Vice President Joe Biden

We have been walking in the cancer on the road to this research for 3-4 years, but only the individual living alone building alone, step by step to move forward, just slow forward.

Now the US President Barack Obama in the State of the Union issued a national cancer plan: to overcome cancer which the vice president I responsible for the implementation. Vice President Biden is actively pursuing. He goes to the cancer centers in the United States every month to preach: "Cancer moon shot".

On June 29, 2016 in the White House to the United States live "national cancer lunar landing plan". It was called the nation scientists to gather wisdom and to overcome cancer.

This international scientific research situation is gratifying, but also the situation is pressing, inspiring. In this case, the government has to be asked to support, ask the government to lead and to guide and to support this unprecedented work for the benefit of mankind.

This is a big deal and it is an unprecedented event for the benefit of mankind.

Therefore, XZ-C proposed: common progress, toward the scientific temple to overcome cancer.

Third, the guidance to act

XZ-C proposed the scientific research plan to build a science city of conquering cancer and launching the total attack. How to implement? How to do it? How to achieve? Now the brief explanation is as the following :

(1), the goal of conquering cancer: reduce the incidence of cancer, improve cancer cure rate, extend the survival time of cancer patients

To achieve:

1/3 can be prevented

1/3 can be cured

1/3 can be treated to relieve pain, is a chronic disease; is the survival with tumor; is to prolong survival

The evaluation criteria for the efficacy of cancer patients should be:

    ①   live a long time, prolong survival time

    ②   good quality of life

    ③   no complications, or less complications

(2) the road of conquer cancer

The way:

    ①   capture cancer and launch a total attack

What is the total attack?

That is, cancer prevention + control cancer + treatment cancer, at the same time it is to launch the total attach and to go hand in hand.

② to build science and technology city to overcome the cancer :

a, how to overcome cancer? It must be the founder of "innovative molecular cancer medical school" and graduate school - and modern high-tech experimental talents

b, how to overcome cancer? It must be founded " Chinese and Western combined hospital with the full process of the preventation and treatment of cancer on the innovative molecular tumor   level."

c, how to overcome cancer? It must be the founder of "Innovative Molecular Cancer Institute" and multidisciplinary and cancer research group.

d, how to overcome cancer? It must be the founder of "innovative molecular tumor nano-pharmaceutical factory"

e, how to overcome cancer? It must create "innovative environmental protection anti-cancer research institute" and carry out the cancer prevention system engineering.

f, how to overcome cancer ? It must be the founder of "Cancer Animal Experimental Center." This is the only way to overcome cancer.

(3) how to prevent? How to control ?How to treat cancer ? It have developed specific measures, feasibility programs, planning, blueprint seeing (Ⅰ) (Ⅱ) (Ⅲ) (Ⅳ) (Part I) in this book.

(4) how to start?

① first to build the hospital with the cancer prevention, control, treatment → the establishment of various disciplines (departments) → the establishment of the school group (study group)

② first to run, teach, research (Section, group) the prevention and control and treatment as a whole dragon and one-stop; the prevention and treatment at the same attention ; there are clinical basis and there are «three early», precancerous lesions.

③ first to build the graduate school, personnel training methods and ways;

To overcome the cancer, the cultivation of multidisciplinary senior personnel is the key; it is to train the personnel through experimental research, clinical practice.

a, first to run graduate tutor course, seminar, training personnel, the above content of how to overcome the cancer to start the total attack is to be discussed and to be studied by the division of the sub-topics for special, special study

b. Talent training program:

Graduate School Recruit graduate students (Ph.D, Master); while working, learning, 100 people, after graduation, all stay in the Science City, so generation of training, it requires results and achievements, patents (not just papers), three years and five years later, it will be talented and the scientific research results will acculated.

- In order to overcome cancer and to launch a total attack , the policy of the prevention cancer + control cancer + treatment cancer at the same attention and same level are is the right way.
- To Create a scientific base to conquer cancer and to launch the total attack----- the Science City, is the necessity way to set up agglutination wisdom and capture cancer. This approach is the right way to overcome cancer.

How to implement?

- It is necessary to establish a pilot area for the Cancer Working Group (station) to explore the experience in prevention, control and treatment.
- This set of cancer planning, program, the total design is applicable to a country, a province, a city reference implementation.
- Because cancer is a disaster for the people of the world, the people of the world, people of all countries, people of all provinces and cities must struggle with them.
- To apply for the International Conference on Oncology in Wuhan, China, November 16-18, 2018, the world's first "Challenging Cancer Summit". To be organized, the United States ... ... global cooperation research organization, once a year to promote the development of Summit Forum.

The Conference Theme:

1, to look forward to the promising prospects of 21st century cancer metastasis, recurrence prevention and treatment;
2, to gather wisdom, capture cancer, launch a total attack, for the benefit of mankind.

To overcome the cancer and launch a total attack is an unprecedented human event, is the forefront of science

- to emphasize on the cancer prevention and cancer control and cancer treatment at the same lever. The way-out of Cancer treatment is in the "three early".
- the emphasis on anti-cancer out of the way is in the prevention, the establishment of the department of the prevention cancer and the department of cancer control and the cancer prevention research institute, because 90% of the cancer is related to the environment and it must be from the big environment, small environment to prevent cancer and from air, water to prevent and from the clothing, food, live to prevent cancer and from changing the living habits, and changing the life to prevent cancer.

(5) XZ-C proposed that it must establish the prevention cancer research institute and the prevention of cancer system engineering in order to conquer cancer and to launch a total attack.

The most prominent of the discovery is that more than 90% of the cancer is caused by environmental factors during the process of that Human beings is in the search for cancer etiology and conditions.

How to implement the creation of the cancer prevention research institute?

Professor Xu Ze XZ-C proposed anti-cancer design, proposed anti-cancer system engineering:

To study the prevention measures of how to reduce or prevent from these carcinogens?

It is because cancer patients cover the world, industrial and agricultural waste water, waste residue, waste gas pollution is also covered the world, therefore, it must be the whole world to conquer cancer and launch a total attack.

Professor Xu Ze suggested:

① **each country, each province, each state should establish the prevention of cancer research institute (or organization), carry out the prevention of cancer system engineering, for their own country, the province, the city to carry out anti-cancer work.**

② **to establish the prevention of cancer regulations, to carry out (some should be legislation)**

③ **I will recommend this project to the World Health Organization to launch anti-cancer operations, the goal is to try to reduce the incidence of cancer.** Capture cancer is the forefront of science, is a worldwide problem; cancer is a human disaster, covering the whole world, people around the world are eager to one day to overcome cancer, for the benefit of mankind.

④ **to promote scientific research ethics; medicine is benevolence and the legislation is the first**

Scientific research ethics: the products should have moral standards.

The standard: it should not harm human health as the standard and as the bottom line.

It should pay attention to the prevention of cancer regulations

The basic ethics: all products should be harmless to people and do not harm people's health, especially for children. (To be beautiful, the flower of the living environment, living environment)

⑤ **health administrative departments is to defend life, to protect health, should lead and guide and support to guide the prevention of cancer measures, the prevention of cancer engineering, the prevention of cancer testing, the prevention of cancer monitoring.**

The summary after guidance

"Condense Wisdom and Conquer Cancer - for the benefit of mankind"

This is a medical monographs with the more complete, more systematic, more comprehensive design and more specific planning of how to overcome the cancer. The whole book content is divided into two parts: ① how to overcome cancer? how to prevent cancer by I see. ② how to overcome cancer? How to treat cancer I see?

1. the book to the length of 40% on the specific programs and planning sand the blueprints of how to prevent cancer. It raised how to overcome cancer? how to prevent cancer by I see .

The target of the study or "target" is located in how to reduce the incidence of cancer.

The current status quo is: the more treatment and the more cancer patients, and the incidence of cancer is continuing rising and the mortality rate is high. The road which walked through for a century is to focus on treatment and to ignore the defense or only treatment and no defense. It was done very little in the prevention work and it almost did not do. The cancer prevention did not attach importance; the prevention did not pay attention so that the incidence of cancer is rising.

How to prevent cancer? Where is the target or goal of the cancer prevention?

It must have a specific prevention cancer object and a clear goal so that it can have operational.

Professor Xu Ze proposed how to prevent cancer I see (a), (b), (c), (d) proposed that it should analyze what causes or which factors lead to an increase in cancer incidence. Currently the more number of patients and the more treatment; the incidence is on the rise and 90% is related to its environment. It should study and explore for the environmental carcinogenic factors (the external environment and the internal environment).

The causes of cancer are related to the carcinogenic factors of the external and internal environment.

If we have a better understanding of the causes of cancer, then in the future it will be able to put forward:

How to prevent which carcinogenic factors? how to monitor which carcinogenic factors? how to clean which carcinogenic factors? so that we can stay away from cancer and prevent cancer.

Therefore, Professor Xu Ze proposed: it should prevent cancer from the big environment and the small environment and it should be from the clothing, food, live and walking to prevent cancer.

2. 60% of the length in this book is the disscussion of how to treat cancer. The study of the target or "target" is located in how to improve cancer cure rate, extends the survival of cancer patients, improve the quality of life and put forward how to cure cancer by I see.

We are taking the new road of cancer treatment in the molecular level of the combination of Western medication and Chinese medication and it is the new road of finding the immune regulation methods and drugs on the basis of new discoveries in animal experiments in our laboratory. After years of animal experiment screening and clinical validation it finally found out this new road of immune regulation of cancer with XZ-C1-10 immune regulation of anti-cancer Chinese medication series.

- From our laboratory experiments it was found that: thymus of the host was acute progressive atrophy and the volume was significantly reduced after the host was inoculated with cancer cells.
- From the above experimental results it was found that thymus atrophy, immune dysfunction may be one of the etiology and pathogenesis of the tumor so the principle of treatment must try to prevent thymic atrophy, promote thymocyte proliferation, increased immune function.
- In order to prevent thymic atrophy and to promote thymocyte proliferation and to increase immune function, we look for from both the traditional Chinese medication and Western medication. Western medication which can improve immune function and promote the proliferation of thymocytes is very rare. So we changed to find from the Chinese medication because the traditional Chinese medication tonic drugs generally have immune regulation.
- After 7 years of laboratory scientific research, we selected XZ-C1-10 immune regulation anti-cancer, anti-transfer traditional Chinese medication with protecting thymus and increasing immune function and protecting bone marrow and hemotesise from the natural drug. on the basis of the success of the animal experiment the clinical validation work was conducted. After 20 years of more than 12,000 cases of clinical application in the cancer specialist outpatient center it achieved the good results.
- After the experimental study, with anti-cancer research of Chinese medication immunopharmacology and the combination of Chinese and Western medication on the molecular level, it walked out of the new path of conquering cancer with XZ-C immune regulation, regulating immune activity, preventing thymus atrophy, promoting thymocyte proliferation, protecting bone marrow hematopoietic function, improve immune surveillance.

3. This medical monograph is the outline of the practical and the applied and the research and the implementation of how to overcome cancer.

This set of scientific research programs and scientific research and design and scientific research planning and blueprint can be used for each country and each province and each of the state as the reference to implement the ambitious of conquering cancer for the benefit of mankind.

The main project of this medical monograph is:

The Main Project

1. To conquer cancer and to launch cancer the total attack: the prevention and the control and the treatment at the same level of the attraction and moving together
2. To create the cancer - related research base with a multi - disciplinary -- - Science City

Two wing works:

A wing - how to prevent cancer - to reduce the incidence of cancer

B wing - how to cure cancer - to improve cancer cure rate

The goals and the aims:

A: to reduce the incidence of cancer

B: to improve cancer cure rate and to extend the survival of patients and to improve the quality of life

If it is implemented and it achieves this total design and planning blue of conquering cancer, it is possible to overcome cancer.

4. The next step is how to implement the work, how to achieve this total design and the programs and the planning and the blueprint.

It should set up the research team of conquering cancer and launching the total attack".

In order to capture cancer and to launch the total attack, the talent is the key and the first thing is to set up research team

The conditions of the research team and the academic members:

Genuine talent; in the cancer research, basic research or clinical work it has academic achievements, academic achievements, monographs, editor, special issue, international papers; has the practical clinical experience and the experimental research results, its direction of the research and academic is to capture cancer.

The leadership leaders who leads and organizes to conquer cancer should support anti-cancer research and support cancer research; the scientists and the entrepreneurs and the leaders and the volunteers of conquering cancer must have both ability and political integrity and medicine is benevolence and the legislation is for the first.

THE SECOND PART
(PART II: CANCER TREATMENT)

Volume V

Walked out of a new way to conquer cancer

The experimental study and anti-cancer research of chinese medication immunopharmacology and molecular level of the combination of chinese and western medication

---- Walked out of the new path of conquering cancer with XZ-C immune regulation and control and the combination of Chinese and western medications on the molecular level.

----Walked out of the new path of conquering cancer with the immune regulation and control of traditional Chinese medications and with regulating the immune activity, preventing thymus atrophy, promoting Thymic hyperplasia, protecting bone marrow hematopoietic function, improving immune surveillance at the molecular level of the combination of Chinese and western medication.

CONTENTS VOLUME V
The basic and clinical

Preface

The experimental surgery is extremely important in the development of medicine, and it is a key to open the medical closed area; the prevention and control methods of many diseases are from conducting after many animal experimental research and achieving a stable effect, then was applied to clinical, and promote the development of medical career.

The laboratory is the key condition for development science and scientific and technological innovation. I deeply appreciate the importance of the laboratory. I was the first college students after the liberation of the college entrance examination, and I didn't have further degree study, nor went aboard for study, but I made a number of international level results. The key is that I have a good lab. In the 1960s, I participated in an open heart surgery in the heart. In the 1980s I established a liver cirrhosis ascites laboratory. In the 1990s I established the Institute of Experimental Surgery in order to capture cancer as the main direction. In my animal laboratory the equipment conditions are better and there are mice, rats, Dutch pigs, rabbits, dogs, monkeys and other animal experiments, a better sterilization operating room where various major surgery such as the chest, abdomen operation can be done and there are animals Postoperative observation room, which can put a variety of design and imagination to achieve results or conclusions through experimental operations.

Therefore, the laboratory is the key condition and the key is to build a good equipment laboratory.

The university teachers should have a dual task on the shoulders, one is to improve teaching; the second is the development of science.

The university teachers should have a good laboratory for scientific research, follow the scientific concept of development, be based on the known science to explore the unknown science, face for the future science and emerging disciplines and marginal disciplines and interdisciplinary, face scientific frontier and strive the innovation and go forward, Increase brick and add watt for the science hall.

In summary, the experimental study and the basic research are very important; if there is no the experimental research and the basic research breakthrough, the clinical efficacy is difficult to improve, it is difficult to put forward the new ideas, the new concepts, and the new theoretical insights. Among them the experiments are the key, and I have a good laboratory, and I was director of the Institute of Experimental Surgery, also the clinical director of surgery which the experimental research, the basic research and the clinical validation are easy to take into account.

The basic research of medicine is very important to the progress of the fight against disease. Experimental oncology is the basic science of tumor prevention research, which has promoted the deepening development of cancer research in China.

We conducted a series of experimental studies on the mechanism of cancer occurrence, invasion and relapse, and we conducted a four-year experimental study in the laboratory. From the experimental study, we found that thymus atrophy, low immune function may be tumor etiology, one of the pathogenesis; how should it prevent thymus atrophy? How to regulate immune function? How to promote immune? How to "protecting Thymus and increasing immune"? it should get on the immune regulation in the molecular level of combining Chinese and Western medicine, walk out of the new path of Chinese characteristics of conquering cancer.

FIRST, WALKED OUT OF A NEW WAY TO OVERCOME CANCER

1. The new discovery of anti-cancer and anti-cancer metastasis

The revelation of anticancer metastasis research:

I am a clinical surgeon, why do I do cancer research? This is due to the petition results of following up a group of cancer patients.

In 1985, I did petition letters for more than 3000 cases of thoracic and abdominal cancer patients which I operated surgery myself.

From the results of follow-up it was found that: the postoperative recurrence and metastasis are the key to long-term effect of surgery.

And therefore it also raised an important question to us: that clinicians must pay attention to and study the prevention and treatment measures of the postoperative recurrenceand metastasis in order to improve the postoperative long-term efficacy. Therefore, it is necessary to carry out the experimental study of the clinical and basic of cancer recurrence and metastasis. If there is no breakthrough in basic research, the clinical efficacy is difficult to improve.

Therefore, we established the Experimental Surgery Laboratory (later in 1991 it established Hubei College of Traditional Chinese Medicine Experimental Surgery to do the research direction for conquer cancer).

We have studied from the following two aspects: one was the animal experimental research: one was the clinical research. After it was successful on the basis of the animal experiments, it was applied to clinical and got the clinical validation. After 28 years of heat and cold hard work and effort, it carried out a series of experimental research and clinical validation work and it has made a series of scientific and technological innovation and scientific research results.

The new discovery:

(1) from the results of follow-up it was found:

① The postoperative recurrence and metastasis are the key to long-term effect of surgery.
② The clinicians must pay attention to and study the prevention and control measures of the postoperative recurrence and metastasis.

(2) from the experimental tumor study it was found:

① The removal of Thymus (TH) can be used to make animal model, and the injection of immunosuppressive agents can also help the establishment of animal model. **The conclusion of the study clearly shows that the occurrence and development of cancer have a definite positive relationship with the immune organ TH and immune organ tissue function, and it is difficult to manufacture animal model without resection of TH.** The repeated experiments are affirmed the experimental results.

② **whether does the immunization decrease first and then easy to get cancer or cancer occurs first and then immune decreases? Our experimental results are: the inferior immune leads to the occurrence and development of the cancer, without the descent of immunologic function, it is not easy to realize the successful inoculation. It is suggested by the experimental results: improving and maintaining the good immunologic function and protecting the good thymus of the central immune organ are one of the important measures for preventing the occurrence of cancer.**

③ in studying the relation between the metastasis of cancer and the immune our lab establishes animal models for liver metastatic carcinoma, which are divided into two groups including Group A applied with immune depressant and Group B not applied with immune depressant. Results: the metastatic lesions in the liver in Group A are obviously more than the ones in Group B. **It is suggested by the experimental results: metastasis is related to the immune and inferior immunologic function or application of immune depressant may promote the tumor metastasis.**

④ When we investigate for how tumor impacts on immune organ, it was found that with the progress of cancer, thymus is showed a progressive atrophy. The thymus of the host meets with the acute progressive atrophy after the cancer cells are inoculated, the cell proliferation is prevented and the volume is obviously shrunk. **It is suggested by the experimental results: the tumor may inhibit the thymus, resulting in the atrophy of the immune organ.**

⑤ Through experiments, we also found that: that if some experimental mice are not successfully inoculated or the tumor is very small, the thymus is not obviously shrunk. In order to understand the relation between the tumor and the atrophy of the thymus, we excise the transplanted solid tumor of one group of mice when it grows up to the size of a thumb. After one month, through anatomy, we find the thymus does not meet with progressive atrophy again. **Therefore, it is inferred by us that maybe the solid tumor produces one kind of unknown factor to inhibit the thymus, which shall be further studied through experiment.**

⑥ **it is proven by the above-mentioned experimental results: the advance of the tumor makes the thymus meet with progressive atrophy, then, can we take some measures to prevent the atrophy of the thymus of the host? Therefore, we further perfect the design to seek for the method or drug to prevent the atrophy of the thymus of the cancer-bearing mice through the experimental study on animal.** So we make the experimental study to recover the function of the immune organ through cell transplantation of the immune organ. We discuss the atrophy of the thymus of the immune organ in preventing the advance of tumor, seek for the method to recover the functions of the thymus and reconstruct the immune, carry out the cell transplantation of foetal liver, spleen and thymus with the mice and establish the immunologic function through adoptive immunity. **It is shown by the results: through the joint transplantation of three groups of cells, namely S, T and L (200 experimental mice), the entire extinction rate of the tumor in the long term is 46.67% and the one with the entire extinction of the tumor get a long survival life.**

⑦ In the experiment to probe into the effects of tumor on the immune organ such as spleen, we find: the spleen can inhibit the growth of the tumor in the early stage of the tumor, however, in the late stage, the spleen meets with the progressive atrophy. It is suggested by the study results: the effects of spleen on the growth of the tumor are embodied into bi-direction, in the early stage, it can inhibit the tumor to a certain extent, however, in the late stage, it fails to inhibit the tumor. The cell transplantation of the spleen can enhance the role of inhibiting the tumor.

In short, from the above series of experiments it was found that thymus atrophy and immune dysfunction may be one of the etiology and pathogenesis of cancer, should be to study further from thymus function and organizational structure, immune dysfunction and how to boost the immune, immune reconstruction, new methods and new ways how to protect Thymus and increase immune function. The following review the structure and function of the thymus and look for cancer treatment.

2. The experimental observation of the thymus tumor effects

Generally it was believed that the body's immune function status affects the occurrence, development and prognosis of cancer, while cancer of the immune status will dampen demand. Both reinforce each other and complex. When doing the animal experiments on the influences of spleen on the tumorous growth, the author have observed that the immune organs thymus, spleen of the cancer-bearing mice have changed a lot. It seems that this process presents a certain law. **In order to study further on the relationship and laws between tumors and spleens or thymus, the following experiments are designed to observe dynamically the changes of conversion rates of thymus, spleen and lymphocyte of cancer-bearing mice in different phases and probe into the relationship between them.**

【Materials and Methods】

(1) Experimental animals and grouping 40 Kunming mice were randomly divided into four groups, rats aged 40 ~ 50d, weighing 15 ~ 18g. Male and female, regardless.

Ⅰ groups: healthy control group, is not healthy mice inoculated with cancer, were killed after thymus, spleen and peripheral blood experiment observation.

Ⅱ group: intraperitoneal inoculation of Ehrlich ascites tumor cells in 0.1 × 107 个, 3d sacrificed after observation.

Ⅲ group: inoculation of tumor cells (ibid.), The first 7 days sacrificed observation.

Ⅳ groups: the first 14 days of the death of tumor cells inoculation observation.

Take Chapter 22 experiments (ie, experimental studies on tumor growth of spleen) in tumor-bearing mice were 100 natural terminally dead after the autopsy results, as advanced tumors thymus, spleen change the outcome of the thymus in advanced tumor-bearing mice The average diameter of (1.2 ± 0.3) mm, average weight (20 ± 5) mg, hard texture. The spleen is withering, average weight (60 ± 12) mg, hard texture, color gray, significantly reduced the growth center, and fibrosis.

(2) Experimental methods for each group of mice were prepared time, dig eye were sacrificed, whole blood specimens from each mouse (with heparin) 1ml, do lymphocyte transformation test, then immediately dissect mice were tumor infiltration range, ascites and the organ involvement and focus visually thymus, spleen, lymph nodes anatomy, complete remove the thymus, spleen, volume with a vernier caliper, and then were weighed with an analytical balance evacuation pathologic examination.

[Results]

(1) mice inoculated with tumor cells at different times the weight of the thymus

Analysis of variance of Table 1, Table 2. Table 1, Table 2 with a graph showing the results, to delineate the thymus weight change curve (Figure 1)

Table 1 Comparison of thymic weights of mice in each group (mg)

Group	Group I Control	Group II on the 3rd after inoculated	Group III on the 7rd after inoculated	Group IV on the 14rd after inoculated	Group On the 25th after inoculated	Group On the 30th after inoculated
Xij	72.8	78.2	90.0	40.0	25.13	16.90
	50.0	83.4	66.0	32.2	29.46	17.00
	56.4	89	85.4	39.8	28.90	19.05
	96.4	68	106.5	23.5	26.77	18.16
	77.4	74.8	51.7	38.0	27.00	16.98
	100.7	95.4	77.8	36.0	28.00	20.01
	87.5	115.0	73.0	46.0	26.78	19.23
	76.8	56.4	60.0	20.0	27.69	18.98
	112.7	43.0	49.4	55	31.37	18.54
	51.0			20	28.90	15.15
åX	781.07	703.2	736.3	350.5	280	180
N	10	9	10	10	10	10
CI	78.17	78.13	73.63	35.05	28.00	18.00
SC²	66261.79	58566.66	57033.75	18467.25	7867.44	6518.612

Table 2 Analysis of variance of table 1

Resources of variation	SS	V	MS	F	P
Between groups within groups	12967.10 11777.12	3 35	4322.36 336.48	12.85	<0.01
Total	24744.22				

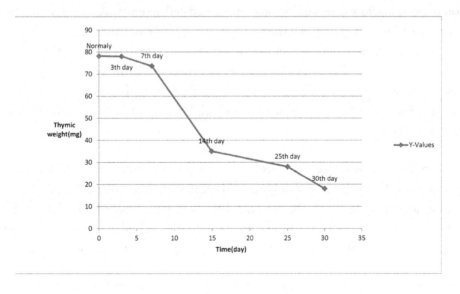

Figure 1 the curve of variation on the thymic weights

From Table 1, Table 2, Figure 1 it can be seen, mice thymus changed regularly, within 7d after inoculation, no significant changes in the thymus eye view, but the weight has started to lighten, 7 days, then was acute atrophy, thymus late to the reduced diameter of each leaf from the normal 5 ~ 8mm to about 1mm, weight reduce the 76.1mg to 20mg, hard texture, function has declined, even lost. Show cellular immune function of tumor progression with growing operations and suppression, causing immune dysfunction, tumor growth has become increasingly fast.

(2) Pathological changes in thymus

Thymus: Thymus presents progressive atrophy during the whole course of disease; on the 3rd day after inoculated with cancer cells, thymus shrinks slightly and the color is gray; on the 7th day, thymic volume shrinks obviously and the cellular proliferation is stopped with reduced mature cells; during the later period of tumors, thymus shrinks extremely and its volume is as big as a sesame with the diameter of 1 mm and hard texture.

(3) The experimental results showed that after inoculation of the tumors, thymus rapidly shrinkle and continue shrinkle during the whole process so that thymus rapidly lost the anticancer immune response. The experiment showed that thymus change its construction after the inoculation of the tumors and shrinkls during the whole process. In the later stage thymus weight decrease from 78.13+13.2 mg to 20+5mg, the diameter of the volume decrease from 5-8mm to 1mm. The cell proliferation clearly decreased.

Due to the thymus atrophy, cell proliferation is blocked, mature cell reduced or depleted, the index declined, the metabolism weakened, the cell viability decreased and thymic hormone secretion also decreased and cellular immune function is inevitably damage, the defense capability in mice is low, namely a large number of transplanted cancer cells grew and reproduced. Similarly the reports by Zhang Tong Wen et al was that while mice had thymus atrophy, it was also accompanied by the proliferation of bone marrow cells was blocked, nucleated cell activity decreased, and it was believed that there is a close relationship between the two. Thus, inhibition of tumor or injury of host immune function is multifaceted, affecting the body's entire immune system. The experiment of lymphocyte transformation rate showed that after inoculation of cancer cells, the lymphocyte transformation rate decreased progressively, until late fall more than 50 percent, also shows that immune effector cells is inhibited. As for why the thymus of mice was inhibited atrophy requires further experimental research and observation.

Thymus also produces a variety of hormones to promote the differentiation of immune lymphoid stem cell maturation. Although thymus is lymphoid organs, but due to the presence of blood thymus barrier, thymus doesn't contact with the antigens directly to play a role in the effect. Therefore there are not tumor-specific antigen stimulation and proliferation of enlargement. The tumors secrete immunosuppressive factors able to act on the thymus, so that thymus is atrophy, dysfunction.

The immune therapy of the tumors is the field which many physicians have great interests.

Since the 1980s, due to the rapid development of immunology and biotechnology which provide an opportunity of tumor immunotherapy, biological response modifiers(BRM) was proposed as fourth treatment in addition to surgery, radiotherapy, chemotherapy which is tumor biological therapy. Using biological modulators to treat cancer may have hoped to promote the development of effective new therapies for immune therapy.

Summary, the host and the tumor are against with each other during the tumor occurrence and development, which exist all the time. In the healthy immune system, our bodyhave ability to limit and to kill the tumor cells. On the other hand, the growth of the tumor produces a lot of influence on the body's immune system which suppresses immune function and promotes tumor development.

3. The shape and the location of Thymus

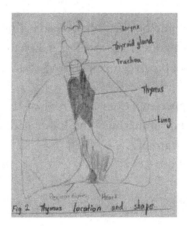

Fig 1. The Thymus location and shape

{Thymus is Upper medial organs and pericardium}

Thymus

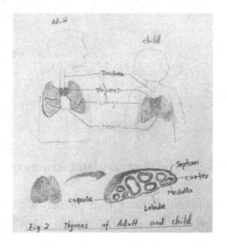

Fig 2. The Thymus of Adult and Child

49

The structure of thymus

1, thymus lobule or leaflets; 2, lobular septum or interval; 3, cortex of thymus ; 4, thymus body; 5, the capsule or film; 6,

Thymus is cone-shaped and can be divided into left and right leaves which are not symmetrical and is soft, elongated flat strip and is connected by connective tissue. The size of the thymus has a large difference in different age groups. Thymus grows fast in late period of embryonic development and neonatal. The period from birth to 2 years old is the best period of development of the thymus weighing 15 ~ 20g. With age, the thymus continues to develop and to increase, but slow during postnatal development. In puberty it reached to 25 ~ 40g. After puberty, the thymus begins to shrink. Thymus in adult still maintain the original shape, but its structure has changed dramatically such as a significant reduction in lymphocytes and thymus tissue is replaced by fat tissue more.

The adult thymus is behind sternum and on the front of mediastinum. Its rear is with the innominate vein and aortic arch adjacent to both sides of the mediastinal pleura and lung. Thymoma and thymic enlargement can compress the above organs corresponding clinical symptoms.

Children thymus is larger with upper end extending root of the neck and with sometimes up to the lower edge of the thyroid gland. Sometimes the lower end can be inserted into the anterior mediastinum up to the front of pericardial.

4. The structure of the thymus

The Thymus Gland

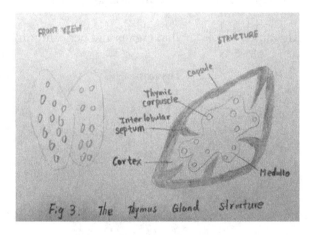

Fig. 3 The thymus gland structure

{Thymus medulla Illustration of the distribution in the medulla of the scattered thymus body (arrow)} (keratinized epithelial cells and debris; epithelial cells; thymocytes are inside)

(1) Capsule: thymus tissue surface is coated with a film, a film composed of dense collagen fibers, elastic fiber and matrix and other substance. Coating of the connective tissue fibers extends into the substance of the thymus. The thymus is divided into many lobules. Leaflets around are the cortex and medulla is in the dark side. There is a mesh stent composed of epithelial cells between these two.

(2) Cortex: thymic cortex is located around the portion of the leaflets by dense lymphocytes and epithelial reticular cells. Lymphocytes near cortex is large which is original cell type. Middle lymphocytes were medium-sized, mostly small lymphocyte is in the inner layer. Scattered macrophages is within the cortex. Hematopoietic stem cell proliferation and differentiation of T lymphocytes process is from shallow to deep.

(3)Medulla: thymic medulla is located deep leaflets composed by epithelial reticular cells and a small number of lymphocytes. Thymus bodies are scattering in the medulla. Small bodies are circular or oval made of several layers of epithelial reticular cells and arranged in concentric circles.

Thymus function

Thymus function is more complex. Thymus is lymphoid organs and has endocrine functions. Some authors will list it in the endocrine system. Its main function is to develop and to manufacture T lymphocytes and thymic hormone secretion. T cells within thymus need a suitable internal environment to develop. Thymic epithelial reticular cells can secrete a variety of solidarity hormones: thymosin, thymopoietin, thymulin, thymic humoral factor(THF) and ubiguitin, etc. These hormones and macrophages within thymus together form a nurturing T cell microenvironment. Thymosin and thymopoietin can promote lymphoid stem cell differentiation to T cells, stimulate T cell proliferation and stimulate hypothalamus to secrete ACTH and LH; thymopoietin can induce T cell differentiation; other hormones can promote early T cell division and have to promote synergy of T cell maturation.

Primitive lymphatic stem cells don't have immune function; later convert into T cells with immune function, then migrate to peripheral lymphoid organs such as lymphoid tissue, lymph nodes, spleen, etc. by blood circulation to be involved in the immune response after antigen activation. Although thymus atrophy and degradation in adult, there is still the ability to secrete thymic hormones. When the body's lymphoid tissue damage, T cells have a significant reduction. In thymic hormone action lymphoid stem cells in thymus can still be converted to T cells.

T lymphocytes

The differentiation and development of lymphocytes in thymus.

The phenotypic changes in T cell differentiation and development:

Two distinct types of thymocytes are produced in the thymus: CD4/CD8. All T cells originate from haematopoietic stem cells in the bone marrow. In the bone marrow haematopoietic stem cells become haematopoietic progenitors; on the way to thymus haematopoietic progenitors are expanded by cell division to generate a large population of immature thymocytes; in the thymus the earlist thymocytes are *double- negative* (CD4⁻CD8⁻) cells, later become *double-positive* thymocytes (CD4⁺CD8⁺); finally mature to *single-positive* (CD4⁺CD8⁻ or CD4⁻CD8⁺) thymocytes. About 98% of <u>thymocytes</u> die during the development processes in the thymus by failing either positive selection or negative selection, whereas 2% matured naïve T cells leave the <u>thymus</u> and begin to spread throughout the body, including the <u>lymph nodes</u>. As the thymus shrinks by about 3% a year throughout middle age, there is a corresponding fall in the thymic production of naive T cells, leaving peripheral T cell expansion to play a greater role in protecting older subjects.

At present it is known that the mature main factors inducing T cell differentiation in the thymus, include: ① thymic stromal cells (thymus stromalcell, TSC) interact directly with thymocytes by adhesion molecules on the cell surface; ② thymic stromal cells secrete a variety of cytokines (such as IL-1, IL-6, IL-7) and thymus hormone-induced thymocyte differentiation; ③ thymus cells themselves secrete a variety of cytokines (such as IL-2, IL-4) on thymocyte differentiation and maturation itself also It plays an important role. **In addition, thymic epithelial cells, macrophages and dendritic cells play a decisive role in the process of thymocyte differentiation, MHC restriction, and the formation of T cell function subsets.**

Especially cellular immunity and T lymphocyte function decreases with age, the structure and function of thymus gradually degenerate in adulthood. Thymus is a central organ of immune system and the base of T lymphocyte differentiation and maturation. Thymic epithelial cells produce and release thymosin which plays an important role in differentiating T lymphocyte precursors into mature T cell immune activity. Thymus is the first organ of the body degradation, and then began a decline after sexual maturity and the ability to produce and secrete thymosin also gradually decreased with age.

Thymus research began in the early 1960s, it was found that closely related to immune function. Miller et al (1960) found that when thymus was removed in animals (neonatal mice), immune function will not develop completely and the number of circulating T cells was significantly reduced. Since 50 years thymus has been recognized as the center of the immune organ and is the first mature organ in the body and the structure and function of the thymus reach a peak while sexual maturity; thereafter with age increase, it is gradually shrinking and degradation and immune function in adult animals is gradually being replaced by the spleen and other lymphoid tissues. The thymus is the core of tissue T lymphocyte development, but it is also the base producing a variety of immune factors (lymphokines, cytokines). Thymosin is the main immune modulators secreting from thymus and now there are a variety of thymosin (peptide) products for the Clinical and Experimental Research. There is a foreign specialized periodicals called "thymus" (thymus) which regularly publishes reports on the thymus research and clinical treatment.

6. Thymus immune function

From the beginning it is believed that it was a single regulatory system independent to other physiological systems. So far it is considered that thymus and the neuroendocrine system are interconnected functional network system. Since the late 1970s Besedovsky (1977) proposed neuroendocrine immune network theory (NIM) which has been recognized as the core guide for thymus and immune function. Thymus and central nervous system and peripheral immune response functions form the system's three-point line connection. Central cerebral cortex, hypothalamus, pituitary is higher regulation center; peripheral lymphoid organs and tissues, cells and cytokines to regulate and implementation units subordinate immune network; intermediate hub is thymus called NIM middle line. NIM path can be divided into three: ① down line that reached down from the central median line to middle line and down line; ② up line from each cytokine feedback information to the central site; ③ middle line access to thymus for the spindle, combined with the spleen and other lymphoid tissue and bone marrow progenitor cell nucleus. Recent studies have shown that the thymus plays an important role in the NIM activities. For example, Fabres (1983) put forward - the concept of "thymic neuroendocrine network", Goldstein AL (1983) that "neuroendocrine - thymus axis" of thought, expression can be described as the thymus special significance in the NIM network.

Thymus starts to degrade after sexual maturity and secreted thymosin and other hormones are also reduced so that T lymphocyte differentiation and immune function decrease. The main reason for human and mammalian aging degeneration has the close relation to atrophy of the thymus.

While Increasing age, thymic atrophy naturally and life is gradually aging, the thymus is an important factor affecting the level of the body's immunity. Experiments show that removal of the thymus in adult rats (2 months) can accelerate its own immune dysfunction and aging. Six months after removal of thymus in rats (2 months) lymphocyte immune activity in spleen decreased, only of 51.6% in the same age without removal of the thymus.

7. Thymus exocrine

Thymic hormone vitality can be detected by available bioassay method. The experiment proved the vitality of the thymus hormone decline with increasing age. With thymic atrophy it decreases. In the animals with removal of the thymus serum cannot be measured. Thymus is the main source of thymic hormone. Thymus hormones are substance secreted by thymocytes regulating immune function.

The thymus is the important organization of body's immune function, secrete and generate thymulin etc, and secrete IL-1 and IL-2 and other interleukins to adjust thymus intrinsic function and viability ingredient; at the same time regulated by the pituitary secretion of prolactin. Now the research about thymus immunomodulator primarily provides evidence indicating that exogenous hormone (such as prolactin, growth hormone, thyroxine, etc.) can rejuvenate the thymus recession and maintain immunomodulatory force. Thymic involution can be reversed which is common developmental prospects of modern immunology and endocrinology.

8. Impact of chemicals on the immune function

Cyclophosphamide (Cy) or hydrocortisone pine (HC) is commonly used in clinical medicine can cause decreased immune function, and other long-term injections can cause the thymus, spleen and lymph node atrophy, and decreased immune function.

In short, Although Cy and HC has a certain inhibition in immune function, after Cy medication is used with 3 W, thymus atrophy; after 6W spleen began to shrink; in 6 ~ 12W proliferation of peripheral blood T lymphocyte decreased significantly.

9. The name and function of the thymus hormone

Since the early 1960s by the famous scientists Good and Miller and others first reported thymus function is "central" organ systemic immune system since the rapid development of cellular immunology. In the early 1970s the hypothesis about the thymus hormone secretion was proposed, several "constructive" but not yet sure of the thymus hormones or hormone-like ingredients have come out, they are extracted from the whole thymus peptides ingredients. Recent studies have shown that thymic epithelial cells (TEC) is to produce thymic hormone component of cells divided into two categories: interleukin-class (Ils) and thymosin class ingredients. Foreign studies have demonstrated that there are four kinds of thymic hormone: (1) thymosin-α; (2) thymulin; (3) thymopoietin; (4) thymichumoral factor (THF). Thymulin is 9 peptide binding component requiring a zinc binding to keep biological activity. Multiple thymus ingredient mostly are extracted from bovine thymus abroad.

10. Immunomodulators: immune enhancers

At present immune enhancers can be divided into several categories by different sources.

The first class of immune enhancers derived from microorganisms

Fungal glucan ingredient containing β-1,3- glucoside chain has demonstrated better clinical effect, they can promote MΦ killing bacteria and tumor cells and induce the release of a single factor (monokine), such as interleukin-1 (IL-1), tumor necrosis factor (TNF), colony stimulating factor (CSF) and the like.

The second largest category of immune enhancer is thymus extract.

Thymus peptides extracted from animal. The world (including our) has a variety of products available which have immunological pharmacological activity, also known as thymic hormone. Thymosin zinc complex (zinc thymulin complex) is the active ingredients secreted by thymic epithelial cells. A variety of other crude thymic extract has clinical effects. Its main role is to enhance T cell activity in vivo, but no effect produce new T cells. In other words, activation of T cells can enhance the body against germs and anti-tumor; and anti-aging vitality animal's immune function subsided. Clinically they are used for the treatment of other chronic infectious diseases and cancer.

The third category of immune agents to promote the development of recombination cytokines since 1980s.

These biologically active factors has achieved significant benefits in clinical treatment, of which the most prominent is rIFN-r, rIFN-α, IL-2 (IL-1 to IL-2), TNF, rCSF (such as GM-CSF). This can be a significant innovations immunity pharmacology or breakthrough, recently appeared monoclonal antibodies (Mabs) and the human gene antibody (H-Ab), these new components can be summarized as recombinant peptide immune substances.

Purification about a variety of immune substances has made significant progress and now we have a variety of effective products available, which indeed has proved clinical usefulness of chemicals is not too much.

11. The Research Progress of Chinese medication polysaccharide anti-cancer immunopharmacology

- Antitumor Study of Wolfberry Polysaccharides(Lycium barbarum polysaccharide, LBP), Polyporus umbellatus Polysaccharides(PUPs), Poria Polysaccharides, Lentinan (Mushrooms Polysaccharide), **Versicolor**(Yunzhi), Ganoderma lucidum Polysaccharides and Tremella Polysaccharides **(White fungus Polysaccharide)**
- Mechanism and Prospect of Anti - tumor Effect of Polysaccharides and the progress of the study on Anti - cancer Immune Chinese Traditional Medications

    Polysaccharides can improve the body's immune surveillance system, including natural killer cells (NK), macrophages (MΦ), cytotoxic T cell (CTL), T cells, LAK cells, tumor infiltrating lymphocytes (TIL), interleukin (IL) and other cytokines to achieve the purpose of the activity of killing tumor cells.

    Although many polysaccharides alone have some anti-tumor effect, two kinds of immune enhancers combining two polysaccharides will be higher effects. Polysaccharides with the use of chemotherapy or radiotherapy may further improve the outcome.

The research overview and progress

Thomas and Burnet's immunological monitoring theory suggests that the in vivo immune system has the effect of eliminating tumor cells produced by cell mutations to maintain a single cell type of each cell. The immune response system of the body, including cellular immunity and humoral immunity, is particularly important for the rejection of the tumor. Immune cells that perform cellular immune functions include natural killer cells (NK), macrophages (MΦ), and recently proposed LAK cells and tumor-infiltrating lymphocytes (TIL), which have an anti-tumor effect of 50 to 100 Times, played a stronger role. If these effector cells are inhibited, it is difficult to exert an immune surveillance system. Elston reported 19 cases with cell immune response in patients with choriocarcinoma, only 3 cases of which was death, and 13 cases were

death in 24 patients who have no immune response or immune response was significantly reduced. All of these indicated that the level of immune function plays an important role in the treatment of cancer. To prevent and control the tumor through enhancing the body's immune function is undoubtedly a bright future of the field of research.

According to the research progress of polysaccharides both at home and abroad and related information it showed that polysaccharides include LBP can play an anti-bacterial, anti-virus, anti-tumor, anti-aging, anti-chemo-chemotherapy side effects and anti-autoimmune diseases; there may also be lower blood pressure, blood fat, anti-vomiting and decreasing blood sugar and other physiological activities. These aspects will also be LBP in-depth research and application development of the important direction.

Compared with other polysaccharides, the composition of LBP is a glycopeptide, the role is strong, the small amount is used and it is water-soluble, stable and easy to absorb by oral etc., and it can be considered a highly effective immune T cell adjuvant. However, LBP is still a crude extract, and it has yet to cooperate with the plant experts to purify and modify LBP including degradation of different molecular weight oligosaccharides and oligosaccharides and sulfated polysaccharides, etc. so that it can further improve the immune activity of LBP and it is expected to find an updated immunologically active drug.

Immune is closely related to aging. Many scholars have found that the main reason for the degradation of cellular immune function in the process of aging is that the thymus is shrinking with age, and it is suggested that the thymus is the biological clock that controls the immune function during aging. LBP is the main part of the immune response to aging - thymus. The main experiments are as follows: ①LBP is mainly selected for thymus T cells; ② Ding Yan and other reports that LBP can promote the number of thymus mature T cells increased, and enhance the "emptying" function, the thymocytes to the peripheral transfer hyperplasia, play thymus Immune center regulation, and enhance resistance to disease and anti-aging effect; ③ our experiment has proved that young mice daily drinking LBP aqueous solution, after six months, the control group of animal thymus atrophy, LBP group thymus atrophy recovery, Has not yet reached the normal level of adulthood. This fact suggests that LBP can reverse the aging of the thymus degeneration. The above can be clearly understood, the relationship between thymus and aging.

12. The characteristics of traditional Chinese medication immunopharmacology

Compared with western immunity pharmacology advantages of traditional Chinese medicine immune pharmacology have their own characteristics or advantages, but also have shortcomings. The advantages of Chinese immunology medications roughly as follows:

The first is the long-term clinical application and have accumulated a lot of herbs to regulate the body immune function, especially having generally dynamic regulation of the immune benefits.

Rich source of traditional Chinese! traditional Chinese medicine is effective medicine during long-term clinical application and have significant pharmacological effects after extraction (including immunomodulatory effects). The research process can save people, save time and have high efficiency.

Secondly, whether single herb or medicine prescriptions contain a variety of active ingredients, unlike Western medicine (synthetic drugs) is a single structure. The roles of traditional Chinese medications are many, in addition to the regulation of immune function, have a certain effect on the overall function of the system and various organs. These effects in turn are interconnected and combined.

Chinese medications regulate immune function by generally tonic that is within the normal range of adjustment, with two-way adjustment as the main feature. Tonics can be called immunomodulatory drugs, causing non-specific immune response.

Tonic medication which there is regulation of immune function, shows the correlation between dose and benefits under the general experimental conditions, in particular a normal healthy animal experiments are obvious. When the animal is low in immune vitality(for example, the animals with removal of thymus, the aging animal or chemotherapy drugs cyclophosphamide under suppression and tumor animals), tonics medications improve immune function even more significant.

Immune pharmacology is an interdisciplinary formed by combining immunology and pharmacology. Traditional Chinese medications immunity pharmacology in our immune pharmacology occupies a special importance. TCM immunity pharmacology can be understood as the new field grafting modern immune pharmacology and TCM.

As early as the 1970s, Professor Zhou Jinhuang have been calling for the creation of integrative medicine pharmacology, clearly put forward the theory of Chinese medicine from starting to study and clarify the role of Chinese Herbal Medicine.

TCM theory has its obvious overall concept emphasizing the balance of the body and maintain balance when internal and external environment change. The body appears syndromes while losing balance and coordination.

Modern medicine also places great emphasis on a stable internal environment. The stable adjustment factors for Internal environment is the three systems of nervous, endocrine and immune systems.

As a system these play their independent regulatory role, but it is also interrelated and influence each other so as to achieve a relatively stable internal environment purposes.

"Nervous, endocrine, immune, regulating network" (NIM Network) is the research focus immunity pharmacology.

Through a lot of research work Professor Zhou Jinhuang developed NIM ideas which was conceived with a wide range of practical significance, is in line with scientific laws of life, but also with traditional Chinese medicine as a whole ideology coincides. Extensive, in-depth study of the role of traditional

Chinese medicine on NIM network on basic theory can greatly develop Chinese medications and make it to the world more quickly.

13. New discoveries from cancer research experiments:

(1) Removal of the thymus (Thymus, TH) can be manufactured bearing animal model for sure;

(2) These results suggest that: the metastasis is related to immune function; immune deficiency may promote tumor metastasis;

(3) It was found that: the host thymus was acute atrophy after inoculation of cancer cells which cell proliferation is blocked and volume was significantly reduced;

(4) It was found that: When solid tumors grow to large thumb, they were removed. A week later there was no further thymus atrophy;

(5) In our laboratory we were looking for immune reconstitution methods by using mice fetal liver, fetal thymus, fetal spleen cell transplantation to reconstitute while exploring to stop thymus atrophy. The results showed that in S, T, L three groups of cell transplantation, recently complete tumor regression was 40%, long-term tumor regression rate was 46.67%.

From the above experimental findings, thymus atrophy and immune dysfunction may be one factor in cancer incidence and pathogenesis, we should start from the body's immune function, especially cellular immunity, T lymphocyte function and immune function of the thymus to explore and seek immune regulation approach in the molecule levels.

In view of the development of Chinese medicine immunity pharmacology, traditional Chinese medicine theory has its obvious overall concept, emphasizing the balance of the body and maintain balance when changes in internal and external environment, loss of balance, the body appeared syndromes.

Modern medicine also places great emphasis on a stable internal environment. Internal environment stable adjustment factors are three systems: nervous, endocrine and immune systems. "Nervous, endocrine, immune regulatory network" (NIM Network) is the research focus immune pharmacology.

There are a lot of traditional Chinese medications regulating the body's immune function, especially having generally dynamic regulation of the immune benefits. During 28 years we have conducted a series of experimental research to find new drugs from natural medications to find new anti-cancer drugs and anti-cancer metastasis, to prevent thymus atrophy and to increase immune anti-cancer medication; looking only inhibit cancer cells without inhibiting normal drugs; from traditional Chinese medication to look for preventing atrophy of the thymus and adjusting the relationship between the host and tumors, preventing recurrence and metastasis drugs.

Existing anti-cancer drugs inhibit the patient's immune function, suppress bone marrow and thymus and immune surveillance was lost so that cancer further develops. Therefore, we must strengthen the research, all the anti-cancer drug used must be able to increase immune function and protect the immune organ, and should not be immune suppression drugs.

14. The research of the action mechanism of XZ-C immunomodulatory anti-cancer medicine

Looking for the new drugs of the anti-cancer, anti-metastasis in natural medicine (TCM) in the experimental work within our laboratory over a long period, a batch of 200 kinds of traditional considered to be "anti-cancer medicine," were screened in the experiments of tumor inhibition in tumor-bearing animal models, the results found that only 48 kinds do have some even better inhibition of tumor proliferation of cancer cells. Optimized combination, and then in vivo anti-tumor experiments in tumor-bearing animal models such as liver cancer, lung cancer, stomach cancer and others to consist of Z-C1 ~ 10 particles, Z-C1 can inhibit cancer cells, but not normal cells, Z-C4 can protect thymus and improve immune function, Z-C8 can protect marrow liters of blood, ZC immune regulation medicine can improve the quality of life of patients with advanced cancer, increase immunity, enhance physical fitness, improve appetite, prolong survival.

With more and deeper researches on traditional Chinese medicine, it has been proved that many kinds of traditional Chinese medicine can regulate and control the production and biological activity of cytokine and other immune molecules, which is meaningful to explain the immunological mechanism of XZ-C traditional Chinese anti-carcinoma medicine for immunologic regulation and control from the level of molecule.

I. Protecting Immune Organs and Increasing the Weight of Thymus and Spleen

That XZ-C traditional Chinese medicine can protect immune organs resulting from the following active principles.

1. XZ-C-T (EBM): Using its 15g/kg and 30g/kg extracting solution (equivalent to 1g original medicine) along with 12.5mg/kg, 25mg/kg ferulic acid suspension to feed the mice for seven days in a raw can increase the weight of thymus and spleen obviously, especially the effects of the group with high dose are more apparent. Intraperitoneal injection of EBM polysaccharide can also alleviate thymus and spleen atrophy obviously caused by perdnisolone.

2. XZ-C-O (PMT) :Extract PM-2, feed the mice with 6g/(kg·d) PMT decoction for successive seven days which can increase the weight of thymus and celiac lymph nodes and antagonize the reduction in the weight of immune organs caused by perdnisolone. Drenching the mouse of 15 months old with 6g/kg decoction (with the concentration of 0.5g/ml) for 14 days can increase the weight and volume of thymus, thicken the cortex and raise cellular density apparently. The combined use of PM and astragalus root can promote non-lymphocyte hyperplasia and benefit the micro environment of thymus.

3. XZ-C-W (SCB):SCB polysaccharide can gain weight of thymus and spleen of a normal mouse. Lavage with it enables cyclophosphane to control the gain in the weight of thymus and spleen.

4. XZ-C-M (LLA):Drench a mouse with LLA decoction for seven days resulting in increasing the weight of thymus and spleen.

5. XZ-C-L:For a 15-month old mouse, its thymus degenerates obviously. Astragalus injectio can enlarge the thymus significantly. The cortex under microscope is thickened and the cellular density increase obviously.

II. Effects on Proliferation, Differentiation and Hematopiesis of Marrow Cells

The following active principles of XZ-C traditional Chinese medicine have effects on hematopiesis of marrow cells.

1. XZ-C-Q (LBP) extracts (PM-2):

(1) Effects on the proliferation of hematopoietic stem cell (CFU-S) of a normal mouse: inject PM-2 with the dose of 500mg/(kg·d)×3d or 10mg/(kg·d)×3d LBP into the experimental mice respectively by venoclysis and kill them in the ninth day. It can be found that the number of spleen CFU-S in the group with administration increases obviously. The number of CFU-S in group PM-2 is 21% higher than that of the control group and it is 36% in the group with LBP.

(2) Effects on colony forming unit of granulocytes and macrophages (CFU-GM): the experimental results indicate that LBP with the dose of 5~30mg/(kg·d)×3d can increase the number of CFU-GM and PM-2 can also strengthen the effect of CFU-GM with the effective dose of 12.5~50mg/(kg·d)×3d. In the early stage of cultivation, most CFU-GMs are units of granulocytes and then units of macrophages increase gradually. In the anaphase units of macrophages take over the dominance.

From the above experiment, it can be found that PM-2 and LBP can promote hematopiesis of normal mice obviously. The experiment proves that during the process of restoring hematopiesis damaged by cyclophosphamide, PM-2 and LBP stimulate the proliferation of granulocytes at first, and then marrow karyocytes multiply; at last these two promote the restoration of peripheral granulocytes.

2. XZ-C-D (TSPG):

Ginsenoside, which is the active principle of ginseng to promote hematopiesis, can bring the recovery of erythrocyte in peripheral blood, haemoglobin and myeloid cell of thighbone in the mice of marrow-inhibited type, increase the index of myeloid cellular division and stimulate the proliferation of myeloid hematopoietic cell in vitro so as to make it into cell cycle with active proliferation (S+G_2/M stage). TSPG can promote the proliferation and differentiation of polyenergetic hematopoietic cells and induce the formation of hemopoietic growth factor (HGF).

3. XZ-C-H (RCL):

Steamed Chinese Foxglove can promote the recovery of erythrocyte and haemoglobin for animals with blood deficiency and accelerate the proliferation and differentiation of myeloid hematopoietic cell (CFU-S) with the effect of predominance and hematosis significantly. Peritoneal injection of rehmannia polysaccharides for successive six days can promote the proliferation and differentiation of myeloid hematopoietic cells and progenitor cells as well as increasing the number of leucocytes in peripheral blood.

4. XZ-C-J (ASD):

ASD polysaccharide has no effects on erythrocytes and leucocytes of normal mice, but for those damaged by radiation, injection of ASD polysaccharide can influence the proliferation and differentiation of both polyenergetic hematopoietic stem cells (CPU-S) and hemopoietic progenitor cells. But its decoction has no obvious effects.

5. XZ-C-E (PEW):

Poria cocos (micromolecule chemical compound extracted from Tuckahoe polysaccharide) is the active principle that can strengthen the production of colony stimulating factor (CSF) and improve the level of leucocytes in peripheral blood inside the mouse's body. It can also prevent the decline in leucocytes caused by cyclophosphamide and accelerate the recovery with the effects better than sodium ferulic which is used to increase leucocytes.

6. XZ-C-Y (PAR):

Its polysaccharide can obviously resist the decline in leucocytes caused by cyclophosphamide and increase the number of myeloid cells to promote the proliferation of myeloid induced by CSF as well as the recovery and reconstitution of hematopiesis for the mice irradiated by X ray. It can also increase the number of hematopoietic stem cells and myeloid cells along with leucocytes.

III. Enhancing Immunologic Function of T Cells

The active principles of XZ-C traditional Chinese medicine and their effects are following.

1. XZ-C-L (AMB):It can raise the percentage of lymphocytes in peripheral blood obviously. The LBP in small dose (5~10mg/kg) can cause the proliferation of lymphocytes, indicating that LBP can promote the proliferation of T cells apparently. 50mg/(kg·d)×7d is the best dose in that it will have no effects if lower than the level and it will bring the effects down if higher than the level. Oral administration of LBP can raise the conversion rate of lymphocytes for the sufferers who are weak and with fewer leucocytes.

2. $XZ-C_4$: It can regulate immune system and active T cells of aggregated lymphatic follicles, as well as stimulate the secretion of hemopoietic growth factor in T cells. Among the crude drugs of $XZ-C_4$, the extract from the hot water of atractylodes lancea rhizome can obviously stimulate the cells of aggregated lymphatic follicles, which is regarded as the base of $XZ-C_4$ immunoloregulation.

IV. Activating and Enhancing NK Cell Activity

Natural killer cell, NK cell is another kind of killer cell in lymphocytes for human beings and mice, which needs neither antigenic stimulation, nor the participation of antibodies to kill some cells. It plays an important role in immunity, especially in the function of immune surveillance as NK cell is the first line of defense against tumors and has broad spectrum anti-tumor effects.

NK cell is broad-spectrum and able to kill sygeneous, homogenous and heterogenous tumor cells with special effects on lymjphoma and leucocytes.

NK cell is an important kind of cells for immunoloregulation, which can regulate T cells, B cells and stem cells, etc. It can also regulate immunity by releasing cytokines like IFN-α, IFN-γ, IL-2, TNF, etc.

The active principles in XZ-C traditional Chinese medicine and their effects are following.

1. XZ-C-X (SDS)

Divaricate Saposhniovia Root can strengthen the activity of NK cells of experimental mice. When combined with IL-2, it can make the activity of NK cell higher, indicating that its polysaccharide can give a hand to IL-2 to activate NK cells and improve the activity.

LBP can strengthen T cell mediated immune reaction and the activity of NK cells for normal mice and those dealt by cyclophosphamide. Peritoneal injection of LBP can improve the proliferation of spleen T lymphocytes and strengthen the lethality of CTL increasing the specific lethal rate from 33% to 67%.

2. XZ-C-G (GUF)

Glycyrrhizin can induce the production of IFN in the blood of animals and human beings and strengthen NK cell activity at the same time. Clinical tests made by Abe show that after intravenous injection of 80mg GL, the raise of NK cell activity reaches 75% among 21 sufferers. Peritoneal injection of 0.5mg/kg GL on mice can strengthen the activity of NK cells in liver.

3. XZ-C-L (AMB)

Its bath fluid can promote NK cell activity of mice both in vivo and in vitro, and can also induce IFN-γ to deal with effector cells under the certain concentration of 0.1mg/ml. Cordyceps sinensis extract can strengthen NK cells activity of the mouse both in vivo and in vitro. Fluids with the concentrations of 0.5g/kg, 1g/kg and 5g/kg can strengthen NK cell activity of mice.

4 Effects on Iterleukin-2 (IL-2)

The active principles in XZ-C anti-carcinoma traditional Chinese medicine and their effects are following.

1. XZ-C-T

EBM polysaccharide can enhance obviously the production of IL-2 for human beings when the concentration is 100ug/ml. At higher concentration (2500ug/ml and 5000ug/ml), it will lead to inhibition. Hypodermic injection of barrenwort polysaccharide for seven days in a row can significantly improve the ability of thymus and spleen of the mouse induced by ConA to produce IL-2.

2. XZ-C-Y

PAR polysaccharide has strong immune activity and is able to promote the production of IL-2. For the mouse bearing S-180 tumor, it can raise the ability of spleen cells to produce IL-2 obviously.

3. XZ-C-D

Ginseng polysaccharide has great promotion on IL-2 induced by peripheral monocytes for both healthy people and sufferers with kidney troubles. The effects are relevant to the dose positively.

IFN are broad-spectrum in resisting tumors and can regulate immunity. It can also inhibit the proliferation of tumor cells and activate NK cells and CTL to kill tumor cells. Meanwhile, IFN can cooperate with TNF, IL-1 and IL-2 to enforce anti-tumorous ability.

The active principles in XZ-C anti-carcinoma traditional Chinese medicine and their effects are following.

1. XZ-C-Z
250mg/kg or 500mg/kg CVQ polysaccharide can improve significantly the level of IFN-γ produced by mouse spleen cells.

2. XZ-C-D
Ginsenoside (GS) and panaxitriol ginsenoside (PTGS) can induce whole blood cells and monocytes of human beings to produce IFN-α and IFN-γ. It can also recover the low level of IFN-γ and IL-2 to the normal.
The IFN potency of ASH polysaccharide on S-180 cell line of acute lymphoblastic leukemia and S$_{7811}$ cell line of acute myelomonocytic leukemia produced after acanthopanax polysaccharide stimulation is 5~10 times more than that of normal control group.

3. XZ-C-E
Hydroxymethyl Poria cocos mushroom polysaccharide has many kinds of physical activity like immunoloregulation, promoting to induce IPN, resisting virus indirectly and alleviating adverse reaction resulting from radiation. Do IFN inducement dynamic experiment on S-180leukaemia cell line by using 50mg/ml Hydroxymethyl Poria cocos mushroom

polysaccharide. The results indicate that its potency to induce interferon at all stages is better than that of normal inducement.

4. XZ-C-G (GL)

It can induce IFN activity. Make peritoneal injection of 330mg/kg GL on mice. IFN activity reaches the peak after 20 hours.

15. The research of which XZ-C4 anticancer Chinese medication induces cytokines

(1) Z-C4 anticancer medicine can induce endogenous cytokines

① Experimental study: Z-C4 has a variety of immune-enhancing effect, but with induced endogenous cytokine closely related.

② Z-C4 inhibit leukocyte, neutrophils and thrombocytopenia role.

③ Z-C4 by interleukin -1β (IL-1β) to produce granulocyte macrophage colony) not only has a direct effect, but also enhances the tumor necrosis factor (TNF), interferon (IFN) and other cytokines, which may be an indirect mechanism.

④ In cancer patients, regulate cellular immune function of Th1 cytokines decreased, while the Z-C4 can rise. Anemia, leukopenia after chemotherapy is curative.

⑤ Experimental analysis found that Z-C4 can not only protect the bone marrow, but also play a direct role in cell differentiation by cytokines.

In short, Z-C4 due to autocrine (autocrne) and the emergence of various cytokines, thereby inducing cell differentiation and natural death. The so-called autocrine, refers to a substance secreted itself in turn act on its own. Looking to the future, Z-C4 may become cancer cells induced differentiation therapy.

(2) Z-C4 inhibit cancer progression, metastasis

Invasion and metastasis of cancer cells obtained in the proliferation of malignant nature of the process, this phenomenon is called malignant progression. Advances in cancer research requires good reproducibility animal model. Thus isolated from mouse fibrosarcoma regression type of cancer QR-32 model made this good reproducibility. QR-32 even though the mice were implanted subcutaneously nor hyperplasia, and will be completely self-limiting; it does not appear input vein metastatic nodules in the lung. However, if the body of foreign substances as gelatin sponge together with QR-32 subcutaneously transplanted into mice, in vivo QR-32 becomes proliferative cancer QRSP.

(3) Z-C1 + Z-C4 immune regulation anti-cancer medicine

Z-C1 + Z-C4 immunomodulatory anticancer medicine has the following characteristics

① Overall improvement in the quality of life of patients with advanced cancer.

② Protect the thymus enhance immunity, protect the bone marrow and enhance hematopoietic function, improve immune and regulatory capacity.

③ Enhance physical fitness, reduce pain, improve appetite.

④ Enhance the therapeutic effect and reduce the side effects of chemotherapy.

16. The experimental and clinical efficacy of XZ-C immunomodulatory anticancer medications

(1) Tumor inhibitory effect of anti-cancer medicine Z-C1 ~ 4 on tumor-bearing hepatoma H22 mice

It was found on H22 mice two weeks, four weeks, six weeks after the using the medication, the inhibition increases with prolonged treatment time, on 6 weeks Z-C4 inhibitory rate reaching 70%, followed by twice repeating the test, results are stable, indicating that the inhibitory effect of Chinese medicine is slow, gradual increase, namely anti-tumor effect and the cumulative medicine dose was positively correlated.

Effect of Anti-cancer medicine Z-C1 or Z-C4 on lifetime of H22 liver cancer tumor-bearing mice:

Experimental results show that anticancer medicine Z-C1, Z-C4 can significantly prolong the survival time of tumor-bearing mice, especially Z-C4 significantly prolong the survival of more than 200%, not only that, Z-C4 also significantly improve the immune function, protect the immune organs, to protect the bone marrow, reducing chemotherapy and radiotherapy drug toxicity, the mice were fed up to 12 service months with no any side effects. The above experimental studies provide a useful basis for clinical applications.

(2) Clinical efficacy On the basis of experimental studies, from 1994 onwards clinical application of various types of cancer, mostly for stage III, IV stage than patients, namely: exploratory surgery unresectable advanced cancer; advanced cancer indications for surgery have been lost persons; after various cancer surgery recently or long-term metastasis or recurrence; a variety of advanced cancer of the liver metastases, lung metastases, brain metastases and have cancer or pleural effusion, ascites carcinoma; various cancer surgery can only do gastrointestinal anastomosis or colostomy and can not be resected: not surgery, radiotherapy, chemotherapy. Systematic observation: after 20 years of clinical application Z-C1, Z-C4 anticancer medicine achieved a significant effect for long-term use and no adverse reactions. Clinical observations demonstrate Z-C1, Z-C4 anticancer medicine can improve the overall quality of life in advanced cancer patients, improve the overall immunity, control cancer cell proliferation, consolidate and enhance the long-term effect. Oral and topical drug to soften ZC, narrow surface of metastatic tumor has a good effect, with intervention or cannula drug pump therapy, can protect the liver, kidney, bone marrow and immune system organs and enhance immunity.

(3) ZC analgesic effect of anti-cancer

Pain in advanced cancer patients is more obvious and painful symptoms, usually pain medication for cancer pain without much effect, narcotic analgesics addiction and dependence; ZC anticancer analgesic cream analgesic effect, and last longer, 298 cases of clinically proven significantly effective rate 78.0%, the total efficiency of 95.3%, re-use, no significant side effects, non-addictive, analgesic effect is stable, pain relief for cancer patients effective treatment methods to improve the quality of life.

Through experimental research and clinical validation, our experience is: Chinese medicine with Chinese characteristics has its unique advantages in terms of cancer treatment, such as a strong overall concept, highlighting the role of conditioning, side effects are mild, can relieve pain, relieve symptoms, significantly improved quality of life of patients, can mobilize immune function and overall disease resistance, improve treatment.

B. Results

(1) The tumor-inhibition effect of Z-C Medicine on Rats bearing hepatic carcinoma H_{22}: in the second week after administration of Z-C_1, the tumor-inhibition rate was 40% and the one in the fourth week was 45% and 58% in the sixth week. The tumor-inhibition rate after administration of Z-C_4 was 55%, 68% in the fourth week and 70% in the sixth week. (P<0.01) the tumor-inhibiting rate after administration of CTX was 45% in the second week, 45% in the fourth week and 49% in the sixth week (See Fig. 1 and 2)

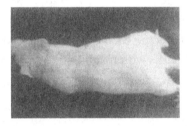 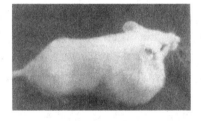

Figure 1 Z-C1, C4 treatment group   **Figure 2 Control group**
30d after inoculation of hepatoma H22   30d after inoculation of hepatoma H22

(2) The effect of Z-C medicine on the survival time of the rats bearing hepatic carcinoma H_{22}: the average survival time of Z-C_1, Z-C_4 and CTX was longer than the one of the normal saline control group (P<0.01); Z-C medicine played a role in obviously prolonging the survival time. Through comparison with the control group, the life elongation rate of Z-C_1 group was 85%, the one of Z-C_4 group was 200% and the one of CTX group was 9.8%. The rats in Z-C_1 and CTX in Group B met with death in 75d. 6 rats bearing carcinoma in Z-C_4 survived after seven months.

(3) Both Z-C$_1$ and Z-C$_4$ medicine improved the immunologic function and Z-C$_4$ obviously improved the immunologic function, increased the white blood cells and red blood cells, without any effect on the hepatic function and kidney function and without damage to the hepatic and kidney section. CTX decreased the white blood cells and reduced the immunologic function with the renal damage to the kidney section. The thymus in the control group was obviously atrophic (Fig. 1-4) while the one of Z-C$_1$ and Z-C$_2$ therapy group was not atrophic but a little hypertrophic (Fig.1-3).

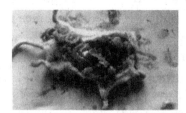

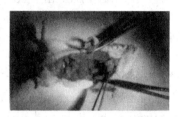

Figure 3 Z-C4 group
30d after inoculation of hepatoma H22
thymus hypertrophy

Figure 4 Control
30d after inoculation of liver cancer H22
marked atrophy of thymus

Pathological section of thymus in the control group: the cortex of the thymus was atrophic, the cells were discrete and the blood vessel met with sludge (Fig. 1-5). The pathological section of the thymus in Z-C$_4$ therapy group displayed that the cortical area of the thymus built up, the lymphocyte was dense, the epithelium reticulocyte increased and the thymus corpuscles increased (Fig. 1-6).

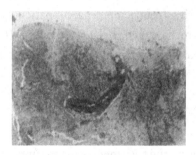

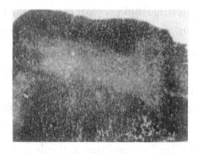

Figure 5 thymic tumor-bearing control group,
HE × 100 lymphocytes decreased cortical atrophy,
Cortex form a lymphocyte empty band

Figure 6 Z-C4 treated thymus

HE × 100 thymic cortex and medulla thickening,
lymphocyte high, intravascular congestion degree intensive

C. Clinical Application

1. Clinical information

(1) Hubei Branch of China Anti-cancer Research Cooperation of Chinese Traditional Medicine and Western Medicine, Anti Carcinoma Metastasis and Recurrence Research Office and Shuguang Tumor Specialized Outpatient Department had treated 4, 698 carcinoma patients in Stage III and IV or in metastasis and recurrence with Z-C medicine combined with western medicine from 1994 to Nov. 2002, among which there were 3, 051 men patients and 1,647 women patients. The youngest one was 11 years old and the oldest one was 86 years old, the high invasion age was 40~69 years. All groups of the patients were entirely subject to the diagnosis of pathological histology or definitive diagnosis with ultrasonic B, CT and MRI iconography. According to the staging standard of UICC, all the cases were entirely the patients in medium and advanced stage over Stage III. In this group, there were 1,021 hepatic carcinoma patients, among which there were 694 primary lesion hepatic carcinoma patients and 327 metastatic hepatic carcinoma patients; there were 752 patients suffering from carcinoma of lung, among which there were 699 patients suffering from the primary carcinoma of lung and 53 patients suffering from the metastatic carcinoma of lung; there were 668 gastric carcinoma patients, 624 patients suffering from esophagus cardia carcinoma, 328 patients suffering from rectum carcinoma of anal canal, 442 patients suffering from carcinoma of colon, 368 patients suffering from breast carcinoma, 74 patients suffering from adenocarcinoma of pancreas, 30 patients suffering from carcinoma of bile duct, 43 patients suffering from retroperitoneal tumor, 38 patients suffering from oophoroma, 9 patients suffering from cervical carcinoma, 11 patients suffering from cerebroma, 34 patients suffering from thyroid carcinoma, 38 patients suffering from nasopharyngeal carcinoma, 9 patients suffering from melanoma, 27 patients suffering from kidney carcinoma, 48 patients suffering from carcinoma of urinary bladder, 13 patients suffering from leukemia, 47 patients suffering from metastasis of supraclavicular lymph nodes, 35 patients suffering various fleshy tumors and 39 patients suffering from other malignancies.

(2) Medications and the methods of drug administration : the treatment aims to support healthy energy to eliminate evils, soften and resolve the hard mass and supplement qi and blood. $Z-C_1$ is the compound, 150ml to be taken on the daily basis, $Z-C_4$ is powder, 10g to be taken on the daily basis. According to the analysis and differentiation of the diseases, anti-cancer powder shall be taken orally and the anti-cancer apocatastasis paste shall be applied externally for the solid tumor or the metastatic tumor. In case of being in pain, anti-cancer aponic paste shall be applied externally. Icterus removal soup or dropsy removal soup shall be taken orally for the patients suffering from icterrus and the ascites.

(3) Therapeutic evaluation: it pays attention to the short-term curative effect and iconography indexes as well as the survival time of long-term curative effect, quality of life and immunologic indexes. Attention shall be paid to the changes in subjective signs in administration of drugs. It will be effective when the subjective signs are improved and last over one month; otherwise,

it will be ineffective. As to the quality of life (Karnofsky Performance Status), it will be effective when it is improved and lasts over one month, otherwise, it will be ineffective. As to the evaluation standard of the curative effect of solid tumor, it can be divided into four levels according to the changes in size of tumor: Level I: disappearance of tumor; Level II: tumor reduces 1/2; Level III: softening of tumor; Level IV: no change or enlargement of level tumor.

Effect of treatment

(1) The symptom was improved, the quality of life was improved, the survival time was prolonged: among the 4,277 carcinoma patients in medium and advanced stage who took Z-C medicine with the return visit over 3 months. It improved the quality of life of the patients in an all-round way, see Table 1.

Table 1 Observation of curative effect on 4 277 patients: fully improving the quality of life of the carcinoma patients in medium and advanced stage

Improvement	Vigor	Appetite	Reinforcement of physical force	Improvement in generalized case	Increase of body weight	Improvement of sleep	The restriction of improvement activity and capability released activity	self servicing normal walking	Resumption of work Engaged in light work
No. of cases (%)	4071	3986	2450	479	2938	1005	1038	3220	479
	95.2	93.2	57.3	11.2	68.7	23.5	24.3	75.3	11.2

In this group, all of them were the patients in medium and advanced stage. After taking the medicine, their symptoms were improved to different extents with the effective rate of 93.2%. With respect to the improvement of the quality of life (as per Karnofsky Performance Status), it rose to 80 scores on average after administration from 50 on average before administration; the patients in this group met with the different metastasis and dysfunction of the organs about Stage III. It was reported by the previous statistic information that the mesoposition survival time of this kind of patients was about 6 months. The longest time among this group of the cases reached up to 11 years; another patient suffering from hepatic carcinoma had taken Z-C medicine for ten years and a half; two patients suffering from hepatic carcinoma met with frequency encountered carcinomatous lesion in the left and right liver and it entirely subsided through secondary CT reexamination after the patient took Z-C medicine for half a year and the state of the disease had been stable over half a year. One patient suffering from double-kidney carcinoma met with the widespread metastasis of abdominal cavity after removal of one kidney, after taking Z-C medicine, he was entirely recovered and began to work again. 3 patients suffering from carcinoma of lung, with the lung not removed through explaraton, had taken Z-C medicine over three years and a half. 2 patients suffering from gastric remnant carcinoma had taken Z-C medicine for 8 years. 3 patients suffering from reoccurrence of rectal carcinoma had taken Z-C medicine for 3 years. 1 patient suffering from metastatic liver and rib of the mastocarcinoma had taken Z-C medicine for 8 years. 1 patient suffering from the recurrent bladder carcinoma after operation of renal carcinoma had not met with the carcinoma for 9 years and a half after taking Z-C medicine. All of these patients were the ones in the medium and advanced stage that could not be operated once more or treated with radiotherapy or chemotherapy. They only took Z-C medicine without other medicines for treatment. Up to today, they are reexamined and get the medicine at the out-patient department every month. Through taking the medicine for a long time, the state of the disease is controlled in the stable state to make the organism and the tumor in balanced state for a relatively long time and get a relatively good survival with tumor, in this way, the symptoms of the patients are improved, the quality of life is improved and the survival time is prolonged.

(2) As to 84 patients suffering from solid tumor and 56 patients suffering from enlargement of upper lymph node of metastatic compact bone, after taking Z-C series medicines orally and applying Z-C3 anti-cancer apocatastasis paste, they met with good curative effects, see table2.

Table 2 Changes of 84 patients suffering from solid tumor and 56 patients suffering from metastatic mode after applying Z-C paste externally

84 cases of physical mass and 56 Lymph nodes on the neck tumor after applying Z-C paste externally.

	Solid tumor				Enlargement of upper lymph node of metastatic compact bone			
	Disappearance	Shrinkage 1/2	Softening	No change	Disappearance	Shrinkage 1/2	Softening	No change
No. of	12	28	32	12	12	22	14	8
cases (%)	14.2	33.3	38.0	14.2	21.4	39.2	25.0	14.2
Total effective rate (%)	85.7				85.7			

(3) 298 patients suffering from carcinoma pain obtained the obvious pain alleviation effects after taking Z-C medicine orally and applying Z-C anti-cancer apocatastasis paste externally, see Table3.

The situation of 298 patients cases of after taking Z-C medicine orally and applying Z-C anti-cancer apocatastasis paste externally

Clinical Symptoms	Pain			
	Light alleviation	Obvious alleviation	Disappearance	Avoidance
No of cases	52	139	93	14
(%)	17.3	46.8	31.2	4.7
Total effective rate (%)		95.3		

17. XZ-C immunomodulatory anticancer medicine is the outcome of the modernization of traditional Chinese medicine

17, XZ-C immunomodulation anti-cancer traditional Chinese medicine is the result of traditional Chinese medicine modernization

XZ-C immunomodulatory anti-cancer medications are not the experience side, nor is the name of the old Chinese side, but the combination of Chinese and Western medicine and traditional Chinese medicine with modern scientific research, are to combine modern medical methods, experimental methods in experimental tumors, and modern pharmacology and medicine efficient methods. After seven years of more than 4000 cancer-bearing animal models, the so-called 200 kinds of commonly used anti-cancer herbs are screened in batches in tumor-bearing animals, then screened out of 48 kinds of anti-cancer effect of good medicine.

Then this 48 kinds of natural medicine are composed of XZ-C1 ~ 10 number which according to the respiratory, digestive, urinary, gynecological, endocrine system are built into animal model of liver cancer, stomach cancer, colon cancer, breast cancer, Kennedy bladder cancer, lung cancer, then tested and selected XZ-C1, XZ-C2, XZ-C3, XZ-C4, XZ-C5, XZ-C6, XZ-C7, XZ-C8, etc. series of immune regulation anti-cancer medicine for in vivo efficacy in tumor-bearing animal experiments and toxicological experiment.

The material basis of the traditional recipe playing its unique clinical efficacy is one of the chemical composition. The changes of quality and quantity of the chemical composition directly affect the clinical efficacy of prescriptions. So only study of the changes of quality and volume of chemical composition of prescription, to find out the main active ingredient preparation, molecular immunology to explore the mysteries of its unique effect can make research tradition reach a new level of prescription.

The formulation of XZ-C immune regulation medicine is Chinese medicine innovation and reform which is not mixed boiling liquid compound, but particles per herb concentrates or powders, which every membrane in every flavor raw pharmaceutical drug retains its original composition, pharmacological effect, molecular weight, constant structure and is made by using modern scientific methods, not the compound to keep the original flavor of each ingredient and function in order to evaluate the efficacy of affirmative action and that smell drugs.

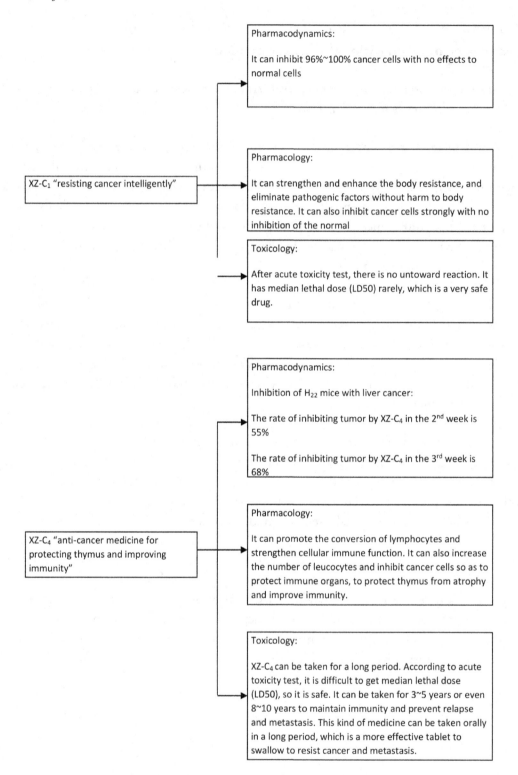

Exclusive research and development of products: XZ-C immunomodulatory anticancer medicine products (Profile)

Independently developed XZ-C (XU ZE China) series of anti-cancer immune regulation medication have significant curative effects and are self-invention, independent innovation and intellectual property rights. They are the results from experimental research to clinical validation, on the basis of success in animal experiments, then applied in clinical practice. There was a large number of clinical cases verification and clinical experience over the years.

Looking from traditional Chinese medication and screening anti-cancer, anti-metastatic investigational new drug:

The purpose is to screen out non-resistance, non-toxic side effects, a high selectivity, long-term oral anti-cancer, anti-metastatic and anti-recurrent cancer medication. To this end, In our laboratory it was conducted the following the screening tests of the new anti-cancer and anti-metastatic drugs from traditional Chinese medications

(A) The method of cancer cells in vitro, the experimental study of Chinese herbal medicine suppressor screening rates:

a. In vitro screening tests: The cancer cells in vitro was observed for sore drugs directly damage cells.

b. The screening test in tube culture of cancer cells: in vitro tests respectively allowing raw and crude drugs of crude product (500ug / ml) to be used and to observe whether there is inhibition of cancer cells or not. 200 kinds of traditional Chinese medicine herbs having anticancer function were screened one by one in vitro screening tests. And under the same conditions with a normal fiber cell culture the toxicity of these cells was tested and compared.

(B) Built cancer-bearing animal model for the screening of anticancer Chinese herbs

In vivo screening test: in cancer-bearing animal model screening Chinese anti cancer herbs, 240 mice were divided into eight experimental groups, each group 30 mice, Group 7 was the blank control group, Group 8 with 5-Fu or CTX was the control group. The whole groups were inoculated with EAC or S180 or H22 cancer cells. 24h later each rat was orally fed by crude drug powder. These medications fed the rats for long term to observe survival time and to calculate inhibition rate.

We conducted experimental studies for four consecutive years in more than 1000 rats each year. A total of nearly 6,000 tumor-bearing animal models were made and autopsy each mice after died to observe liver, spleen, sheets, pituitary gland, kidney and to get pathological anatomy with a total of 20,000 slices to explore to find out whether There may be slight carcinogenic pathogens and the establishment of tumor micro-vessels beds and microcirculation was observed with the microscope in 100 tumor-bearing mice.

Through experimental study we first found that Chinese medication TG had a significant effect on inhibiting tumor angiogenesis. Now it has been used as anti metastasis in more than 80 patients in clinic treatment.

Experimental results: In our laboratory animal experiments after screening 200 kinds of Chinese herbal medicine, 48 kinds of medications with certain and excellent inhibitory effect on cancer cells and inhibition rate of more than 75-90% were selected. 152 kinds with no significant anti-cancer effects were screened-out.

Screening out of 48 kinds of traditional Chinese medications with having good tumor suppression rates, and then optimized the combination and repeated tumor suppression rate experiments in vivo, and finally developed XU ZE China1-10(XZ-C1-10) immunomodulatory anticancer Chinese medication with Chinese characteristics.

$Z-C_1$ could inhibit cancer cells, but does not affect normal cells; $Z-C_4$ specially can increase thymus function, can promote proliferation, increased immunity; $Z-C_1$ can protect bone marrow function and to product more blood.

Clinical validation: Based on the success of animal experiments, clinical validation was conducted. Namely the oncology clinics and the Research Group of combined Chinese with Western medicine for anti-cancer and anti-metastasis and recurrence were established. The patient medical records were retained and the regular follow-up observation system were established to observe the long-term effects. From experimental research to clinical evidence, the new questions were discovered during the new clinical validation process, then went back to the laboratory for the basic research, then applied the results of a new experiment for clinical validation. Thus, the experiment to the clinics, the experiment again and the clinical experiment again, all experimental studies must be clinically proven in a large number of patients observed 3--5 years, or even clinical observation of 8 to 10 years. According to evidence-based medicine, the long-term follow-up assessment information had gained and they have been verified indeed to have a good long-term efficacy. The efficacy of the standard is: a good quality of life, longer survival. XZ-C sectional immune regulation anti-cancer medicine was made after a lot of applications in advanced cancer patients verification and achieved remarkable results and can improve the quality of life of patients with advanced cancer, enhance immune function, increase the body's anticancer abilities, increased appetite and significantly prolong survival.

In the chinese herbal medications many of them are the immune enhancer and the biological reaction regulator and the tonic medications; many can strengthen the body immune and have anti-cancer function. The two major global diseases that threaten human life are cancer and AIDS. The former is immunocompromised, the latter is immune deficiency. **At present, the world scientists agree that tumor formation is summarized as three processes: the first step, carcinogenic factors act on the body, interfere with cell metabolism; the second step, disrupting the genetic information within the nucleus, causing cell cancer; the third step, cancer cells escape the body Immune alert defense system; the body's immune defense capability is internal causes and the external causes have the action and the function through the internal factors. Cancer cells must be escaped from the alarm system monitoring in the body, breaking the body's immune line, to develop into a tumor. Therefore, trying to improve the body immune function is the key of the measures of the anti-cancer and the prevention of cancer. How to improve immune function? Chinese herbal medication has the extremely important advantage; there are many immune herbal preparations and there are a lot of drug sources and it should be an important anti-cancer and prevention cancer resources and it organizes the research and performs the development.**

The prevention and treatment of malignant tumors in the world are in progress. Each country focuses on a large number of experts and scholars with the experimental research and clinical experience to study and try to overcome cancer.

We should have advantages in our country areas to play the advantages of our country and to catch up with the international advanced level.

In the field of cancer research, the traditional Chinese medication is the advantage of our country. To play this advantage in the function of the field of cancer research and to explore and to develop the prevention of the cancer and anti - cancer Chinese herbal medications and to play this advantage of the study should be a strategic significance of the international significance.

On the road of human conquest cancer the research and the excavation and the development of effective and reproducible anti-cancer anti-cancer new Chinese herbal medication preparations must be promising and can be excavated into effective treasure and must be carried out the strict and objective and realistic and scientific and repetitive research with the strict scientific methods and the modern experimental surgical methods. All experimental studies must be rigorously and clinically proven in a large number of patients who demonstrate that there is a good curative effect and that the standard of efficacy is good quality of life and prolonged survival.

A series of products of XZ-C immunoregulation anti-cancer traditional Chinese medicine

1. **XZ-C1+4: for all kinds of cancer**
2. **XZ-C1: has the stable and significant anti-cancer effects, the inhibition rate up to 98%, no harmful to normal cells.**
3. **XZ-C4: protection of thymus and increase of immune function, promote the thymus proliferation, increase the immune function XZ-C8: protection of bone marrow and production of blood, increase T cells, and anti-metastasis**
4. **Lung cancer: XZ-C1+XZ-C4+XZ-C7**
5. **Breast cancer: XZ-C+XZ-C+XZ-C+ mushroom**
6. **Esphogus cancer: XZ-C1+XZ-C4+XZ-C2**
7. **Stomach cancer: XZ-C1+XZ-C4 or +XZ-C5**
8. **Liver Ca: XZ-C1+XZ-C4+XZ-C5 + Mushroom+ Red ginseng**
9. **Bile cancer: XZ-C1+XZ-C4+XZ-C5 + Capillaris**
10. **Pancrease cancer : XZ-C1+XZ-C4+XZ-C5+XZ-C9**
11. **Colon and rectal cancer: XZ-C1+XZ-C4+XZ-C5**
12. **Kidney and bladder cancer: XZ-C1+XZ-C4+XZ-C6**
13. **Cervical and ovary cancer: XZ-C1+XZ-C4+XZ-C5+ Lms+ MDS**
14. **Lymphma: XZ-C1+XZ-C4+XZ-C2+ Dai Dai**
15. **Leukemia: XZ-C1+XZ-C4+XZ-C2+XZ-C8+ barge pole**
16. **Prostate cancer:XZ-C1+XZ-C4+XZ-C6**

Comments: A series of XZ-C immune regulation anti-cancer traditional medications have been verified and tested for 20 years in Shuguang tumor special out-patient center on 12,000 of middle or later stage cancer patients. On clinical application they can change the symptoms, the patients have the good spirit and appetites are good, the life quality is improved, and they significantly prolong the survival time.

Face the future of medicine, look forward, after 20 years of long and hard work, practice the scientific concept of development, face the frontiers of science, for innovative, forward. To fight against cancer, it must come from the clinic, through experimental study, go to the clinic in order to solve practical problems of patients; must be realistic, with the facts, to speak with the data; must constantly self-transcendence, self-advancement; scientific research should emancipate the mind in bondage, get rid of the traditional old ideas, based on independent innovation, original innovation; our decades of research line is to find the problem → to ask a question → research a question → solve problems or explain the problem, the road is so came step by step, difficult journey, we hope out with Chinese characteristics, innovative road proprietary anti-cancer metastasis.

Our medical oncology research model is based on patient-centered, discovery and questions from clinical work, on the basis of in-depth study of animal experiments, and then turned to the clinical application of basic research results to improve the overall level of health care, and ultimately benefit patients.

SECOND, THE INTRODUCTION - "PATHFINDER"

- After more than 20 years the new way of conquering cancer walked out!
- The research revelation of walking out of a new way -----Pathfinder

Where is the road direction of conquering cancer? - where is the road? Where are you going? How to find this way?

We walked out of a new way of cancer treatment!

We are taking a new path of combining Chinese and Western medication: it is the new road on the molecular level of combining Western medication and Chinese medication; it is the new way to find immune regulation methods and drugs on the basis of new discoveries in animal experiments in our laboratory; after years of animal experiments and clinical validation, it finally was found out this new road of XZ-C immunoregulation anti-cancer traditional Chinese medication series.

Why should we take the new path of combining Chinese and Western medication? Why should we walk on the new road in the molecular level of combining Western with Chinese medication? Why should we look for a new way to look for immunomodulatory drugs?

The road which we are looking for was such came over step by step came. After the long process of more than 20 years of clinical validation, it didn't have this understanding at the beginning, but it was the gradual understanding step by step exploring and coming over.

We are taking the new way of the combination of Chinese and Western medication in the molecular level of combining Western medication and Chinese medication

The new road of anti-cancer "Chinese-style anti-cancer"

The combination of Chinese and Western medication is Chinese medication characteristics and advantages; the goal of the combination of Chinese and Western medication should combine the innovation and the aims should improve the treatment effect. The standard of efficacy of cancer patients should be: a long survival time; a good quality of life, and fewer complications.

For 28 years we have walked out of the new path of conquering cancer which is the traditional Chinese medication with immune regulation, the regulation of immune activity to prevent thymus atrophy and to promote thymic hyperplasia and to protect bone marrow hematopoietic function and to improve immune surveillance at the molecular level of combining Chinese medications with Western medications the new path of cancer.

Our Institute of Experimental Surgery is based on the study of cancer as the research direction and the main task to conquer the cancer of this major issue of joint research and takes the road of combining traditional Chinese and Western medication at the molecular level of combining Chinese with Western medication research, and it based on animal experimental research and in clinical practice to achieve the combination of Chinese and Western medicine, and then in the anti-cancer and anti-cancer metastasis theory it has developed and innovated.

It adheres to the combination of Chinese and Western medication with innovative scientific research work. It should be persevere and let go and adhere to the road of independent innovation with Chinese characteristics as so to promote the 21ˢᵗ century modern theory of oncology new development.

It strives to take the path of innovation with our characteristics of anti-cancer metastasis and to take the road of Chinese medication modernization and promote the molecular level of combining Chinese with Western medication and merge international medication modernization. We have walked out of the road of conquering cancer with XZ-C immune regulation and the molecular level of combining Western medication with Chinese medication----- "Chinese-style anti-cancer" new road.

- "Chinese-style anti-cancer" is the monograph title which Tang Zhaoyou academician published in April 2014 on the wisdom of Sun Tzu's tactics for anti-cancer strategy and tactical thinking.
- I think the combination of Chinese and Western medication is just a way and is a means, why should the combination of Chinese and Western medication? How to combine Chinese and Western medication? What is the goal of combining? Academician Wu Xianzhong proposed : the goal of the combination of Chinese and Western medication should be combined with innovation.

   What is the goal of combining innovation? What is the achievement hope of combining innovative?

- I think the goal of combining innovation is to improve the effectiveness of treatment and benefit the patient. The effect of cancer patients should be: a long survival time and a good quality of life and less complications.
- the fruits of combining the innovation should be innovative "Chinese medication " innovation "Chinese-style anti-cancer".

If this sentence goes on the sentence analysis, it should be:

The subject: Combination of Chinese and Western medication

The predicat: combine and innovate
The object: innovation "Chinese medication" and innovation "Chinese anti - cancer"
Subject (S) + Verb predicate verb(V) + Object object(O)

This is a complete sentence and has purpose and the method and the result so that I quoted Tang Zhaoyou academician the created word "Chinese anti-cancer". It is also the innovative new road of our 28 years of the scientific journey of ideological understanding and scientific thinking of anti-cancer and anti-metastasis research.

Find the way - to find where the way direction is:

For 20 years the road that we are looking for is such came over step by step :

- The revelation by findings of follow-up results:
  (1) - looking for the road of the research of the prevention and treatment of cancer recurrence and metastasis
  (the method and the medication and the technology and the basic theory)

- The discovery through experimental findings:
  (2) - looking for the path to prevent thymus atrophy and to promote thymic hyperplasia and to increase the immune path
  (Method, medicine, technology, basic theory)
  (3) - looking for the path of immune reconstruction
  (Method, medicine, technology, basic theory)

- Through the understanding of the new concepts and the new theory which was proposed and related to cancer metastasis from the anti-cancer metastasis study the revelation is that : the key to cancer treatment is anti-metastasis and is how to destroy the cancer group cells in the way of metastasis.
  (4) - looking for the way to eliminate cancer cells on the way of metastasis
  (Method, medicine, technology, basic theory)

- Through the above findings it was found that : we basically found the path of immunoregulation therapy, and gradually established XZ-C immunomodulation therapy.

We think it is one of the ways which leads to conquer cancer. In order to explore the cause and pathogenesis and pathophysiology of cancer, a series of animal experimental researches were carried out. From the experimental results the new discoveries and new revelation are that : thymus atrophy and immune dysfunction are one of the causes and pathogenesis of cancer. Therefore, Xu Ze put forward one of the causes and pathogenesis of cancer may be thymus atrophy and central immune organ damage and immune dysfunction and immune surveillance capacity decline and immune escapes at the international conference.

No matter how complex the mechanisms behind cancer, the mechanisms of immunosuppression are the key to cancer progression. The removal of immunosuppressive factors and the recovery of immune system cells on the identification of cancer cells may be effective against cancer.

By activating the body's anti-tumor immune system to treat the tumor, the next major breakthrough in cancer is likely to come from this. The prospect of immune regulation therapy is is gratifying.

In 1985 I carried out a petition for more than 3000 cases of chest, general cancer patients after radical surgery which I did. The results showed that most of the patients have the recurrence and metastasis after 2 to 3 years, and some even after a few months. This makes me realize that although the operation is successful, but the long-term efficacy is not satisfactory. The postoperative recurrence and metastasis are the key factor affecting the long-term efficacy of surgery. Also it prompted us that to prevent postoperative recurrence and metastasis are the key to extend the survival time. Therefore, the basic research must be carried out. If there is no breakthrough in basic research, clinical efficacy is difficult to improve. So we established the Institute of Experimental Surgery and from the following three aspects it spent 24 years doing a series of experimental research and clinical validation work.

The First, to explore the mechanism of the pathogenesis and invasion and recurrence and metastasis and to carry out the experimental research of the effective measures of the regulation of invasion, recurrence and metastasis.

We conducted a full four years of laboratory experiments in the laboratory and it is the clinical and basis research. The research topics are clinical questions. It was to explain these clinical problems or to solve these clinical problems with the experimental studies.

From the experimental tumor study it was found that :

(1) The resection of thymus (Thymus, TH) can be made to produce animal models;
(2) The experimental results suggest that metastasis and immune function are related and immune dysfunction may promote tumor metastasis;
(3) The results showed that the after the host was inoculated with cancer cells, Thymus had acute progressive atrophy and cell proliferation was blocked and Thymus volume significantly reduced;
(4) The experimental results found that: when the mice transplanted solid tumors grow to the size of thumb and then were removed. A week later the anatomy revealed that thymus was no longer atrophic;
(5) In our laboratory the experimental research of the prevention of tumor progression on the immune organ thymus atrophy and looking for immune reconstruction method and it used the mice fetal liver, fetal thymus, fetal spleen cell transplantation to reconstruct its immune function was done. The results showed that in the S, T, L three groups of

cells combined transplantation, the recent tumor complete rate of regression was 40% and the long-term tumor complete regression rate was 46.67%.

In our laboratory experimental results it was found that: in the tumor-bearing mice the thymus was atrophic atrophy and volume reduction, cell proliferation is blocked, and the mature cells decreased. To the late stage of the tumor, the thymus is extremely atrophic and the texture becomes harder.

From the above experimental study it was found that thymus atrophy and immune dysfunction may be one of the pathogenesis and mechanism of the tumor. Therefore, it must try to prevent thymic atrophy, promote thymocyte proliferation, increased immune function. It should be from the body's immune function, especially cellular immune, T lymphocyte function and thymus immune regulation function, at the molecular level to explore and to seek immunoregulation methods and the effective drug research.

It should further in-deep study from the thymus function and tissue structure, immune dysfunction and how to promote immune, so that immune reconstruction, how to "protecting Thymus and increasing immune function "to find the new ways of cancer treatment and new methods.

The Second, the experimental study of finding the new anti-cancer and anti-metastasis and anti-recurrence drug from the natural medication.

The existing anti-cancer drugs can kill both cancer cells and the normal cells and have the severe adverse reactions. Through in the Dutch mice in vivo tumor inhibition experiments, from the natural drug it was to find the new drugs which only inhibit the cancer cells without affecting the normal cells. We spent a total of three years tasting 200 kinds of Chinese herbal medications which are the commonly used traditional anti-cancer prescription and reported anti-cancer prescription in the use in vivo tumor inhibition. The results of screening are 48 kinds of good anti-tumor effect, but also a better role in traditional Chinese medications.

The research of which was done from the research traditional Chinese medication to find and to screen the new drugs of anti-cancer, anti-metastasis:

The purpose is to screen out the intelligent drugs of the anti-cancer and the anti-metastasis and the anti-recurrence with no the drug-resistant and the non-toxic side effects and the high selectivity which can be used by the long-term oral route.

To this end, our laboratory conducted the following experimental study screening the new anti-cancer, anti-transfer drug from the Chinese medications:

(1). The screening experimental study with the cancer cells in vitro culture method screening anti-cancer and anti-metastasis medication from of Chinese herbal medications:

In vitro screening test: the use of cancer cells in vitro culture to observe the direct damage to cancer cells.

In vitro tube screening test: in the culture of cancer cells in the tube the raw and crude drugs (500ug / ml) were placed to observe whether it inhibits the cancer cells. 200 kinds of traditional Chinese medicine herbs having anticancer function were screened one by one in vitro screening tests. And under the same conditions with a normal fiber cell culture the toxicity of these cells was tested and compared.

(2) the experimental study on the tumor suppressing rate of Chinese herbal medication in the tumor-bearing animal models which were made

In vivo, 240 mice were divided into 8 groups, 30 rats in each group, 7 group was blank control group, 8 group was treated with 5-FU or CTX as the control group. The whole group of mice was Inoculated with EAC or S180 or H22 cancer cells. After 24 hours of inoculation, each mouse was orally fed with the crude drug powder and the traditional Chinese medication was screened for a long time. The survival time and toxicity were observed. The survival rate was calculated and the tumor inhibition rate was calculated.

In this way, we conducted seven consecutive years of experimental study, but also carried out 3 years of the experimental research pathogenesis and metastasis and recurrence mechanism in the tumor-bearing mice and the experimental study of exploring how the tumor caused the death. Each year used more than 1,000 tumor-bearing animals model; in 4 years the total of nearly 6000 tumor-bearing animal models was used. After each mouse died, the liver, spleen, lung, thymus, kidney had the pathological anatomy and the total of more than 20,000 slices were made to explore whether there were carcinogenic small pathogens or not; with microcirculation microscopy it was to observe 100 tumor-bearing mice tumor microvascular establishment and microcirculation.

Through the experimental study, in the country we found for the first time that the traditional Chinese medication TG has a significant effect on the inhibition of tumor microvascular formation, has been used in more than thousands of cases of clinical anti-metastasis therapy and had great treatment effect.

The experimental results: In our laboratory through animal experiments 200 kinds of Chinese herbal medications were screened, 48 kinds of them which were screened out have the certain, even excellent on the inhibition of the proliferation of cancer cells and the inhibition rate was 75 to 90% or more. After some of the anti-cancer traditional Chinese medication which were commonly used in vitro, in vivo tumor experiment, the inhibition rate does not have anti-cancer effect, or little effect. This group was selected by animal experiments and 152 kinds of these medications with no obvious anti-cancer effects were gotten rid of.

48 Chinese medication with good anticancer rate were selected out from this experiment and then it did the optimal combination and then repeated the inhibition rate experiments in vivo,

and finally developed with China's own characteristics of the immune regulation of anti-cancer Chinese medications XU ZE China 1- 10 formulation (XZ-C1-10).

XZ-C1 can significantly inhibit the cancer cells, but does not affect the normal cells; XZ-C4 can promote thymic hyperplasia and increase immune; XZ-C8 can protect the marrow to protect bone marrow hematopoietic function.

The Third, where should a new way of immune regulation and treatment be searched

In order to try to prevent thymic atrophy, promote thymocyte hyperplasia, and to increase immune, we looked for both from the traditional Chinese medication and Western medication. There are rare drugs which can improve the immune function and promote thymus hyperplasia in western medication so we changed to look for from the Chinese herbal medication.

(1) why was it to find the medications which can promote thymus hyperplasia and prevent thymus atrophy and enhance immune function from the Chinese medication? It was because the traditional Chinese tonic drugs generally contain the role of immune regulation.

① Many of chinese medication and polysaccharides medication and tonic medication have the role of immune regulation.
Chinese medication of regulating the role of immune function is generally the benefit and the benefit and tonic types of traditional Chinese medications generally have the effect of regulating immune activity. Tonic drugs can be called immunomodulatory drugs, causing non-specific immune response.

Tonic types of traditional Chinese medictions have to regulate the role of immune function in the general experimental conditions show the correlation between dose and benefit, especially in normal healthy animal experiments are more obvious. When the animal is in a low level of immune activity (such as removal thymus animals, aging animals or chemotherapy drugs cyclophosphamide inhibition and tumor animals), tonic drugs can improve immune function more significantly.

② In recent years, Chinese medication polysaccharide anti-cancer immunization research progresses quick. A large number of immunopharmacological studies have been carried out at the molecular level.
Polysaccharides can improve the immune system, including natural killer cells (NK), macrophages (MΦ), killer T cells (CTL), T cells, LAK cells, tumor infiltrating lymphocytes (TIL), interleukins (IL) Other cytokine activity to achieve the purpose of killing tumor cells. Many olysaccharides alone have a certain anti-tumor effect, but the two immunostimulants, including the combination of two polysaccharides will be more effective.

Chinese medications and Western medications have their own strengths, each has shortage; it should take the long complement each other. Compared Traditional Chinese medicine immunopharmacology with Western medicine immunopharmacology, each has its own characteristics or advantages, but also has its own shortcomings. The advantages of traditional Chinese medication immunology is as follows:

A large number of righting traditional Chinese medication has the function of regulating the immune function of the body, especially the traditional Chinese medication is the benefit of regulating the immune activity.

The source is rich in traditional Chinese medication and all of them are the effective medications with the long-term clinical treatment. After it was the extraction it can become effective ingredients and has a significant pharmacological effects (including immunomodulatory effects); the study process saves time and labor with high efficiency.

(2) why is it to find immune regulation drugs from the Chinese medication? It is because of the progress of Chinese medication immunopharmacology research

In view of the development of traditional Chinese medicine immunopharmacology, TCM theory has its obvious overall view, emphasizing the balance of the body in the internal and external environmental. If it changes from maintaining balance into the loss of balance, the body appears the disease.

In modern medication it also emphasizes the stability of the internal environment. The factors which adjuct the stability of the environment in the body are the three systems: the nervous, the endocrine and the immune system. "Nerve, endocrine, immune regulation network" (NIM network) is the current research focus of immunopharmacology.

Traditional Chinese medicine has a large number of prescription drugs which have to regulate the role of immune function, especially tonic medicine commonly used to regulate the effectiveness of immune activity. In 28 years our laboratory conducted a series of experimental studies, from the natural drug to find the new chinese drugs with anti-cancer and anti-cancer metastasis and preventing thymus atrophy and increasing immune function; Looking for anti-metatasis and anti-recurrence new drugs; finding the drugs which only inhibit cancer cells and not inhibit the normal cells ; from traditional Chinese medication to find the new drugs which prevent thymus atrophy, adjust the relationship between the host and tumor regulation and prevent recurrence and metastasis.

The existing chemotherapy anti-cancer drugs inhibit the immune function of patients, inhibit bone marrow hematopoietic function, inhibit the thymus, inhibit bone marrow so that the host develops the loss of immune monitoring, and then further develop cancer. Therefore, it is necessary to strengthen the research so that all the anti-cancer drugs used must be able to increase immune and to protect the immune organs and it should not inhibit the immune function.

(3) why is it from the Chinese medication to find the medications which are to promote thymic hyperplasia, to prevent thymus atrophy and to enhance immune? It is because in our anti-cancer, anti-cancer metastasis research process it gradually found and realized that the theory and concept of Chinese anti-cancer, anti-cancer metastasis medications and the treatment is similar and even very consistent.

A). Chinese medication theory

1, In Chinese medicine treatment it is thought of that righteousness is not true, not into the evil, the treatment must be righteousness and tonic Qi.

And the development of a series of traditional Chinese medicine supplements. Its essence is to maintain the overall functional balance and enhance disease resistance. In modern scientific language, the main role of tonic drugs are to enhance the immune function.

Chinese medicine treatment is emphasizing righting and it is the equivalent of Western medicine to raise immune.

2, Chinese medicine is righting to Quxie and in Western medicine research the treatment principle of cancer is to raise immune, thereby enhance the immune surveillance to eliminate the cancer cells on the metastasis way. These two are very consistent.

3, The blood stasis in Chinese medicine treatment is commonly used the principles of treatment so that the blood stasis drugs are commonly used.

Traditional Chinese medication has many blood stasis medications and has the certain effective, lasting effect, long-term oral, suitable for anti-cancer drug use, because anti-cancer and anti-transfer drugs must be long-term oral medication.

Chinese medicine has many blood stasis medicine, for the application of anti-cancer clot and bolt, anti-cancer clot and bolt, anti-cancer metastasis.

B).The new concept of Anti - cancer and Anti - cancer Metastasis research

1, In our experimental study it was found: in the tumor model Thymus atrophy and immune dysfunction. It must try to prevent thymic atrophy and promote thymocyte proliferation and increase immune; it must seek to enhance the immune drugs to enhance immune.

Therefore, the theory of Chinese medicine and the concept of our study of "cancer metastasis treatment of new concepts and new methods" is very consistent.

The righteousness and solid in Chinese medication which we think of is the equivalent of Western medicine to enhance immune and to enhance the body resistance.

2, the traditional concept of Western medicine that cancer is the continuous division of cancer cells, proliferation, the target of treatment must be cancer cells (Quxie).

We study the "new concept of cancer metastasis therapy and new methods" that the treatment of cancer, cure should be controlled rather than kill.

We protect the thymus, improve immunity, improve immune surveillance, control the transfer of cancer cells and traditional Chinese medicine to help the concept of Qishen have similar.

3, we study the "new concepts and new methods of cancer metastasis therapy" that the blood cells in the blood cells gathered in the heap, peripheral cellulose, platelets and a small amount of white blood cells around the formation of small tumor thrombus. This tumor can be transported to other parts of the blood flow, or in situ after a certain period of time, piercing the local upper wall, in the blood vessels around the real organs and cells adhesion, division, proliferation, the formation of metastases.

We in the anti-cancer metastasis study, recognize the need for the transfer of cancer cells within the group or small tumor thrombi for Wai, chase, resistance, cut, anti-coagulation, anti-cancer bolt is the focus of anti-cancer.

How to eliminate the transfer of cancer cells, tumor thrombus, must be anti-thrombosis, anti-coagulation, improve blood rheology, Western medicine called anticoagulation, improve blood rheology, Chinese medicine called blood stasis, the two are very consistent.

The Fourth, clinical validation work

(1) After seven years of laboratory scientific experiments XZ-C immunoregulation anti-cancer, anti-transfer Chinese medication are selected from the natural drugs and composed with preventing Thymus an increasing immune function and protecting bone marrow and activating blood circulation and remove stasis ; based on the successful animal experiments the clinical validation work was conducted.

(2) Since 1985, one side of the tumor-bearing mice with tumor-bearing experiments, one side in the clinic clinical validation of efficacy.
But the patient is small, and the clinic without medical history (medical records are issued to the patient) can not accumulate scientific research information, we must take the road of scientific research cooperation.

(3) to form the anti-cancer research collaboration group, take the scientific research cooperation, joint research road and to establish the dawn cancer specialist clinic.

(4) to restore the outpatient medical records, fill out a complete and detailed outpatient medical records, in order to obtain clinical validation of the complete information, easy to analyze, statistics, is conducive to clinical research outpatient to improve the quality of medical care.

(5) to retain outpatient cases withregularly followed up, and a brief analysis of the case of diagnosis and treatment after the experience and lessons learned in order to long-term observation of long-term efficacy.

(6) Tumor specialist outpatient medical records are the table format including all the relevant medical information and related epidemiological data in order to facilitate the statistical analysis of its possible risk factors.

(7) The summary of the medical records and the outpatient medical records are written for the referral of more than 1 year of cases and has a large table analysis in which contains the outpatient medical records in the table of the content, both concise and thorough, dawn Cancer specialist Outpatient examination has been 20 years, a large table has accumulated nearly 10,000 cases of outpatient clinical data for outpatient clinical research.

(8) from experimental research to clinical research, and from clinical to experimental. Collaborative group has experimental research base and clinical application validation base, the former in the medical laboratory, the latter in the dawn of cancer specialist outpatient department, from experimental to clinical, that is, on the basis of successful experimental research applied to clinical, but also in the clinical application process Found that the new problems, and then further the basic experimental study, and then the new experimental results applied to clinical validation, such as outpatient patients with liver cancer with portal vein tumor thrombus, renal cell carcinoma patients with inferior vena cava tumor thrombus, some CT reports, some surgery Resection of specimens of the pathological biopsy report, in fact, cancer is in the transfer of cancer cells in the group, is the third manifestation of cancer in the human body, found the cancer bolt problem, we began to carry out the experimental study of tumor thrombosis, Looking for anti-cancer bolt and dissolved tumor thrombus of the new approach, the results we found four kinds of Chinese medicine to help dissolve cancer thrombus, and find out its active ingredients.

So that the experiment → clinical → re-experimental → re-clinical, continuous rise, after 12 years of clinical practice experience, awareness also continue to rise, sum up practice, analysis, reflection, evaluation and rise to theory, put forward new ideas, new thinking, Treatment ideas.

(9) the clinical efficacy observation: on the basis of experimental research, from 1994 on the clinical use of various types of cancer, mostly III, IV or more patients, that can not resect the advanced cancer; Or distant metastasis or recurrence; a variety of advanced liver metastases, lung metastasis, brain metastases, bone metastases or cancerous pleural effusion, cancerous ascites; all kinds of cancer palliative resection, exploration can only do stomach Chest anastomosis or colostomy and can not be removed; should not be surgery, radiotherapy, chemotherapy and other patients. XZ-C immunoregulation anti-cancer traditional Chinese medicine by 20 years of clinical application, systematic observation, and achieved remarkable results. Long-term use no adverse reactions. Clinical observation shows that XZ-C immunosuppressive medicine can improve the quality of life of patients with advanced cancer, improve the immunity of the body, control the proliferation of cancer cells, consolidate and enhance the long-term effect of postoperative or postoperative chemotherapy.

(10) Oral, topical XZ-C drugs to soften, reduce the body surface metastases have a better effect, with intervention or intubation drug pump treatment, to protect the liver, kidney, bone marrow hematopoietic system and immune organs, improve immunity. Dawning Cancer specialist outpatient department 1994-1995 treatment of stage III, IV or metastatic cancer 4698 cases were long-term referral or follow-up.

(11) service XZ-C immunomodulation of traditional Chinese medicine in patients with advanced cancer quality of life evaluation: the group were advanced patients, after taking the symptoms improved the effective rate of 93.2%, the mind improved 95.2%, appetite improved 93%, physical enhancement 57.3 %, A comprehensive improvement in the quality of life of patients with advanced cancer.

(12) Efficacy evaluation: both the importance of recent efficacy and imaging indicators, more emphasis on long-term efficacy of life, quality of life and immune indicators, the goal of patients to live a long time, good quality of life. Medication should pay attention to changes in symptoms, symptoms improved for more than 1 month for the effective, otherwise invalid; attention to the spirit, good appetite, quality of life (card score) increased.

From experimental research to clinical validation, in the clinical validation process to find new problems, and back to the laboratory for basic research, and then the new experimental results applied to clinical validation. For example, the experimental - clinical - re-clinical - all clinical studies, must be clinically proven, in a large number of patients who observe 3 to 5 years, or even clinical observation of 8 to 10 years, according to evidence-based medicine, Visit and assessable information to prove that there is a good long-term efficacy, efficacy of the standard is: good quality of life, long survival XZ-C immunoregulation anti-cancer traditional Chinese medicine preparation after a large number of patients with advanced cancer application validation, and achieved remarkable results. XZ-C immunomodulatory medicine can improve the quality of life of patients with advanced cancer, enhance immunity, enhance the body's anti-cancer ability, increase appetite, significantly prolong survival.

The Fifth, the research of the mechanism of XZ-C immune regulation anti-cancer traditional Chinese medication

A.) XZ-C immunomodulation of traditional Chinese medication can improve the quality of life of patients with advanced cancer, enhance immune function, enhance the body's anti-cancer ability, increase appetite and significantly prolong survival. The introduction is as the followings:

With the deepening of traditional Chinese medicine research, it is known that many traditional Chinese medicine regulates the production and biological activity of cytokines and other immune molecules. At this time, the immunological mechanism of XZ-C immunoregulation anti-cancer traditional Chinese medicine is described from the molecular level. There is a very important significance.

1, XZ-C anti-cancer traditional Chinese medication can protect the immune organs, enhance the weight of thymus and spleen.

2, XZ-C anti-cancer traditional Chinese medication has a significant role in promoting the bone marrow cell proliferation and hematopoietic function.

3, XZ-C anti-cancer traditional Chinese medication has enhanced T cell immune function and has a significant role in promoting T cells proliferation.

4, XZ-C anti-cancer traditional Chinese medication has the significant enhancement on the production of human 1L-2.

5, XZ-C5 anti-cancer traditional Chinese medication has a strong and enhanced role on NK cell activity and NK cells have the broad-spectrum anti-tumor effect and can kill heterogeneous tumor cells.

6, XZ-C anti-cancer traditional Chinese medication has enhanced the role in LAK cell activity and LAK cells can kill NK cells sensitive and insensitive solid tumor cells and has the broad-spectrum anti-tumor effect.

7, XZ-C anti-cancer traditional Chinese medication has the role of promoting tumor necrosis factor (TNF). TNF is a cytokine which can directly cause tumor cell death and its main biological role is for killing or inhibiting tumor cells.

B.) Biological response modifier (BRM) and BRM-like Chinese medicine and tumor treatment

1, the biological response regulator (BRM) has opened up a new field of tumor biotherapy and the current BRM tumor treatment is as the fourth program by the medical profession attention.

Oldham founded in 1989 the biological response modifier (BRM), that is BRM theory, on the basis of this in 1984 it was put forward the fourth treatment of cancer treatment (four modality of cancer treatment) - biological therapy. According to BRM theory, under normal circumstances, tumor and body defense in a dynamic balance between the occurrence of tumor and even invasion, metastasis, is entirely caused by the imbalance of this dynamic balance. If the state has been adjusted to artificially adjusted to the normal level, you can control the growth of the tumor and make it subside.

Specifically, BRM includes the following anti-tumor mechanisms:

① to enhance the effect of host defense mechanism, or to reduce the immunosuppression of tumor-bearing host, in order to achieve the immune response to cancer.

② to offer the bioactive substances with the natural or genetic reorganization to enhance the host's defense mechanism.

③ to modify the tumor cells to induce a strong host response.

④ to promote the differentiation and the mature of tumor cells so that cancer cells can be the normal cells.

⑤ to reduce the toxic side effects of cancer chemotherapy and radiotherapy to enhance the tolerance of the host.

2, the BRM-like effect and efficacy of XZ-C immunomodulatory anti-cancer traditional Chinese medication

XZ-C immune regulation anticancer medications have the functions and curative effects similar to BRM after four years experimental research and 16 years clinical research which are the drugs similar to BRM selected from traditional Chinese medicine and are from the screening of Chinese medicine resources to explore the role of BRM-like drugs. XZ-C is the durgs that XU ZE in China professor selected from two hundreds of the anticancer herbs after the experiments. At first the culturing tumor were done. The in vitro was done One by one to select and abserve the direct damage to tumor cells in the culture setting and the control groups of the rate of the anticancer are the chemotherapyxxxx and the normal culture tube cells. The results are to select the a series of the medicine of the anti-cancer proliferation, then made the animal modes which 200 drugs were used on one by one. These experiments of the analysis and evaluation are steps by steps, scientific, practical and strict, etc. The results proved that48 of them have the excellent tumor inhibition effects, however the rest 152 of the tumors anticancer medicine are all common old anticancer medicine which proved no anticancer or less inhibition of the tumors in the animal models during these medicine selection experiments.

Through the above experiments, XZ-C immunoregulatory anti-cancer metastasis of Chinese medicine with better tumor inhibition rate has the advantages of improving immunity, increasing thymus weight, protecting thymus function, improving cell immunity, promoting bone marrow cell proliferation, protecting bone marrow function, Increase the number of red blood cells and white blood cells, enhance T cell function, activation of immune cytokines, improve blood flow in the immune surveillance.

the main pharmacological effects of XZ-C immunoregulation anti-cancer traditional Chinese medication is anti-cancer and increasing immune function and its anti-cancer mechanism is :

1).activing the host immune system to promote the host immune function to reach the immune respond to the tumors.

2). Activing the host immune factors of the anticancer systems to strengthen the host immune function and improve the immunce surviellence of the host immune systems.

3).protecting the thymus and bone marrow,improve the immune system, and stimulate the bone marrow function to reduce the inhibition of the bone marrow and increase the white blood cell and red blood cells etc.

4). Reduction of the side effects of the chemotherapy and radioactive therapy to increase the tolerance of the hosts.

5). can increase the thymus weight gain, so that the thymus is not atrophy due to thymus atrophy while the progress of cancer.

As the mentioned above, the mechanism of XZ-C immunoregulation for anti-cancer traditional Chinese medicine is basically similar to that of BRM, and clinical use has the same therapeutic effect as BRM. Therefore, XZ-C immunomodulatory anti-cancer traditional Chinese medicine has BRM-like effect and efficacy. So that it makes the combination of today's advanced molecular theory of oncology and ancient Chinese herbal medicine resources in the molecular level of Western medicine; based on the BRM theory as a bridge, it merges with the international modernization of advanced theory and practice of oncology.

3, XZ-C1 + XZ-C4 immunoregulation anti-cancer traditional Chinese medication

XZ-C1 + XZ-C4 immunomodulation anti-cancer traditional Chinese medicine has the following characteristics:

(1) to improve the quality of life of patients with advanced cancer.

91

(2) to protect the thymus to improve immunity, protect bone marrow, enhance hematopoietic function, improve immunity and regulation.

(3) to enhance physical fitness, reduce pain, improve appetite.

(4) to enhance the treatment effect and reduce the adverse reactions of chemotherapy.

The Sixth, XZ-C immune regulation and control anti-cancer traditional Chinese medications are the results of modern Chinese medications

XZ-C immunoregulation anti-cancer traditional Chinese medication is not the experience side, nor is the old Chinese medicine side, but the combination of traditional Chinese medication and western medications and the traditional Chinese medicine modernization of scientific research, is the combination of the study methods with the modern medical methods, experimental experimental methods and modern pharmacology. After 7 years more than 4000 tumor-bearing animal model, 200 kinds of commonly used anti-cancer Chinese herbal medication which the literature describes, in batches of animal experiments screening, were tasting in vitro and by tumor-bearing animal tumor inhibition rate, then 48 kinds of anti-cancer effect of traditional Chinese medication were screened out.

XZ-C immunomodulation of traditional Chinese medicine preparation is the innovation and reform of traditional Chinese medicine preparation, it is not a mixture of decoction of the compound preparation, but each grain of the particles concentrated or powder, each agent in the drug every taste still maintain its original ingredients, pharmacology Role, molecular weight, structural formula unchanged, made with modern scientific methods, rather than the combination, to maintain the original flavor and function of each flavor unchanged, easy to evaluate, sure the role of the herbs and efficacy.

The above series of studies, we spent four years to explore the mechanism of cancer metastasis and the law, looking for an effective method of anti-cancer metastasis; and spent three years from 200 kinds of traditional anti-cancer Chinese herbal medicine through a rigorous scientific model The results showed that 48 kinds of XZ-C immunoregulatory anti-cancer and anti-metastatic traditional Chinese medicine with good tumor inhibition rate were screened. In this experimental study based on the clinical application of 20 years more than 10,000 cases, advanced cancer patients, and achieved good results. From clinical to experimental, but also from the experimental to clinical, the implementation of basic and clinical combination, take the molecular level of Western medicine, to be out of a Chinese characteristics of anti-cancer, anti-transfer of new roads.

The Seventh, Take the road of XZ-C immune regulation and control and the combination of chinese and western medication at the molecular level of overcoming cancer

The combination of Chinese and Western medications is the advantages and characteristics of Chinese medicine; the goal of the combination of Chinese medications and Western medications should be combined with the goal of innovation; the goals combined with innovative should be to improve the treatment effect. Cancer patients should be the standard of efficacy: long life, good quality of life, fewer complications.

Adhere to the combination of Chinese and Western medication innovation direction should be sustained.

Mr. Lu Xun once said that in the world it is no way to go and of more people go, it is the way. For 28 years we have walked out of the new path of a traditional Chinese medication immune regulation and the regulation of immune activity to prevent thymus atrophy, and to promote thymic hyperplasia, protect bone marrow hematopoietic function, improve immune surveillance, at the molecular level of the combination of chinese and western medication to overcome of cancer.

To achieve the combination of innovation, improve the efficacy of high-level combination of Chinese and Western medicine goals, it is not only to implement the theory of traditional Chinese medications and modern medical practice, but also to use the experimental research to clarify the theory of traditional Chinese medication, modern molecular theory of traditional Chinese medicine immunopharmacology... ... modern theory of oncology theory, and then in theory and clinical practice there are the development and innovation, so as to improve the treatment effect and so that patients benefit.

Our Institute of Experimental Surgery is based on the study of conquering cancer as the research direction and the main task, around this major issue of joint research to tackle the cancer, take the path of the combination of Chinese and Western medication and the study at the molecular level of Chinese and Western medicine which is based on animal experimental research, And in the clinical practice verification of clinical practice to achieve the combination of Chinese and Western medication, and then in the anti-cancer, anti-cancer metastasis theory it has developed, innovation:

- Chinese medication is the righteousness and is not true, and the evil can not into; the treatment must be righteousness, attention to righting. In Western medicine it is considered that the tumor is immune dysfunction, must be "protection of thymus and increase immune function" to enhance immune function.

Chinese medicine emphasizes righting and is the equivalent of Western medicine to increase immune function, these two are very consistent.

- Chinese medicine treatment, not only attach importance to righting, but also attention to Quxie, that is righting or righting to Quxie; Western medication raises immune function, improves immune surveillance, thus eliminate the transfer of cancer cells; the treatment concept is similar or The two are very consistent.

- Traditional Chinese medication treatment of activating blood and being stasis is a common principle. In the anti-cancer metastasis study, it is recognized that it must stop the cancer cells in the transfer way and must stop the blood clot and have anticoagulation to improve blood flowing rheology, Chinese medicine treatment of activating blood circulation is very consistent with The treatment of siltation in the Western medication; the two anticancer treatment of cancer treatment are the similar or the two are very consistent.

Adhere to Chinese and Western medicine combined with innovative scientific research work, should be persevere, and let go, adhere to the road of independent innovation with Chinese characteristics, to promote the 21st century modern theory of oncology new development.

Take the road of modern chinese medication to promote the molecular level of Chinese and Western medicine, and international medicine modernization, and strive to take our characteristics of anti-cancer, anti-cancer transfer path.

It is now the second decade of the 21st century, should be the combination of Chinese and Western medicine innovation era, more than 30 years, we have been to improve the clinical efficacy of cancer this major disease as the main direction, perseverance and persistence and never giving up and never dismay and then it has published three research books. The third monograph "New Concept and New Method of Cancer Treatment" has been translated into English by the American medicalian Bin Wu and the English version has been published internationally. To study the related theory of anti-cancer and anti-metastasis, to develop the morden anticancer and anti-metastasis drugs; XZ-C immunocompromised anti-cancer traditional Chinese medicine preparation series (XZ-C1-10) have been carried out the experimental study and the combination of basic and clinical and the combination of medicine and drugs and the combination of the ancient Chinese herbal medicine and traditional Chinese medicine immunology, molecular biology, cytokology ; it is to Chinese and Western complement and to combine with innovation.

Efforts to take the new and innovation path of our characteristics of anti-cancer transfer path and to take the road of modern medicine, promote the molecular level of Chinese and Western medicine, and to merge with international medicine modernization. We have walked out of a XZ-C immune regulation, the molecular level of Western medicine combined to overcome the cancer path.

The excavation, development of prevention of cancer and anti-cancer new Chinese medication preparations

Prevention and treatment of malignant tumors in the world are in progress, all of the countries are focused on a large number of the experts and scholars with the experimental research ability and clinical experience to study trying to overcome cancer.

We should play the advantages of our country with our country advantage areas and catch up with the international advanced level.

In the field of cancer research the traditional Chinese medication is the advantage of our country. To play this advantage in the field of cancer research and to explore the development of Chinese herbal medication with the prevention of cancer and anti – cancer and to play this advantage of the study should be a strategic vision of international significance.

First, the reason and the background

1. At present, in addition to the study of synthetic drugs, each country in the world also study the herbal medication or earthwork in the country, the region and the national. Scientists are now returning to nature to find new drugs for cancer. At present the experts and scholars are dong the study of immune response in the treatment of biological response modulators; in the United States and the English the United States it is studying LAK cell lymphokine-activated killer cells (1ymphokine actviated killedinea), interleukin-2 (Interleukin. -2), Japan's OK a 432, the principle is T cells, B cells, lymphocyte immunity and so on.

   China in this field has many natural drugs (unilateral, prescription, earthwork, folk side), such as rutus polysaccharide K, lentinan, Ganoderma lucidum polysaccharides, ginseng polysaccharides, Hericium polysaccharides and many other natural plant herbs contain a variety of histones, Polysaccharides, etc., which have the good role in biological anti-modifier, are cancer immunotherapy drugs. Many of the unilateral and the prescription contain such these drugs, scattered in the civil or in some out-patient trial and did not do the correct research and verification, and need to further explore and to develop and to study in the laboratory with experimental research in modern science and technology, strictly, Scientific, objective, realistic by people with lofty ideals. This is our unique and valuable natural wealth, and may be the gold deposits to overcome the cancer. Foreign scientists also attach great importance to the study of folk, earth, herbs. China has a wealth of natural medicine resources, and thousands of years of traditional medical experience, which is our research and capture cancer a major advantage. It should be further researched, with the modern scientific and technological methods, and doed the experimental research, sorting, induction, excavation, development to product the new anti-cancer Chinese herbal medication preparations.

2. Many Chinese herbal medicine is immune enhancer, biological reaction regulator, tonic, many can strengthen the body immunity and anti-cancer. The two major global diseases that threaten human life are cancer and AIDS. The former is immunocompromised, the latter is immune deficiency. At present, the world scientists agree that tumor formation is summarized as three processes: the first step, carcinogenic factors act on the body, interfere with cell metabolism; the second step, disrupting the genetic information within the nucleus, causing cell cancer; the third step, cancer cells escape the body Immune alert defense system, the body's immune defense capability is internal, external causes through internal factors. Cancer cells must be escaped from the body of the alarm system monitoring, breaking the body's immune line, to develop into a tumor. Therefore, trying to improve the body immunity

is the key anti-cancer anti-cancer measures. How to improve immunity, Chinese herbal medicine is an extremely important advantage, there are many immune herbal preparations (such as ginseng, Astragalus, Cordyceps sinensis, etc.), a rich source of medicine, should be an important anti-cancer, anti-AIDS resources, Organizational research, development.

In the late 1980s, the new understanding of cancer, the new theory of "seesaw", put forward the international first four kinds of therapy that bioimmune therapy (surgery, radiotherapy, chemotherapy for the first three methods). Has been the above, so that Chinese herbal medicine can be included in the fourth kind of therapy, Chinese medicine anti-cancer, anti-cancer can be raised to an extremely important position, rising to the 21st century, urgent research, urgent development of cutting-edge disciplines.

On the road of human conquest cancer, research, excavation and development of effective and reproducible anti-cancer anti-cancer new Chinese herbal medicine preparations, must be promising, can be excavated into effective treasure, must be carried out with strict scientific methods, modern experimental surgical methods Strict, objective, realistic, scientific and repetitive research. All experimental studies must be rigorously clinically proven in a large number of patients who demonstrate that there is a good curative effect, and that the standard of efficacy is good quality of life and prolonged survival.

Second, the research and the outlook

After many scientists work hard to explore, the anti-tumor botanical research and development has developed a number of Chinese and Western medication with highly educated low toxicity and the exact effect so that the treatment of malignant tumors from The state of terror of the past "chronic death" up to today which can generally cure more than 1/3 of the results. Of course, this is mainly due to the development of modern medicine, and the new anti-tumor drug research and development play a pivotal role in this development, especially the active ingredients from the natural and having effective and small toxic side effects Is to become the focus of today's human research.

Looking at the research and development of antitumor drugs in recent decades, people all feel the profound changes in their changes. Especially since the 1980s, with the development of science and technology, people's understanding of the causes, physiological and biochemical and pathological status of malignant tumors has deepened, and brought new ideas to the research and development of anti-tumor drugs, especially the computer Assisted drug design, combined chemistry and a large number of drug screening methods to make its drug extraction, screening, structural transformation, synthesis more reasonable, a variety of new formulations, new drugs have come out. At the same time, the administration system, the structure of the receptor and the mechanism of functional regulation have become very active in the field of pharmacy. Looking back at recent years of change, looking to the prospect of the future, many pharmaceutical industry experts predict that antitumor drugs, especially from natural anti-tumor drugs research and development, will have great development in the 21st century.

China is a treasure house of huge drugs, the development and utilization of natural medicine has a long history, brilliant achievements. Especially in recent decades, the use of modern science and technology and analytical testing methods, the traditional Chinese medicine research will be more extensive and in-depth, so that many traditional drug applications more scientific and rational, and theoretically find its application Basis.

Derived from the natural anti-tumor activity of the drug, relative to the chemical synthesis of drugs, has many irreplaceable advantages, in addition to less adverse reactions to the human body, but also can effectively reduce the environmental pollution caused by the pharmaceutical industry.

Today, mankind is increasingly concerned about its own living environment, drug research in the field of bio-genetic engineering at the same time, anti-Pu Guizhen, return to nature, will achieve the 21st century, high-tech development of medicine and natural resources development and utilization of the perfect combination.

THIRD, THE INNOVATION CONTENT OF THE RESEARCH THERAPY OF THE NEW CONCEPT AND NEW METHODS OF CANCER METASTASIS TREATMENT

After more than 60 years of clinical experience in surgical oncology practice and 30 years of laboratory research I carried out careful sorting and summarizing and then it was formed an unique new understanding and new concept of cancer metastasis and proposed new methods and new technology of anti-metastatic cancer therapy. Its main contents include: ① cancer in the body exists in three forms; ② the whole process of two points and One Line of Carcinoma Development ③ cancer metastasis" eight steps and three-stages "theory; ④ the third field of human anti-cancer metastasis treatment;⑤cancer metastasis treatment "trilogy"; ⑥ independently developed XZ-C immunomodulatory anticancer Chinese medications.

The following series of new understanding, new theories, new concepts have not yet been mentioned so far in the literature and textbooks. After lessons and experiences of half century practice and 10 years of experimental research and analysis, reflection and waking up it converses to real theory which founded new concepts and all of which have independent innovation and creative and original intellectual property rights.

一. Theoretical Innovation Content (Introduction)

All of the following of the new concept of cancer anti-metastasis therapy is my exclusive theory system, and independent intellectual property rights of the independent innovation and original innovation.

(一).Xu Ze first found and put forward a new theory or a new theoretical proof in the international community: the existence form of cancer in the human body there are three forms of the expression, and the third form of the existence of the human body is as the group of cancer cells on the way of metastasis.

XU ZE's new concept of cancer metastasis treatment: the existence form of cancer in the human body has three forms: one existence form is the primary cancerous lesion; the second form is metastatic cancer lesion: the third form is the cancer cell group on the routing of metastasis. The first two forms of expression may be visible, touched, or through the endoscope to see, but also through the imaging to see the stalls: the third form of expression is the cancer cells on the way of metastasis which is invisible, cannot be touched, or cannot be found with the endoscope, B ultrasound, CT,

MRI and so on, and these millions of potential, hidden, swim cancer cells which are on the way of metastasis are the greatest enemy of threatening life of the cancer patients.

The goal of the cancer treatment or the "target" should be directed against the cancer in the human body in three forms, namely: (1) one of the goals of treatment for the primary lesion; (2) the second target treatment of cancer is for metastasis Cancer foci; (3) the three of the target of cancer treatment should be for cancer cells in the group on the routing of metastasis.

This new doctrine or new theoretical understanding proven nor recognized will lead to a series of changes, renewals and updates of the chain-like tumor diagnosis and treatment:

(1) changes and updates on the understanding of the concept of cancer treatment;
(2) changes and updates of the goals or "target" awareness on cancer treatment;
(3) changes and updates on cancer diagnostic methods;
(4) will cause significant changes and updates of the research and development on the search of the new drug of anti-cancer and anti-metastasis;
(5) will cause significant changes and updates on cancer treatment models and methods;
(6) will inevitably lead to the changes and updates of the research of cancer metastasis and recurrence from the cell level of the cytopathology of the microscopic oncology to the molecular level oncology of the molecular biology, gene expression.

Why should it is suggested that the third existence form of cancer expression in the human body is cancer cells, cancer cell populations and micro-being on the way of metastasis in the process of multi-step, multi-factor? This question has not yet been known, has not attracted enough attention, but no specific discussion of strategies, countermeasures and methods of how to conduct diagnosis and treatment. Since This third form of existence have not yet been mentioned, not yet known, and not yet paid attention to, in fact, to annihilate and to block and to interfere and to cut off the new route of treatment model are the key to anti-cancer metastasis.

To overcome the cancer should be updated thinking to change the concept; the cancer treatment should have a comprehensive cancer treatment concept

About the main existence forms of cancer in the human body there are two main manifestations of the concept, there are two different understandings:

(1) the traditional concept of cancer treatment think of that there are two forms of expression;

The first form of expression - primary foci;
The second form of expression - the metastasis foci.

The target or goal of the traditional cancer therapeutic is to aim on these two forms,
The first one is to aim on the first form of expression - the primary foci;
The Second one is to aim on the second form of expression - metastatic foci.

This traditional concept of treatment was used for more than 100 years, the treatment target or "target" is for these two forms of expression - primary foci or metastatic foci. The two "targets" are treated in isolation, and the dynamic relationship between the two, causality, subordination is not considered; however how the primary foci is formed to metastasize the foci and how to stop its metastasis is not involved. Therefore, the traditional concept of cancer therapy that cancer in the human body has only two existence forms of expression which this understanding is not comprehensive, incomplete and defective; therefore, according to this understanding and the implementation of treatment only for these two forms - primary foci and metastatic foci ignores the cancer cells in transit or on the way of metastasis. It is well known that metastasis is the biological and biological behavior of malignant tumors. The difference between benign tumor and malignant tumor is that the former does not transfer and the latter can have metastasis, and anti-metastasis is the key to cancer treatment. It cannot control the transfer of cancer cells without blocking cancer cells on the way of metastasis, and thus it is difficult to obtain the possibility of cancer complete treatment.

(2) Xu Ze new concept of cancer treatment has three forms of cancer in the human body, and there are three forms of existence:

The first form of expression - primary foci;
The second form of expression - metastatic foci;
The third form of expression - cancer cells, cancer cells group on the way of metastasis and microvascular thrombus metastasis.

The goal or "target" of treatment is also for these three manifestations:

One for the first manifestation - primary foci;
Two for the second form of expression - the second foci;
Three for the third manifestation - the cancer cell population on the way of metastasis.

This new concept that cancer exists in the human body for the performance of the three forms is relatively complete and more comprehensive, clarified the dynamic relationship, causal relationship and affiliation among these three forms, is a complete new concept of cancer therapies, and is a comprehensive explanation of the whole process of cancer development and how to control the whole process of cancer cell metastasis. This new theory will bring the dawn of conquering cancer.

(二). Xu Ze first mentioned another new theory or new theoretical understanding in the international community: the two points and one line "theory in the whole process of cancer development. It was considered that both at home and abroad cancer treatment now only recognize and pay attention to two points and ignore a line. In fact, the treatment of cancer not only should pay attention to two points, but also should pay attention to the one front line, and to cut off the line is the key to anti-cancer metastasis.

What is called as two points and one line? Two points, that is, for the metastasis starting point, the primary foci; and the metastasis end, metastatic foci. A line that is a long routing between the two points of the primary lesion and metastatic foci which cancer cells travel a long distance to the distant organs. (see Figure 1)

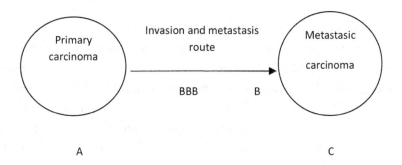

Fig.1 Sketch Map of Two Points and One Line of Carcinoma Development

Note: A. Primary carcinoma, the starting point of metastasis; B. Invasion and metastasis route; C. Metastasic carcinoma, the end point of metastasis

Whether it is the starting point of the primary foci, or the end of the metastatic foci, when the growth of the foci to a certain size, it will become a new source of cancer metastasis. This metastasis focus can have metastasis again and becomes the starting point of the second round of transfer. So the transfer can continue to develop slowly, and ultimately endanger the patient's life. (See Figure 2)

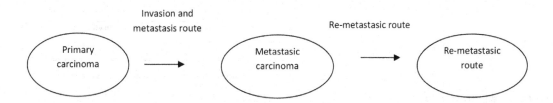

Fig. 3-2 Sketch map of re-metastasis of metastasic carcinoma

Note: A' is the new starting point; B' is the re-metastasic route; C' is the new end point

Traditional treatment is often only focus on the 'two points', but ignored the "line"

XC ZE new concept of treatment cancer should pay attention to "two points", but also to cut off the one front line.

Through the analysis of the experimental data of laboratory study of searching the metastasis rules and the clinical data of anti-cancer metastasis recurrence research tumor specialist outpatient large number of metastatic cases, we summed up the cancer cell transfer process, quite some similar to the infectious disease process:

1. the three major elements of infectious diseases; (1) a source of infection; [2] transmission pathways: (3) susceptible population. The transfer of cancer cells also have: (I) the metastasis source; (2) transfer pathways; (3) the organ or tissue with easy implanting.

2. the countermeasures of the treatment of infectious diseases are: (1) isolation of patients with infectious diseases; (2) cut off the transmission pathways; (3) to enhance immune function of the susceptibility of people. XU ZE believes that the treatment of cancer metastasis can also adopt a similar principle: (I) treatment of primary foci; (2) cut off the transfer pathway, the intervention, blocking and killing of metastasis cancer cells: (3) to enhance the body Immune function surveillance and to improve the body's anti-cancer power. However, the control of infectious diseases (such as the control of SARS) is in the community of macro-environment in the epidemiological control, and control of cancer cell metastasis is only the intervention of cancer cells metastasis in the condition of the host organ visceral microcirculation. The above treatment scheme is summarized in Figure 3.

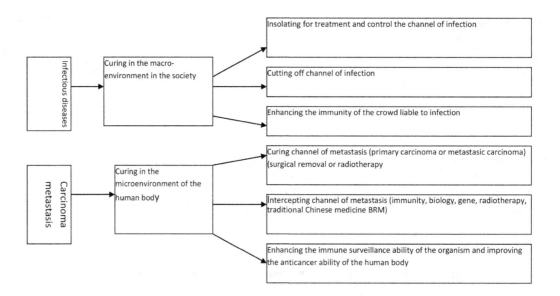

Fig. 3-3 Therapeutic method of infectious diseases and carcinoma metastasis

To sum up, it can be seen that XU ZE New Concept of Carcinoma Treatment pays attention not only to the surgical removal, radiotherapy and chemotherapy of primary carcinoma and metastasic carcinoma but also to intercepting and killing the cancer cells in the route of metastasis. This new theory called "Two Points and One Line" has the following important significance:

(1) Making the goal or target of anti-metastasis more clear and specific;

(2) Further supplementing an perfecting the countermeasures or strategy of traditional carcinoma therapeutics;

(3) Emphasizing that the anti-metastasis shall pay attention not only to "Two Points" but also "One Line". Only the cancer cells in the route of metastasis are cut off, can the curative effect of carcinoma treatment can be improved.

(4) Making the people relatively clearly understand the metastasis of carcinoma, putting forward a new theoretic basis, which is advantageous for the clinicians to reasonably design and make use of the existing various therapeutic methods and probe into the new therapeutic methods.

(5) Opening up a new field for fundamental experimental research and clinical practice research of carcinoma.

(二). The first time Xu Ze proposed anti-cancer metastasis therapy "three steps" in the international community

1. Try to break each step during each metastasis step

First, the concept of each transfer step is clarified so that the "target" of the treatment is more specific. In order to scientifically design to block each metastasis step, each break, you must clearly understand the concepts of each metastasis steps, and after the "target" of each step is clear, it can be operational, to study and explore the prevention and treatment strategies of each step. From the treatment strategy to consider, after in-depth analysis, I further summarized the "eight steps" of cell metastasis as "three stages."

The first stage is the separation of cancer cells from the mother tumor, into the stage before entering the blood vessels:

The second stage for the cancer to pierce through the blood vessels into the blood circulation of the stage;

The third stage is the stage that cancer cells are piercing out from the blood vessels to implantation and the formation of the metastasis foci in the target organ tissue.

In order to scientifically design the blockade for each transfer step, we design and formulate the control strategies of each stage according to the molecular mechanism of "eight steps" and "three stages", and call it as "three steps" of XU ZE anticancer metastasis Treatment.

2, the three major countermeasures of Xe ZE anti-cancer metastasis of (ie, three steps)

(1) The first step of anti-cancer metastasis

This stage of cancer cell metastasis through: in this stage, the metastatic process of cancer cells is as follows: cancer cells falling from the primary carcinoma---adhering to the stroma outside the cells---degrading ECM to open up a road for cancer cells---carrying out cell movement via the adherence of degraded stroma or the degraded stroma for adherence---then arriving at the external wall---degrading basement membrane of blood vessel---doing Amoeba movement, firstly stretching out the pseudopodium---then passing through the wall.

Prevention and cure countermeasures: this stage is the intervention and repression countermeasure before the cancer cell falls from the primary carcinoma and enters the blood vessel. In this stage, the therapeutic "targets" are mainly anti-adherence, anti-degradation, anti-movement and anti cancer cell attack. The therapeutic goal is to prevent the cancer cells from entering the blood vessel so as to realize the goal of "turning the enemy back at the border".

(2) The second step of anticancer metastasis

in this stage, the metastasis process of cancer cell: it will pass through the wall and enter the blood circulation. Most of the cancer cells in the circulation will be damaged and killed by the immunological cells in the circulation or the strong blood impact force and shearing force, the tiny minority of the survived cancer cells form the micro-cancer embolus, adhering to the endothelial cell of the micrangium, degrading the basement membrance and passing through the blood vessel. Prevention and cure countermeasures: in this stage, the "target" of therapy of carcinoma metastasis is to protect and enhance the immunologic function of various immunological cells in the blood circulation, activate the immunological cytokine and resist adherence (homogenous adherence of cancer cells and cancer cells, alloplasmatic adherence of cancer cells with blood platelet and so on), resist movement, resist aggregation of blood platelet, resist high coagulation and resist cancer embolus.

Therapeutic goal: activating the immunological cell, protecting function of thymus organization, improving immunity, protecting the bone marrow and producing the blood and promoting the cancer cells floating in the blood circulation to be captured, phagocytized, surrounded and annihilated and intercepted by the immunological cell group.

The second step is the main battlefield to kill off the cancer cells floating in the blood circulation as well as the main countermeasures to interfere and repress the carcinoma metastasis.

(3) **The third step of anti carcinomatous metastasis**: the metastasis process of the cancer cell in this stage: the cancer cell escapes the monitoring of the immunological cell in blood circulation and the annihilation of the immunological cell, passes through the wall and anchors itself in the organs with agreeable local microenvironment for settlement, in this way, the new blood capillary of tumor forms and then it gradually forms the metastatic carcinoma.

Prevention and cure countermeasures: the interference and repression countermeasures, mainly aiming at improving the histogenic immunity of the local microenvironment and regulating the local microenvironment to make it adverse to the survival and nidation and repress the angiogenesis factor and the new angiogenesis.

To sum up, space allocation of Xu Ze Three Steps of Therapy of Carcinoma Metastasis is in the blood circulation and the time allocation is in three different stages. It attaches importance to improvement of the host immunity. It can be summed up and concluded as Table 10-1

Table 1. Xu Ze Three Steps of Therapy of Carcinoma Metastasis

Metastasis stage of cancer cell	Metastasis process	Prevention and cure countermeasures
The stage before the cancer cell intrudes the circulation First step of anti metastasis	Separating the cancer cell from the primary cancer→degrading ECM→adherence and de-adherence→movement→before entering the blood vessel.	● anti-adherence ● anti-degradation ● anti-movement ● anti stroma metal protease
Transportation stage of cancer cell in blood circulation Second step of anti-metastasis	The cancer cell group and micro cancer embolus float in the blood circulation and are damaged due to being phagocytized and captured by the immunological cell and be subject to the shearing force of the blood.	● enhancing and activating various immunological cells in circulation, improving the immunologic function as the main battlefield of killing off the cancer cells in the routing of the metastasis
The stage in which Cancer cell escapes the blood circulation and anchors "target" organ Third step of anti metastasis	After cancer cell escapes from the blood vessel, it anchors the organ for nidation, forms the new blood vessel and forms the metastatic lesion.	● anti-adherence ● anti-aggregation of blood platelet ● anti cancer embolus ● TG ● Inhibiting angiogenesis factor ● Inhibiting angiogenesis ● Improving immunological regulation ● Improving the immunity of local microenvironment.

The metastatic lesion is not the terminal. When the metastatic lesion grows up to a certain size, it has the cancer cells separated, intruded and transferred, in this way, it will become a new original place of the cancer cell metastasis. At this moment, the primary lesion and metaststic lesion will become the original place of the ablation and metastasis of the cancer cells via blood metastasis. Therefore, the more and larger the metastatic carcinoma is, the more the cancer cells in the blood circulation are. The number of the immunological cells in the blood circulation of the body of the patient is far insufficient for controlling a large number of cancer cells falling from the carcinoma lesion and entering the blood circulation. The immunologic function of the organism will be severely unbalanced, even the immunologic function will break down, resulting in the hematogenous dissemination. At this time, the organism of the patient will meet with the functional crisis of the immunologic cells. As to how to perfect and deal with this situation, there are only two methods, one is foreign aid and another is endogeny. The foreign aid is the transplantation of stem cell and the endogeny is bioremediation, immunological therapy, genetherapy, molecular biological therapy, treatment by Chinese herbs, Z-C immunologic regulation therapy by Chinese herbs and BRM therapy.

㈣ Xu Ze first proposed anti-cancer metastasis of the third field in the international community

What is anti-cancer metastasis therapy in the third field? All of the third existence form of cancer in the human body -- - is cancer treatment the way, can be called the third field of anti-cancer treatment.

The first form of existence of carcinoma in a body is the primary lesion and all the therapies aiming at the primary lesion are called the first field of anti-carcinoma-metastasis; the second form of existence of carcinoma in a body is the metastatic lesion and all the therapies aiming at the carcinoma metastasis (radiotherapy, chemotherapy, intervention and some local therapeutic programs) are called the second field of anti-carcinoma-metastasis. Now it is recognized and put forward by us that the third form of existence of carcinoma in a body is the cancer cell in routing of metastasis, then, all of the therapeutic methods aiming at the cancer cells in routing of metastasis are called the third field (or the third battlefront) of anti-carcinoma-metastasis by us for the moment.

1. Necessity of putting forward the third field of anti-carcinoma-metastasis

why do the patients meet with reoccurrence or metastasis after standardized radical treatment of the carcinoma? Now that the radical primary carcinoma is removed and the radical regional lymph node is cleaned down, why do the patients meet with the reoccurrence and metastasis after operation in a short time? Where are the residual cancer cells incubated? How many? What is its movement rule? Through repeated meditation, the author has been aware that these cancer cells may be beyond the regional lymph node; or some cancer cells enter the blood circulation through lymph path; or some cancer cells are extruded into the blood circulation in operation. These cancer cells are in routing of metastasis and they are potentially and slowly metastatic, some are monitored, phagocytized and captured by the immunological cells in the blood circulation and some are in dormancy. Some form the metastatic lesion rapidly. However, some patients' metastatic lesions formed slowly, lasting several months even 1~2 years, the cancer cells in the routing of metastasis were in rest and sleep state.

The above-mentioned cancer cell in the routing of metastasis is actually the third form of existence of carcinoma in a body and it is absolutely necessary to take measures pioneer the third field for carcinoma therapeutics.

2. Probability of intercepting the cancer cells in routing of metastasis

The formation of metastatic lesion is the most important turning point. Before metastasis, the carcinoma is only a local problem and good curative effect can be obtained with the local therapeutics.

However, when it is metastatic, the local therapeutics cannot cure the patient any more. Therefore, the therapeutics for metastasis is most important. In this stage, there are thousands of cancer cells entering the blood circulation everyday, however, only less than 0.01% of the cancer cells become the metastatic lesions finally. Therefore, it is necessary and possible to carry out the therapeutics for metastasis through intercepting or killing off the cancer cells in routing of metastasis; if appreciate measures are taken to activate the immunological cells in the blood, improve the immunological surveillance of the immunological cells and activate the immunological cell factors, it is possible to intercept the cancer cells in routing of metastasis.

How to intercept and kill off the cancer cells in routing of metastasis?

The patient suffering from carcinoma has low immunologic function, especially the low immunologic function of cells with the development of tumor day by day. However, many studies have shown that, although the tumor-bearing host may be a systemic immune deficiency, but in general have a normal I cell response. In animal experiments and clinical studies can stimulate an effective anti-cancer response. The key is how to break through the inhibition of the tumor to the immune system and activate the effective immunological reaction especially the one based on T cell.

How to effectively regulate the immunologic function of the host and improve the local immune micro-environment so as to be advantageous to the anti-cancer effect of the host, is an important and effective measure to prevent the metastasis and reoccurrence of the carcinoma after operation and eliminate the residual cancer cells as well as the important content of integrated therapeutics of the carcinoma.

3.Circle system has lots of immune surveillance cells

The cancer cells are intercepted, captured and killed off by the immunological cells in the blood circulation, therefore, it can be said that the blood circulation is the main battlefield of killing off the cancer cells in the routing of metastasis and the immunological cells are the effective strength to kill off the cancer cells.

The circulation system owns lots of immune surveillance cells, which can kill, wound and phagocytize the cancer cells with heterosexual antigen, together with the impact force and the shearing force of the blood stream, the single adrift cancer cell cannot survive. In order to escape from the interception of eth immunological cells, the cancer cells will be adhesive to the blood platelet on the inner wall of the blood vessel and endothelial cells will meet with ameba movement in the inner wall of the blood vessel and it will pass through the blood capillary and settle in the new viscera, gradually forming the new metastatic lesion.

4. The specific programs of Xu ZE anti-cancer treatment

According to the biological behavior of modern oncology about carcinoma metastasis and the theory of reoccurrence and metastasis, in the past years, this lab has been finding the new drug for anti-carcinoma-metastasis from the natural herbs. In the experimental study of tumor-bearing animal body, the method of traditional Chinese herbs combined with western medicine is adopted by us to interfere and intercept each link of the metastasis steps. And a series of Z-C immunoregulation anti-metastasis program and measures was researched and developed:

Z-C-TG anti-angiogenesis; Z-C-AS lysis; Z-C-MD anti-invasive blood vessels, piercing blood vessels;Z-C-LM antigenicity,Z-C-Ind anti-PGE2: VA and Z-C-CA calcium channel blockers;Z-C-GB anti-adhesion; Z-C-TIMP anti-drug;Z-C, only inhibit cancer cells, we do not kill normal cells;Z-C4 chest lifting, Z-C8 marrow care:Crowy bile into a lymph node. The comprehensive measures of the above treatment program in our anti-cancer cooperative group out-patient practice have achieved good results.

The carcinoma metastasis is a multi-step and multi-link complicated process, the measures for anti-carcinoma-metastasis shall be comprehensive and they are assorted with each other. Do not rely on one drug or one method, through scientific design, aiming at the metastasis step, we take the different therapeutic methods and countermeasures, see Table 1, which aims at the metastasis step to realize the same goal of anti-metastasis.

Table 2 New Mode of Anti-Carcinoma-Metastasis in XU ZE New Concept
(Therapeutic Method and Countermeasures Aiming at Carcinoma Metastasis)

Metastasis step	Therapeutic method	Z-C immune regulation medicine and its role
Hyperplasia of primary cancer	Operation, radiotherapy and chemotherapy	$Z-C_1$ inhibiting cancer cells $Z-C_4$ protecting chest and improving immune $Z-C_8$ protecting bone marrow and hematogenesis
Growth of new blood vessel of tumor	Inhibiting growth of blood vessel	Z-C-TG anti blood vessel formation Z-C-CA anti-adhesion
Invading basement membrance	Anti-adhesion, anti-movement Inhibiting activity of hydrolase	Z-C-K (LWF) anti-adhesion Ind anti PGE2 Z-C-MD anti movement
Passing through blood vessel or lymph	Anti-adhesion, anti-movement Inhibiting activity of hydrolase	Z-CMD anti-invasion blood vessel Z-C-K (LWF) $Z-C_{1+4}$ immune regulation

		Z-C-K (LWF) anti adhesion
In the blood of circulation system	Anti-agglomeration of blood platelet, anti- agglomeration, biological reaction regulation BRM	Z-C-N (CZR) anti agglomeration of blood adhesion Z-C-LM Z-C-ASP cancer dissolve plug $Z\text{-}C_{1+4}$ immune regulation
Formation of cancer plug	Anti-thrombus, invigorating the circulation of blood and removing blood stasis	Z-C-K (NSR) anti-cancer plug Z-C-N (CZR)
Passing through blood vessel	Anti-adhesion, anti-movement and anti activity of aminopeptodrate enzyme	Z-C-MD anti out-invasion of blood vessel
Formation of metastatic lesion	Operation, radiotherapy and chemotherapy	$Z\text{-}C_{1+4}$ immune regulation Z-C-TG inhibiting growth of blood vessel
Metastasis of lymph node	Lipide dissolve medicament	Crow gallbladder emulsison fat carrier Entering lymph node

（五）XU ZE new concept and new model of cancer treatment

1. To strengthen immunotherapy and to improve the side effects of chemotherapy

(1) The side effects of the traditional chemotherapy: when chemotherapy is made on cancer, it usually inhibits immunologic function and hematopoiesis function of the bone marrow, descends WBC and PLT and damages liver and kidney function as well as gastroenteric function, leading to the side effects such as nausea, emesis, abdominal distension, anorexia and so on. See Figure 4.

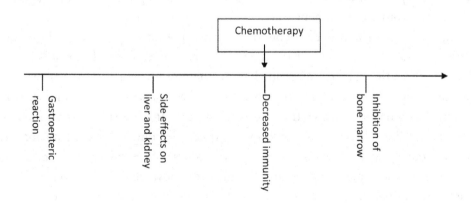

Fig. 4 Side effects of traditional chemotherapy

(2) Thecountermeasures of Xu Ze's new concept: the method to improve the side effects of chemotherapy is to strengthen the supporting therapy and take effective measures to protect the host. Among the traditional Chinese medicine for immunological mediation, $XZ\text{-}C_4$ can protect thymus thus and improve immunity; $XZ\text{-}C_8$ can protect hematopoiesis function of the bone marrow and generate more stem cells; XZ-C medicine for immunity mediation can strengthen physical strength of cancerous patients. See Fig. 5.

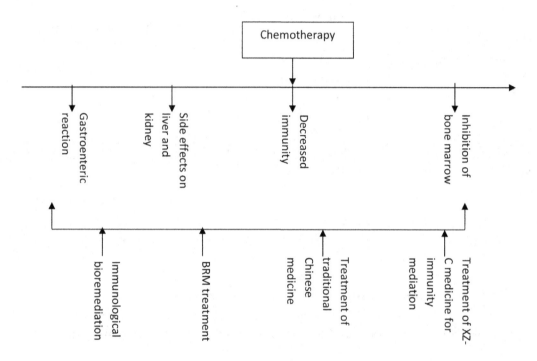

Fig.5 Countermeasures for side effects of chemotherapy

2. Changing intermittent treatment into continual treatment

1. Traditional intravenous chemotherapy is an intermittent therapy, that is to say, after the drug for chemotherapy is applied for 3-5 days, it is necessary to apply the chemotherapeutic drug for the second course of treatment when WBC and PLT return to normal after 3-4 weeks. The drug for chemotherapy shall not be continually applied during the intermission between the first and the second course of treatment, whereas the cancel cells are still continually and uninterruptedly proliferated and divided in the intermission and increase at the speed of geometrical progression. In addition, because of the inhibition of immunologic function caused by chemotherapeutic drug, the cancel cells escape from or are free of the immunological surveillance, their proliferation and division are quickened during the intermission between these two courses, in other words, the longer the course of treatment of chemotherapeutic drug, the more the combined drug and the more the dose, the more serious of the attack against immunity of the human body, resulting in lack of immunological surveillance, and even resulting in reoccurrence and metastasis in chemotherapy, and shrinkage of tumor firstly before continual enlargement later (see Fig. 6). These cases occur commonly, how to

treat them? It is held by us that the following model should be adopted for a continuous immunological therapy in the intermission between two courses of treatment.

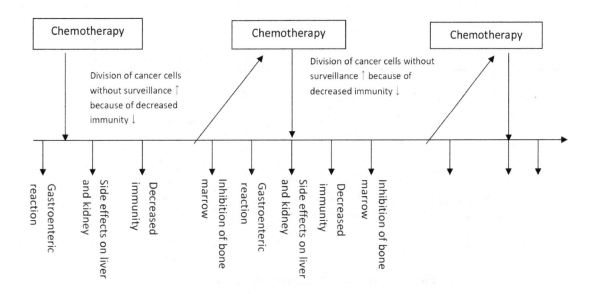

Fig. 6 Easy reoccurence of tumor without treatment in the intermission

(2).Xu Ze's new concept and model of cancer treatment is a continuous treatment. It adopts traditional Chinese medicine for immunological mediation, namely $XZ\text{-}C_1 + XZ\text{-}C_4$, or BRM for treatment during the intermission. $XZ\text{-}C_1$ was screened through the experimental study on tumor-bearing animals over 7 years and has been proven by a sixteen-year clinical verification that it has only inhibited the cancel cells rather than normal ones and that it can benefit spleen and stomach. $XZ\text{-}C_4$ can protect thymus from atrophy, prevent immunity from decreasing and make it better. Continual treatment in the intermittence with XZ-C medicine can control proliferation of caner cells and also protect the function of immune organs such as thymus.

The combination of chemotherapeutic drug and XZ-C medicine can decrease teh side effects from chemotherapy and strengthen chemotherapy effects against the loss of immunological surveillance as well meanwhile. See Fig. 7.

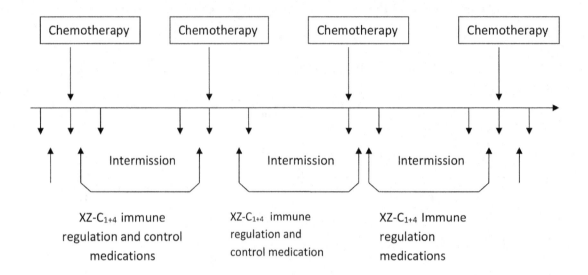

Fig. 7 Continual treatment in the intermission

The occurrence and development of tumor depends on the relationship between immunologic function of the host and the intrinsic biological characteristics of tumor. Similarly, the invasion and metastasis of cancer also rests with the relationship, namely, carcinoma would be put under control in case of the balance between biological characteristics of tumor cells and impacts of the host on the inhibition factors; otherwise, the cancer would grow up.

Traditional radiotherapy and chemotherapy are inclined to weakening immunologic function and lead to a worse unbalance between both of them.

Xu Ze's new model of cancer treatment aims to improve the immunity of patients as much as possible, to make immune increase reach the balance, and thus inhibit tumor growth and strengthen immunological surveillance.

VOLUME VI

For more than 30 years it has been walked out of a new way to overcome cancer; It has formed the theoretical system of XZ-C immune regulation of cancer treatment which has experienced the clinical application and observation and verification.

CONTENTS VOLUME VI

Preface

Why do I get the title "Embark on a new way to overcome cancer"? The origin of the title is due to the guidelines and revelations from several experts, scholars, seniors and teacher letters :

Wu Min academician mentioned on July 2, 2001: "The overall impression is that the model from the clinical to the experiment and from experiments to clinical is good, taking the road of combining Chinese and Western is very correct, and sincerely wish you continue to move forward and walk out of a new way to overcome cancer."

On February 22, 2006 Tang Zhao academician mentioned: "...... Chinese medicine and biological therapy are the most promising two anti-metastasis ways, particularly in traditional Chinese medicine, I hope you get out of the characteristic antimetastatic road."

On March 22, 2006 Liuyun Yi academician said: "...... I agreed to your questions and ideas of overcoming cancer in the book very much ...... hope you make a breakthrough in Chinese medicine contribution so that the majority of patients get benefit and so that Chinese medicine develops further and our medical career can reach world levels."

January 9, 2006 Wu Xian academician mentioned: "...... tumor is hard bone to hoe, but it should continue to bite down, but fortunately we are very happy to support, only if effective, whether it is in the treatment of tumors and body, or reduce the radiation and chemical reaction "and on April 10, 2012 the letter mentioned:." ...... I think you walked out a very unique street, traditional Chinese medicine to apply formulations, methods taking medications, pharmaceutical composition, innovations of XZ-C series of drugs, developed your own patents, which should continue down this road."

We thank them for their guidance and help for our research work, scientific thinking, research objectives, research route, research guidelines, research methods. Our research work has been to follow the guidance in the direction of their efforts. In here I give my great gratitude to Wu Min, Tang Zhao, Wu Jiang Zhong, Liuyun Yi and other academicians.

Our 28 years (1985 - present) cancer research work in animal studies, clinical basic research, clinical validation has made a series of scientific and technological innovation, scientific research. After 20 years of hard work, XZ-C Immune Regulation anti-cancer therapy has formed and a new way to overcome cancer has taken out.

20 years of experimental and clinical research in this series has been enthusiastically supported and cordially guided by international renowned foreign scientists and medical dean of general surgery QiFaZhu academician. 1990 State Science and Technology to the author at presenting "eight five" key scientific and technological project (further explore the anti-cancer herbal liver cancer, gastrointestinal cancer, cancer, experimental and clinical studies of anti-metastatic precancerous lesions on) application, Academician Qi instructions on expert advice: "Study how to prevent cancer metastasis and metastasis is currently a very important topic, the experimental study to investigate prevention methods in clinical practice is feasible, is beneficial to the people's work." In my teacher Qiu Yuanshi rigorous scientific study style under the influence and guidance, we completed the initial project work above, hereby express my gratitude.

Scientific literature must have nutritional feeding. In 1986 when we have just established a legitimate animal model experimental surgical laboratory to manufacture cancer metastasis experimental research, we see Professor Gao Jin's book "invasion and metastasis - basic research and clinical", see Tang Zhao academician monograph "HCC metastasis, basic and clinical recurrence," which theories of two books make us suddenly understanding, also encouraged and facilitated our experimental work and clinical verification from the other sides. Professor Tang Zhaoyou in his monograph that read: "The next important goal of primary liver cancer study - Prevention of recurrence and metastasis," and said: "The transfer of further recurrence has become a bottleneck to improve the survival rate of liver cancer, is the most important fight against cancer One of the difficulties." This theoretical literature has given us to update thinking, innovative wisdom and courage, but also strengthened the confidence and determination of our experimental group work. In here I gave Tang Zhao academician and Professor Gao Jin my extend gratitude.

For seven years, we used more than 6000 tumor-bearing animal models one after another to explore a fundamental problem. Selecting 200 kinds of Chinese herbal flavor carried by tumor-bearing animal model experiments in vivo anti-tumor screening were completed by my graduates such as Dr.Zhu Siping master, Dr. Zou Shaomin, Dr. Li Zhengxun Master, Master Dr.Liu Liling, etc., who conducted and completed a lot of painstaking experimental work. Hard work! day and night! they made a contribution to prevent the development of cancer tumor experiments. Here are my sincere thanks.

(1) THE CONCEPT OF CANCER THERAPY

(Introduction)

1) Traditional concept is that cancer cells keep dividing and proliferation and its treatment goal must be to kill cancer cells **so that traditional concept of cancer therapeutics is based on killing cancer cells**. In order to achieve cure, it must be to kill the last cancer cell so that people used to expand operations, intensive chemotherapy and radical radiotherapy, but the results are not satisfactory.

2) New model of cancer therapy is that: **cure should be regulated, not by killing**. The last step of cure of cancer cells should be to mobilize action to control the reproduction of the host, rather than the elimination of the last of the cancer cells.

(The unfolded introduction)

1, the concept of traditional cancer therapy
2, the new concept of cancer treatment

1. The concept of traditional cancer therapy

The concept of traditional therapies that cancer is the continuous division of cancer cells, proliferation, the treatment goal must be to kill cancer cells. Therefore, the goal of the traditional three treatments are based on the killing of cancer cells.

The traditional treatment of cancer is based on the principle that the last cancer cell must be killed or eliminated. Therefore, people have adopted the expansion of surgery, chemotherapy and radical radiotherapy. But the result is not ideal. In the early 1960s, the scope of tumor surgery was expanding and developed a series of radical surgery. After years of practice proved to expand the scope of surgical resection, such as breast cancer, lung cancer, liver cancer, pancreatic cancer, did not change the patient without cancer survival and overall survival. In the 1980s, intensive chemotherapy and radical radiotherapy failed to improve the quality of life or prolong survival, but because bone marrow hematopoietic function and immune function had severe inhibition it was increasing the number of life-**threatening complications. Therefore, it is necessary to establish a new mode to**

probe into the cancer, strive for opening a new way and renew the concept from the clinical and experimental data.

In short, the traditional concept of cancer is based on cell division, proliferation, cancer cells is the culprit, therefore, the target of the traditional cancer therapy targets cancer cells, the goal is to kill cancer cells.

2. The new concept of cancer treatment

Cure should be done by regulation rather than by killing

The assumptive new mode of cancer therapeutics includes some new examples and its predominant idea holds that cancer is a kind of disease, the regulation and signal transmission among the cells are disrupted instead of loss and the carcinogenesis is a continuous entity with possibility of reversion.

The understanding of the cancer by the new mode is based on information transfer and regulation and control. It is convinced that the canceration is a process of evolvement step by step, however, it holds that they may be potentially reversed. **The new model of cancer believed: heal should be adopted through regulation and non-destruction.**

Note: "monograph" - "new concepts and new methods of cancer treatment" (the book author Xu Ze (XU ZE) professor of the third monograph)

It is indicated by the clinical and experimental experience that the tumor keeps a certain response relation with the host. When the tumor results from the unbalance of regulation and control instead of the autonomy of the tumor, some clinical phenomena can be easily understood. Clinically, it is known by us that the cancer cells can make adaptive response to the environment of the host at high level. The long-term application of immunosuppressant may induce the tumor, when the immunosuppressant is suspended, the tumor can be entirely released. Although the factors inducing the tumor have not been proven, the reaction of host determines the final results. The kidney transplantation tumor with metastasis to the lung will be entirely released after suspension of the antirejection therapy. It looks as if the pregnancy improves the relation between the tumor and the host. Now people have focused on killing the tumor, developed so many therapeutic methods and developed many anti-cancer cytotoxic drugs in the past half a century, however, they cannot prevent the attack and metastasis of tumor. Viewed from the data, the cytotoxic drugs as the assistant of radiotherapy after operation also cannot prevent the reoccurrence and metastasis of the cancer because most of them severely inhibit the immunity even the non-immunological part of the host reaction. When people increase the concentration and dosage of the chemotherapeutic drugs to make them more aggressive to the cancer cells (such as intensified radiotherapy), we right lead the mechanism of long-term survival or healing to the more dangerous way, even bring about the artificial or iatrogenic immunologic function breakdown.

Viewed from molecular biology, the cancer results from the change in DNA structure. It is the unbalanced differentiation of the cells caused by the genetic information that introduces the normal nucleic acid to the cancer cells via the genetic engineering, inducing the tumor cells to differentiate to the normal cells. Shanghai Tumor Research Institute had extracted RNA from the normal hepatic cells, then incubated and cultivated it together with the liver cancer cells to correct the abnormal genetic activities of the liver cancer cells through the regulation and control reaction of normal liver RNA so as to make it reversed to the normal cells. The scientists now are looking for the bioactive substances related to the genetic information, for example, the normal mRNA can induce the cancer cells to reverse to the normal cells.

The precondition of adopting the cytotoxic drugs to treat the tumor is the understanding that the it is not only possible but also necessary to kill the last cancer cell until it is proven by the clinic application and the lab that the tumor has been entirely eliminated, as is the prerequisite of healing the patient suffering from the tumor. However, according to our experience over 20 years, this argumentation is contradictory. Some clinical cases show that killing can shrink or subside the tumor, however, it cannot directly heal the tumor. Although the dosage of cytotoxic drug is increased and most of the cancer cells are subsided, the survival rate of the patient is not improved. Soon after, it will reoccur and the tumor will be enlarged.

All the obviously healed patients do not seem to adopt the mode of killing the cancer cells. For example, the treatment of tumor with platinum-based drug seems to be related to the induced cell differentiation. The action of interferon and interleukin to the sensitive cells is realized by the regulation and control mechanism. As to the levamisole as the adjuvant for carcinoma of large intestine, it is deemed that its effects are from the change in host reaction.

We had tried out best to kill the cancer cells to treat the cancer before, however, no great achievements had been made. Later, enlarged radical operation, intensified chemotherapy and radical radiotherapy were adopted. However, the results were not ideal and they could not improve the survival quality of the patient suffering from cancer and the survival time of the patient suffering from cancer after operation.

In the recent 50 years, the treatment of cancer by traditional Chinese medicine has made great achievements. A large number of data indicate that the cancer cells can coexist with the host and they may not always damage the host. In the recent 16 years, among 12000 patients suffering from metaphase and advanced cancer treated by Shuguang Tumor Research Institute and Wuchang Shuguang Tumor Special Clinic, some reoccurrence and metastasis patients, such as the patients with anastomotic stoma reoccurrence cancer and gastric carcinoma that cannot be ablated or treated through radiotherapy and chemotherapy, after taking Z-C medicine for a long time over 3-5 years, the conditions are controlled and stabilized, they can survive with tumor (coexist with the tumor) and take care of themselves, the survival quality is good and the survival quality is obviously prolonged.

It is deemed by us that undoubtedly we should kill the foreigners invading the body, however, as to the cancer cells, we shall make a differential treatment just because they are only the variant tissues in the normal body of the host, here we reaffirm that the cancer shall be treated through regulating the control over them by the mechanism instead of the necessary and impossible killing-off of all cancer cells.

Since we have a new cognition of the cancer concept, then, the concept of cancer therapeutics shall renew the thought, the understanding and the concepts and innovate the therapeutic theory and technology.

In view of the experience and lessons of the author over half a century, now we should research the urgent problems in the current cancer study, seek for the breakthrough for clinical research from the weak link of the modern medicine and find the breakthrough of prevention and control from the invasion, reoccurrence and metastasis, look for the anti-reoccurrence and anti-metastasis drugs from the chemical drugs and the natural herbs and deepen the new understanding of the cancer concept at the molecular level, genetic level, integrated treatment level and targeted treatment.

(2) THE CAUSE AND THE DEVELOPMENT MECHANISM OF CANCER

(Introduction)

To explore the etiology and pathogenesis and pathophysiology of cancer, we conducted a series of animal experiments, from the experimental results to analyze and to think so that we get the new discoveries and new thinking and the **new revelation: thymus atrophy and immune dysfunction are one of the cause and the pathogenesis of cancer so that Xu Ze (Xu ZE) professor at the international conference put forward one of the cause and the pathogenesis of cancer may be thymus atrophy, central immune function damage, immune function, immune surveillance ability to fall and immune escape.**

After investigation, this is the first time to be put forward in the international community. (See this in Volume V in this book)

(brief introduction)

Thymic atrophy and immune dysfunction may be one of the causes and pathogenesis of cancer

1, the new discovery of the experimental study of cancer etiology and pathogenesis and pathophysiology

2, to explore the method of the prevention of tumor progression and thymic atrophy and the immune reconstruction

1, the new discovery of the experimental study of cancer etiology and pathogenesis and pathophysiology

Nearly 16 years the author conducted a series of animal studies to search for the etiology, pathogenesis and pathophysiology of cancer, to explore mechanism of cancer invasion, recurrence, metastasis, and to find effective measures to control.

Experimental Surgery is extremely important in the development of medical science and is a key to open the box medicine. Many diseases control methods are achieved after many experiments the stability of the results of animal studies only after clinical application. So, I established Experimental Surgery Laboratory conducting experiments in cancer research, cancer cell transplant purposes, establishing tumor animal model, carrying out the following series of experiments in cancer research: ① to explore the experimental study of cancer etiology, pathogenesis and pathophysiology; ② To explore mechanisms and laws of cancer recurrence, metastasis; ③ investigate the relationship between the tumor and immune and immune organs and between immune organs and tumor ; ④To investigate method of curbing tumor progression, progressive atrophy of immune organs and of immune reconstitution;⑤ looking for effective measures of regulating cancer invasion, recurrence and metastasis.

From cancer experimental research the author and his colleagues conducted a full four-year experimental cancer research in order to explore the cancer etiology, pathogenesis, invasion, metastasis mechanism to find the regulation, intervention invasion, recurrence, metastasis and effective measures.

Experiment 1: in this lab thymus (TH) was removed and then the cancer-bearing animal model was made. **It is proven by the study conclusions: the occurrence and development of the cancer has remarkably affirmative relation with the thymus of the immune organ of the host and its functions.**

Experiment 2: Does the inferior immune lead to the cancer or the cancer lead to the inferior immune at all? Our experimental results: the inferior immune leads to the occurrence and development of the cancer, without the descent of immunologic function, it is not easy to realize the successful inoculation. **It is suggested by the experimental results: improving and maintaining the good immunologic function and protecting the good thymus of the central immune organ are the important measures for preventing the occurrence of cancer.**

Experiment 3: in studying the relation between the metastasis of cancer and the immune, this lab establishes animal models for liver metastatic carcinoma, which are divided into two groups including Group A applied with immune depressant and Group B not applied with immune depressant. Results: the metastatic lesions in the liver in Group A are obviously more than the ones in Group B. **It is suggested by the experimental results: metastasis is related to the immune and inferior immunologic function or application of immune depressant may promote the tumor metastasis.**

Experiment 4: When making experiments to probe into the effects of tumor on immune organ, this lab finds that the thymus meets with progressive atrophy with the advance of the cancer. The thymus of the host meets with the acute progressive atrophy after the cancer cells are inoculated, the cell proliferation is prevented and the volume is obviously shrunk. **It is suggested by the experimental results: the tumor may inhibit the thymus, resulting in the atrophy of the immune organ.**

Experiment 5: we also find through experiment that if some experimental mice are not successfully inoculated or the tumor is very small, the thymus is not obviously shrunk. In order to understand the relation between the tumor and the atrophy of the thymus, we excise the transplanted solid tumor of one group of mice when it grows up to the size of a thumb. After one month, through anatomy, we find the thymus does not meet with progressive atrophy again. **Therefore, it is inferred by us that maybe the solid tumor produces one kind of unknown factor to inhibit the thymus, which shall be further studied through experiment.**

Experiment 6: it is proven by the above-mentioned experimental results: the advance of the tumor makes the thymus meet with progressive atrophy, then, can we take some measures to prevent the atrophy of the thymus of the host? Therefore, we further perfect the design to seek for the method or drug to prevent the atrophy of the thymus of the cancer-bearing mice through the experimental study on animal. So we make the experimental study to recover the function of the immune organ through cell transplantation of the immune organ. We discuss the atrophy of the thymus of the immune organ in preventing the advance of tumor, seek for the method to recover the functions of the thymus and reconstruct the immune, carry out the cell transplantation of fetal liver and fetal spleen and fetal thymus with the mice and establish the immunologic function through adoptive immunity. **It is shown by the results: through the joint transplantation of three groups of cells, namely S, T and L, the entire extinction rate of the tumor in the long term is 46.67% and the one with the entire extinction of the tumor get a long survival life.**

Experiment 7: in the experiment to probe into the effects of tumor on the immune organ such as spleen, we find: the spleen can inhibit the growth of the tumor in the early stage of the tumor, however, in the late stage, the spleen meets with the progressive atrophy. **It is suggested by the study results: the effects of spleen on the growth of the tumor are embodied into bi-direction, in the early stage, it can inhibit the tumor to a certain extent, however, in the late stage, it fails to inhibit the tumor. The cell transplantation of the spleen can enhance the role of inhibiting the tumor.**

Experiment 8: **it is suggested by the results of the follow-up survey: control over the metastasis is the key to cancer treatment.** Now it is well known that the cancer cell metastasis has multiple steps and links. In order to try to interrupt one link so as to prevent the metastasis, we consider the formation of the regenerative blood vessel of tumor is one of the links in which the metastatic cancer cells can nidate, root and grow into the cancer node or not. In 1986, this lab was making the microcirculation study and we observed the formation of the blood capillary of transplanted tumor node of cancer-bearing mice and its flow rate and flow with the micro-circle microscope; then we tried to seek for the drugs for prevention of the formation of the tumor blood vessel from the natural herbs, observed the formation process of the regenerative blood vessel with Olympus micro-circle microscope photograph system and counted the flow rate and flow of the arteriole and venule, found Common Threewingnut Root acetic ether extract (TG) from the traditional Chinese herbs and carried out the blood vessel inhibition test. It was found from the results: in the first day of inoculation there was no regenerative blood vessel and in the second day it was found that the fine micro regenerative blood vessel grew up. TG can reduce the density of the regenerative blood capillary of the tumor.

Experiment 9: we also found from a large batch of tumor-bearing animal models in the lab that the more the hypodermically inoculated solid tumor of some cancer-bearing experimental mice, the more different the cancer cells of the central tissue of the transplanted solid tumor from the peripheral cancer cells. The center of the node is mostly aseptically necrosed or liquefied its periphery is still surrounded with active cancer cells. Therefore, in the clinical treatment, we adopted the measures to treat the aseptic necroses.

2. Discussion methods of preventing cancer progression and thymic atrophy and of rebuilding the immune function

One of the etiology and pathogenesis of tips from the experimental study is that cancer may be thymus atrophy, thymocyte proliferation is blocked, the thymus dysfunction, immune dysfunction, resulting in immune escape of malignant cells.

Now that along with the progress of the tumor, thymus atrophy occurs, then how to prevent thymus from shrinking? Through animal studies we looked for the way or drugs to prevent mice thymus atrophy and eventually adopted immune organs cell transplantation to restore the immune organs, and achieved exciting results.

In 1986, I got enlightened from the discussion in the satellite meeting of one international micro-circulation academic conference to seek for the micro-circulation drug from the natural herbs and then transplanted the adoptive immune from the biological cells to reconstruct the immune and then sought for a kind of drug from the natural herbs of traditional Chinese herbs that can activate the cytokine, enhance the immunological surveillance, inhibit the tumor and prevent the atrophy of the thymus. All drugs must be subject to the animal experiment and clinical verification. **As a result, we made the cancer-bearing animal model and made the in vivo tumor-inhibiting screening experiment on the cancer-bearing animal with over 200 kinds of natural traditional Chinese herbs one by one within seven years. Finally, the anti-cancer immune-regulating TCM with relatively good tumor-inhibiting rate had been screened. From experimental screening to clinical observation and verification and then to further screening and concentration from the angle of immunopharmacology of TCM, we prepared XZ-C1-10 medicine, which can promote the thymus hyperplasia, prevent the thymus atrophy, improve the immune, protect the bone marrow and promote the function of lymphocyte T and cytokine, with relatively high tumor-inhibiting rate. XZ-C1-10 medicine only inhibits and kills the cancer cells, does not affect the normal cells and can be used for oral administration for a long time. Since cancer is a kind of chronic disease, the division, proliferation and clone of the cancer cells is a long, sustainable and progressive process, so it's better to select the orally administered traditional Chinese herbs with long-term curative effects, without toxin and with slow release. The treatment of cancer with traditional Chinese herbs is carried out after the pathogenic factors are judged on the human body. It shall kill the cancer cells as well as improve the immunologic functions of the organism as well so as to strengthen the anti-cancer capability of the organism, as a result, some refractory cancer with wide metastasis can be controlled, the life of the patient is prolonged, the pain of the patient is reduced, which opens up a new way to further probe into the treatment of the cancer.**

Therefore, based on the enlightenment from the study results of a series of animal study regarding pathogenic factors and pathophysiology of the cancer by this lab, we put forward:

that thymus resection leads immunologic deficiency, then leads descent of immunological surveillance ad immunologic escape may be one of the pathogenic factors of the cancer and one key of the pathogenesis. It is the new progress of tumor theory in 21st century, offering direction and basis to the cancer therapeutics in 21st century and offering theoretical basis and experimental basis of the immune regulation and control targeted therapy of the cancer. The new finding, enlightenment and thinking is the original innovation and it has not been mentioned in the textbooks and literatures at home and abroad.

One of the pathogenic factors mentioned above by will lead to a series of reform and innovation of cancer therapeutics, for example, the reform and innovation of the cognition of cancer therapeutic concept, the reform and innovation of cognition of cancer treatment objective or target; the one of cancer diagnostic procedure and curative effect judgment standard, the one of cancer treatment way and treatment mode and the one of research and development of anti-metastasis drug.

Study on New Concept and Way of Treatment of Carcinoma

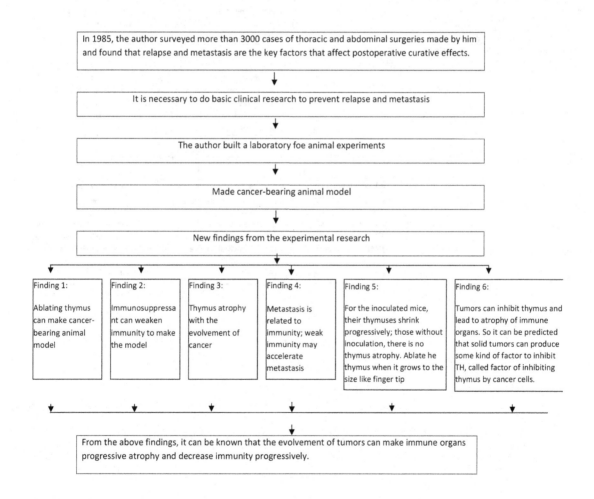

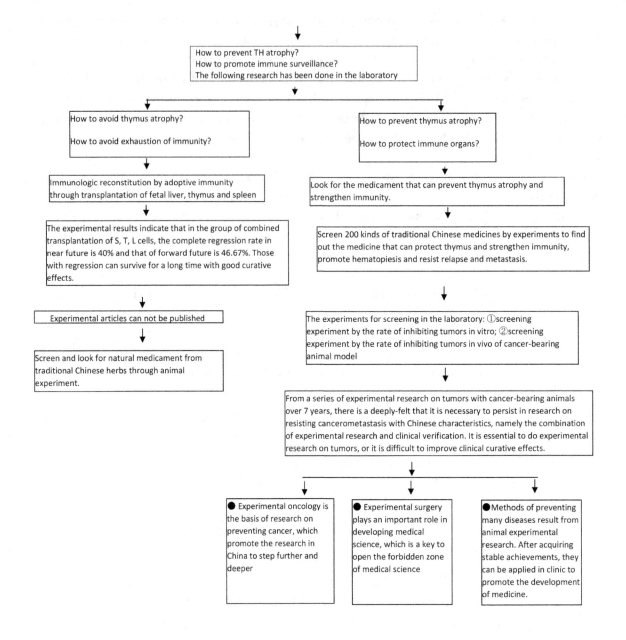

(3) THE THEORETICAL BASIS AND EXPERIMENTAL BASIS OF CANCER TREATMENT (PROFILE)

As a result of laboratory experiments it was found that: the mice bearing thymus was atrophic atrophy, and central immune function damage, decreased immune function, immune monitoring is low, **so the treatment principle must be to prevent thymus atrophy, promote thymic hyperplasia, To protect bone marrow hematopoietic function, improve immune surveillance, control malignant cells immune escape.**

Based on the above research on the cause and pathogenesis of cancer, the new theory and new method of XZ-C immunoregulation therapy are put forward. The author after 16 years of specialist specialist outpatient clinic more than 12,000 cases of advanced cancer patients with clinical validation, it was confirmed that the principle of treatment of thymus protection and increasing immune function is reasonable, the effect is satisfactory.

XZ-C (XU ZE China) immunomodulatory therapy is first proposed by Professor Xu Ze in 2006 in his monograph "New concepts and new methods of treating cancer metastasis," which he believes under normal circumstances, the body's defense was in a dynamic equilibrium between host and cancer; cancer occurs while this dynamic balance was lost. If the state has been adjusted to offset the normal level, it can control cancer growth and make it subside.

As we all know, the incidence of cancer development and prognosis depends on the comparison of two factors, namely, the biological characteristics of cancer cells and the defense capability of cancer cells in host organism itself, **such as the balance between the cancer and host which can be controlled. If both are imbalance, the cancer will develop.**

Under normal circumstances, the host organism itself against cancer cells have a certain capacity of constraints; **but in cancer these constraints are subject to different levels of defense suppression and damage so as to lead to the loss of the immune surveillance of cancer cells, immune escape occurred and to further develop cancer cells and metastasis. (See Volume 5 in this book)**

Brief introduction

Theoretical Basis and Experimental Basis of "Protecting Thymus and Increasing immune function" of XZ-C Immunomodulation Therapy

1, the revelation of the animal experiment
2, it should protect, regulate, activate the body's anti-cancer immune system
3, the research overview of the bio-regulator-like immune regulation of anti-cancer Chinese medication
4, the biological response regulator-like effect and efficacy of XZ-C immunoregulation of traditional Chinese medication class

1, the revelation of the animal experiment

It is found by this lab that the cancer-bearing rats are confronted with the progressive atrophia and damage to the central immune organ, which shall be protected to protect the thymus so as to improve the immunity.

Based on the above-mentioned enlightenment from the results of experimental study on the pathogenic factor and pathogenesis of carcinomatosis by this lab, the new theory and new ways of XZ-C targeted therapeutics of immunity regulation and control initiated by Professor Xu Ze have the theoretical and experimental basis because the findings from the experimental study by this lab indicate that the cancer-bearing rats are confronted with progressive atrophia, damage to the central immune organ, descent of immunologic function and inferior immunological surveillance, so its curative principles shall be based on prevention of progressive athophia, promotion of thymus hyperplasia, improvement of immunity, protection of hematopiesis function of bone marrow, improvement of immunological surveillance and control over the immunologic escape of the canceration cells.

As is now well known, the immune organs include the central immune organs and peripheral immune organ, the former includes the thymus and the bone marrow and the latter includes the spleen and the lymph node. It is validated by the literature and the work in this lab that when the cancer comes, the tumor will produce a factor inhibiting the immune organ, which is temporarily called thymus-inhibiting factor by us and inhibits the thymus, causing the thymus to be progressively atrophic and inhibiting the functions of the central immune organ, in this way, the immunologic function descends and the immunological surveillance of the tumor is lost or weakened, resulting in the further progress of the tumor.

Therefore, the therapeutic theory of the curative principles of thymus protection for immunity improvement and bone marrow protection for hematogenesis initiated by us is reasonable and scientific and has the theoretical and experimental basis. The clinical verification and observation of over 12000 patients suffering from metaphase and advanced cancer in Shuguang Tumor Special Clinic over 16 years, has indicated that the curative principle of thymus protection for immunity improvement and bone marrow protection for hematogenesis initiated, clinically verified, observed by us over 16 years through clinical application is correct and reasonable and the curative effects are satisfying and worth of the patients' confidence.

XZ-C therapeutics of immunity regulation and control was initiated by Professor Xu Ze in 2006 in his monograph New Concept and New Way of Treatment of Cancer Metastasis. He holds that the cancer and the defense of the organism are in the dynamic balance in the normal conditions and the occurrence and development of the carcinomatosis is caused by the disturbance of the dynamic balance. If the disturbed state can be artificially regulated to the normal state, it can control the growth of cancer and subside the cancer.

As is now well known, occurrence, progress and development and treatment prognosis of the cancer are determined by the contrast of two factors: biological characteristics of the cancer cells and the inhibition and defensive capability of the host organism to the cancer cells, if both of them are in balance, the cancer can be controlled; otherwise, the cancer will advance.

Under the normal conditions, the host organism has a certain capability in inhibiting the cancer cells, however, the inhibition and defensive capabilities are suppressed and damaged to different extent, resulting in the loss of the immunological surveillance and the immunologic escape of the cancer cells, leading to development and metastasis of the cancer cells.

2, it should protect, regulate, activate the body's anti-cancer immune system

In discussing the principles of cancer treatment, we should study what the body of anti-cancer immune cell series are, which anti-cancer cytokine series are, which anti-cancer gene series are, and which humoral immune series are.

(1) What are the anti-cancer immune cells in the human body that may be activated and enhanced for cancer cell metastasis

(1) Cytotoxic lymphocyte (CTL): it plays a primary role in anti-tumor immunity, CTL in the human body includes CD_3 and CD_8, and CTL has a high content in peripheral blood and spleen and a certain content in thoracic duct, thymus and bone marrow. Under a certain condition, it can produce IL-2, IL-4 and IFN to activate other anti-cancer immunological cells and lethal macrophages, NK cells and lethal B cells to jointly exert the anti-tumor role.

(2) Natural killer cell (NK cell) with the anti-tumor role: NK cells are a group of broad spectrum anti-cancer cells. They do not rely on the antibody or the thymus to kill the activity and their main role is to surveil and remove the canceration cells in the human body. It is found by the clinical observance that the ones with activity insufficiency of NK have obviously increased incidence rate of malignant tumor. NK cells are an important part in the organism with anti-cancer immunological surveillance function in the early stage.

(3) LAK cells: LAK cells are the most important cancer cells in the modern biological therapeutics and peripheral mononuclear cells in the human body can remarkably kill so many kinds of tumor cells in the human body with the induction of IL-2. LAK cells have a wider anti-cancer spectrum than NK cells while LAK cells can kill the tumor cells that cannot be killed by NK cells.

(4) Macrophage (MO): it plays an important role in anti-tumor immunity in the human body.

(2) What anti-cancer cytokines in the human body can be activated, enhanced to anticancer metastases?

(A) Interferon (IFN): Interferon can be resistant to cell differentiation and has immunomodulatory function. On some tumor cells with anti-proliferative effect, its anti-cancer effect may be related to immune regulation. It enhances NK cell and MΦ cell activity.

(B) Interleukin-2 (IL-2): It is a T cell growth factor, has a strong immune regulation function, can promote T cells, NK cells and monocyte activation, but also promote IFN-a, TNF The release.

(C) Tumor necrosis factor (TNF): its role in cells is cytotoxic effect, and can affect the tumor microvessels, and ultimately lead to tumor necrosis of the central site.

(3) other

In recent years, with the rapid development of molecular biology, molecular immunology, molecular immunological pharmacology and gene engineering, the foundation of molecular level of "anti-cancer organ" and the clinical study are continuously expanded and deepened, its outlook of anti-cancerometastasis is very attracting.

At present, the study on immunotherapy of anti-cancer molecular biology is mainly centralized on "four sub-systems" of "anti-cancer organ", namely "anti-cancer cellular therapy", "anti-cancer cytokine therapy", "anti-cancer gene therapy" and "anti-cancer anti-body therapy".

The basic characteristics of these molecular biological and immunological therapies are as follows: all pharmaceutics of molecular biological and immunological therapies are the inherent substances in the organism and fundamental differences from radiotherapy and chemotherapy are: it has no progressive damage to the normal histiocytes of the organism, especially the cells and the functions of the immune system and the structure and the function of the hemopoietic system of the bone marrow and plays a role in regulation and reinforcement of immunological reaction. As is now well known, radiotherapy and chemotherapy are entirely different from it, the chemotherapy is a kind of non-selective traumatic therapy, killing the cancer cells as well as the normal cells at the same time, which damage the normal histiocytes of the organism, resulting in severe damage to the hemopoietic system and the immunological structure and function, with the severe consequence.

The biotherapy is a kind of therapy stabilizing and balancing the vital mechanism by means of the regulation on biologic reaction. The American scholar Oldham (1984) initiated biological regulation and mediation (BRM) theropy and then initiated the concept of tumor biotherapy based on the therapy.

3, the research overview of the biological regulator of immune regulation of anti-cancer Chinese medication

Through study on animal experiments by us for 4 years and the clinical verification by the tumor special clinic over 16 years, it is indicated that XZ-C medicine has the roles and curative effects similar to BRM and it is screened from the traditional Chinese herb resources with role similar to BRM.

XZ-C medicine is screened from 200 kinds of traditional Chinese herbs through experiments by Professor Xu Ze (ZU ZE-China, Z-C) in the lab. Firstly, we adopt the culture in vitro of cancer cells and screen 200 kinds of traditional Chinese herbs in vitro one by one, observe the experimental study on the direct damage to the cancer cells in the culture tube by each drug and make the check experiment on tumor-inhibiting rate between the chemotherapy drug CTX and the control group of normal cells in the culture tube. Finally, we select a batch of herbs with a certain tumor-inhibiting rate of proliferation of cancer cells. Then we further establish the tumor-bearing animal model and carry out the experimental study on the 200 kinds of traditional Chinese herbs for the in vivo tumor-inhibiting rate of the tumor-bearing animal model and screen, analyze and evaluate the herbs scientifically, objectively and strictly one by one. It is proven by the results that only 48 kinds of herbs have relatively good tumor-inhibiting rate and another 152 kinds of traditional Chinese herbs are the traditional Chinese herbs commonly used by the herbalist doctors, through experimental screening of tumor-inhibiting rate in vivo by the tumor-bearing experiment, it is proven that they have no anti-cancer role or the tumor-inhibiting rate is very slight.

The screening by this lab is mainly the in vivo tumor-inhibiting experiment of the tumor-bearing animal model. The in vivo chronic experiment on every traditional Chinese herb is observed by one experimental group for 3 months, after screening, 48 kinds of traditional Chinese herbs are selected and then 2 and 3 kinds of dried medicinal herbs are arranged in groups to carry out the tumor-bearing experiments in vivo on the tumor-bearing animal and then it is found by us that the tumor-inhibiting effect of a single dried medicinal herb is not better than the one of the dried medicinal drug compound through tumor-inhibiting experiments. It seems that the single dried medicinal herb only play a role in inhibiting the proliferation of the tumor while the dried medicinal herb compound can inhibit the proliferation of the tumor-bearing rats and play a role in regulating and controlling the organism, enhancing the physical power, improving the immunity, promoting the generation of tumor-inhibiting cytokines, protecting the normal cells and promoting the anti-cancer cytokines as well.

Based on the screening of the single traditional herbs through the in vitro experiments and the tumor-inhibiting experiment screening on the tumor-bearing animal model over 4 years, through experimental optimization and combination and then experiment, this lab finally recombines Z-C$_{1-10}$

compound of anti-cancer, anti-metastasis and anti-reoccurrence through immunity regulation and control and finally it is subject to the clinical verification. Since 1992, we have established the cooperation group to carry out the clinical verification. Up to today from then on, through the clinical verification and observation of over 12000 patients suffering from the cancer in Shuguang Tumor Special Clinic over 16 years, the condition has been stable and improved, the symptom has been improved, the survival quality has been improved and the survival time has been obviously prolonged. So the lesions of many patients suffering from metastasis have been stabilized and have not further spread, as to some patients after operation cannot receive the chemotherapy due to the descent of leucocytes, the metastasis has been controlled after taking the medicine and no metastasis occurs again. Good curative effects have been obtained.

4. The Similar BRM Functions and Effects of XZ-C Medications

Biological response modifier (BRM) is first put forward by Oldham in 1982 to describe BRM. It refers to the ability of regulating the organism's response or reply to surface "attack" by biological response modifier.

The cells and humoral factors of the organism's immunity system are under subtle control, the organism's ability of response or reply will be affected significantly in case of imbalance. Biological response modifier is used to restore the unbalanced organism to normal balance, fulfilling the purpose of preventing diseases.

BRM opened the new field for biological treatment of tumor. At present, BRM is widely recognized in the medical circle as the fourth model of tumor treatment.

BRM is designed to regulate the immunologic function of the organism and restore the function of immune system of the contained organism. Such drug has manifold function mechanisms, but all of them exert regulating functions by activating the organism's immune system.

Biological response modifiers, most of which drive from microorganisms and plants, were previously referred to as immunopotentiator, immunostimulant, immunologic cordial or immunomodulator, now collectively named as biological response modulator or modifier(BRM).

The author screened out XZ-C medicine with good inhibition rate through in vivo experiment on mice inoculated with tumor. It has the functions of improving immunity, protecting centrum immune organ thymus, improve cellular immunity, protecting thymus tissue, protecting hematogenesis of bone marrow, increasing the number of akaryocyte and leukocyte, activate immunologic cytokine, the main pharmacological action of XZ-C improving the immunological surveillance in blood is protecting thymus and improving immunity. 48 types of immunologic drugs with high inhibition rate are screened out by four-year animal experiment, among which 26 types are identified through immune and cytokine level detection as capable of enhancing phagocytic function, or enhancing cellular immunity, or enhancing humoral immunity, or enhancing thymus weight, or promoting proliferation of bone marrow cells, or enhancing T cell function, or enhancing LAK cytoactive; or inhibiting blood platelet coagulation and resisting embolus; or resisting tumor poison and metastasis; or removing free radical. The anticancer mechanism of the above XZ-C medicine is:

Activating the organism's immunocyte system, promoting the enhancement of the host's defense mechanism and effect, achieving the capacity of immune response to cancer.

Activating immune cytokine system of anticancer mechanism of the organism, enhancing the host's immune defense mechanism and improving immunological surveillance of immunocyte of the organism's blood circulation system.

Protecting thymus and improving immunity, protecting bone marrow for hematogenesis, stimulating hematogenesis of bone marrow, promoting recovery of marrow inhibition, increasing leukocyte and akaryocyte.

Mitigating toxicant and side effects of chemotherapy and radiotherapy, enhancing the endurance of the host.

Cancer progress is caused by imbalance between biological characteristics of cancer cells and the organism's pharmaceutical capacity for cancer, XZ-C medicine is used to improve immunity and make them regain balance.

Regulating directly the growth and differentiation of tumor cells.

Increase the volume and weight of thymus, keeping thymus from progressive atrophy, for thymus will go through progressive atrophy when cancer evolves.

Stimulating the host's immune response to anticancer, enhancing the organism's anticancer ability, strengthening the sensitivity of cancer cells to the organism's anticancer mechanism, favorable for killing cancer cells on the way of metastasis.

XZ-C medicine can enable the host to make powerful immune response to cancer cells, achieving the purpose of treating cancer. XZ-C medicine can trigger the following immune responses of the host: enhancing regulation or restoring the host's immune response to tumors; stimulating inherent immunologic functions of the host, activating the host's immune defense system; restoring immunologic functions.

As described above, XZ-C medication has similar function mechanism to BRM, can have the same treatment effects with BRM in clinic application.

(4) THE PRINCIPLES OF CANCER TREATMENT

(Introduction)

Theory guides clinic: carry out the treatment in an all-round way aiming at the cancer cells and the host synchronously.

Cancer treatment should change their concepts to establish a comprehensive treatment concept. I believe that cancer treatment should overcome the current one-sided treatment concept targeted only killing cancer cells and change concepts to establish a comprehensive treatment concept. Traditional therapies target alone and only kill cancer cells, but ignore the host itself constrain cancer cells. Therefore, while we advocate the establishment of a comprehensive concept of treatment focus on both tumors and the hosts. It is necessary to establish a new treatment model in order to obtain better therapeutic effect.

After pondering the author presents the impact of cancer occurrence and development of the "Theory of Balance" concept.

If the only goal of cancer treatment is to kill cancer cells, but for one aspect, for one-sided treatment, it is impossible to overcome cancer. The goal of treatment should be for both host and cancer cells, both kill cancer cells and protect the host to enhance immune function and to protect thymus, to nurse marrow and blood, and enhance the host ability to anti-cancer, which is the concept of comprehensive treatment, will be possible to overcome cancer.

How to build a comprehensive concept of cancer treatment?

The goal of cancer comprehensive treatment concept is on both tumor and host which the scheme of the clinical treatment of cancer should be on cancer research from both cancer biological characteristics and the response of host organism.

(1) Must pay attention to a set of inherent human anticancer systems which should fully play its role in the immune system, enhancing immune surveillance and preventing escape of malignant cells.

(2) While chemotherapy is used, improving the immune function of the host should be done. To kill cancer cells cannot simply rely on chemotherapy drugs, but must also rely on the body's

cancer-fighting ability to destroy residual cancer cells after chemotherapy because of the limited ability of cytotoxic chemotherapy to kill cancer cells.

1) Time of chemotherapy e is limited and transient effects and time which patients administered chemotherapy to kill cancer cells is only effective about 1-5 days of intravenous injection and its role is to kill cancer cells, which it's just short Time to kill me (1-5 days) and not "once and for all". After 5 days the cancer continues to divide and to proliferate. While chemotherapy ends, efficacy will disappear so it can only relieve short-term improvement in a few weeks, after which you must also rely on the host immune function of cancer-fighting ability.

2) Chemotherapy is "double-edged sword" which is not only to kill cancer cells but also to kill the host bone marrow hematopoietic cells, to decline boost the immune function; therefore, while chemotherapy is used, host immune function must be protected, restored or enhanced.

3) After radiotherapy and chemotherapy cancer cells continue to divide and to proliferate, to clone so that the host need to rely on its own anticancer ability to suppress tumor long-term growth.

Since radiotherapy and chemotherapy all contribute to decreased immune function, therefore, I propose radiotherapy or chemotherapy, should be used with simultaneously immunotherapy, biotherapy, XZ-C immunomodulatory anti-cancer traditional Chinese medicine which is reformed into immunotherapy and chemotherapy and/or immunotherapy and radiotherapy.

(3) Improve the host immune function to inhibit tumor progression. Treatment of cancer in the short term is to rely on chemotherapy drugs to kill cancer cells ;in the long term it should rely on the host's immune function, immune surveillance to destroy the remaining cancer cells so that the concept of a comprehensive treatment must enhance host immune function to inhibit tumor progression.

Professor Xu Ze holds: the treatment of cancer shall get rid of the one-sided treatment outlook of simply killing the cancer cells and we should update the idea, change the concept and establish the treatment outlook in an all-round way. Since the cancer is opposite to the cancer cells and the host, the impaired anti-cancer force of host leads to the occurrence and development of the tumor while the intensive anti-cancer force of the host can control the development of the cancer, just like the "teeter-totter", as one falls, another rise. Therefore, the treatment of cancer is not only to kill the cancer cells, but also to protect the host and does not harm the host so as to enhance the anti-cancer force of the host and establish the cancer treatment outlook in an all-round way.

I. The objective of traditional therapy is relatively simple, just to kill the cancer cells, which is only one aspect of cancer treatment.

The traditional cancer therapy holds that the cancer is the continual division and proliferation of the cells, so the cancer cells are the arch criminal. Its treatment objective must be to kill the cancer cells. Objective of chemotherapy: to kill the cancer cells, only to kill the cancer cells.

Objective of radiotherapy: to kill the cancer cells, only to kill the cancer cells.

Why the traditional therapy with the objective of simply killing the cancer cells cannot reduce the death rate? Why it cannot prevent recurrence and metastasis? Why it only can play a role in a short-term remission? Why it only can remit the cancer but cannot heat the cancer patients? Is it real that the cancer cannot be cured? Or only simple radiotherapy and chemotherapy cannot cure the cancer? What is the problem in chemotherapy and radiotherapy? What are the defects and the disadvantages? Or is the therapeutic strategy with the objective of simply killing the cancer cells wrong? Are the cancer cells killed in chemotherapy? How many cancer cells are killed? How many cancer cells are remained in the body of the patient? Whether is the chemotherapy drug sensitive or not? Whether does it have drug tolerance? All of these things are remained unknown. Whether it is presented that the traditional therapy does not conform to the actual conditions of the biological characteristics of the cancer cells? It only kills the cancer cells while ignores the host.

II. The objective of traditional therapy ignores the resistance and inhibition of the host itself to the cancer

Actually, the occurrence and development of the tumor, is dependent on the immunologic function of the host and the biological characteristics of the tumor, namely the balance between the biological characteristics of the tumor cancers and the influences of the host on the confinement factors, if both of them are balanced, it is controlled; otherwise, it will be developed.

In the past half a century, the researchers at home and abroad had been focusing on the test on cancer cells to seek the drugs to kill the cancer cells, their ideas were affected by the mode of antibiotics killing the bacteria so as to kill the cancer cells. However, they did not know that they were two entirely different things: the antibiotics only kill the bacteria install of the normal cells and they can be used to make experiments on drug susceptibility while the chemotherapy drug can kill the cancer cells as well as the normal cells, however, it cannot be used to make the experiments on drug susceptibility. **The objective of the traditional therapy only pays attention to radiotherapy and chemotherapy killing cancer cells and ignores the anti-cancer system of the host.** The human body itself has a complete set of anti-cancer cell system while radiotherapy and chemotherapy ignore the anti-cancer cells in the host (NK cell group, K cell group, LAK cell group, macrophage group and TK cell group), the reaction of anti-cancer cell sub-systems IFN, IL-1 and TNF; ignores the reaction of cancer-inhibition gene and cancer-inhibition transfer gene in the host (cancer gene and cancer-inhibition gene as well as cancer transfer gene and cancer-inhibition transfer gene exist in the human body) and ignores the reaction of nervous body fluid system and the incretion system in the host. These organs and their affectois play an important role in adjustment, balance and stabilization of the host organism. These intrinsic anti-cancer factors in the human body shall be protected and activated by all means.

III. Professor Xu Ze proposes the objective or target of cancer treatment should establish the treatment outlook in an all-round way aiming at the cancer cells and the host synchronously.

Since the traditional therapeutic mode with the objective of simply killing the cancer cells has not settle the problem in the past half a century, it is necessary to establish a new treatment mode, update the idea and open a new way.

Through deep consideration and analysis, Professor Xu Ze proposes the concept of "balance theory" affecting recurrence and development of cancer:

Biological characteristics of cancer

Restriction capability of host on it

if both of them are balanced, it is controlled;

otherwise, it will be developed

Therefore, the objective or target of the cancer treatment must aim at the cancer and the host.

Namely treatment of

① host---immunity---biological factor, cytokine and traditional Chinese medicine for immune regulation and control target of cancer

②carcinoma---cancer cells---operation, radiotherapy and chemotherapy

Professor Xu Ze holds: if the treatment objective or target only kills the cancer cells, it only focuses on one side, which is unilateral. If the treatment objective or target only focuses on the immune regulation and control, it only stresses on one side, which is unilateral. The above-mentioned treatment outlook is unilateral and is not comprehensive and it is impossible to conquer the cancer. If the treatment objective or target focuses on both the host and the cancer, which can kill the cancer cells, protect the host, strengthen the immunity, protect the chest and the bone marrow, produce the blood and enhance the anti-cancer capability of the host, which is an all-round treatment outlook and it is possible to conquer the cancer.

As to the concept of current traditional therapy, the treatment objective or target only killing the cancer cells is the unilateral treatment outlook, which does not protect the anti-cancer force of the host, but damages the immunity of the host, therefore, it cannot conquer the cancer. It is necessary to establish cancer treatment outlook in an all-round way, that is to say, the objective or target is to focus on both the host and the carcinoma, which not only kills the cancer cells but also strengthen the immunity of the host, conforming to the actual conditions of the biological characteristics of cancer cells, so it is possible to conquer the cancer.

Through reviewing and reflecting the experience and lessons from clinical tumor surgery over 54 years, Professor Xu Ze holds: in order to conquer the cancer, it is necessary to simply kill the cancer cells as well as strengthen the immunity of the host to inhibit the tumor, bring the anti-cancer organ functions of the human body into play and exert their anti-cancer capability to make the anti-cancer resistance of the host stronger, in this way, it can inhibit the tumor for a long time and prevent its development to realize the cancer-bearing survival. Its treatment objective:

1. To control occurrence and development of the tumor, firstly the host shall be taken into consideration, stressing on how to strengthen the anti-cancer capability of the host to inhibit occurrence and development of the tumor.

2. Strengthen the anti-cancer force of the host to inhibit the development of the tumor so as to realize the cancer-bearing survival and prolong the survival period.

3. Try to make the anti-cancer force of the host stronger to inhibit the development of the tumor for a long time to make it stable and dormant, in this way, it will not be developed, resulting in the long-term cancer-bearing survival and becoming a chronic disease.

IV. How to establish the cancer treatment outlook in an all-round way? Stressing on killing the cancer cells as well as strengthening the anti-cancer immunity of the host

The objective or target of cancer treatment outlook in an all-round way aims at both the tumor and the host and research the clinical treatment scheme of cancer from the biological characteristics of the cancer cells and the reaction of the host organism. And then, how to realize the objective?

1. It must be made clear that the human body has a complete set of anti-cancer organ, so it is necessary to bring the reaction of the immune system into play, enhance the immune surveillance and prevent the escape of canceration cells. In fact, the radiotherapy and the chemotherapy cannot kill off all of the cancer cells, the remained cancer cells will be continually divided, proliferated and cloned in geometrical progression, such as one into two, two into four, in this way, it leads to recurrence and metastasis.

2. Radiotherapy and chemotherapy must pay attention to improvement of the immunologic functions of the host synchronously. In order to kill the cancer cells, it cannot simply rely on the chemotherapy drug, it is necessary to rely on the anti-cancer capability of the organism to eliminate the remained cancer cells, why? Because the cytotoxic drug for chemotherapy has limited capability to kill the cancer cells, in addition, the drug effect only lasts a short period.

(1) The chemotherapy reaction time is limited and momentary and the chemotherapy drug cannot kill off the cancer cells once and for ever, it only has the drug effect on killing the cancer cells in the days of intravenous injection for chemotherapy, after chemotherapy, the drug effect disappears and it has no reaction again and it only has the drug effect within 2-3 months even though the chemotherapy is made 4 times even 6 times, after that, it must rely on the anti-cancer capability of the immunologic functions of the host.

(2) The chemotherapy is a two-sided sword, which kills the cancer cells as well as the hematopoietic cells and immunological cells of the bone marrow, promoting the decrease of the immunologic function, therefore, it is necessary for the chemotherapy to recover or strength the immunologic functions of the host.

(3) After radiotherapy and chemotherapy, the remained stem cells of tumor are still continually divided, proliferated and cloned, so it is still necessary to improve the anti-cancer capability of the host to suppress the development of tumor for a long term.

Therefore, Professor Xu Ze proposes the current radiotherapy or chemotherapy should be combined with immunological therapy, biological therapy and XZ-C anti-cancer medicine for immune regulation synchronously. It is necessary to reform it to immune + chemotherapy and immune + radiotherapy.

3. How to improve the immunologic functions of the host to suppress the development of tumor for a long time? Viewed from a short term, the radiotherapy kills the cancer cells with chemotherapy drugs, viewed from a long term, it shall rely on the immunologic functions and the immune surveillance of the host to eliminate the remained cancer cells. So the treatment outlook in an all-round way must stress on protecting the chest and improving the immunity to improve the immunologic functions of the host so as to suppress the development of the tumor.

The cancer is a kind of general disease, so it is necessary to research the cancer and consider the clinical treatment scheme from the biological characteristics and behaviors of the cancer. The immune system is specially suitable for eliminated the remained cancer cells, especially the cells in resting stage of the stem cells of the tumor which are difficult to be eliminated by radiotherapy or chemotherapy, which is helpful to prolong the cancer-free survival time. Radiotherapy and chemotherapy only can kill a part of the cancer cells instead of all cancer cells, the rest cancer cells are slowly eliminated by the immunological cells of the host organism, so it is difficult to conquer the cancer by radiotherapy and chemotherapy.

Immunological therapy of tumor is an important part of biological treatment of the tumor and it is the key of the treatment outlook in an all-round way. Biological treatment of tumor is based on biological response modifier (BRM), namely BRM theory created by Oldham in 1982. Based on this, Oldham put forward four modality of cancer treatment of tumor treatment in 1984, namely the biological treatment. According to BRM theory, in normal conditions, the tumor and the defense of the organism are in dynamic balance, the occurrence, invasion and metastasis of the tumor are entirely caused by the maladjustment of the dynamic balance. If the maladjusted state can be artificially adjusted to the normal level, it can control the growth of the tumor and make the tumor extinct.

The biological treatment is to adjust the biological response through supplementing, inducing or activating the intrinsic biological active cells (or) factors with cell toxic cytoactive in BRM system in the body in vitro. The biological treatment is different from the three largest traditional therapies, including operation, radiotherapy and chemotherapy, the radiotherapy and the chemoyherapy targets directly attacking the tumor.

The biological treatment of the tumor mainly includes: (1) adoptive infusion of immunologic living cells; (2) application of lymphokine/cytokine; (3) specific active immunity, including tumor vaccine and monovalent vaccine.

The cells and the humoral factors of the organism reaction system are in delicate regulation and control, when they are unbalanced, the reaction or response capability of the organism will be remarkably affected, the adoption of biological reaction moderator is to recover the unbalanced organism state to the normal state so as to realize the objective of preventing the tumor.

The biological reaction moderator is to moderate the immunologic function of the organism, recover the suppressed functions of the immune system of the organism. The reaction mechanism of the drugs is to activate the immune system of the organism to bring its regulation function into play, most of them are from microorganism and the plants.

V. Immune regulation and control therapy is the key of the all-round cancer treatment

It has been proven by 4-year's experimental study and 30 year's clinical verification that XZ-C medications have the similar reaction and curative effect to BRM and it is the one with the similar reaction to BRM screened from the resources of Chinese traditional herbs.

XZ-C medications were screened through experiment by Professor Xu Ze in China (XU ZE-China, XZ-C) in the lab from 200 kinds of Chinese herbal medicines. Firstly we adopted the culture in vitro of cancer cells, screened 200 kinds of Chinese herbal medicines one by one in vitro, observed the direct damage to cancer cells by the medicines in the culture tube through experimental study and did the testing experiment of tumor-suppression rate with the normal cells cultured with chemotherapy drug CTX and in the test tube as the control group. Finally, we selected a batch of drugs with the rate of tumor-suppression of the proliferation of cancer cells. Then we further created the tumor-bearing animal model and did the experimental study on 200 kinds of Chinese herbal medicines for in vivo tumor-suppression rate and then screened, analyzed and evaluated them one by one scientifically and objectively. It was proven by the experimental results that only 48 kinds of medications had relatively good tumor-suppression rate.

Application principles of XZ-C medicine:

BRM and XZ-C medicine with similar reaction to BRM can strengthen immunological reaction of the organism, strengthen the immune surveillance reaction of the organism and they have relatively good effects when the cells meet with catastrophe or the tumor is very small. Through surgical operation or radiotherapy or medication, it will realize the best curative effect when the tumor is minimized.

As to the patient losing the opportunity of operation, with bad body condition, not withstanding radiotherapy and chemotherapy, the immunological therapy has a certain curative effect and reduces the symptom and prolongs the survival time.

After radical excision of the tumor, in order to reduce the recurrence and metastasis, XZ-C medicine can be administered for treatment; when large tumor is excised with operation, in order to eliminate the remained cancer cells and the ones that may be spread remotely, XZ-C medicine can also be administered.

If the tumor cannot be excised, the chemotherapy or the radiotherapy can be made firstly to kill a large number of tumor cells, after the tumor load in the body is reduced, XZ-C medicine can be administered for treatment.

In a word, the host is opposite to the host and the contradiction exists all along the whole process of occurrence and development of the tumor. When the functions of the immune system of the organism are complete, the organism can restrain and eliminate the tumor through cellular immunity and humoral immunity reaction. On the other hand, the growing tumor has so many effects on the immune system of the organism, inhibiting the immunologic functions of the organism and promoting the development of the tumor.

So the cancer treatment scheme must aim at the host and the tumor synchronously. The theory shall be used to guide the clinic; at the same time, the all-round anti-cancer treatment shall be made aiming at the cancer cells and the anti-force forces of the host to treat and to establish the outlook in an all-round way.

(5.) CANCER TREATMENT MODALITIES

The new mode combinations multidisciplinary treatment of cancer

Cancer treatment requires a scientifically designed treatment programs, the occurrence of cancer is a disease lose the ability to hang between the immune and tumor development in the balance, loss of immune surveillance, the further development of the tumor, treatment is necessary to restore the balance between stability.

Cancer Treatment requires a "multidisciplinary treatment program". This program is an organic integrated treatment must comply with the actual situation of the patient's condition.

Combinations multidisciplinary treatment must have a reasonable theoretical basis, it must be comprehensive therapy concept; the new knowledge which a host can affect the tumor progress and transfer has important theoretical value and clinical significance. During making the plans of anti-cancer invasion and metastasis, the two aspects from the tumor and host should be considered, which is theoretical basis for discipline and methods.

Based on the above analysis, when the diagnosis and treatment and the research of drug formulation are being done and it is to make the anti-cancer and anti-metastatic strategies, it should be considered from two angles to the tumor and the host. This is probably only fundamentally change the current the principle of one-sided treatment programs to kill cancer cells, thereby establishing a comprehensive treatment concept that should be followed.

How to combine multidisciplinary treatment? At first, we should transform the idea and update the approach, establish treatment outlook in an all-round way, arrange intervention, regulation, control and treatment measures in the whole course of disease, i.e. the whole process of cancer occurrence, development, recurrence and metastasis. Now we comprehensively divide the responsibilities of the main treatment methods of all disciplines commonly used at present and coordinate them organically as overall therapy and short-term therapy:

① Overall therapy. In radical surgery the main tumor has been removed and lymph node was dissected, then carried throughout the long course of treatment or biological therapy, immunotherapy, cytokines, gene therapy, XZ-Cimmunomodulatory anti-cancer traditional Chinese medicine, combining Chinese and Western medicine treatment of immune regulation in order to enhance the whole process of anticancer immunity, regulation or control of recurrence and metastasis in the host. It can be used in the whole cancer therapy.

② short-term treatment. Radiotherapy and chemotherapy, only intermittent treatment, or are used short-term to kill the cancer cells, rather than not Full course or long course of treatment, can not "once and for all", because of medication bombs that kill the cancer cells for 3-5 days, followed by no action to kill cancer cells, after a short remission, cancer cells continue to divide, proliferate recurrence, metastasis, because cancer cells can kill 4 cycles or six weeks the public for a long time may develop resistance.

Over the entire treatment and short-course treatment strategy are aimed at the tumor and host two angles to consider, which may fundamentally change only kill cancer cells from the current one-sided treatment concept.

Short-term therapy only in cancer patients in the whole course of a short stage, it should be for the adjuvant treatment (or vice-axis), because it unilaterally against cancer, not long-term, not excessive.

Traditional radiotherapy and chemotherapy for cancer but this factor is limited, one-sided, not comprehensive, and therefore difficult to overcome cancer. Because cancer is a result of the regulation process imbalance, we must address both host and tumor factors, response of the host to determine the final outcome. Cure should by regulation rather than a single killer.

Full treatment from cancer development, recurrence, metastasis, overall disease progression whole process is aimed at the tumor and host two factors to radical surgery foci entity, biological therapy, immunotherapy, gene therapy, cell factor treatment, XZ-C immune regulation medicine and other treatment to improve the host organism anticancer force, this scientific organic integrated comprehensive treatment, is reasonable, in line with cancer pathogenesis, pathophysiology of science, in line with the biological characteristics of cancer cells and biological behavior, therefore, may overcome cancer.

Therefore, the full course of treatment should be used as a cancer treatment spindle, which is the ultimate solution. The short-term treatment should be as countershaft cancer treatment, only palliative, only compatible with the full course of treatment.

Cancer treatment modalities(In the detail)

New Combinational Mode of Multi-disciplinary Comprehensive Treatment

1. The Reason why we put forward the new treatment mode of scientific organic integration
2. How to carry out organic, integrated and multi-disciplinary treatment scheme

3. It was proposed the specific scheme for new combination mode of comprehensive multi-disciplinary treatment.

Professor Xu Ze holds the combination of multi-disciplinary comprehensive treatment must have reasonable theoretical basis, and the new recognition that the host affects tumor progress and metastasis is of important theoretical value and clinic guiding significance. Two factors including tumor and host shall be considered in formulating anti-carcinoma and anti-metastasis strategies and making comprehensive treatment. Organic integration of discipline, method, technology and medicine with reasonable theoretical basis must be the treatment outlook in an all-round way.

At the beginning of 21st century, carcinoma treatment has entered into the era of multi-disciplinary comprehensive treatment.

Current situation of comprehensive treatment: it takes three traditional therapies as the main body. In most cases, the way of comprehensive application depends on the clinical department for initial diagnosis. Most patients are initially diagnosed in chemotherapy department, in which case they will be subject to chemotherapy firstly and then radiotherapy. If the patients are initially diagnosed in radiotherapy department, then they will be subject to radiotherapy followed by chemotherapy. If the patients are initially diagnosed in surgery department, they will be subject to operation with the presence of operation indications, followed by chemotherapy or radiotherapy, and will be subject to radiotherapy or chemotherapy with the absence of operation indications. The result of such comprehensive treatment is that many patients still fail to prevent recurrence and metastasis, and some even promote the failure of immunologic function.

Biotherapy, immunotherapy, differentiation-inducing therapy, cytokine therapy and immunologic regulation and control therapy of Chinese medicine combined with western medicine have not been incorporated into the treatment scheme of most tumor therapist.

I. The Reason why we put forward the new treatment mode of scientific organic integration

The study on carcinoma therapeutics must be based on tumor biology, both of which must be consistent with each other. Unit now, in the early years of 21st century, the tumor biology has developed into the level of molecular biology, cytokine and gene while the theoretical basis of the traditional cancer therapeutics has been still remaining the cellular level over 50 years which is based on the unceasing proliferation aiming at killing off carcinoma cells. Traditional radiotherapy and chemotherapy aims at killing cancer cells, so cytotoxic drug is used, but the effect is poor which requires increasing the dosage and adding several medicines for combination. In the recent decade, the trend of research on antitumor drugs and status of clinical application indicate the clinical application of traditional anticancer drugs was subject to more limitations due to great side effects, low targeting, the patients' tolerance to drugs, etc.

It can be deemed that the research on anticancer drugs has entered a new stage, facing updating of theories, technologies and ideas. The traditional idea and working method are merely aiming at simply eliminating cancer cells by cytotoxic drug as the theoretical basis is under attack.

Since 1980s, with the rapid development of medical molecular, molecular immunology, immunopharmacology, TCM immunopharmacology and cytokine, new bio-therapeutics has emerged, driving the advancement of cancer therapeutics. Biotherapy, immunologic therapy, differentiation inducer, biological reaction regulator, immunological regulation and control TCM at molecular level combined with western medicine are coming out in succession. New tumor vaccine development and gene therapy in recent years presents a more fascinating prospect.

The author holds that cancer therapy needs a scientifically designed treatment plan. In case of cancer, further development of tumor is contributed to imbalance between anticancer immunocompetence and tumor development of the organism and the absence of immune surveillance. Hence, both of them must be recovered to balance and stability through therapy.

II. How to carry out organic, integrated and multi-disciplinary treatment scheme

1. Professor Xu Ze proposes that carcinoma treatment needs a scientifically designed "organic, integrated and multi-disciplinary treatment scheme". And the scientifically designed organic integration must be consistent with the actual conditions of the patient:

(1) **Biological characteristics and behaviors of cancer cells, which means that the malignant cells in the organism will be continually progressively divided, proliferated and cloned once becoming cancer cells, from one to two, two to four......throughout the whole course of cancer occurrence, evolvement, metastasis and recurrence. Hence, treatment measures must stress on control and treatment in the whole course, rather than a certain stage of the course of disease.**

(2) Cancer is in continual evolvement. Cancer cells are featured in uncontrolled infinite proliferation; their canceration results from imbalance in control. A response relationship must be kept between tumor and host, **and the response of the host determines the final results.**

(3) According to the biological behaviors of cancer cells, multiple-step and multi-link of cancer cell metastasis and its "eight steps", "three stages" and "two points and one line", intervene and intercept cancer cells on the way to metastasis and adopt a new, scientific, organically integrated treatment mode in an all-round way.

2. The combination of comprehensive multi-disciplinary treatment must have reasonable theoretical basis, that is to say, an all-round treatment outlook and the new recognition of host affecting tumor progress and metastasis must be of great theoretical value and clinical guiding significance. In working out the strategies of anticancer attack and metastasis and selecting comprehensive treatment, we should consider adopting which discipline, method, technology and medicine to realize the organic integration with reasonable theoretical basis in light of tumor and host.

What is the primary determining factor during occurrence, development and metastasis of cancer? Is it tumor or host? Is it immunological anticancer competence of the host organism or attack and metastasis competence of cancer cells? In the past half century, the research has focused on cancer cell itself, all countries aim at the way of killing the cancer cells. Therefore, traditional treatment is killing cancer cells, which is the single objective. Despite some remarkable progresses, they all fail to solve the problem radically, just addressing secondary symptoms rather than primary ones.

In recent years, more attention is shifted to host factor. Our lab has spent four years in experimental study on tumor origin, pathogenesis, pathologic physiology and cancer attack and metastasis mechanism to explore anticancer immunocompetence and tumor interaction and to seek the control effects on cancer cell attack and metastasis. Hence, Professor Xu Ze proposes the "balance" theory which holds that cancer will evolve if the relation between the biological characteristics of cancer cells and the immunological anticancer competence of the host organism is unbalanced; it will be under control and stabilized if the balance is recovered. Thus the treatment must be targeted at two aspects, namely host and tumor, so as to recover them to a balanced and stable state.

Through experimental exploration of the interaction, interrelationship between host and tumor coupled with clinic practice experience and lessons, we analyze whether cancer cells or host determines the occurrence, development and metastasis and recurrence of cancer. What is behind the death of cancer? Why cancer tumor causes death? **Our current understanding is that the death of tumor patients is mainly contributed to metastasis and recurrence, but how recurrence and metastasis leads to death? According to our preliminary analysis, consideration and understanding, it is contributed to complication and immunologic failure.** So the final result shall be considered as both tumor itself and host.

According to analysis and understanding in our lab, poor immunological function of host

organism $\xrightarrow{\text{plus some factor causing cell mutation}}$ malignant mutation of cells $\rightarrow$ most of them are phagocytized by immunologic cells of the organism $\longrightarrow$ the rest malignant cells will be continually divided, proliferated and cloned $\longrightarrow$ tumor formation of metastasis and then have widespread metastasis.

Professor Xu Ze holds: based on the findings of experimental study in our lab and the data of clinic verification and clinic observation, it is the interaction between cancer cells and host microenvironment and anticancer immunological competence that finally determines cancer progress and that whether and when the metastasis lesion can be formed. The revelation of this regulatory mechanism of interaction is of great theoretical value and clinical significance. **As regards formulation of anticancer metastasis strategies and development of new medicines, we should consider tumor and host factors, which provide theoretical basis for seeking effective intervention methods and developing new medicines. XZ-C medicine developed by us for immunological enhancement through thymus protection and hematopoiesis through spinal marrow protection takes strengthening host factor as the theoretical and experimental basis.**

Based on the above analysis, the strategies of diagnosis, treatment, medicine development, anticancer control, antimetastasis should be considered from the perspectives of tumor and host. This may be deemed as the principle of radically changing the current partial treatment scheme with the single aim of killing cancer cells and establishing the treatment outlook in an all-round way previously described.

III. Professor Xu Ze proposes the specific scheme for new combination mode of comprehensive multi-disciplinary treatment Advocated

How to combine multi-disciplinary for comprehensive treatment?At first, we should transform the idea and update the approach, establish treatment outlook in an all-round way, arrange intervention, regulation, control and treatment measures in the whole course of disease, i.e. the whole process of cancer occurrence, development, recurrence and metastasis. Now we comprehensively divide the responsibilities of the main treatment methods of all disciplines commonly used at present and coordinate them organically as per overall therapy or short-term therapy.

1. Overall therapy: mainly based on radical operation treatment, tumor removal and lymph node elimination are followed by biotherapy, immunotherapy, cytokine therapy, differentiation inducement, gene, immunotherapy with Chinese medicines combined with western medicine, XZ-C medicine in a long term or the whole course, to strengthen anticancer immunocompetence of the host, regulate or control recurrence and metastasis. They can be used in the whole course of cancer disease.

2. Short-term therapy: mainly based on radiotherapy and chemotherapy as the primary form, which is in phases or intermittent, or killing cancer cells suddenly in a short course, but not and cannot cover the overall course or a long course. In this case, the duration of cancer cell elimination can be only four cycles or six cycles, longer duration will produce drug resistance.

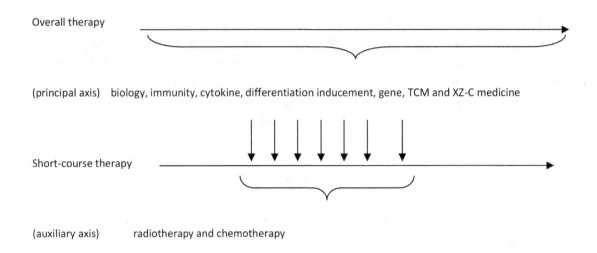

Figure schematic diagram of the combination mode of multi-disciplinary comprehensive treatment

(1) When working out the strategies of the above overall therapy and short-course therapy, we should take tumor and host into account, which may thoroughly change the partial treatment merely killing cancer cells at present. Currently, radiotherapy and chemotherapy only aim at cancer cells, which are partial and incomplete, and fail to consider treatment approaches in light of tumor and host as described above. Apart from this, radiotherapy and chemotherapy will also injure and kill hematopoietic cells and immunological cells of the bone marrow of the host, undermining the immunological function of the host and damaging the host.

(2) Short-course therapy just covers a short stage in the whole course of disease for cancer patients, so it should be deemed as an adjuvant therapy (or referred to as auxiliary axis), for it merely aims at a single aspect of cancer cells.

① Biological characteristics of cancer cells. Cancer stems from malignant mutation of a single cell, the cancer cells are progressively divided and proliferated, from one to two, from two to four…… Cancer is a development process rather than a form or entity. Therefore, the therapy to kill off cancer cells cannot eliminate all cancer cells. As long as several cancer cells remain, they can be continually divided, proliferated and recurred. Moreover, chemotherapy cannot injure tumor stem cells, which are bound to constant division, proliferation, resulting in cancer cells. Hence, the treatment method solely relying on killing cancer cells fails to comply with biological characteristics and biological behavior of cancer cells.

② **The effective time of cytotoxic drug is limited. It is only effective during the period of application, and ineffective beyond the period, so it cannot be done once and for all. Its effective time is limited, so the remaining 10^{6-7} cancer cells still need to be eliminated by immunological competence of the host. Moreover, tumor stem cells will continue** to form cancer cells. Therefore, radiotherapy and chemotherapy can only relieve the condition for several months but cannot heal it.

③ Chemotherapy killing cancer cells is only the first order kinetics, its lethality is limited and it can only kill 10^{6-7} cancer cells.

④ Chemotherapy drug is a double-edged sword. Apart from killing cancer cells, it can also kill normal cells, hematopoietic cells and immunological cells of the bone marrow of the host, causing drop in immunological function of the host.

Traditional chemotherapy and radiotherapy are only targeted at the factor of cancer cell tumor, which is limited, partial and incomplete, thus it is difficult to conquer the cancer. Because canceration process is the result of regulation imbalance, it must be targeted at host and tumor, and the reaction of the host decides the final result. It should be cured by regulation instead of injury alone.

(3). Overall therapy. It covers the whole course of cancer disease from cancer occurrence, development, recurrence, metastasis, progress, targeted at these two factors, i.e. tumor and host. It applies radical operation to remove cancer lesion entity, and applies biotherapy, immunotherapy, gene treating cytokine, immunological regulation TCM and so on to the host, so as to improve anticancer competence of the organism. **Such scientific and organic integration is targeted at two aspects, i.e. cancer cells and host. It is an all-round treatment outlook, which is comprehensive, reasonable and scientific, complies with pathogenesis, pathological physiology, biological characteristics and biological behaviors of cancer cells, and is likely to conquer cancer.**

Therefore, **overall therapy should be the principal axis of cancer treatment, with operation treatment as the main form, biotherapy, immunotherapy, gene therapy, and differentiation inducement therapy, TCM immunological regulation therapy, improving immunity by chest protection and hematogenesis by bone marrow protection distributed and applied in the whole course of cancer treatment. It is a scientific, reasonable and all-round treatment outlook and a radical method.** Short-course therapy should be auxiliary axis of cancer treatment, with chemotherapy and radiotherapy as the main form. It is only designed to kill off cancer cells and should be combined with overall therapy.

Xu Ze holds: the new mode of multi-disciplinary comprehensive treatment described above has a reasonable theoretical basis, comply with the realities of the patient's condition and is rational and scientific.

1. The experience and lessons of clinic treatment practice demonstrate killing cancer cells cannot control cancer or overcome cancer. It is partial and incomplete to merely target at one aspect of cancer cell.
2. The objective or target of cancer treatment should be both host and tumor. As regards which is the main side and who decides the final destiny of the cancer patient, both tumor itself and host should be considered.

3. We must update the approach and transform the idea, fist establish a treatment outlook in an all-round way, scientifically arrange intervention, regulation and treatment measures with the whole course of cancer occurrence, development, recurrence and metastasis.

4. **We should work out design and arrangement of "principal axis" and "auxiliary axis" new treatment mode, which is appropriate and scientific, with theoretical basis and in line with the realities of the patient.**

5. We must orient human firstly, manage to eliminate toxicant and side effects of radiotherapy and chemotherapy as possible, increase patient safety, study the toxicity and safety of each medicine and technology, which must have appropriate theoretical basis guiding clinic practice.

In short: cancer treatment, whether in early, middle or late stage, requires multi-disciplinary comprehensive treatment and appropriate theoretical basis guiding clinic practice.

In the last two decades, there are many reports on cancer treatment by tradition Chinese medicine. Its prospect is of concern. Especially with further research on medicine and immunology, it has been recognized that confusion of immunological system is closely related with occurrence and development of tumor. Traditional Chinese medicine has its own characteristics and advantages in treating tumor by regulating immunological function of the organism. Immunological regulation of traditional Chinese medicines and the development of Chinese medicine immunomodulator will be concerned and favored across the world. If combined with operation, radiotherapy and chemotherapy, SZ-C medicine can give full play to its immunological regulation function during treatment, obviously prolong survival time and improve survival quality, displaying characteristics and advantages of traditional Chinese medicine. Its disadvantage lies in that it cannot cause evident change on tumor itself.

Since the methods above are different in action mechanism and effects of cancer treatment, and have their own disadvantages, thus it is necessary to evaluate the advantages and disadvantages of the therapies, "gains" and "losses" of the patients, for example, what are the advantages and disadvantages of adopting this therapy, what will the patients gain or lose? We can draw from the advantages of each therapy to offset their disadvantages, combine the therapies in an organic and appropriate way, forming a comprehensive plan of cancer treatment. Only in this way can we significantly reduce toxic and side effects of the medicine, improve survival quality of the patients and prolong overall survival time. Over the past 30 years, Shuguang Tumor Clinic has applied the comprehensive treatment mainly involving operation +XZ-C medication to more than 12000 cancer patients at middle and late stage. Most of them have achieved the effects of improving survival quality, stabilizing disease lesion, controlling metastasis, existence with tumor and significantly prolonging life.

(6.) THE PRINCIPLES OF ANTI-CANCER METASTASIS TREATMENT

- The key to conquer cancer is to anti-metastasis;
- The basic principle of cancer therapy is anti-metastatic;
- The main features of the new concept of cancer treatment is namely to control metastasis

It has been seen from the clinical medical practice in about 100 years that the three traditional therapeutics including operation, radiotherapy and chemotherapy have made relatively good curative effects in treating the malignant tumor and so many patients have obtained CR/PR curative effects throaty radiotherapy and chemotherapy and the tumor has been obviously shrunk. However, it is a pity that the tumor meets with reoccurrence, enlargement and metastasis later. Although radiotherapy or chemotherapy is made again, the curative effects on most patients are extremely bad and they die of metastasis and reoccurrence.

The author summarizes the experience and lessons positive and negative from the clinical practice cases over 60 years, forms the following new understanding, puts forward the new theoretical concept and launches the new therapeutic strategies through combining the long-term experimental study with the clinical practice.

1. The key to conquer cancer is to anti-metastasis

Anti-cancerometastasis is the key to overcome the cancer because the metastasis is the first cause of the death caused by cancer.

In the past one century from 20ᵗʰ century, the goal of tackling the key problem is to kill the cancer cells aiming at the primary carcinoma lesion and metastatic carcinoma lesion. Although the efforts have been made for a century, the cancer mortality has been always taking the first place. **The main reason why the mortality is so high is the metastasis. Obviously, the previous traditional therapeutics cannot reduce the stubbornly high mortality. The first cause of its failure is that the goal cannot target the metastasis and control the metastasis.**

So far, the uppermost problem of cancer treatment is still how to prevent the metastasis. If the metastasis of cancer cannot be successfully solved, the cancer treatment cannot get a great-leap-forward development. Therefore, one of the goals of cancer treatment in 21ˢᵗ century is anti-metastasis.

The above-mentioned problems impel us to update the thoughts and change the ideas to open a new road to find the new therapeutics for preventing metastasis and overcome the cancer while improving the curative effects of the traditional therapeutics as per the traditional ideas. Therefore, we proposed a new treatment mode for anti-cancerometastasis after the analyzing and understanding the immune state of the host and the multiple steps and links of cancerometastasis based on the biological characteristics of the cancer and the biological behaviors of the cancerometastasis.

The academician of Liver Cancer Research Institute of Fudan University, Tang Zhaoxian, raised in *On Clinical Research on Carcerometastasis* on Nov. 9, 2007: "if the cancerometastasis is not studied, the improvement of curative effects is a soap bubble".

Great attention has been paid to the tumor metastasis since 1990s in the world. Metastasis Research Society was established, Clinical and Experimental Metastasis was issued. Cancerometastasis Research Society was established in Tokyo, Japan.

The study on metastasis in China starts relatively late, Professor Gao Jin published *Cancer Invasion and Metastasis------Fundamental Research and Clinic* based on a large quantity of rich experimental data in 1996, which was the first monograph on cancerometastasis and was excellent in both the pictures and their accompanying essay. In 2003, the academician Tang Zhaoxian published his monograph Foundation and Clinic of Metastasis and Reoccurrence of Liver Cancer and he raised in the monograph: "the next important goal of study on primary liver cancer is to prevent and control reoccurrence and metastasis", in addition, he said: "metastasis and reoccurrence have become one bottle-neck of further improving the survival rate of liver cancer and one of the most important difficulties in overcoming the cancer". These monoprahies accelerate the attention to and study on the metastasis by the scholars in China. In 2006, Professor Xu Ze published New Concept and New Way of Treatment of Cancer Metastasis and put forward some theoretical innovations, which was granted with "Three-One-Hundred Original Book" by General Administration of Press and Publication of the People's Republic of China.

2. The basic principle of cancer treatment is anti-metastatic

(1).Aiming at the biological behaviors of the cancer cells, that is, the unique behaviors of invasion and metastasis

Metastasis is a malignant behavior. It is well known that the fundamental difference between the benign tumor and the malignant tumor is that the former meets with metastasis while the latter does not meet with the metastasis. If we can take measures to prevent the metastasis of the cancer cells, is the malignant tumor becoming the benign tumor? 85%~95% of the patients die of the metastasis of the cancer. In case of no metastasis, most of the patients will not die. In case that the metastasis does not happen or it is controlled, the cancer is not so terrible. Therefore, the principle of treatment of cancer is to prevent the metastasis, design the therapeutic scheme and intervention scheme of anti-metastasis, research and develop the anti-metastasis drug, try to obstruct

and intercept the cancer cells in metastasis and cut off or block one or more links of metastasis so as to control the metastasis.

(2) How to prevent metastasis? The biological characteristics and behaviors of the cancer cells are invasion and metastasis. The reason why the cancer is malignant is mainly the wide harm of invasion and metastasis to the human body. Over a century, the goals of the three traditional therapies have been always aiming at the primary lesion cancer and metastatic carcinoma lesion and ablating the primary carcinoma lesion by operation or treat the metastatic carcinoma lesion with radiotherapy and other local treatment. It is commonly held that the primary carcinoma lesion and the metastatic carcinoma lesion can be seen or touched and they are local, so they can be treated with operation or radiotherapy. Reviewing and reflecting the clinical practice for 54 years, I had made so many radical operation on chest and abdomen based on the above-mentioned understanding, however, after the follow-up survey of 3000 patients after operation made by me in 1985, I was discerning and apprehending quickly and completely that how to prevent the reoccurrence and metastasis after operation is the core to determine the long-term curative effects of the cancer. The primary carcinoma lesion or the metastatic carcinoma lesion may be represented locally while the remote metastasis is systemic.

Since 1970s, in view of the high reoccurrence and metastasis rate of the cancer after operation, in order to control the reoccurrence after operation, the assistant chemotherapy after operation has been adopted, even the chemotherapy before operation (for example, on breast cancer) has been made, however, the results have not been so satisfactory and the assistant chemotherapy after operation on the patients cannot prevent the reoccurrence and metastasis. As to some cases, the chemotherapy is intensified, resulting in adynamia of immunologic function. All these issued shall be seriously and calmly thought, reviewed, analyzed and reflected by the clinicians so as to find how to prevent the reoccurrence and metastasis to treat the cancer.

In the recent 20 years, the understanding of the molecular metastasis mechanism of cancer has made great progress, however, there have been no actually effective measures for preventing the metastasis of the cancer cells at home and abroad. Although some new anti-cancer drugs have come out in recent years, the curative effects cannot be improved to our satisfaction. The reason why some cancer cells cannot be radically cured by the exploration in the middle and late stage is that the lymph node meets with the remote metastasis. It is important and key to inhibit the cancerometastasis so as to reduce the death rate of cancer and improve the curative effects.

The goal of tackling the key problem is relatively simple, just to kill the cancer cells, which does not entirely conform to the actual condition of the biological characteristics of the cancer at present, for example, the invasion behaviors of the cancer cells, metastasis link and multi-step, molecular biological mechanism of metastasis, immunoreactivity of the organism and inducement of reoccurrence and reoccurrence after incubation for several months even several years. Now it is known by the people at present that the anti-cancer drug does not always prevent the metastasis or kill the cancer cells.

Therefore, it is held by the author that now it is key to prevent the metastasis so as to overcome the cancer and it is core to study how to prevent the metastasis so as to cure the cancer.

3. The main features of the new concept of cancer treatment namely is to control the metastasis

Killing cancer cells in human body should resort to two kinds of force: one is foreign force from operation, radiation therapy and chemotherapy, the other is intrinsic force from patient's autoimmunity. Although medication, operation and therapeutic techniques are important to patient's therapy, intrinsic immunity of human body is more important. Many problems must depend on patient's self force and power to be solved, such as nutrition problem, it is hard to attain the object if the patient organism can't absorb and utilize despite given sufficient nutriment. Take healing of incision as another example, it must rely on patient's intrinsic healing function and exogenous factor can only influence or accelerate its healing.

Intrinsic immunity of human body can kill cancer cells. Literature material shows that a tiny tumor (1-8g) can release several millions or hundreds of thousands of cancer cells to blood within 24h, but most (99.99%) of them will be killed by human body immune system can kill cancer, only less than 0.1% can survive and grow to metastatic carcinoma. The data from our own laboratory show that Kunming mouse can kill 99% of cancer cells by its autoimmunity within 24h when injected 10^5 S_{180} malignant cells to caudal vein. More cancer cells will be killed if the mouse takes XZ-C-$_1$ and XZ-C$_4$ immunization regulation and control traditional Chinese medicine. Anti-cancer Metastasis Lab of Wuhan Shuguang Tumor Special Clinic has implied XZ-C$_1$ and XZ-C$_4$ to patients regularly in recent 10 years, it is shown by clinical data statistics that certain amount of cancer cells in metastasis can indeed be killed.

Human body has certain anti-cancer ability and there is a complete anti-cancer mechanism and system in host body with the anticancer effect of anticancer cell cluster (NL cell cluster, K cell cluster, LAK cell cluster, macrophage cluster and TK cell cluster), the anticancer effect of anticancer cytokine system, FN, IL-2, TNF and LT, and the effect of anti-oncogene and inhibiting cancer metastasis gene, and the effects of the neurohumoral and endocrinohumoral functions. **In the human body these anti-cancer systems and their functions have the effects for the regulation and stabilization of the body anticancer systems; therefore, it must be protected, activated and brought into play.**

The generation and development of cancer is close related to immunologic hypofunction of the body. The carcinoma can directly infringe immune organ to worsen or inhibit immunologic function and can release immunosuppressive factor to bring down the immunity of host or to induce the intracorporeal suppressor cell to increase. The Thymus of host has been inhibited in case of cancer and chemotherapy inhibits bone marrow, just like one disaster after another. Traditional therapy neglects the intrinsic anticancer ability of human body and the anticancer force of anticancer cell, anticancer cytokine, antioncogene and anti-metastasis gene in anticancer system, in this way, the whole central immune organ shall be damaged and can not be effectively protected, which is why the curative effect of traditional therapy can't be improved.

Consequently, the author suggests attaching great importance to exerting and relying on the intrinsic force of anticancer system of the host.

The main characteristics of Xu Ze's cancer therapeutics: to control over metastasis and to protect the immune function of the patient instead of simply killing the cancer cells.

(7.) NEW CONCEPT OF TREATMENT OF CANCER METASTASIS

The aiming on treatment of the cancer group on the metastasis way

Cancer in the body exists in the main form

    a.   in the conventional cancer therapeutics it thinks there are two forms;

    b.   Inthe new concept of cancer treatment it thinks that there are three forms;

    c.   The research and understanding of the process about there is the third form of cancer in the body;

    d.   The goal of cancer treatment should be the third existing form.

After 60 years of clinical experience in surgical oncology practice and 10 years of laboratory research I carried out careful sorting and summarizing and formed an unique new understanding and new concept of cancer metastasis and proposed new methods and new technology of anti-metastatic cancer therapy.

Its main contents include: ① cancer in the body exists in three forms; ② the whole process of two points and One Line of Carcinoma Development ③ cancer metastasis" eight steps and a three-stage "theory; ④ the third field of human anti-cancer metastasis treatment (5) metastasis treatment "trilogy"; ⑥ independently developed XZ-C immunomodulatory anticancer Chinese medication.

The following series of new understanding, new theories, new concepts have not yet been mentioned so far in the literature and textbooks. After lessons of half century practice and 10 years of experimental research, analysis, reflection and wake up, it converses to real theory which founded new concepts and has become distinctive anti-metastatic cancer in therapy theoretical system and have independent innovation and creative and original intellectual property rights.

1. Traditional cancer therapeutics that there are two forms

There are two forms of cancer existing in human body: one is the primary lesion of primary tumor and another is the metastatic node or metastases.

The goal or target of treatment of traditional cancer therapeutics aims at these two existing forms, namely the primary tumor or metastatic tumor just because no matter the primary tumor or metastatic tumor is composed of cancer cell while the goal of treatment is to kill the cancer cell.

The main reason for the failure of conventional therapy is recurrence and metastasis.

2. XU ZE New Concept of Cancer Treatment Holding Three Forms Exist

The author first published an new theory which the third form of cancer group which exists in our body is the cancer cells on the route of metastasis.

The author holds that the cancer existing in the human body has three forms: the first one is the primary lesion of primary tumor; the second one is metastatic node or metastatic tumid lymph node; the third one is the cancer cell and cancer cell group and micro-metastasis in metastasis routing which the main reason for the failure of conventional therapy is recurrence and metastasis.

It is just this cancer groups or slight cancer embolus in metastasis routing which is the main reasons for the postoperative metastasis and recurrence.

In operation, the third group of cancer cell and micro-metastasis in metastasis routig which cannot be seen by eyes, for example, in radical operation for carcinoma of stomach, the phyma of stomach cancer and metastatic tumid lymph nodes can be seen by us, however, whether the cancer cell exists in the vein of stomach wall or portal vein blood stream cannot be seen? And how many cancer cells exist? And where the cancer cells in the vein blood stream go? Whether the cancer cell groups touched and extruded into the vein flood stream arrive at the stomach vein or the portal vein even the portal vein branch in the anus? It is impossible to not touch the cancer tumor in operations research and abscission of tumor of stomach cancer and cleaning down of lymph node, since the operation by hand necessarily makes a large number of cancer cells extruded and exfoliated, flowing into the blood circulation through out-neoplasm vein and rushing into the blood stream of portal vein, however, which cannot be seen by the operation doctor. These cancer cells rushing into the blood stream of portal vein will flow into the portal vein system. . Generally, the various immunological cells in the portal vein will carry out the immune surveillance over the cancer cells in the blood circulation of the portal vein and will phagocytize them. However, in a short time, the immunological cells in the portal vein system cannot phagocytize these cancer cells rushing abruptly. After a period of time, some cancer cells escape the immune surveillance, the cancer cells surviving after impact of blood stream may implant in the sinus hepaticus, the blood vessel produces and forms the intrahepatic metastasis.

The phenomenon as well as a fact has not been thought and discovered that is a dynamic manifestation of the cancer cell existing in the human body. **The anti-cancer metastasis and recurrence lab of this experimental surgical research institution, through analysis and research of the metastasis rule of over 10000 clinic patients suffering from cancer, has been aware of this phenomenon and find it, that is to say that the essence of the metastasis is the cancer cells in the metastasis routing and the goal of anti metastasis and the target of treatment should aim at the cancer cells in metastasis routing, namely the third manifestation of cancer existing in human body; in the past, since the people had not been aware of this point, they only cured the primary lesion and metastasis and tried to shorten or eliminate it, but not knew that the shrinkage of the tumor did not mean that it did not metastasis. The traditional therapy of treatment fails in reoccurrence and metastasis in a long term.**

3. The process of the research and understanding of Cancer in the body of a third form

(1) Where are metastasis cancer cells?

Since it is cognized by us that the key to cure the cancer is to anti-metastasis, how to realize the anti-metastasis? And how to cognize the detailed process, step and mechanism of the metastasis of cancer cells? How these cancer cells move? What is their movement rule? Where is the weak link of the cancer cell in metastasis routing? Which link(s) should be stricken or blockaded? The goal of striking the cancer metastasis must be objictified.

(2) The experimental study tracked the fate and the role of the way in the metastasis cancer cells

In order to settle the above-mentioned problems, the experimental surgical anti-metastasis and recurrence lab was established by us to carry out the fundamental research of experimental tumor, implant the cancer cells, establish the animal model of tumor and develop a series of experimental tumor research: probing into the mechanism and rule of cancer invasion and metastasis; probing into the relationship between the tumor and immunity and the immune organ as well as the one between the immune organ and the tumor; finding the effective measures to regulate and control the invasion and metastasis of cancer. This lab has spent 3 years in the experimental research on the animal model of cancer metastasis and the experimental observation for observing and tracing the fortune and rule of the cancer cells in the metastasis routing.

In animal experiments cancer cells could not be found in mice blood 48h after 10^5 cancer cells were injected. **These injected cancer cells are eliminated completely**? Through analysis and presumption, it is possible that some cells transfused into the circulation system are killed because they do not adapt the environment or they are damaged due to the impact of the rapid blood stream or are obstructed by the impediment micro-circulation, however, most of the cancer cells entering the blood circulation, are mainly the immunizing ability of the mouse, which are killed by a large number of immunological cells in the blood circulation of the mouse. Therefore, in the treatment of anti-metastasis, the treatment of cancer cells and cancer cell groups in the metastasis routing must protect the immunizing ability of the host body and it is necessary to try to mobilize, recover and activate its immunologic function of the immune system, instead of striking, damaging and reducing or avoiding striking, damaging and reducing the immunizing ability and functions of immune system of the host body as much as possible. How to try to protect, mobilize and activate the immune functions of the host to deal with the cancer cells in metastasis routing is an important anti-metastasis strategy.

(3) Where do the transfer of cancer cells present and what is the form of the cancer existence?

Some new approaches through the animal experiment and some experimental achievements are obtained. However, it is difficult to verify many experimental results just because that the clinical verification must last 3~5 years before the long-term curative effect can be evaluated. Usually, good effect is obtained in the experimental research, however, it is difficult to observe the remarkable clinical effect just because that the subject investigated in the lab is the mouse while the clinical object is the patient, the experimental results are not always be applied to clinic and it must be subject to the clinical verification and observation for 3~5 years even 8~10 years before the long-term reoccurrence and metastasis of cancer can be understood.

Why the patients meet with the occurrence even wide metastasis and spreading where-after or before long even after the primary lesion or metastasis of these patients are appropriately even satisfactorily cured? Where these metastasis and reoccurrence cancer cells exist in which form? What causes the difference in metastasis time from several months to several years? We remain perplexed despite much thought. Where are these cancer cells hidden in the human body? Why are they so pertinacious? The popular explanation of the patients' families is that "the cancer is alive and it can move". The author realized and found that the forms of the cancer cell in human body were not only the primary lesion and metastasis; the third manifestation, namely the cancer cell and cancer cell group exist in the metastasis routing. The third manifestation has been not mentioned in the literatures and teaching books up to today. Just because that the people have not cognized it, resulting in ignore of the special manifestation of the cancer cell in the metastasis routing.

(4) How cancer cells can survive during the metastasis way?

Many patients are subject to the comprehensive treatment such as radiotherapy and chemotherapy over the primary lesion or metastasis tumor by means of various traditional therapeutic methods, the cancer cell meets with metastasis chronically and duratively, **thus where these cancer cells exist or hide?** Through research, it is deemed by us that **these cancer cells has slow or quick metastasis speed in the metastasis routing;** under a certain conditions, **they may meet with dormancy and rest in GO stage; sometimes, the cancer cells are active, entering the cell cycle.** The so-called "condition" may be relevant to the factors such as the cancerous protuberance and local micro-environment of the host; it also be related to the cyto-dynamics of the cancer cells. **In facts, these thousands of cancer cells in metastasis routing are most dangerous. They are the hidden enemy;** the cancer cells with metastasis potential surviving in the metastasis routing will slowly and gradually form the new metastasis. They are in the active and slow attack. However, the presently traditional therapeutic method is to wait for the new metastasis and then cure it.

The reason why the cancer cells survive in the metastasis routing is because that it can escape the immune surveillance of the immunological cell in the blood circulation. If the cell toxicant chemotherapy is used to cure the metastasis, it is possible to kill many immunological cells, resulting in further weakening the immune surveillance of the immunological cells in the blood circulation of the patient and surviving of more cancer cells in the metastasis routing due to escaping the immune surveillance, forming more new metastasis.

4. Target for cancer therapy should be the three existing forms

Cancer treatment goal or "target" should aim on the three existing forms of cancer in the body, namely treatment for primary lesions; the second goal of treatment for tumor foci; the third goal of treatment for the cancer cell group on the metastasis route.

(I) To aim on the cancer cell group on the metastasis routing is the key to anti-cancer metastasis

Presented at the human n the third manifestation is being transferred during the multi-step, multi-factor fine the way cancer cells, cancer cells and micro-thrombus metastasis group because this issue has not yet been recognized and did not cause enough attention, but did not specifically discuss how their diagnosis, treatment methods and countermeasures. In fact, the key to anti-cancer metastasis was to surround and annihilate the cancer cells, blocking or interference and, cutting off the transfer of new treatment modalities way.

(2)To aim on cancer cells on the metastasis routing will cause change and renewal of cancer diagnosis and treatment.

The new doctrine or a new theoretical understanding, upon demonstration confirmed, may cause a chain reaction like tumor treatment changes and updates, such as changes in cancer treatment in understanding the concept and updated target for cancer therapy or "target" change and renewal of understanding, to change and update on cancer diagnosis method of looking for anti-cancer, anti-metastasis caused major changes and updates on the research and development of new drugs for cancer treatment modalities and major changes in treatment methods and updates as well as cancer metastasis, recurrence study, pathological cells from the cell level to change and update oncology molecular biology, gene expression at the molecular level oncology.

(3) To aim on cancer cells on the metastasis routing will bring new hope for the fight against cancer

① conventional cancer therapeutics think there are two forms: The first manifestation is the primary cancer,; the second is the manifestation of tumor foci. This traditional therapeutic concept, followed the more than 100 years, the treatment goal or "target" is for the two forms - the primary tumor or metastatic foci. Isolated treat these two "target" on the dynamic relationship between the two, a causal relationship, affiliation is not taking into account. As primary foci is how to form a tumor foci, and how to stop its transfer. Therefore, the traditional concept of cancer therapeutics is incomplete, imperfect, flawed, because it ignores the way cancer metastasis, and cancer metastasis is the most important biological characteristics and biological behavior. There is no way for the transfer of cancer cells is blocking, you can not control the transfer of cancer cells, it is difficult to obtain cancer treatment all the more possible.

② The author provides new concept of cancer which there are three forms: The first manifestation is the primary foci; the second is the manifestation of tumor foci; third manifestation is being transferred on the way cancer cells, cancer cells Group and micro thrombus metastasis. This new concept is more complete and more comprehensive, it illustrates the dynamic relationship between the three, garden fruit relationships and dependencies is a complete new concept of cancer therapeutics, fully explain the whole process of cancer development and how control the whole process of transfer of cancer metastasis, this new doctrine proposed to combat cancer brought new hope.

(4) According to the cancer metastasis pathway to design the new anti-metastatic therapy mode and to annihilate interdiction

In summary, cancer treatment includes not only surgery for resection of the primary tumor and the implementation of the first two forms, surgery or radiotherapy or chemotherapy for the treatment of metastatic immunity stoves, should also include a third form of treatment for the goal or target, that is shifting the way for red cell carcinoma group, conducted surround and annihilate interdiction, enhance host immune surveillance, interference prevents cancer metastasis. By transfer pathways of cancer cells, multi-step transfer of line, multi-factor, multi-link molecular transfer mechanisms, design of new anti-metastatic treatment modalities, for cancer intervention and interdiction of new treatments.

Metastasis cancer group or micrometastases on the routing, although no clinical manifestations, but it does exist, only to enter the molecular biological level, the gene level, molecular level of immunity in order to find and recognize, over expression of various tumor markers such as now it already could be undertaken the molecular immunology and genetically modified micro-metastasis detection. Individual cancer cells (ITC) existing in the blood and bone marrow can be detected at the molecular level; the new detection of new molecular targets, indicators of immune molecules, cytokines, tumor markers will continue to emerge; we believe that in the near future we will reach the early diagnosis of pre- cancer and micrometastases.

(8.) HOW TO STOP CANCER CELLS METASTASIS? CANCER METASTASIS TREATMENT TRILOGY

- To understand cancer cell metastasis steps so that the treatment goal will be more specific;
- More specifically, trying to break each step;
- Three measures of anti-cancer metastasis treatment ("trilogy")

1. To understand cancer cell metastasis steps so that the treatment goal will be more specific

As to how to make clearer the extremely complicated dynamic and continuous biological process of carcinoma metastasis with multi-step and multi-element, through repeated thinking and carefully analysis, we summed up and put forward Eight Steps of Metastasis of Cancer Cells in the aforesaid. Based on Eight Steps, we tried to make clearer and more particular of the concept of extremely complicated dynamic and continuous biological process of carcinoma metastasis with multi-step and multi-element with respect to understanding. In order to take scientific measures to obstruct and intercept each metastasis step and destroy it one by one, it is necessary to make clear the concept of each step in the metastasis process. Only when the target of each step is made clear, can the prevention and cure countermeasures be carried out, researched and probed into.

In the above, we have mentioned "Three Stages" of carcinoma metastasis and illuminated it in details. The reason why "Three Stage" is put forward is that one of the keys to therapy of cancer is to anti metastasis, however, at present, the understanding of the concept of metastasis is still ambiguous and it is not clear and particular. People only understand the severity of the harm of the metastasis to the patients, however, it lacks of effective prevention and therapeutic countermeasures with clear concept and detailed profile. In order to take scientific measures to obstruct and intercept each metastasis step, based on the Eight Steps, Three Stages and the molecular mechanism of carcinoma metastasis, we try to establish the preventive and therapeutic countermeasures for each stage and called it Xu Ze Three Steps of Therapy of Carcinoma Metastasis.

2. More specifically, trying to break each step and Trying to Get a Good Idea about the Object

The basic process of carcinoma metastasis is: the cancer cell falling from the primary tumor---degrading the basement membrance---migrating into blood capillary and small vein---survived cancer cell adhering to endothelial cell of blood capillary or basement membrance under the exposed endothelium---passing through wall---growing up in the remote target organ and forming the metastatic carcinoma, which is an extremely complicated, dynamic and continuous biological process, composed of several relatively independent but interlocked steps. In each step, a series of molecular biological events will happen between cancer cells, and between the cancer cells and the host cells, finishing the whole metastatic process and finally forming the metastatic carcinoma.

That is to say, it is necessary for the cancer cells to be subject to and finish the whole metastatic process before forming the metastatic carcinoma. any failure of each step will result in the stop of the whole metastatic process, which presents that if we take measures to destroy the metastatic steps one by one and carry out the strategy and tactics of obstruction and interception of the cancer cells in the routing of the metastasis, it is certainly possible to break or intercept the metastatic routing and intercept and kill the cancer cells in the routing of metastasis.

Xu Ze New Concept and Mode of Therapy of Carcinoma and Carcinoma Metastasis are to try to intercept one or several steps or links of the above-mentioned metastatic process so as to control the metastasis.

In order to realize the above-mentioned objectives, what measures shall be taken by us for anti metastasis? With which theory? Which technology and which drug? In which step or in which stage and link to intercept the cancer cells in the routing of the metastasis?

3. Three measures of anti-cancer metastasis treatment ("trilogy")

1. First step of anti carcinomatous metastasis:

①In this stage, the metastatic process of cancer cells is as follows: cancer cells falling from the primary carcinoma---adhering to the stroma outside the cells---degrading ECM to open up a road for cancer cells---carrying out cell movement via the adherence of degraded stroma or the degraded stroma for adherence---then arriving at the external wall---degrading basement membrane of blood vessel---doing Amoeba movement, firstly stretching out the pseudopodium---then passing through the wall.

② **The countermeasures of prevention and cure:**

This stage is the intervention and repression countermeasure before the cancer cell falls from the primary carcinoma and enters the blood vessel. In this stage, the therapeutic

"targets" are mainly anti-adherence, anti-degradation, anti-movement and anti cancer cell attack.

③The therapeutic goal is to prevent the cancer cells from entering the blood vessel so as to realize the goal of "turning the enemy back at the border".

2. Second step of anti carcinomatous metastasis:

①In this stage, the metastasis process of cancer cell: it will pass through the wall and enter the blood circulation. The cancer cell will be interweaved in various blood cell components including blood plasma and blood or will be adhered to cancer cell group together with homo-cancer cell, or will be adhered to slight cancer embolus together with the alloplasm such as blood platelet and white blood cell and float in venous system→turn back to the right ventricle→circulate→enter pulmonary vein→turn back to left ventricle together with the venous blood, some cancer cells can stay in the pulmonary microcirculation blood vessel (forming the pulmonary metastasis lesion), some will enter the pulmonary vein→turn back to the left ventricle via the pulmonary microcirculation. The cancer cell, interweaved in the blood, enters the aorta and then jets into the small artery of the parenchymatous viscera and then enters the microcirculation of each organ (especially the parenchymatous organ, such as liver, kidney, brain and porotic substance of bone through the impact force and vertex flow and pump flow of the heart valve blood. Most of the cancer cells in the circulation will be damaged and killed by the immunological cells in the circulation or the strong blood impact force and shearing force, **the tiny minority of the survived cancer cells form the micro-cancer embolus, adhering to the endothelial cell of the micrangium, degrading the basement membrane and passing through the blood vessel.**

In this stage, the cancer cell will contact various immunological cells in floating in the blood circulation and cannot survive possibly due to being captured and phagocytized by various immunological cells in the blood. Few survived cancer cells will be adhered to the endothelial cell of the blood vessel due to escaping from the monitoring of the immunity in the blood circulation.

②Prevention and cure countermeasures: in this stage, the "target" of therapy of carcinoma metastasis is to protect and enhance the immunologic function of various immunological cells in the blood circulation, activate the immunological cytokine and resist adherence (homogenous adherence of cancer cells and cancer cells, alloplasmatic adherence of cancer cells with blood platelet and so on), resist movement, resist aggregation of blood platelet, resist high coagulation and resist cancer embolus.

③Therapeutic goal: activating the immunological cell, protecting function of thymus organization, improving immunity, protecting the bone marrow and producing the blood and promoting the cancer cells floating in the blood circulation to be captured, phagocytized, surrounded and annihilated and intercepted by the immunological cell group.

The second step is the main battlefield to kill off the cancer cells floating in the blood circulation as well as the main countermeasures to interfere and repress the carcinoma metastasis.

3. Third Step of anti carcinomatous metastasis:

①the metastasis process of the cancer cell in this stage: the cancer cell escapes the monitoring of the immunological cell in blood circulation and the annihilation of the immunological cell, passes through the wall and anchors itself in the organs with agreeable local microenvironment for settlement, in this way, the new blood capillary of tumor forms and then it gradually forms the metastatic carcinoma.

②**Prevention and cure countermeasures: the interference and repression countermeasures, mainly aiming at improving the histogenic immunity of the local microenvironment and regulating the local microenvironment to make it adverse to the survival and nidation and repress the angiogenesis factor and the new angiogenesis.**

To sum up, space allocation of Xu Ze Three Steps of Therapy of Carcinoma Metastasis is in the blood circulation and the time allocation is in three different stages. It attaches importance to improvement of the host immunity. It can be summed up and concluded as Table and the figure as the following:

Table Xu Ze Three Steps of Therapy of Carcinoma Metastasis

Metastasis stage of cancer cell	Metastasis process	Prevention and cure countermeasures
The stage before the cancer cell intrudes the circulation First step of anti metastasis	Separating the cancer cell from the primary cancer→degrading ECM→adherence and de-adherence→movement→before entering the blood vessel.	● anti-adherence ● anti-degradation ● anti-movement ● anti stroma metal protease
Transportation stage of cancer cell in blood circulation Second step of anti-metastasis	The cancer cell group and micro cancer embolus float in the blood circulation and are damaged due to being phagocytized and captured by the immunological cell and be subject to the shearing force of the blood.	● enhancing and activating various immunological cells in circulation, improving the immunologic function as the main battlefield of killing off the cancer cells in the routing of the metastasis

The stage in which Cancer cell escapes the blood circulation and anchors "target" organ Third step of anti metastasis

After cancer cell escapes from the blood vessel, it anchors the organ for nidation, forms the new blood vessel and forms the metastatic lesion.

- anti-adherence
- anti-aggregation of blood platelet
- anti cancer embolus
- TG
- Inhibiting angiogenesis factor
- Inhibiting angiogenesis
- Improving immunological regulation
- Improving the immunity of local microenvironment.

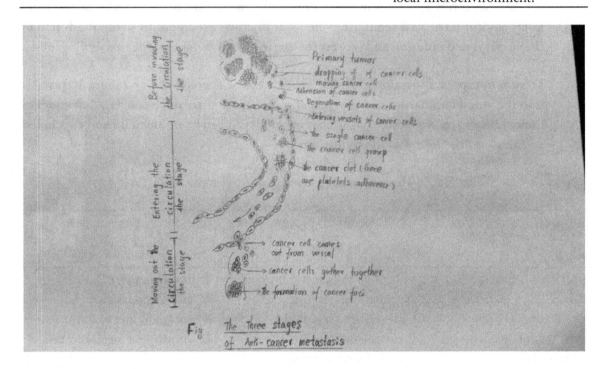

Figure The three stages of anti-cancer metastasis

(9.) CANCER TREATMENT METHODS AND DRUGS

Outline

XZ-C immunomodulatory anticancer medicine are from traditional Chinese herbal medicines which are selected 48 kinds of anti-tumor Chinese herbal medicine with better inhibitory rate. After made up into the composition of the compound, and then tested by inhibiting cancer-bearing mice tumor experiments in cancer-bearing mice experiments, the compound inhibitory rate inhibition rate is much greater than single herbs. XZ-C1, XZ-C4 God grass, agrimony, Shu Yang Quan etc 28 Chinese herbal medicines, of which XZ-C1-A, XZ-C1-B 100% inhibit cancer, 100 percent don't kill normal cells, with righting improvment of the role of the body's immune function. From our experiments XZ-C pharmacodynamics, study results show: they has a good inhibitory rate on Ehrlich ascites carcinoma, S182, H22 hepatocellular carcinoma; there are obvious synergy and toxicity attenuation; experiments also demonstrated that the immune XZ-C the regulation of traditional Chinese medicine have significantly improved immune function.

After the acute toxicity test in mice, no obvious toxicity, no significant side effects for long-term oral clinical taking (2--6 years). XZ-C can significantly reduce the toxicity while oral immune regulation medicine during chemotherapy. Intermittent oral XZ-C drugs make leukocytosis, hemoglobin increased while Chemotherapy. Advanced cancer patients, mostly weakness, fatigue, loss of appetite, after taking XZ-C immunomodulatory anticancer medicine 4-8-12 weeks, more significantly improved appetite, sleep, relieve pain, gradually recuperate.

The experiments have been carried out in the research and clinical validation work.

The Experimental studies

Our laboratory conducted the following new cancer screening experiment study from traditional Chinese medicine, anti-metastatic drugs:

I. In vitro screening test: the use of cancer cells in vitro was observed for cancer drugs directly damage cancer cells. Cultured cancer cells in a test tube, were placed raw meal drug products (500ug / ml) to observe whether there is inhibition and inhibition rate of cancer cells.

2. In vivo antitumor screening test: manufacture cancer-bearing animal model for the screening of Chinese herbs for cancer-bearing animal experiments suppressor rate, batch experiments with 240 mice were divided into eight experimental groups, each group 30, para. 7 group was the control group, Group 8 with 5-Fu or CTX as the control group. The whole group of mice were inoculated with EAC or S180 or H22 cancer cells inoculated 24h, the crude product by oral feeding crude drug powder, long-term feeding the herbs screened each mouse was observed survival inhibition rate was calculated.

Our experimental study for four consecutive years, with more than 1000 per year tumor-bearing animal models, four years made a total of two tumor-bearing animal models, mice each were carried out after the death of the liver, spleen, lung, thymus, 'kidney pathological anatomy, in the 20000 times slices.

3. **Results**: In our laboratory animal experiments after screening 200 kinds of Chinese herbal medicine, the selected 48 kinds indeed carry, even excellent inhibition of cancer cells, the inhibition rate of more than 75-90%. The group of animal experiments made screening test 152 had no significant anti-cancer effect.

The Clinical Vertification:

On the basis of successful experiments on animals to clinical validation

1). Methods: built oncology clinics and combination Research Group of anti-cancer, anti-metastasis and anti-recurrence, keeping the medical records, built perfect follow-up and observation system to observe the long-term efficacy and clinical validation. From experimental study to clinical verification means the clinical application on the basis of successful experimental study. Then new problems are found during the clinical application, which need fundamental experimental studies. Afterwards new experimental results are applied to clinical verification. Experiments → clinic → experiments once more → clinic once more, recurrent ascent continuously; through eight-year clinical practical experiences, knowledge also continues to improve. Summation, analysis, reflection and evaluation ascend to theory, putting forward new knowledge, new concept, new thought, new strategy and new therapeutic route and scheme.

Clinical criteria are: good quality of life, longer survival.
Results: XZ-C immunomodulatory anticancer Chinese medicines have significant treatment effect after applying through a lot in advanced cancer patients treated with observation,

2). **Clinical information**

(1) Hubei Branch of China Anti-cancer Research Cooperation of Chinese Traditional Medicine and Western Medicine, Anti Carcinoma Metastasis and Recurrence Research Office and Shuguang Tumor Specialized Outpatient Department had treated 4, 698 carcinoma patients in Stage III and IV or in metastasis and recurrence with Z-C medicine combined with western medicine from 1994 to Nov. 2002, among which there were 3, 051

men patients and 1,647 women patients. The youngest one was 11 years old and the oldest one was 86 years old, the high invasion age was 40~69 years. All groups of the patients were entirely subject to the diagnosis of pathological histology or definitive diagnosis with ultrasonic B, CT and MRI iconography. According to the staging standard of UICC, all the cases were entirely the patients in medium and advanced stage over Stage III. In this group, there were 1,021 hepatic carcinoma patients, among which there were 694 primary lesion hepatic carcinoma patients and 327 metastatic hepatic carcinoma patients; there were 752 patients suffering from carcinoma of lung, among which there were 699 patients suffering from the primary carcinoma of lung and 53 patients suffering from the metastatic carcinoma of lung; there were 668 gastric carcinoma patients, 624 patients suffering from esophagus cardia carcinoma, 328 patients suffering from rectum carcinoma of anal canal, 442 patients suffering from carcinoma of colon, 368 patients suffering from breast carcinoma, 74 patients suffering from adenocarcinoma of pancreas, 30 patients suffering from carcinoma of bile duct, 43 patients suffering from retroperitoneal tumor, 38 patients suffering from oophoroma, 9 patients suffering from cervical carcinoma, 11 patients suffering from cerebroma, 34 patients suffering from thyroid carcinoma, 38 patients suffering from nasopharyngeal carcinoma, 9 patients suffering from melanoma, 27 patients suffering from kidney carcinoma, 48 patients suffering from carcinoma of urinary bladder, 13 patients suffering from leukemia, 47 patients suffering from metastasis of supraclavicular lymph nodes, 35 patients suffering various fleshy tumors and 39 patients suffering from other malignancies.

3). **Medicine and medication**: the treatment aims to protect thymus and increase immune system, protect bone marrow so that improve the immune surveillance and to control cancer cells escape. From traditional Chinese medicine the treatment aims are to support healthy energy to eliminate evils, soften and resolve the hard mass and supplement qi and blood. XZ-C_1, XZ-C_2, XZ-C_3, XZ-C_4, XZ-C, XZ-C_6, XZ-C_7, XZ-C_8, ...XZ-C_{10}, according to different kinds of cancers, disease conditions, metastasis situations and according to disease syndrome, choose the above medications. According to the analysis and differentiation of the diseases, anti-cancer powder shall be taken orally and the anti-cancer apocatastasis paste shall be applied externally for the solid tumor or the metastatic tumor. In case of being in pain, anti-cancer aponic paste shall be applied externally. Icterus removal soup or dropsy removal soup shall be taken orally for the patients suffering from icterrus and the ascites.

4. **Curative results : The symptom was improved, the quality of life was improved, the survival time was prolonged**

(1) Among the 4,277 carcinoma patients in medium and advanced stage who took Z-C medicine with the return visit over 3 months, the case history had the specific observation record of the curative effect, see the following table:

The observation of curative effect on 4 277 patients: fully improving the quality of life of the carcinoma patients in medium and advanced stage

Improvement	Vigor	Appetite	Reinforcement of physical force	Improvement in generalized case	Increase of body weight	Improvement of sleep	The restriction of improvement activity and capability released activity	self servicing normal walking	Resumption of work Engaged in light work
No. of cases (%)	4071	3986	2450	479	2938	1005	1038	3220	479
	95.2	93.2	57.3	11.2	68.7	23.5	24.3	75.3	11.2

In this group, all of them were the patients in medium and advanced stage. After taking the medicine, their symptoms were improved to different extents with the effective rate of 93.2%. With respect to the improvement of the quality of life (as per Karnofsky Performance Status), it rose to 80 scores on average after administration from 50 on average before administration; the patients in this group met with the different metastasis and dysfunction of the organs about Stage III. It was reported by the previous statistic information that the mesoposition survival time of this kind of patients was about 6 months. The longest time among this group of the cases reached up to 11 years; another patient suffering from hepatic carcinoma had taken Z-C medicine for ten years and a half; two patients suffering from hepatic carcinoma met with frequency encountered carcinomatous lesion in the left and right liver and it entirely subsided through secondary CT reexamination after the patient took Z-C medicine for half a year and the state of the disease had been stable over half a year. One patient suffering from double-kidney carcinoma met with the widespread metastasis of abdominal cavity after removal of one kidney, after taking Z-C medicine, he was entirely recovered and began to work again. 3 patients suffering from carcinoma of lung, with the lung not removed through explaraton, had taken Z-C medicine over three years and a half. 2 patients suffering from gastric remnant carcinoma had taken Z-C medicine for 8 years. 3 patients suffering from reoccurrence of rectal carcinoma had taken Z-C medicine for 3 years. 1 patient suffering from metastatic liver and rib of the mastocarcinoma had taken Z-C medicine for 8 years. 1 patient suffering from the recurrent bladder carcinoma after operation of renal carcinoma had not met with the carcinoma for 9 years and a half after taking Z-C medicine. All of these patients were the ones in the medium and advanced stage that could not be operated once more or treated with radiotherapy or chemotherapy. They only took Z-C medicine without other medicines for treatment. Up to today, they are reexamined and get the medicine at the out-patient department every month. Through taking the medicine for a long time, the state of the disease is controlled in the stable state to make the organism and the tumor in balanced state for a relatively long time and get a relatively good survival with tumor, in this way, the symptoms of the patients are improved, the quality of life is improved and the survival time is prolonged.

(2) As to 84 patients suffering from solid tumor and 56 patients suffering from enlargement of upper lymph node of metastatic compact bone, after taking Z-C series medicines orally and applying Z-C3 anti-cancer apocatastasis paste, they met with good curative effects, see the following table :

The Changes of 84 patients suffering from solid tumor and 56 patients suffering from metastatic mode after applying Z-C paste externally

	Solid tumor				Enlargement of upper lymph node of metastatic compact bone			
	Disappearance	Shrinkage 1/2	Softening	No change	Disappearance	Shrinkage 1/2	Softening	No change
No. of cases (%)	12	28	32	12	12	22	14	8
	14.2	33.3	38.0	14.2	21.4	39.2	25.0	14.2
Total effective rate (%)	85.7				85.7			

298 patients suffering from carcinoma pain obtained the obvious pain alleviation effects after taking Z-C medicine orally and applying Z-C anti-cancer apocatastasis paste externally, see the following table:

	Pain			
Clinical menifetation	Light alleviation	Obvious alleviation	Disappearance	Avoidance
No of cases	52	139	93	14
(%)	17.3	46.8	31.2	4.7
Total effective rate (%)		95.3		

5. Exclusive research and development of products: XZ-C immunomodulatory anticancer medicine products (Profile)

Independently developed XZ-C (XU ZE China) series of anti-cancer immune regulation medicine preparation, from experimental research to clinical validation, in animal experiments on the basis of success in clinical practice, clinical experience over the years a large number of clinical cases verification, a significant effect. The results are self-invention, the Department of independent innovation and intellectual property rights.

Looking from traditional Chinese medicine, and screening anti-cancer, anti-metastatic investigational new drug:

The purpose is to screen out non-resistance, non-toxic side effects, a high selectivity, long-term oral anti-cancer, anti-metastatic and anti-recurrent cancer drug. It is well known now for the world's anti-cancer agent does inhibit proliferation of cancer cells, but it only kill cancer cells but also kill normal cells, especially the bone marrow of immune cells, a host of serious damage, because of chemotherapy cytotoxic and non-selectivity. And traditional chemotherapy can suppress the immune function and inhibit bone marrow function. Traditional intravenous chemotherapy treatment is interrupted, the cancer cells cannot be treated during the gap period which cancer cells continued proliferation and division. Although chemotherapy drugs can inhibit the proliferation of cancer cells, but because of its toxic side effects when cancer has not yet been eliminated, administration had to stop. After treatment, cancer cell proliferation up again, and began to have resistance. When resistance, this dose would not work so as to increase the amount executioner. However, if the dose is increased, it may endanger the lives of patients. If the chemotherapy drug resistance has been given, then the cancer is not only ineffective; Contrary to killing only patient's normal cells so cancer cells resistance to cancer drugs and toxics of cancer drugs on the host side effects is a long vexing problem. And we are looking for new drugs, the purpose is to avoid these drawbacks.

According to the theory of cell cycle, anticancer agents must be able to continue long applications so that cancer foci can bath in anti-cancer agents long lasting time, and is available without stopping to prevent their cell division and to prevent recurrence and metastasis. It must be long years, have been conducting long-term, it is best to long-term oral drugs to control existing foci and prevent nascent cancer cells to form. Due to large toxicity the currently used anticancer medication cannot long continuous use, but only short cycle applications. Existing anticancer medication has suppressed immune function, bone marrow suppression, suppression thymus, bone marrow suppression side effects. The formation and development of cancer is due to the patient's immune system to reduce lost immune surveillance, therefore, all anticancer medications should be increased immunization, protection immune organs, immune suppression and should not use drugs.

To this end, we conducted the following experiment laboratory screening of new anti-cancer research from the traditional Chinese medicine, anti-metastatic drugs:

(A) The method of cancer cells in vitro, the experimental study of Chinese herbal medicine suppressor screening rates:

In vitro screening tests: The cancer cells in vitro was observed that the drugs directly damage cells.

The screening test in culture tube: in the cancer cell culture tube respectively allowing raw and crude drugs of crude product (500ug / ml) to be used and to observe whether there is inhibition of cancer cells, we believe that 200 kinds of traditional Chinese medicine herbs have anticancer function performed one by one in vitro screening tests. And under the same conditions with a normal fiber cell culture to test the toxicity of these cells, and then compared.

(B) Building cancer-bearing animal model for the screening of Chinese herbs for cancer-bearing animal experimental tumor suppressor rate

The inhibition test in vivo screeing test: each batch experiments with mice 240, divided into 8 groups, each group 30, the first group was the control group 7, group 8 with 5-Fu or CTX control group, the whole group of small mice was inoculated with EA C or S 180 or H22 cancer cells. After inoculation 24h, each rat oral feeding crude product of crude drug powder, long-term feeding the screened the herbs, observed survival, toxicity, computing prolong survival rate calculated suppression sores.

So, we conducted experimental study for four consecutive years, and has conducted a 3-year incidence of tumor-bearing mice and transfer mechanism, the experimental study of the mechanism of relapse, and experimental studies to explore how cancer causing death of the host each year with more than 1,000 tumor-bearing animals model, made a total of nearly four years, 6000 tumor-bearing animal models, mice each were carried out after the death of the liver, spleen, lung, thymus, kidney pathological anatomy, a total of 20,000 times slice to explore to find out whether There may be slight carcinogenic pathogens, with microcirculation microscope 100 tumor-bearing mice were tumor microvessels bell establish and microcirculation.

Through experimental study we first found in China a medicine to inhibit tumor angiogenesis TG had a significant effect, more than 80 cases have been used in clinical treatment of patients Hang metastasis being observed.

Results: In our laboratory animal experiments screened 200 kinds of Chinese herbs and screened48 kinds of certain and excellent herbs with inhibition of cancer cell proliferation, inhibition rate of more than 75 to 90%. But there are some of commonly used Chinese medicine which consider to have the anticancer roles, after animal in vitro and in vivo inhibition rate anti-cancer screening, showed really no effect, or little effect which 152 kinds of medications having no anti-cancer effect had removed from the phase-out of animal experiments.

Screening out of this real 48 kinds of traditional Chinese medications with having good tumor suppression rates, and then optimized the combination and repeated tumor suppression rate experiments in vivo, and finally developed immunomodulatory anticancer Chinese medication XU ZE China1-10 with Chinese own characteristics China (ZC_{1-10}).

$Z-C_1$ could inhibit cancer cells, but does not affect normal cells; $Z-C_4$ specially can increase thymus function, can promote proliferation, increased immunity; $Z-C_1$ can protect bone marrow function and to product more blood.

The Clinical validation: Based on the success of animal experiments, clinical validation was conducted. Namely the establishment of oncology clinics and Western medicine combined with anti-cancer, anti-metastasis, recurrence Research Group, **retained patient medical records, to establish a regular follow-up observation system to observe the long-term effect**. From the experimental research to the clinical evidence and to find the new questions during the clinical validation process and then went back to the laboratory for basical research, then applied the new experimental results for the clinical validation. Thus, the experiment to the clinical and to the experiment again and to the clinical again; **all experimental studies must be clinically proven in a large number of patients observed 3--5 years, or even clinical observation of 8 to 20 years**, according to evidence-based medicine it has the long-term follow-up assessment information, **It was verified indeed that there is a good long-term efficacy and the efficacy of the standard is: a good quality of life, longer survival**. XZ-C immune regulation anti-cancer medications have the verification after a lot of applications in advanced cancer patients and have achieved remarkable results. **XZ-C immune regulation anti-cancer medication can improve the quality of life of patients with advanced cancer, enhance**

immune function, increase the body's anticancer abilities, increased appetite and significantly prolong survival. The brief introduction is the following:

(C) XZ-C immunomodulatory anticancer Chinese medication Mechanism of Action

With the deepening of traditional Chinese medicine research, it is known to produce a lot of traditional Chinese medicine and biological activity of cytokines and other immune molecules having a regulatory role, this time to clarify XZ-C from the molecular level immunomodulatory anticancer Chinese medication immunological mechanisms very important.

1. XZ-C immunomodulatory anticancer Chinese medication can protect immune organs, increasing the weight of the spleen and chest pay attention.

2. XZ-C immunomodulatory anticancer Chinese medication for hematopoietic function of bone marrow cell proliferation and significant role in promoting.

3. XZ-C immunomodulatory anticancer Chinese medication on T cell immune function enhancement effect on T cells significantly promote proliferation.

4. XZ-C immunomodulatory anticancer Chinese medication for human IL-2 production has significantly enhanced role.

5. XZ-C immunomodulatory anticancer Chinese medication activation of NK cell activity and enhance the role, NK cells with a broad spectrum of anticancer effect, can anti-xenograft tumor cells.

6. XZ-C immunomodulatory anticancer Chinese medication for LAK cell activity can enhance the effect, LAK cells are capable of killing of NK cell sensitive and non-sensitive solid tumor cells, with broad-spectrum anti-tumor effect.

7. XZ-C immunomodulatory anticancer Chinese medication to induce interferon and pro-inducing effect, IFN has a broad-spectrum anti-tumor effect Wo immunomodulatory effects, IFN can inhibit tumor cell proliferation, IFN can activate the skin to kill cancer cells and OIL cells.

8. XZ-C immunomodulatory anticancer Chinese medication for colony stimulating factor can promote credit enhancement, CSF not only involved in hematopoietic cell proliferation, differentiation, and in a host of anti-tumor immunity plays an important role

9. XZ-C immunomodulatory anticancer Chinese medication can promote tumor necrosis factor (TNF) role, TNF is a class can directly cause tumor cell death factor, its main biological role is to kill or inhibit tumor cells.

D. Bilogical response modification(BRM), traditional chinese anticancer medicine similar to BRM and tumor treatment

1. Biological reaction modification (BRM) explores the new field of the tumor biological therapy. Currently BRM as the fourth methods of the tumor treatment gets widely attention in the world.

Oldham in 1982 built BRM theory. Based this in 1984 he advanced the fourth modality of cancer treatment-----biological therapy again. According to this, in the normal condition, there is the dynamic equilibrium between the tumor and the body. The development of the tumors, and even invasion and metastasis, completely is caused by the loss of this equilibrium. If this unbland situation is adjusted to the normal level, the tumor growth can be controlled and will disappear.

The anticancer mechanism of BRM in details as the following:

1.) mprove the host defence abilities or decrease the immune inhabitation of the tumors to the host to reach the immune response to the tumors.

2.) Look for the biological active things in natural or gene combination to enhance the host defense abilities.

3.) Reduce the host response induced by the tumor cells

4.) Promote the tumors to division and mature to become the normal cells

5.) Reduce the side effects of the chemotherapy and redio therapy and enhance The host toleration.

2. XZ-C immune regulation anticancer medicine have the functions and curative effects similar to BRM

After four years experimental research and 30 years clinical research which are the drugs similar to BRM selected from traditional Chinese medications.

XZ-C is the drugs that XU ZE in China professor selected from two hundreds of the anticancer herbs after the experiments. At first the culturing tumor was done in vitro ; 200 kinds of chinese herbs were tested one by one to observe the direct damage to tumor cells in the culture setting; the control groups for the inhibition rate test were the chemotherapy CTX and the normal cultured cells. Eventually, the a series of the medications with the anti-cancer proliferation were selected, then it was made the animal mode in which 200 drugs were used one by one to analyze and evaluate the inhibition rate of anticancer steps by steps, scientific, practical and strict, etc. The results proved that 48 of them have the excellent tumor inhibition effects, however the rest 152 of anticancer medication which are all common old anticancer medication were proved that there were no anticancer or less inhibition of the tumors in the animal models during these medication selection experiments.

XZ-C medications with excellent anticancer functions and selected on the tumor animal models can improve immune function, protect central immune organ functions such as thymus and bone marrow, and improve the cell-mediated immune functions, increase the red blood cells and white blood cells number, activate the immune factors, improve the immune surviellence in the blood etc.

The main pharmacology functions of XZ-C anticancer immune regulation medication are to increase immune functions. XZ-C anticancer immune regulation medications have the following functions as :

1.) Activate the host immune system to promote the host immune function and to reach the immune respond to the tumors.

2.) Activate the host immune factors of the anticancer systems and to strengthen the host immune function and to improve immunce surviellence of the host immune systems.

3.) Protect thymus and bone marrow, improve the immune function, and stimulate the bone marrow function and to reduce the inhibition of the bone marrow and to increase the white blood cell and red blood cells etc.

4.) Reduce the side effects of the chemotherapy and radioactive therapy and to increase the tolerance of the hosts.

5.) Increase thymus weight and stop atrophy of thymus because thymus goes on atrophy when the tumor grows.

As the above statement, the basic mechanism of XZ-C is similar to BRM and the clinical application is similar to those of the BRM.

(A) XZ-C1 "Smart grams cancer"

The main components are eight Chinese herbs.

Anticancer pharmacology

1. Detoxification, increasing blood circulation, righting, dispelling evil without injury, strong inhibition of cancer cells and inhibition of cancer cell metastasis without inhibition of normal cells.

2. In anti-cancer in vivo tests in mice, they have inhibitory activity in the mice Ehrlich ascites tumor cells which there had been significant differences in the control group.

3. Can prolong survival of mice bearing cancer, increased the survival rate of 26.92%.

4. The main prescription drugs Z-C1-A and Z-C1-B has a stable and significant anticancer effects, 100% inhibition of cancer cells, cancer cell mitotic reduced and degenerated and necrosed seriously and epithelial cells or fibroblasts is no impact in the administration group. XZ-C1-D extract have inhibitory activity on human cervical cancer cells, on mouse sarcoma s180 inhibition rate was 98.9%, several other ingredients also have a strong anticancer effect.

5. Z-C1 Herbs inhibition effect on Mice bearing H22 hepatoma tumor: z-c1 drug inhibition rate was 40 percent in the second week, the first four weeks was 45%, the first six weeks of 58%; in the control group CTX medication first two weeks inhibition rate was 45%, the first four weeks inhibition rate was 45%, 49% for the first six weeks.

6. Z-C1 medicine influence on survival in mice bearing H22: life-prolonging rate was 85% in z-c1 group; life extension was 9.8% in CTX control group ; in Z-C1 group Thymus did not shrink; however thymus shrank in Control group.

Clinical application

1. Indications: esophageal cancer, stomach cancer, colorectal cancer, lung cancer, breast cancer, liver pain, bile duct cancer, pancreatic cancer, thyroid cancer, nasopharyngeal cancer, brain tumors, renal cancer, bladder cancer, ovarian cancer, cervical cancer, various sarcoma and a variety of metastasis, recurrent cancer.

2. Usage: after taking z- c1 continuously 1 - 3 months, the patients felt better. This medication can be taken for long-term and can be taken one dose every other day after three years; can be taken two doses weekly after 5 years to retain immune function and cytokine long-term stable at a certain level.

Toxicity Test

ZX-C1 can be used for long-term. The acute toxicity test showed that when adult mice was fed a dose 104 times (10g / Kg body weight), respectively, in 24, 48, 72, 96 hours of observation, 30 purebred mice didn't die. The median lethal dose (LD5O) didn't have any number so that it is a rather safe prescriptions.

In the oncology clinic it has been used for many years and some patients have taken more than three to five years and more than 8 to 10 years in order to maintain immunity and to stop recurrence. It can be taken for long-term and it is quite safe oral cancer.

(B) XZ-C2

Ingredients: 9 kinds of anticancer herbs

Anticancer pharmacology

1. Animal experiments show that it can prolong L7212 mouse (mouse leukemia) survival, well-behaved compared to the control group, there were statistically significant.
2. Can improve inhibition rate in the L7212 in mice
3. Z-C1-A and Z-C2-B on mouse sarcoma (s180) has a strong inhibitory effect.

Application

Indications: leukemia, upper gastrointestinal cancer, tongue, larynx, nasopharynx cancer, cervical cancer, bone metastasis, esophagus cancer or gastric ulcer anastomotic recurrence narrow (no longer surgery). It has general effect on Acute leukemia lymph and has obvious efficiency of each of the other type of leukemia. It has a more significant effect on Bone metastasis

Usage: one capsule Qid generally or two capsules tid
Leukemia 3 capsules tid after meal and seven days for a course.

(C) XZ-C3 topical pain Patch

Prescription Content: kaempferol, turmeric, etc. 14 flavors
Anticancer pharmacology

1. Detoxification, anti-inflammatory pain, qi Sanjie pain;
2. Increasing the blood circulation, reducing swelling and pain, played a total of detoxification, swelling and analgesic effect, while the most prominent role in cancer treatment is to stop pain.
3. For point application, applicator than simply pain, can better play the efficacy and achieve rapid pain relief purposes.

Clinical application

Indications: liver cancer, lung cancer pain, back pain from pancreatic cancer, bone pain, neck and supraclavicular lymph nodes metastasis.

Usage: A total of research and go take honey, mix, stir into a paste backup, lung disease spreads in milk root point (nipple straight down 5, 6 ribs), liver cancer spreads on the door hole (milk midline 6-7 rib room), treated and covered with gauze and tape securely, severe pain 6h for a second, lesser pain, 12h replacement of 1: continuous use to relieve pain or disappeared.

Experience: Treatment of 84 cases of liver cancer, lung cancer pain patients, have analgesic effect, general medicine three times, will receive different levels of pain relief, 3 to 7 days after a significant analgesic effect, some basical pain.

(D) ZX-C4 anticancer medication of protecting thymus and increasing immune function (5g / bag)

Ingredients: including 12 valuable herbs
Anticancer pharmacology

1. To promote lymphocyte transformation, enhancing immune function, increased white blood cells, inhibit cancer cell, Warming blood.

2. Ehrlich ascites tumor cells transplanted into the abdominal cavity of mice, one day after transplantation and 7 Days 2 times for chemotherapy drugs in mice, while serving z -c4 (2g / kg) per day is significantly enhanced the effectiveness of chemotherapy drugs effect.

3. To suppress leukopenia and weight loss induced by chemotherapy medicinal MMC

4. While serving Z-C4, it was found to inhibit cancer cells in terms of improving the effect of intravenously injected anticancer chemotherapy drugs than simply using more than three times in cancer-bearing mice.

5. Chemotherapy drugs for cancer-bearing mice can damage special thymus, spleen and other immune organs, but after adding the service z-C4, thymus, spleen and other organs completely don't shrink, showed z-C4 have effects on the immune organ protective nature function.

6.ZX-C4 extract in Ehrlich ascites disease mouse prolonged the mice life span of up to 167.1%, the average survival time of mice in the control group 15.2 days, and z-c4 administration group is 25.4 days, while reticuloendothelial system function in mice showed significantly higher.

7. Z-C4 allows the chemotherapy drugs cisplatin quickly to mitigate its effects, can enhance the effectiveness of cisplatin. z-C4 can be 100% inhibition of cisplatin toxicity chloroplatinic day conventional dose amount that is human can be. z-c4 not resist cisplatin Chen Hang crazy. z-C4 can protect the kidney, the renal damage cis-platinum chlorine hardly occurs. Z-C4 has highly promising anticancer drug.

8.Z-C4 patients after cancer surgery have a significant effect, gastrointestinal, liver, pancreas and other ulcer disease after radical: all manifestations of physical decline, decreased immunity, fatigue, burnout, loss of appetite and anemia, after 1 a 2 weeks from the beginning can be oral or tube feeding, oral Z-C4 granules, 7.5 g daily, before meals three times a blunt, 12 weeks, during which can be chemotherapy or immune therapy.

9. Z-C4 medicine antitumor effect in mice bearing hepatoma H22:XZ-C 4 first two weeks of medication inhibition rate was 55%, the first four weeks inhibition rate was 68%, the first six weeks inhibition rate was 70% the control group, CTX (cyclophosphamide) Week 2 inhibitory drugs was 45%: the first four weeks inhibition rate of 49%.

10. z-C4 medicine for liver cancer H22 bearing mice survival, z-C4 group extend survival rate 200%, CTX group life span was 9.8%.

11. Z-C4 can significantly improve immune function, can increase white blood cells and red blood cells, liver and kidney function had no effect on the liver, kidney slices without damage. CTX cause leukopenia, reduced immune function, kidney sections have kidney damage.

12. Z-C4 treated group Thymus do not shrink and slightly hypertrophy, CTX thymus control group significantly shrink. Z-C4 on mouse sarcoma (S180) has a strong inhibitory effect.

Clinical Application:

Indications: various types of cancer, sarcoma, a variety of advanced cancer, metastasis, recurrence of cancer, radiotherapy, chemotherapy, post-operative patients. It can be applied all kinds of cancer, especially dizziness, weakness, fatigue, lazy words, less gas, spontaneous sweating, heart palpitations, insomnia, blood deficiency were more applicable.

Z-C4 medicine was used before surgery and after starting the medication and medication every four weeks to do a clinical and laboratory tests, for 20 weeks. Test items: conscious and objective symptoms, body weight, total protein and albumin, total cholesterol, dielectric, ALT AST blood and platelets, lymphocytes, T cells and B cells, r globulin, urinary protein.

Treatment Results: ① increase in the number of lymphocytes, inhibit the role of leukopenia; ② no impact on liver function; ③ protect the kidney function, kidney damage is not so; ④ can significantly reduce the chemotherapy and radiotherapy-induced rash, stomatitis etc; ⑤ postoperative, after chemotherapy, effective physical recovery after radiotherapy, can increase appetite, improve the general malaise and weight gain.

ZX-C4 reduce side effects of radiotherapy and chemotherapy and improve the overall state of the patient after surgery. It is a very valuable rehabilitation medication.

Experience: Modern medicine for the treatment of advanced cancer presents a variety of methods, but there are still some problems, it is still not convinced that the combined use of chemotherapy for advanced disease if certain effective drugs. Even if effective, but it also brings serious side effects, may be considered modern medical treatment for cancer is to kill cancer cells, is offensive, while the Chinese places to enhance the body's own functions to draw even tone pull eliminate cancer. To this end, it should find a way to reduce or eliminate symptoms, improve or treat the disease with few side effects, the treatment can prolong life, and Z-C4 being has the features and advantages.

Through experiments ZX-C4 has the role of enhanced anticancer effect ; promote B cell mitosis role; the catch into the effects of radiation damage hematopoietic system recovery; the promotion of the role of phagocytic cells; thymus increased protective immunity, protection of bone marrow Blood role.

Toxicity Test

Z-C4 can be used long-term. Acute toxicity experiments showed that the median lethal dose (LD50) can not do, is safe and herbs, has been used in the specialist clinic for many years, some patients long-term use three to five years, or even take 8-10 years to maintain immunity, prevent cancer recurrence and metastasis. This anticancer and antimetasatasis medication can be taken by oral for long-term oral and is quite safe.

(5) The following XZ-C various immunomodulatory anticancer medicine series and the experimental and clinical contents are too many and too long so that here only gave names and profiles were omitted.

1. XZ-C5:for liver cancer
2. XZ-C6: for bladder cancer
3. XZ-C7: for Lung cancer
4. XZ-C 8: protect bone marrow and increase blood, attenuated toxics of radiotherapy and chemotherapy
5. XZ-C9:pancreas cancer, prostate cancer.
6. XZ-C10: for brain tumor

All of above of a variety of cancer anticancer, antimetastasis, recurrent research Chinese medicine are based on the experimental study and applied by specialist in outpatient clinics more than 20 years and achieved good results.

Our research Chinese medications for cancer complications in out-patient center of cancer treatment:

1. Anticancer eliminate water soup for pleural effusion and ascites
2. Drop yellow soup for liver cirrhosis and jaundice
3. Anticancer soup after surgery for postoperative recovery
4. Starvation soup for cancer loss of appetite
5. Through Quiet soup for anastomotic stenosis
6. Adhesiolysis soup for adhesions after surgery for cancer

Above all research product formulations. Observation by cancer specialist clinic over the years this big boy patient, have achieved good results, reduce patient suffering, improve the survival quality first, extended survival term.

Summary table of the main pharmacological effects of Z-C immune regulation anticancer Chinese herbal medicine (anti-cancer and increasing immune)

	Increased white blood cells	Enhanced phagocytosis	Enhance cellular immune	Enhance humoral immune	Enhanced hematopoietic function	Improve gastrointestinal function	Enhance the weight of the thymus	Promote bone marrow cell proliferation	Enhanced T cell function	Enhanced NK cell activity	Enhanced LAK cell activity	Enhanced IL-2 activity levels
Z-C-A-APL												
Z-C-B-SLT												
Z-C-C-SNL												
Z-C-D-PGS	+	+	+	+	+	+	6	+	+	+	+	+
Z-C-E-PCW		+	+				2	+	+			+
Z-C-F-AMK		+	+	+	+	+	5			+		+
Z-C-G-GUF		+	+	+		+	4				+	+
Z-C-H-RGL	+		+		+		3		+	+		+
Z-C-I-PLP	+	+	+	+	+	+	6		+	+		
Z-C-J-ASD	+	+	+	+	+		5	+	+	+		+
Z-C-K-LWF		+	+				2					
Z-C-L-AMB	+	+	+	+	+		5	+	+	+	+	+
Z-C-M-LLA	+	+	+	+			4	+		+		
Z-C-N-CZR		+					1					
Z-C-O-PMT	+	+	+	+	+	+	6	+	+	+		
Z-C-P-STG							0					
Z-C-Q-LBP	+	+	+	+	+		5		+	+	+	+
Z-C-R-NSR		+					1	+			+	
Z-C-S-GLK	+	+	+	+	+		5			+		+
Z-C-T-EDM	+	+	+	+	+		5	+		+		+
Z-C-U-PUF		+	+	+			3		+	+	+	
Z-C-V-ABB							1		+	+	+	
Z-C-W-SCB	+						1	+				
Z-C-X-SDS							0			+	+	+
Z-C-Y-PAR							0			+	+	+
Z-C-Z-CVQ							0					

Enhance the level of interferon IFN activity	Enhanced TNF activity levels	Enhanced CSF colony stimulating factor	Antagonistic WCBYC ↓	Inhibition of platelet coagulation and antithrombosis		Antitumor	Anti-metastasis	Antiviral	Anti-cirrhosis	Liver protection	Eliminate free radicals	Protein synthesis	Anti-HIV	
						+	+							
						+	+							
						+	+							
+	+	+	+		9	+	+	+			+	+		20
+	+	+	+		7	+	+	+				+		12
			+		3	+		+		+				11
				+	3	+		+		+		+		11
+		+			5	+					+			10
				+	3	+		+					+	12
+	+		+	+	8	+				+				15
	+			+	2	+	+							5
+					7	+		+				+		5
					2	+						+		5
	+			+	2	+	+							5
		+			4	+		+	+	+	+	+		16
					0	+								1
	+	+	+		8	+	+				4			16
			+		3	+	+		+	+				8
+	+		+		6	+	+			+		+	+	16
+		+	+		6	+		+			+			14
					3	+				+				8
	+				4	+								6
			+		2	+				+	+			5
					3	+								4
	+	+			5	+								6
+					1	+								2

(10.) THE RESEARCH ON NEW CONCEPT AND WAY OF TREATMENT OF CARCINOMA

Professor Xu Ze is the only one to research on and develop the particular experimental program of XZ-C traditional Chinese medicine for immunologic regulation and control of anti-cancer and anti-metastasis.

Goal: to find out and pick up the traditional Chinese herbs for anti-cancer and anti-metastasis.

Purpose: to pick out the "intelligent anticancer drugs" that can be taken orally during a long period with high selectivity but without drug resistance and untoward reactions

Approach: from experimental research to clinical research, applying the successful animal experiments to clinical practice.

Methods: the author has done the screening test on 200 kinds of traditional Chinese herbs that were thought to have anti-cancer effects by traditional Chinese medicine with the expectation to find out new anti-cancer and anti-metastasis drugs.

The particular experimental program on the immunologic function of XZ-C traditional Chinese anti-carcinoma herbs for immunologic regulation and control on the level of molecule:

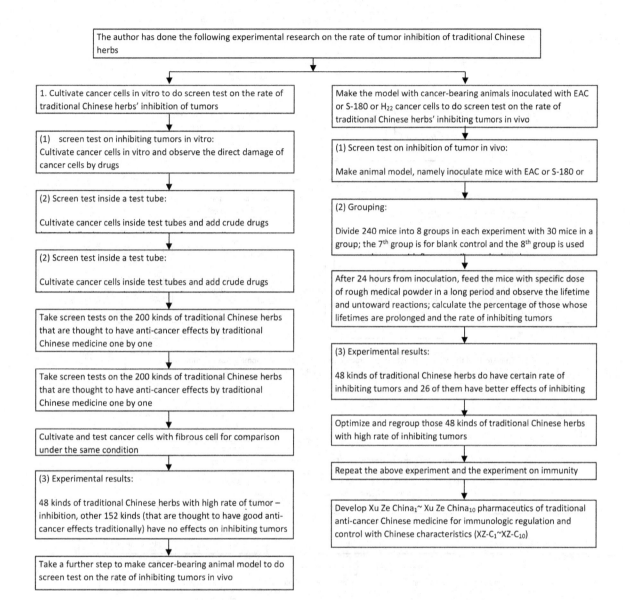

The author has done the following experimental research on the rate of tumor inhibition of traditional Chinese herbs

1. Cultivate cancer cells in vitro to do screen test on the rate of traditional Chinese herbs' inhibition of tumors

(1) screen test on inhibiting tumors in vitro:
Cultivate cancer cells in vitro and observe the direct damage of cancer cells by drugs

(2) Screen test inside a test tube:
Cultivate cancer cells inside test tubes and add crude drugs

(2) Screen test inside a test tube:
Cultivate cancer cells inside test tubes and add crude drugs

Take screen tests on the 200 kinds of traditional Chinese herbs that are thought to have anti-cancer effects by traditional Chinese medicine one by one

Take screen tests on the 200 kinds of traditional Chinese herbs that are thought to have anti-cancer effects by traditional Chinese medicine one by one

Cultivate and test cancer cells with fibrous cell for comparison under the same condition

(3) Experimental results:
48 kinds of traditional Chinese herbs with high rate of tumor – inhibition, other 152 kinds (that are thought to have good anti-cancer effects traditionally) have no effects on inhibiting tumors

Take a further step to make cancer-bearing animal model to do screen test on the rate of inhibiting tumors in vivo

Make the model with cancer-bearing animals inoculated with EAC or S-180 or H_{22} cancer cells to do screen test on the rate of traditional Chinese herbs' inhibiting tumors in vivo

(1) Screen test on inhibition of tumor in vivo:
Make animal model, namely inoculate mice with EAC or S-180 or

(2) Grouping:
Divide 240 mice into 8 groups in each experiment with 30 mice in a group; the 7th group is for blank control and the 8th group is used

After 24 hours from inoculation, feed the mice with specific dose of rough medical powder in a long period and observe the lifetime and untoward reactions; calculate the percentage of those whose lifetimes are prolonged and the rate of inhibiting tumors

(3) Experimental results:
48 kinds of traditional Chinese herbs do have certain rate of inhibiting tumors and 26 of them have better effects of inhibiting

Optimize and regroup those 48 kinds of traditional Chinese herbs with high rate of inhibiting tumors

Repeat the above experiment and the experiment on immunity

Develop Xu Ze China$_1$~ Xu Ze China$_{10}$ pharmaceutics of traditional anti-cancer Chinese medicine for immunologic regulation and control with Chinese characteristics (XZ-C$_1$~XZ-C$_{10}$)

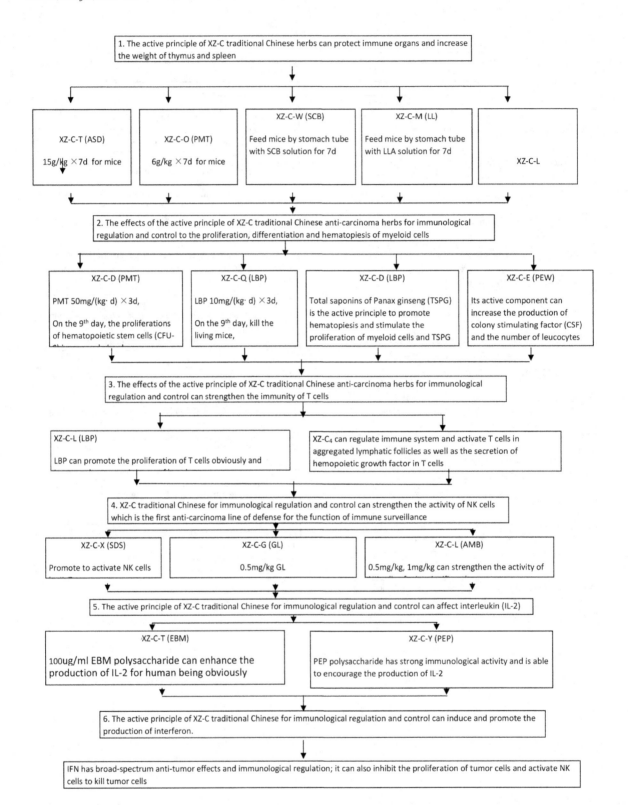

1. The active principle of XZ-C traditional Chinese herbs can protect immune organs and increase the weight of thymus and spleen

| XZ-C-T (ASD)

15g/kg ×7d for mice | XZ-C-O (PMT)

6g/kg ×7d for mice | XZ-C-W (SCB)
Feed mice by stomach tube with SCB solution for 7d | XZ-C-M (LL)
Feed mice by stomach tube with LLA solution for 7d | XZ-C-L |

2. The effects of the active principle of XZ-C traditional Chinese anti-carcinoma herbs for immunological regulation and control to the proliferation, differentiation and hematopiesis of myeloid cells

| XZ-C-D (PMT)

PMT 50mg/(kg· d) ×3d,

On the 9th day, the proliferations of hematopoietic stem cells (CFU- | XZ-C-Q (LBP)

LBP 10mg/(kg· d) ×3d,

On the 9th day, kill the living mice, | XZ-C-D (LBP)

Total saponins of Panax ginseng (TSPG) is the active principle to promote hematopiesis and stimulate the proliferation of myeloid cells and TSPG | XZ-C-E (PEW)

Its active component can increase the production of colony stimulating factor (CSF) and the number of leucocytes |

3. The effects of the active principle of XZ-C traditional Chinese anti-carcinoma herbs for immunological regulation and control can strengthen the immunity of T cells

| XZ-C-L (LBP)

LBP can promote the proliferation of T cells obviously and | XZ-C$_4$ can regulate immune system and activate T cells in aggregated lymphatic follicles as well as the secretion of hemopoietic growth factor in T cells |

4. XZ-C traditional Chinese for immunological regulation and control can strengthen the activity of NK cells which is the first anti-carcinoma line of defense for the function of immune surveillance

| XZ-C-X (SDS)

Promote to activate NK cells | XZ-C-G (GL)

0.5mg/kg GL | XZ-C-L (AMB)

0.5mg/kg, 1mg/kg can strengthen the activity of |

5. The active principle of XZ-C traditional Chinese for immunological regulation and control can affect interleukin (IL-2)

| XZ-C-T (EBM)

100ug/ml EBM polysaccharide can enhance the production of IL-2 for human being obviously | XZ-C-Y (PEP)

PEP polysaccharide has strong immunological activity and is able to encourage the production of IL-2 |

6. The active principle of XZ-C traditional Chinese for immunological regulation and control can induce and promote the production of interferon.

IFN has broad-spectrum anti-tumor effects and immunological regulation; it can also inhibit the proliferation of tumor cells and activate NK cells to kill tumor cells

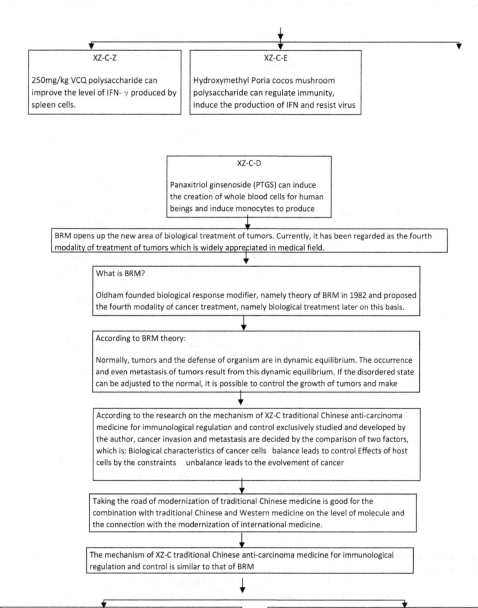

XZ-C-Z

250mg/kg VCQ polysaccharide can improve the level of IFN- γ produced by spleen cells.

XZ-C-E

Hydroxymethyl Poria cocos mushroom polysaccharide can regulate immunity, induce the production of IFN and resist virus

XZ-C-D

Panaxitriol ginsenoside (PTGS) can induce the creation of whole blood cells for human beings and induce monocytes to produce

BRM opens up the new area of biological treatment of tumors. Currently, it has been regarded as the fourth modality of treatment of tumors which is widely appreciated in medical field.

What is BRM?

Oldham founded biological response modifier, namely theory of BRM in 1982 and proposed the fourth modality of cancer treatment, namely biological treatment later on this basis.

According to BRM theory:

Normally, tumors and the defense of organism are in dynamic equilibrium. The occurrence and even metastasis of tumors result from this dynamic equilibrium. If the disordered state can be adjusted to the normal, it is possible to control the growth of tumors and make

According to the research on the mechanism of XZ-C traditional Chinese anti-carcinoma medicine for immunological regulation and control exclusively studied and developed by the author, cancer invasion and metastasis are decided by the comparison of two factors, which is: Biological characteristics of cancer cells   balance leads to control Effects of host cells by the constraints   unbalance leads to the evolvement of cancer

Taking the road of modernization of traditional Chinese medicine is good for the combination with traditional Chinese and Western medicine on the level of molecule and the connection with the modernization of international medicine.

The mechanism of XZ-C traditional Chinese anti-carcinoma medicine for immunological regulation and control is similar to that of BRM

The effects of biological response modifier include the following:

(1) To strengthen the defense mechanism of host cells or to weaken the immunodepression of cancer-bearing host cells so as to achieve immune response
(2) To add natural or biological active substance with genetic recombination to strengthen the defense mechanism of host cells
(3) To modify tumor cells and induce the strong response of host cells
(4) To promote the proliferation and mature of tumor cells and normalize them
(5) To alleviate untoward reaction of radiotherapy and chemotherapy and strengthen the resistance of host cells

The main pharmacological action of XZ-C traditional Chinese anti-carcinoma medicine is to resist cancer and strengthen immunity, whose mechanism is similar to that of BRM

(1) To activate the system of immune cells and strengthen the defense mechanism of host cells to achieve the immune response to cancer cells
(2) To activate the system of immune cytokine of the organismal anti-cancer mechanism to improve immune surveillance
(3) To protect thymus and strengthen immunity and to protect hematopiesis of marrow
(4) To alleviate the untoward reactions of radiotherapy and chemotherapy
(5) To augment thymus and gain the weight to prevent its progressive

The current molecular oncology combines with the traditional Chinese herbs to realize the combination of Chinese and Western medicine on molecular level. With BRM theory being the bridge, traditional Chinese medicine connects with international advanced theory

Treatment of tumors by biological response modifier (BRM) and analogous BRM traditional Chinese medicine

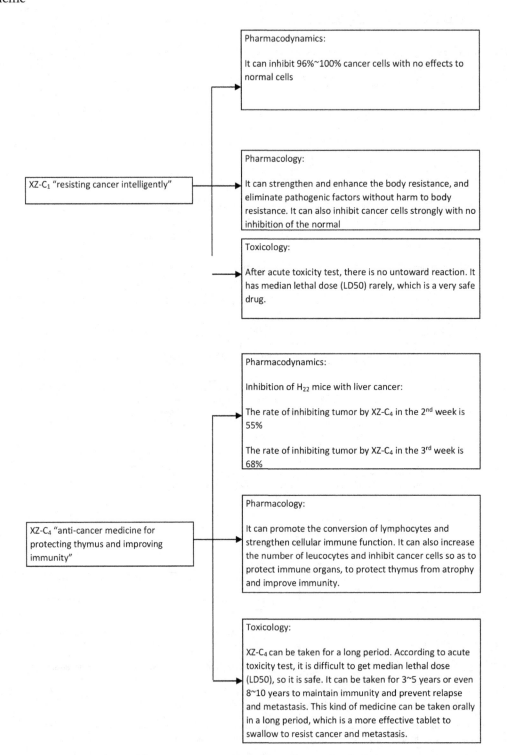

The research on New Concept and Way of Treatment of Carcinoma

The clinic verification:

The animal experiment of XZ-C traditional Chinese medicine for immunological regulation and control has been successful, so it can be applied to clinic to verify its curative effects.

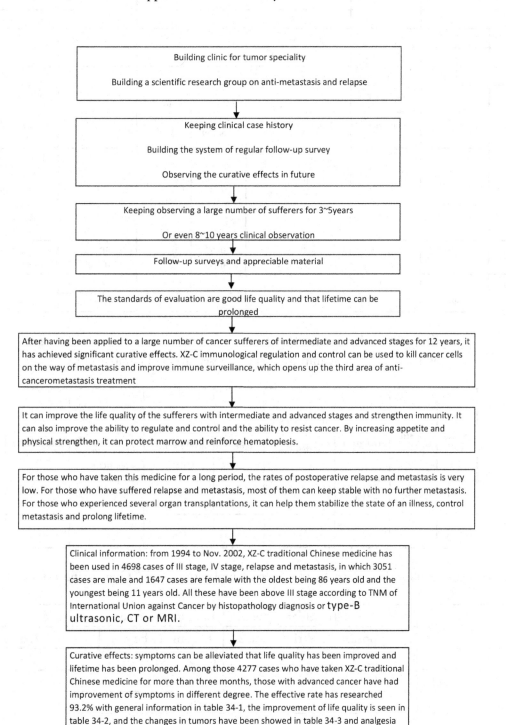

Building clinic for tumor speciality

Building a scientific research group on anti-metastasis and relapse

Keeping clinical case history

Building the system of regular follow-up survey

Observing the curative effects in future

Keeping observing a large number of sufferers for 3~5years

Or even 8~10 years clinical observation

Follow-up surveys and appreciable material

The standards of evaluation are good life quality and that lifetime can be prolonged

After having been applied to a large number of cancer sufferers of intermediate and advanced stages for 12 years, it has achieved significant curative effects. XZ-C immunological regulation and control can be used to kill cancer cells on the way of metastasis and improve immune surveillance, which opens up the third area of anti-cancerometastasis treatment

It can improve the life quality of the sufferers with intermediate and advanced stages and strengthen immunity. It can also improve the ability to regulate and control and the ability to resist cancer. By increasing appetite and physical strengthen, it can protect marrow and reinforce hematopiesis.

For those who have taken this medicine for a long period, the rates of postoperative relapse and metastasis is very low. For those who have suffered relapse and metastasis, most of them can keep stable with no further metastasis. For those who experienced several organ transplantations, it can help them stabilize the state of an illness, control metastasis and prolong lifetime.

Clinical information: from 1994 to Nov. 2002, XZ-C traditional Chinese medicine has been used in 4698 cases of III stage, IV stage, relapse and metastasis, in which 3051 cases are male and 1647 cases are female with the oldest being 86 years old and the youngest being 11 years old. All these have been above III stage according to TNM of International Union against Cancer by histopathology diagnosis or type-B ultrasonic, CT or MRI.

Curative effects: symptoms can be alleviated that life quality has been improved and lifetime has been prolonged. Among those 4277 cases who have taken XZ-C traditional Chinese medicine for more than three months, those with advanced cancer have had improvement of symptoms in different degree. The effective rate has researched 93.2% with general information in table 34-1, the improvement of life quality is seen in table 34-2, and the changes in tumors have been showed in table 34-3 and analgesia in table 34-4

The clinic application verification:

The general information about 4277 cases of relapse and metastasis

		Liver cancer	Lung cancer	Gastric cancer	Cardia Cancer	Rectal and anal cancer	Colon cancer	Breast cancer	Cancer of pancreas
Cases		1021	752	668	624	328	442	368	74
Male: Female		4:1	4.4:1	2.25:1	3.1:1	1:1	2.1:1	All female	3.2:1
Focus	primary	694(68.8%)	699(93.9%)	-	-	-	-	-	-
	metastatic	327(31.2%)	53(6.1%)	-	-	-	-	-	-
General parts of metastasis		from lung (2%) from gorge (27.2%)	lymph nodes metastasis in clavicle (11.6%)	from liver (23.8%) from lung (3%)	from clavicle (13.1%)	rate of relapse (14.8%)	from liver (16.0%)	lymph nodes metastasis in clavicle (17.5%)	from liver (11.7%)
		from cardia (19.5%) from recta (31.2%)	from brain (3.1%) from marrow (4.6%)	from peritoneum(29.1%) from clavicle (6.1%)	from liver (8.3%)	from liver (7.0%)	from peritoneum (6.0%)	lymph nodes metastasis in armpit (15.0%) from bone (5.0%)	behind peritoneum (39.1%)
Age (year)	popular (%)	30-39 (76.2)	50-69 (71.6)	40-49 (73.4)	40-69 (80.4)	40-49 (75.2)	30-69 (88.0)	40-59 (65.9)	40-59 (70.0)
	youngest	11	20	17	30	27	27	29	34
	oldest	86	80	77	77	78	76	80	68

The life qualities of the sufferers with advanced cancer among the 4277 cases
with comprehensive improvement in observation of curative effects

	Spirit	Appetite	Physical strengthen	Improvement of general situation	Gain in weight	Improvement of sleep	Improvement of mobility and alleviation of movement restriction	Living by oneself and ambulating normally	Recovery of the ability to do light muscular work
Cases with improvement	4071	3986	2450	479	2938	1005	1038	3220	479
Percentage (%)	95.2	93.2	57.3	11.2	68.7	23.5	24.3	75.3	11.2

The changes in metastatic nodes after the external application of XZ-C medicine among 56 cases

	The enlargement of lymph nodes in cervical clavicle			
	Disappear	Shrink by 1/2	Become to be soft	No changes
Cases	12	22	14	8
Percentage (%)	21.4	39.2	25.0	14.2
Total effective rate	85.7			

The situation of analgesia after oral administration and external
application of XZ-C medicine among 298 cases

Clinical performance	Analgesia			
	Alleviated lightly	Alleviated obviously	Disappear	No effects
Cases	12	22	14	8
Percentage (%)	21.4	39.2	25.0	14.2
Total effective rate	85.7			

On the aspect of improving life quality (according to KPS)
The average score is 50 before administration; it increases to 80, even 90 or 100

Analysis of lifetime: it is difficult to compare clinical sufferers as their stadiums and degrees are different. In this group, all sufferers are above third stage with different organ transplantations and dysfunctions. According to former statistics in this sort, the medium lifetime is about six months. In this group, the longest case is 14-years with the average lifetime of other cases being more than 1 year.

Analysis of prolonging lifetime:

without surgeries, radiotherapies and chemotherapies, cases that have been taking XZ-C traditional Chinese medicine for immunological regulation and control solely for 5 years are: ① Di, central type carcinoma of lung in left top lung accompanied by metastasis in left lung, has been taking $XZ-C_1+XZ-C_4+XZ-C_7$ for 5 years; ② Huang, with esophageal carcinoma has been taking this medicine for 5 years; ③ Huang with cancer in the middle place of oesophagus has been taking this medicine for 5 years; ④ Huang, with primary massive type cancer has been taking this medicine for 5 years; ⑤ Qi, primary liver cancer, has been taking this medicine for 5 years.
Typical cases whose cancer can not be cut off by exploratory surgeries and can not use radiotherapies and chemotherapies to treat, have been taking XZ-C traditional Chinese medicine for immunological regulation and control for 4 years: ① Cheng, with tumors after abdominal distention which can not be cut off by exploratory surgery, has been taking this medicine for 4 years; ② Fang, with cancer of pancreas which can not be cut off by exploratory surgery, has been taking XZ-C medicine for 7 years; ③ Li, with primary massive type liver cancer that can not be cut off by exploratory surgery in Tongji Hospital, has been taking XZ-C medicine for 4 years; ④ Ke, with primary liver cancer that can not be cut off by exploratory surgery in the PLA general hospital, has been taking XZ-C medicine for 5 years.

Immune pharmacology of XZ-C Immune regulation anti-cancer medications

Compared traditional Chinese immune pharmacology with Western immune pharmacology, they have their own characteristics and advantages. Traditional Chinese medications through clinical experience accumulated a large of medications which have the role in regulating the immune function, especially beneficial traditional Chinese medications generally having dynamic regulation of the immune benefits.

Whether single herb or drug prescription will have a variety of active ingredients, and unlike Western medicine (synthetic drugs) is a matter of a single structure. Traditional medications are multifaceted roles. In addition to the regulation of immune function, traditional medications have certain roles on each function of the whole systems.

XZ-C traditional Chinese medicine immunomodulator have a major role in regulate cell-mediated immune (Cellular imnune) including cytokines or lymphokines and traditional Chinese medicine has the main role in the stem cells immune such as the thymus, gonads and lymphatic systems and T, B cells and various cells factors.

There have been a few ancient medicine concepts through righteousness and no evil, which constitute an integral part of traditional Chinese medicine and its essence of this theory is a few two-dimensional three functional balance, enhance resistance to disease. In fact, its main role is to enhance immune function. Immune pharmacology is an emerging interdisciplinary, a bridge contact between pharmacology and immunology. XZ-C immunomodulatory agents have obvious immune function.

The scope of Clinical application of XZ-C immunoregulation anti-cancer traditional Chinese medications XZ-C1-10 anticancer metastasis and recurrence

(1) **For a variety of distant metastatic cancer, such as liver metastases, lung metastases, bone metastases, brain metastases, abdominal lymph node metastasis, mediastinal lymph node metastasis, malignant pleural effusion, cancerous ascites, XZ-C Immune regulation of anti - metastatic therapy can be applied according to the transfer step, to intervene, block the transfer of cancer cells, to extend life.**

(2) **For the patients who completed a variety of radiotherapy and chemotherapy treatment course, XZ-C1-4 immune regulation of traditional Chinese medicine can be used to consolidate long-term efficacy and prevent recurrence.**

(3) **For the patients who have chemotherapy, the reaction is serious and can not continue, XZ-C immunoregulation treatment to anti-metastasis, recurrence can continue to be applied.**

(4) In the elderly or frail with other diseases who can not put, chemotherapy, XZ-C immune regulation of anti-metastasis and anti-recurrence treatment can be applied.

(5) On the patients who surgical exploration can not cut down the tumor XZ-C immune regulation treatment can be used.

(6) For the palliative surgery XZ-C immunoregulation anti-transfer therapy can be applied.

(7) After a variety of radical mastectomy, XZ-C immunoregulation treatment of traditional Chinese medicine anti-recurrence, metastasis should continue to serve to improve the long-term effect after radical operation.

(11.) FORMED XZ-C TREATMENT OF THE THEORETICAL SYSTEM

After 20 years of self-reliance, hard work, Professor Xu Ze completed national science and technology commission of the application of "eight five" basic and clinical research and technological topics. Series of nearly one hundred scientific research papers summarized the information and several books were published. This book collected and summarized his formed theoretical system of XZ-C cancer Therapy which the theoretical basis and experimental evidence and clinical observation verification were undergoing for cancer treatment.

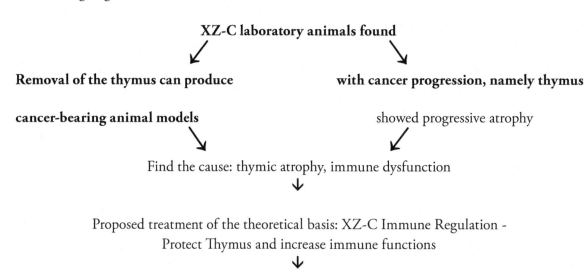

XZ-C laboratory animals found

Removal of the thymus can produce / **with cancer progression, namely thymus**

cancer-bearing animal models / showed progressive atrophy

Find the cause: thymic atrophy, immune dysfunction

Proposed treatment of the theoretical basis: XZ-C Immune Regulation - Protect Thymus and increase immune functions

Exclusive development of products: XZ-C immunomodulatory agents 1-10

Clinical validation:
18 years, outpatient follow-up observation of the more than 12,000 cases of advanced cancer patients, and more able to improve the quality of life and prolong survival, satisfactory

Theoretical System XZ-C cancer therapy

The comparation between XZ anticancer theropy concepts and the traditional concepts

	XZ anticancer therapy	Traditional anticancer therapy
The principles	Improve the immune function to get rid of the cancer cells	Kill the cancer cells
Cancer Pathogenesis	Thymus shrink Immune function decreases	no
The experimental results and evidences	Improve the immune functions And increases the immune functions	no
The therapy rules	Build up enter pictures	Partially and only kill the cancer cells.
The therapy models	The enter therapy: surgery and bioimmunology The short therapy: radiotherapy and chemotherapy because of the side effects so that it is not good to be used too long and too strong	Chemotherapy+ radiotherapy
The therapy medications	XZ-C improve the immune functions, which combined the western and Chinese tradition medicine together on the molecular level.	Has the cell toxicities(kill the cancer cells and the normal cells)
The side effects	No	More side effects, some have the more toxicities, even the immune function failure. The radiotherapy damage is perminant.
The therapy effects	To improve the life qualities and to extend the survival times	Several months of recovery, then recurrence and development again.
The medical costs	Cheaper than radioactive and chemotherapy	Cost more money.
The prospects	It is very safe and a new way against the cancers.	The therapy effects is only 5% and have limit future.

Note: Xu Ze, etc on his reform and innovation of research on treatment of cancer.

CONDENSE WISDOM AND CONQUER CANCER

--- for the benefits of mankind

How to conquer cancer? and how to prevent cancer?and
how to treat cancer? by my opinion

(Volume VII)

Innovation must be challenge to and reform the
traditional concept and then can develop

CONTENTS VOLUME VII

Preface

I am a clinical surgeon, why do I study cancer? This is due to the results after the letter petition of a group of cancer patients.

In 1985, I made the petition for more than 3,000 cases of chest and abdominal cancer patients after I operated; the results: it was found that most of the patients were the recurrence or metastasis after 2-3 years, and some even after a few months, 1 year.

From the results of follow-up it was found: postoperative recurrence and metastasis are the key to long-term effect of surgery.

And therefore also it raised an important question to us: that clinicians must pay attention to studying the postoperative recurrence and the prevention measures to improve postoperative long-term efficacy. Therefore, it is necessary to carry out the experimental study of the clinical basis of recurrence and metastasis. If there is no breakthrough in basic research, the clinical efficacy is difficult to improve.

So we established the Experimental Surgery Laboratory (later established in 1991, Hubei College of Traditional Chinese Medicine Experimental Surgery, research direction for the capture of cancer).

We have studied from the following two aspects: one for animal experimental research; one for clinical research. After success in animal experiment basis it was applied to clinical, and conducted the clinical validation. After 28 years of cold and hot hard work, it was carried out a series of experimental research and clinical validation work, has made a series of scientific and technological innovation and scientific research achievement.

Through the experience of experimental study and clinical practice, combined with half a century to the traditional therapy clinical medical practice case review, analysis, evaluation and self-reflection, summed up their 58 years of clinical medical success and failure of both positive and negative experience, then had the following new discoveries, new thinking, new knowledge, new treatment concepts.

A new discovery of Anti - cancer, anti - cancer metastasis research

一 . A new discovery

1, from the results of the follow-up it was found:

(1) the postoperative recurrence and metastasis are the key to long-term efficacy of surgery.

(2) the clinicians must pay attention to studying the prevention and control measures of the postoperative recurrence and metastasis.

2, from the experimental tumor study it was found:

(1) In our laboratory the removal of thymus (Thymus, TH) in mice can produce animal model; the injection of immunosuppressive agents can also help the establishment of animal model. The study was conducted that: the occurrence and development of cancer and the host immune organs thymus and its function has a clear relationship.

(6) We explored the effects of tumor on the immune organ impact. It was found that with the progress of cancer the thymus showed progressive atrophy (600 tumor-bearing animal model mice); after the host is inoculated with cancer cells the thymus is acute Atrophy.

(3) ... (6) ... ... (delecting slightly)

3, through the review of clinical practice cases and the analysis and evaluation and reflection of the postoperative adjuvant chemotherapy case, it was found that there are problems:

(1) in some patients the postoperative adjuvant chemotherapy failed to prevent recurrence;

(2) in some patients the postoperative adjuvant chemotherapy failed to prevent metastasis;

(3) in some patients chemotherapy promotes immune failure.

4, from the clinical practice case to analysis and to reflect why chemotherapy failed to prevent cancer recurrence and metastasis

From the role of chemotherapy drugs in the cancer cell cycle to analyze and reflect; from the chemical drugs to suppress the overall immune function to analyze and reflect; from the drug resistance of chemotherapy to analyze and reflection it was found:

(1) there are some important errors in the current chemotherapy;

(2) There are several major contradictions in current chemotherapy.

5, through clinical medical practice case to review and to analysis and to evaluate and to reflect it was found the following problems:

"The analysis and evaluation and questioning of systemic intravenous chemotherapy for solid tumors";

"The review and analysis and review of the three major treatments for cancer";

"The chemotherapy to be further research and improvement."

二. update thinking, update awareness

Through the review and analysis and evaluation and self-reflection of seven years of experimental observation of the live animal and sixty years of specialist outpatient treatment in more than 6,000 cases, and it also summed up the success and failure of both positive and negative experience and lessons learned why the traditional therapy did not significantly reduce the death Rate? why did not it control relapse and transfer? What is the problems of the traditional concept of traditional therapy? So I gradually realize that the current cancer traditional therapy may still have some problems such as:

1, the traditional chemotherapy suppresses immune function and inhibits bone marrow hematopoietic function;

2, the traditional intravenous chemotherapy is intermittent treatment and in intermittent period cancer can not be treated. While cancer cells are in the intermittent, cancer cells continue to proliferate and divide;

3, the traditional therapy damage the host, because the chemotherapy cell poison as a "double-edged sword", both kill cancer cells and kill normal cells;

4, the traditional therapy target only focus on chemotherapy can kill cancer cells, while ignoring the host itself on the resistance of cancer control, because the occurrence and development of the tumor depends on the level of host immune function and the biological characteristics of the tumor itself, that decision The biological characteristics of the tumor cells and the host of the constraints on the impact of the two potentials; if it is the balance, cancer is controlled; if the two is imbalance, cancer is progress. Traditional radiotherapy and chemotherapy are to promote the decline in immune function and it is possible to make the two potential more imbalance;

5, the traditional therapy damage the central immune organs; in cancer patients thymus has been inhibited, and chemotherapy also inhibit bone marrow, as "snow plus frog, worse" so that the entire central immune organs were damaged and failed to effectively protect;

6, the traditional therapy is for injury therapy and has a certain blow for the patient resistance to disease, but do not give the effectively protection;

7, the traditional therapy ignored the body's own anti-cancer ability, and ignores the body's own anti-cancer ability, ignores the host anti-cancer system anti-cancer cell system (NK cells, K cells, LAK cells, macrophages), anti-cancer cells Factor gene (1FN-1L2-. ThF, LT and other factors) anti-cancer gene system (Rb gene, P53 gene), ignores the body's anti-cancer mechanism and its influencing factors, ignores the body's own anti-cancer internal factors which are not activated, mobilized, but it only blindly kills cancer cells;

8, The goal of the traditional radiotherapy and chemotherapy is relatively simple and is just to kill cancer cells. And it is not consistent with the current understanding of the biological behavior of cancer cells and biological characteristics of the actual situation. For example, cancer cell invasion behavior: metastasis and multiple steps; relapse incentives, latent months, or years and recurrence. It is now recognized that anticancer drugs are not necessarily resistant to metastasis and anti-transfer drugs do not have to kill cancer cells.

三. challenge the status of cancer treatment, reform can develop.

How to do? Both the above problems, we should further study the basic experimental research and clinical research, deepen the reform, should update thinking, update awareness, update observation, in the reform forward, try to the innovation. Innovation must challenge to the traditional concept, to overcome its shortcomings, to correct its shortcomings so that it is become the more perfect. Innovation must challenge the status quo and beyond the status quo. Innovation also is to find another way and it is to find a new way to overcome cancer.

1. THE ANALYSIS, EVALUATION AND QUESTIONING OF THE SOLID TUMOR SYSTEMIC INTRAVENOUS CHEMOTHERAPY

- *Analysis and questioning of the route of intravenous chemotherapy for solid tumor*
- *Analysis and questioning of the method of calculating the dose of solid body intravenous chemotherapy*
- *Analysis and evaluation of the efficacy of systemic intravenous chemotherapy for solid tumors*

Through reviewing, reflecting, summarizing and analyzing the experience in success and lessons from failure, I have gradually realize that systemic intravenous chemotherapy on solid tumor may be confronted with some important problems, which are worthy of reflection, evaluation and re-discussion.

Why the chemotherapy does not prevent the recurrence and metastasis and get the expected curative effects? Through repeated reflection, we doubt: whether it is reasonable and scientific or not to use route of administration of intravenous chemotherapy to treat the malignant tumor in stomach, intestines, liver, gallbladder, pancreas and pelvic cavity and so on. We think deeply about the route of administration, especially the one for the malignant tumor in the abdomen and find that it is necessary to research and discuss the route of administration over again, the same to calculation of the dose and the evaluation standard of curative effects.

I. Analysis and doubt of the route of administration for systemic intravenous chemotherapy of solid tumor?

The present chemical chemotherapy for tumor is mainly the systemic intravenous chemotherapy, the standard scheme of chemotherapy in the world, the united scheme or the single-agent scheme is mostly the systemic intravenous chemotherapy, the same to the treatment of leukemia, malignant tumor of the blood system, tumor of the lymphatic system, solid tumor, tumor of the abdominal cavity, malignant tumor of stomach, intestines, liver, gallbladder and pancreas and to the assistant chemotherapy after operation or perioperative assistant chemotherapy.

1. Analysis of route of administration and medication of cytotoxic drug for intravenous chemotherapy for solid tumor:

In systemic intravenous chemotherapy, the intravenous drip enters the blood circulation, flows back to the right ventricle via venous blood, and then enters the arteria pulmonalis, after it is oxygenated with blood in lung, it flows into left ventricle via pulmonary vein and then is transfused into the aorta via bender and enters the systemic artery system for systemic circulation. Then it is distributed to the systemic organs with the arterial blood in viscera. At this moment, the chemotherapy drug enters the extracellular tissue fluid via interspace of capillay wall and then comes into play after entering the cancer cells.

As to the systemic intravenous chemotherapy, after the drug is distributed by the systemic blood, only a tiny minority of cytotoxic drug for chemotherapy enters the external organs of tumor cells and a tiny minority of drug enters the cancer cells, with slight curative effects.

Intravenous injection of chemotherapy drug via forearm vein →right ventricle →pulmonary artery→ oxygenation of pulmonary alveoli→ pulmonary vein→ aorta →systemic artery system (the drug is transported to the systemic viscera and is distributed in the whole body) →arteries of viscera→ veins of viscera →venae cavae→ right ventricle→ recirculation as above.

Analysis: as above-mentioned, the drug is spread in the whole body and distributed to all viscera, in this way, the systemic viscera obtain the cytotoxic drug, however, the body surface area or volume of the solid tumor only accounts for a very little ratio of the systemic body surface area or volume, for example, even through one carcinoma of stomach as large as one adult's fist, accounts for a very little ratio of the volume of an adult. Therefore, the carcinoma of stomach as large as one adult's fist obtains a tiny minority of cytotoxic drug in the chemotherapy of systemic intravenous injection, resulting in very little curative effects or roles. Meanwhile, most of the cytotoxic drug for chemotherapy is transported to the normal histiocytes of the viscera (including heart, liver, spleen, lung, kidney, brain, bone marrow, blood, lymph and immune organ), all of which receive the cytotoxic drug for chemotherapy, resulting in side reaction. The more the times of chemotherapy, the larger the dosage, the more the drug combination, the more serious of the accumulative side reaction, even resulting in loss of immunologic function and endangering the life. The patient takes a risk of endangering the life, however, does it have curative effects on the cancerous protuberance? The carcinoma of stomach as large as a fist only can obtain a very tiny minority of dose for chemotherapy entering the cancer cells as per the body surface area, in this way, the curative effects are very little and it is impossible to realize the good curative effects.

Some patients think by mistake that the large side reaction represents the curative effects, the larger the reaction, the better the curative effects, therefore, they mistake that the reaction kills the cancer cell, but they hardly realize that the reaction kills the normal cells: it is the reaction that kills the active normal cells with normal proliferation, such as bone marrow cells, immunological cells and mucous membrane cells of the stomach and intestine and the hair, resulting in decrease of white blood cells and decrease of blood platelets. Meanwhile, no one knows whether the cancer cells are killed by the chemotherapy and how many cancer cells are killed. However, it is known that it kills the normal cells just because the decrease of white blood cells and blood platelets only indicates the completion of the chemotherapy, no one knows whether it has curative effects or not.

Therefore, we analyze the reason why the chemotherapy cannot prevent the recurrence and metastasis is possibly that the route of systemic intravenous chemotherapy does not realize the curative effects you hope and expect, the local cancer lesion is applied with a tiny minority of dose, since a very tiny minority of drug enters the external tissue fluid of the cancer cells and only a minute of dose can enter the cancer cells and takes curative effects.

An example of 5-FU, the common chemotherapy drug: 5-FU intravenous chemotherapy 1000mg/d x 5=5000mg, 85% is catabolized by DPD enzyme in the liver without any therapeutic effects; some of the rest 15% is excreted through the kidney in form of drug prototype, some enters the cells and takes curative effects through anabolism. Given the latter is 8% and the locality with easy recurrence and metastasis of carcinosis accounts for 5% of the volume of the whole body, the effective availability of 5-FU is only:

5000mg x 8% x 5%=20mg (0.4%).

In another word, when intravenous drip is used for systemic chemotherapy, chemotherapy drug 5-FU infused via intravenous drip is 5000mg, after distributed in the whole body by the viscera, the available 5-FU really reaching the cancer lesion is only 20mg, that is to say, only 0.4% of the drug reaches the cancer lesion and is utilized. The drug takes the curative effects in the cancer cells. The rest, namely 99.6% of the chemotherapy drug takes the untoward reaction in the normal cells. In other words, only 0.4% of the chemotherapy drug plays a role in killing the cancer cells while 99.6% of the chemotherapy drug kills the normal cells of the patients with active proliferation, namely bone marrow cells, epith epithelial cells of mucous membrane of the stomach and intestine, hair, white blood cells, blood platelets and immunological cells and so on, resulting in degression of immunologic function, inhibition of hematopiesis of bone marrow cells, emesis, alopecia and obvious decrease of white blood cells and blood platelets.

According to the reports of the literatures, the metabolic pathway of 5-Fu:

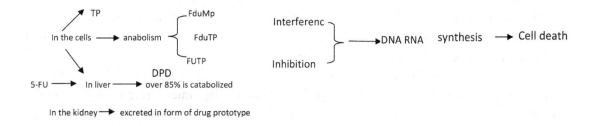

In systemic intravenous chemotherapy, how many chemotherapy drugs can reach the cancer cells and play a role in killing the cancer cells? With an example of the above-mentioned 5-FU, the patient is intravenously injected with 5000mg in 5 days, however, the one really reaching the cancer cells and playing a role is only 20mg, only accounting for 0.4% of the injected chemotherapy drug, the rest of the injected chemotherapy drug, namely 99.6% has the side effects on the normal cells with active proliferation in the whole body in clinical menifetation, namely bone marrow cells, epithelial cells of mucous membrane of the stomach and intestine and immunological cells, the systemic side reactions include arrest of bone marrow, reaction of gstrointestinal tract and toxic reaction of heart, lung and liver; the local toxic reactions include toxic reaction of skin and alopecia and so on.

In systemic intravenous chemotherapy, how does the cytotoxic drug for chemotherapy work from blood to cancer cells intravenously transfused? The chemotherapy drug is distributed and applied in the whole body, finally the chemotherapy drug enters the external tissue fluid of the cells via the interspace of capillay wall and then comes into play after entering the cancer cells.

In systemic intravenous chemotherapy, after the chemotherapy drug enters the vein, the drug is necessarily distributed in the body fluid, among the moisture in the human body, about 5% is blood, 15% is the external tissue fluid of the cells and 40% is intracellular fluid. The chemotherapy drug in blood is circulated and utilized in the whole body and distributed with the blood in the viscera. When the chemotherapy drug is in the external tissue fluid, it is absorbed and metabolized respectively by the viscera. When the chemotherapy drug enters the cells, the drug takes curative effects in the cancer cells while it takes side reaction in a large number of normal cells.

As above mentioned, we should objectively and calmly analyze the advantages, the disadvantages, the gain and the loss of the route of administration of systemic intravenous chemotherapy for the solid tumor? Which are the advantages? And the disadvantages? What the patient gains? And losses? All of which shall be seriously reflected, analyzed and evaluated.

2. It shall be discussed and doubted whether the route of administration of cytotoxic drug to kill the cancer cells of the solid tumor and the systemic intravenous drip are reasonable and scientific or not?

The above-mentioned systemic intravenous chemotherapy is used for all types of leukemia, leucoma and malignant tumor in the blood system, which is reasonable just because the malignant tumor of the blood system and the malignant tumor cells of the malignant leucoma of the lymphatic system are distributed in the systemic blood system or lymphatic system, in this way, they shall be applied with drug through the intravenous drip, which is reasonable and scientific just because there are so many cases and experience in successful treatment.

However, as to the carcinoma for solid tumor, the drug entering the tumor is minute, it plays a minor role in killing the cancer cells, it has obvious side reaction in damaging the systemic proliferative cells. The chemotherapy drug transfused through the route of administration to solid tumor only can kill a tiny minority of cancer cells while most of it kills the normal proliferative cells of the host, resulting in pains from the side reaction of chemotherapy undertaken by the patients.

At present, there are so many solid malignant tumors adopting the systemic intravenous administration route for the assistant chemotherapy after operation or perioperative assistant chemotherapy. Through intravenous drip, the chemotherapy drug enters the right ventricle via the caval vein, enters the lungs via pulmonary artery, enters the left ventricle through the pulmonary vein and then is distributed in the whole body through the aorta, in this way, the chemotherapy drug reaching the cancer lesion is very little, most of the drug is distributed in the whole body and kills the normal cells, especially the immunological cells, hematopoietic cells of bone marrow, causing the patients to be severely damaged; meanwhile, it does not play a remarkable role in the solid tumor. Over half a century, it has been all the same, although it has not taken the expected effects, so many patients have suffered from the pains from the side reaction of the chemotherapy drug widely killing the normal cells. The clinicians should seriously reflect, analyze and evaluate the route of administration, which is unadvisable, unreasonable and unscientific. We shall try to apply the drug to the specific locality instead of applying drug in the whole body and we shall research it and try to correct, reform and innovate it.

2. Analysis and doubt of calculation method of the dose of systemic intravenous chemotherapy drug for solid tumor

1. Based on the above-mentioned systemic intravenous administration route, the medication is calculated as per the calculation method of leukemia, since the leukemic cells are distributed in the systemic circulatory system, the administration must cover the systemic blood system. The malignant lymphocytes of leucoma is also distributed in the systemic lymphatic system, the administration must also cover the systemic lymphatic system, the blood system and the lymphatic system are distributed in all organs, tissues and skin in the whole body, therefore the administration shall be calculated as per body surface area or volume. This kind of route of administration, calculation of dose, pharmacokinetics and bioavailability is reasonable and scientific, which conforms to the distribution of the cancer cells.

2. Since the systemic intravenous chemotherapy has taken good curative effects and experience in all types of leukemia, leucoma, epithelioma of chorion, some malignant moles, blastocytoma Wilms tumor and so on, it has been widely applied to the solid tumor of the viscera in the whole body and the assistant chemotherapy after operation, although we have accumulated much experience and obtained some achievements, we have not had our wish fulfilled just because the death rate has been not reduced, the recurrence and metastasis has been not prevented, indicating it is unreasonable to apply the calculation method to dose of the leukemia and it does not conform to the actual conditions of the solid cancer, therefore, its reasonableness and scientificalness shall be doubted and it shall be further researched for reforming and innovation.

3. Since the carcinoma of the solid tumor is restricted to the viscus before remote metastasis, it is necessary to distribute the drug to the viscus in chemotherapy, however, the drug for systemic intravenous chemotherapy is distributed in the whole body, it necessarily needs relatively more dose. However, the chemotherapy drug is the cytotoxic drug, large dose necessarily leads to large toxicity, which cannot be withstood by the patient, so the calculation of dose for systemic intravenous chemotherapy cannot be calculated as per pharmacodynamics namely how much dose is needed to kill a certain number of cancer cells, but as per the

tolerance dose of the patient to the cytotoxic drug just because the patient cannot withstand it if it exceeds the tolerance dose of the cytotoxic drug as the too large toxicity will endanger the life. In the recent 30-40 years, the systemic intravenous chemotherapy is widely used to the solid tumor or the assistant chemotherapy after operation and there have been various international chemotherapy standard schemes. the schemes and the guides indicate the kind of drug, the dose mg/m², from which day to which day, iv or others, indicating how many days are a cycle. The schemes are universal, no matter the side of the solid tumor, no matter whether the solid tumor is ablated or not, the schemes are all the same, the same to the calculation of the dose, which are not individualized. Since the dose determined for each scheme is determined as per the tolerance dose of the cytotoxic drug undertaken by the patient instead of the effective dose. It is calculated as per the distribution of the systemic intravenous chemotherapy in the whole body, therefore, the calculation of the dose for solid tumor and the assistant chemotherapy after operation is not reasonable and scientific just because the normal tissues of the viscera shall not be killed by the cytotoxic drug, which shall be seriously analyzed, individualized, further researched and reformed.

3. Analysis, evaluation and doubt of curative effect evaluation criteria of systemic intravenous chemotherapy for solid tumor

The evaluation criteria of curative effects on solid tumor at present include:

1. Size of tumor: it shall be measured in every examination.

   (1) Shrinkage of measurable volume of tumor and/or metastatic lesion: indicating the degree of shrinkage with the arithmetic product of the max. diameter (cm) and its diameter (cm) of the tumor;
   (2) As to the tumor with immeasurable size, the method for improvement of disease is the calcification of osteolytic tumor again, as to the celiac tumor that cannot be easily measures shall be expressed with the estimated shrinkage value.

2. Remission stage: the remission stage shall begin from the treatment. In both checks in the treatment stage, the tumor grows up once again, the arithmetic product of its orthogonal diameters increases over 25%. The remission stage is calculated in days, weeks or months.

3. Evaluation criteria of size of solid tumor

   CR (complete remission; evidently effective): the tumor disappears entirely, lasting over 4 weeks;
   PR (partial remission; effective): the arithmetic product of two diameters of the tumor is shrunk to over 50%;
   MR (middle remission): the tumor is shrunk to over 25% and below 50%;
   NC (or S, stable, unchanged): the tumor is shrunk to below 25% and enlarged to below 25%;
   PD (or P, progressive; deteriorative): the tumor is enlarged to over 25% or new lesion appears.

Analysis and discussion

1. The above-mentioned curative effect criteria of systemic chemotherapy for solid tumor is summarized in three points: size of tumor, remission and remission period.

Chemotherapy and radiotherapy only kill the differentiated and matured tumor cells rather than the stem cells of the tumor accounting for 0.1%~1.0% of the tumor cells. The remained stem cells of tumor are differentiated and proliferated once again, forming new tumor, with the clinical menifetation of recurrence and metastasis of tumor as well as the failure of treatment, resulting in death of the patient.

At present, although the chemotherapy drug for clinical application can shrink the tumor, the effects are commonly temporary and it cannot obviously prolong the life of the patient. Therefore, the curative effect evaluation criterion is referred to as remission, the remission stage is calculated in days, weeks or months, for example, the complete remission only means the tumor disappears entirely, lasting over 4 weeks, indicating it may recur after 4 weeks. What is meant by remission? I understand it as follows: we rope an animal, then untie it for two hours and then rope it again, in this way, the untying is referred to as remission, the two hours of untying is the remission stage, obviously, remission is not the treatment objective of the patient, the patient is hospitalized for chemotherapy, undertaking the pains and the risks from the side reaction of the cytotoxic drug for chemotherapy, only getting a temporary remission at most, which is apparentlyteh requirements and treatment objective of the patient hospitalized for chemotherapy, which shall not be the objective of clinical treatment.

2. Why chemotherapy only can play a role in remission? Because:

(1) The cytotoxic drug for chemotherapy only can kill the differentiated and matured cancer cells rather than the undifferentiated or immature stem cells or the ones to be differentiated and matured, the chemotherapy drug kills the differentiated and matured cancer cells at this time, however, after a time, the undifferentiated and immature cancer cells are gradually differentiated and matured, the tumor cells are uninterruptedly and progressively divided, proliferated and cloned, one is divided into two, and two into four, in this way, it is multiplied in form of geometric progression, at the same time, the period of effectively killing cancer cells of the patient through chemotherapy drug is only 1~5 days of intravenous drip, that is to say, it only lasts 5-6 days for taking the effects on killing the cancer cells, the so-called cycle of 3-4 weeks only means that the white blood cells and the blood platelets with bone marrow inhibited can be recovered within 3-4 weeks and withstand the second chemotherapy.

(2) Since the chemotherapy drug only can kill the differentiated and matured cancer cells rather than the undifferentiated stem cells of the tumor or the ones being differentiated, the chemotherapy only can merely alleviate the symptoms, but it cannot treat the root cause, it only can be regarded as the assistant treatment, but not as the radical treatment because the principles of chemotherapy do not conform to the biological characteristics and behaviors of the cancer cells. Although chemotherapy can temporarily shrink the tumor, it cannot obviously prolong the life and one of the reasons why the treat fails is that the tumor cells loss the drug resistance, maybe another reason is the existing therapeutic methods cannot

213

effectively kill the stem cells of the tumor, the treatment of cancer through chemotherapy may be said that "no prairie fire can destroy the grass, it shoots up again with the spring breeze blows". Why? Because the grass is burn, but the root is remained, only some matured cancer cells rather than the stem cells of tumor to be differentiated and matured are killed, the stem cells of tumor will be continually divided and cloned in form of geometrical progression.

(3) The judgment of the curative effects on tumor shall not regard the size of the tumor as the standard: the objective of existing tumor chemotherapy and radiotherapy is mainly to reduce the volume and number of the tumor cells just because they often determine the curative effects by means of the capability of shrinking the tumor, in fact, "the big" does not mean "the bad" and "the small" does not mean "the good". The clinic judgment of chemotherapy at present, no matter the clinic or the sickroom, is mainly based on CT and MRI as well as space occupation, as a matter of fact, the space occupation is not the size of the solid tumor because the peripheric tissue of the solid tumor may affect the space occupation. I am a surgeon and I have been engaged in medicine practice for 54 years and performed over 5000 radical and abscission operations for cancers at breast or abdomen. The size of the tumor seen in the operation has not been always consistent with the one reported in CT and MRI. In addition, although some solid tumors are as large as a fist even larger than a fist, when they are incised, the cancer cells inside is not dense while there are so many interfibrillar interstitial tissues; although some solid tumors are only as large as a table tennis, when then are incised, there are so many highly malignant cancer cells inside, the latter is more malignant than the former. Therefore, I think "the big" does not means "the bad" and "the small" does not means "the good", which cannot be regarded as the standard. We also find from a large batch of tumor-bearing animal models in the lab that although the hypodermically inoculated experimental tumors of some tumor-bearing experimental mice are very large, the cancer cells of the central tissue of the transplanted solid tumor are unlike to the peripheral cancer cells, the mode center is mostly aseptically necrotic or liquefied while its periphery is the active cancer cells, although its volume is increased, the malignancy is low.

This topic is the core content in Chapter 11 in my third book "new concepts and new methods of cancer treatment" Chapter 11 which put forward the "analysis and questioning of solid tumor systemic intravenous chemotherapy, solid tumor systemic intravenous chemotherapy drug pathways were analyzed." Take the chemotherapy drug 5-Fu as an example:

5-Fu intravenous chemotherapy 100rng / d * 5 = 5000mg, 99.6% of the chemotherapy cytotoxic effect of intravenous drip systemic chemotherapy work on the patient's normal cells, only 0.4% of the drug to reach the foci, So its role is minimal, very little effect, too much damage to the patient. So it is put forward that : is it reasonable? Is it science?

Through this analysis and demonstration, this route of administration is unwise and unreasonable and unscientific, there is damage to the patient. Should be corrected, should be reformed, should be reformed. However, this reform will be involved in the chemotherapy in the various levels of the hospitals, involved the world's hospital oncology chemotherapy work, and should be reformed.

At present, all countries in the world, the provinces and cities around the province of the Department of Oncology and Chemotherapy are so, the solid tumor of the body intravenous chemotherapy need to get the common comments and to be a consensus, to have the gradual reform, involving very deep, very wide.

This paper is the first time in the international community that to raise this problem and the drawbacks, pointing out its shortcomings of **the use of traditional chemotherapy in the world for more than 40 years of traditional chemotherapy** - systemic intravenous chemotherapy systemic distribution, this paper is the first in the world to raise this problem, pointing out its shortcomings of the route of administration and Contradiction, that it is detrimental to the patient, and the first time in the academic community to evaluate its unreasonable, unscientific, will cause the world, the whole Chinese oncology vibration, causing tens of thousands of cancer patients shocked. (See Chapter 11, P76) (here is the first published in this book as a new doctrine for independent innovation).

2. THE CENTURY REVIEW AND ANALYSIS AND COMMENT OF THE THREE TRADITIONAL TREATMENT OF CANCER

Three traditional cancer treatments : surgical treatment, radiotherapy and chemotherapy have been for nearly a hundred years. How are the results of these treatment? **It should conduct some centuries review and evaluation for their efficacy, from theory to practice, to the efficacy; in the future can the three major treatment be relied on to overcome cancer? how are its prospects assessed? The evaluation criteria are: reduce morbidity, reduce mortality, prolong survival, improve quality of life, reduce complications.**

We should stop and calm down and collate, analyze, review, reflect, sum up the success and failure of both positive and negative experience and lessons. What are the results? What lessons are there? Did the patient benefit? Whether is it to prolong life and reduce the pain? you should carefully analyze the successful experience, conscientiously sum up the lessons of failure, find out the problems, find out the experience and lessons.

Should it think about why traditional therapy did not significantly reduce mortality? Should it think about why traditional therapy does not control recurrence and transfer? Should it think about why the three treatment has been nearly a hundred years, and now the cancer mortality rate is still the number one and the first in the city of China and township residents?

I entered the Tongji Medical College for 63years and has been 60 years for cancer surgery clinical medical work and experienced and witnessed the three traditional treatments for half a century. Deeply it is thought about how to evaluate the efficacy of these treatments with the century.

What are the treatment effects of cancer patients? It is often considered to be: patients with long survival time and the good quality of life, the improved symptoms and fewer complications.

The above three traditional major means of cancer has made a brilliant contribution for the human cancer treatment,however, until the two decades of the 21st century, cancer is still rampant; the more treatment ; the more patients; the incidence of cancer continues to rise and it has high mortality and it remains the first cause of death in China's urban and rural areas. Although the patient has undergone the regular and systemic radiotherapy and / or chemotherapy after surgery, it has not been able to prevent the recurrence of cancer cells.

Why did not traditional treatment significantly reduce mortality? Does it suggest that traditional therapies do not meet the biological characteristics of cancer cells? What is the problem with traditional radiotherapy and chemotherapy? What is the traditional concept of cancer therapies? What is theoretically or conceptual problem? How can its concept or understanding of the shortcomings be corrected so that it can be the more perfect?

The review of the traditional concept

The traditional concept of cancer is the continuous division of cancer cells, proliferation; the target of treatment must be cancer cells, therefore, the traditional three treatment goals is to establish on the basis of the traditional model of killing cancer cells.

The principle basis of the current cancer is based on the following premise, that is, in order to achieve cure, it must kill the last cancer cell or the last cancer cell is killed or eliminated. Therefore, people use the expansion surgery, chemotherapy and radical radiotherapy; but the results are not ideal. In the early 1960s, the scope of tumor surgery is expanded and developed a series of radical surgery. After years of practice it is proved that to expand the scope of surgical resection, such as breast cancer, lung cancer, liver cancer, pancreatic cancer, etc failed to improve its cancer-free survival and overall survival. In the 1980s, the intensive chemotherapy and radical radiotherapy did not improve the quality of life or prolong survival, but because of severe inhibition in bone marrow hematopoietic function and immune function, it is increasing the number of life-threatening complications.

Therefore, it makes us realize that the three treatment means must be further studied and improved: the problems and drawbacks of the surgery and radiotherapy and chemotherapy should be analyzed and commented.

The reviews of surgical treatment:

Comments 1: Surgery is the effective treatment of malignant tumors, even if the cancer treatment has developed the multidisciplinary treatment today, surgery is still one of the most important and the most common means the treatment of malignant tumors and is an important part of a multi-disciplinary comprehensive treatment.

Comment 2: Surgical treatment is the main treatment of solid tumors, but the "radical surgery" design ineeds to be further studied and improved to reduce postoperative recurrence and metastasis. It should pay attention to intraoperative "tumor suppression technology" to reduce or prevent intraoperative cancer cell shedding, planting, transfer. It should pay attention to surgical operation light, stable, accurate, to reduce intraoperative promotion of cancer cell metastasis and reduce cancer cells spread from the tumor vein. To prevent postoperative recurrence and metastasis must start from surgery. It must pay attention to the non-tumor technology and to prevent the transplant and implant metastasis in the incision and drainage sites.

Comments 3: after a century of historical evaluation the solid tumor surgery is still the most important and the most reliable and it is the main treatment method which can rely on and is the main science and technology and the main treatment method for conquering cancer in the future.

Radiotherapy:

Comment 1: radiotherapy to be further studied and improved, the current radiotherapy on the patient's radiation damage protection is poor, whether for radiation diagnosis or radiation therapy, the hospital attention to the physician's protective measures, did not attach importance to the patient's protective equipment, So that patients suffer from radiation damage.

Comment 2: radiation therapy is killing cancer cells at the same time, but also killing a large number of normal tissue cells so that patients are suffering from the torture of the radiation therapy complications, the quality of life decreased, the radiotherapy and toxic effects and damage are generally persistent and irreversible, and therefore it must pay attention to the prevention of the complications of tumor radiotherapy.

Comments 3: Since the 20th century, the goal of cancer treatment is aimed at primary cancer and metastases cancer cancer cells. Despite the efforts of a century, the mortality rate of cancer still accounts for the first rate of human disease mortality, the main reason for such a high mortality rate is the transfer.

The original traditional therapy failed to reduce the long-term high mortality rate, the main reason for its failure is not for the transfer, control transfer.

Radiotherapy is the topical treatment and cancer metastasis is the systemic problems, which is a major contradiction. How to play a role in anti-metastatic therapy must be carefully considered and studied in depth.

Today, the most important problem of cancer treatment is how to resist the transfer. If you can not solve the problem of cancer metastasis, cancer treatment can not move forward. Therefore, one of the goals of cancer treatment in the 21st century should be how to prevent metastasis, but radiotherapy for local treatment, nasopharyngeal carcinoma, laryngeal cancer, lymphoma, cervical cancer, etc. have achieved good results, but it can not be anti- The

Chemotherapy:

<u>Chemotherapy need to be further studied and improved.</u> Does postoperative adjuvant chemotherapy prevent recurrence? Whether to prevent the transfer? How can we help prevent postoperative recurrence and metastasis, which is worthy of our in-depth thinking, research, so should come up with our own data and experience to carry out further research and refinement.

Through the review, reflection, it was summed up the analysis of successful experience and failure of the lessons, people gradually realize that in the current real truncation systemic intravenous chemotherapy there are some important problems and drawbacks worth pondering and analysis and evaluation and re-discussion.

<u>The problems and disadvantages of systemic intravenous chemotherapy</u>

<u>The Analysis and evaluation and questioning of the route of systemic intravenous chemotherapy for solid tumors</u>

The current status of tumor chemotherapy is mainly systemic intravenous chemotherapy; this systemic intravenous chemotherapy route of administration is:

Chemotherapy Cell toxic drugs → Elbow Vein → Upper Venous Vein → Right Heart → Left Heart → Aorta

↓

Spray to the whole body

↓

1.Cancer lesions get about 0.4% of the doses of the medications

2. the normal tumor-free organs and tissues (brain, heart, liver, lung, kidney, bone marrow … …) of the body recieved about 99.6% of the dose

Comment 1: Comment on the route of administration of systemic intravenous chemotherapy

This route of administration was not fixed-point targeted administration, but through the heart pump to the chemotherapy cell poison with the blood spray to the body so that cytotoxic has the whole systemic distribution and so that the normal organs (brain, Lung, kidney, bone marrow) of the body obtain chemotherapy cytotoxic and are damaged, leading to toxic side effects. It is very unreasonable, very unscientific, the result is:

① very few foci cancer can get the medications, only about 0.4%, minimal effect (due to cancer foci accounted for a very small proportion of the body surface area)

② 99.6% of the cytotoxic drugs are killed to the normal body of normal cells, causing brain, heart, liver, lung, kidney, bone marrow, gastrointestinal system, hematopoietic system, immune system, endocrine system toxicity.

All of these toxicity reactions are caused by the treatment design and unreasonable route of the drug administration and can be avoided.

③ the current hospital chemotherapy drugs were not for drug sensitivity test, if the drug is resistant, then the whole chemotherapy are to kill normal tissue cells! Especially to the inhibition of bone marrow hematopoietic cells and immune cells! On the foci it is no effect! (it is in vain of that is done once a chemotherapy!)

④ so does every chemotherapy kill cancer cells? It does not know how much to kill? It does not know, and it can only be said to have once chemical work.

Therefore, this route of administration is unreasonable, unscientific, easily lead to iatrogenic side effects.

How to do? Should change the route of administration, to target organ tissue chemotherapy within the pathways, the drug directly to the "target organ", so the dose is very small, the effect is certain, no side effects, is conducive to the patient.

<u>Comment 2: the dose calculation of the assessment of solid body tumor intravenous chemotherapy</u>

① because the whole body intravenous chemotherapy is not targeted delivery, but systemic coverage, systemic distribution, it is necessary to have a large amount of cytotoxic drugs, and the need for multi-drug combination is likely to make a very small area of cancer foci may reach ease Of the required dose. So the dose slightly larger, then toxic side effects increase, so this dose calculation is unreasonable.

② This is the experience and methods of leukemia treatment extended to the solid tumor treatment, the guiding ideology is the whole body surface area of administration, it is unwise, unreasonable.

why?

Because leukemia cells are distributed in the systemic blood circulation system, the treatment of the "target" also exists in the systemic blood circulation system, so the use of systemic intravenous chemotherapy is reasonable, wise, but also in line with targeted therapy.

However, solid tumors are confined to an organ whose target "target" should be an organ suffering from cancer and should be targeted at the target organ's intravascular route. It should not use the leukemia treatment experience of the body surface area calculated medication, it is unwise, unreasonable.

But now solid tumors are all having systemic intravenous chemotherapy, according to the body surface area to calculate dose, in order to achieve the purpose of cancer shrinkage, the inevitable need is to increase the amount of chemotherapy cells poisoning, it will lead to more toxic side effects and complications, damage the patient.

How to do?

It should change the route of administration and change into target organ intravascular chemotherapy; this dose is very small, the effect is certain, no side effects, and is conducive to patients.

<u>Comment 3: The Evaluation and evaluation of the evaluation criteria for the efficacy of systemic intravenous chemotherapy</u>

The current assessment of the efficacy of solid tumors are: a, tumor size; b, remission: the general use of days, weeks, months to express.

①why the evaluation of the standard as a mitigation?

At present, the clinical use of chemotherapy drugs can shrink the tumor, but the effect is usually temporary, and can not significantly extend the patient's life. Therefore, the efficacy evaluation criteria are called "mitigation". Generally with days, weeks or months to calculate, such as complete remission which is completely disappeared tumor only sustains more than 4 weeks, that is, 4 weeks later it may recur and progress.

What is mitigation? Play one by one to explain the relief, with a rope to tied up an animal, and then let it loose rope tied for 2 hours and then tied up. This release rope even if the ease of relaxation 2 hours is the remission period.

Obviously, remission is not the purpose of patient treatment; the patient is hospitalized for chemotherapy, suffering the toxicity and risk of toxic effects from chemotherapy, however it only obtains a brief remission, which is clearly not the patient to hospital treatment requirements and treatment purposes, but not the purpose of clinical care.

Mitigation, as the name suggests is palliative treatment, palliative is unable to rule, but the temporary effect, the patient to bear the pain and risk of chemotherapy cytotoxic toxicity, only for a temporary effect, ease.

② why chemotherapy can only alleviate?

a, the effective time to kill cancer cells of the patients with chemotherapy to kill is only 3-5 days of the intravenous infusion which have the role of killing cancer cells, and then there is no the role of killing cancer cells, it is only a short time to kill about (3-5 Day), cannot once and for all, after 3-5 days the cancer cells continue to split and go on proliferation, so it can only alleviate a short time, can not be cured, so it is ease (CR, PR) - As the name suggests, to ease is not cured and it is only the short time,that is, several weeks to get better, after this short time better, then can develop further and increase and metasatasis, therefore, to ease (CR, PR) is not the ultimate goal of treatment and not the desired purpose of the patient and the family, the patient is suffering the possible risk of the toxicity from the treatment of chemotherapy and the drug, but it only may be short-term relief. (As the following Figure 1)

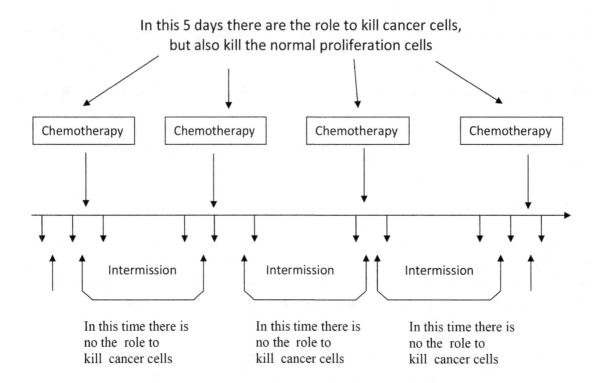

Fig1. The killing time peroid of chemotherapy

So chemotherapy can not be cured and can only alleviate and can only treat the symptoms and cannot treat the reason and can only adjuvant therapy and can not cure.

So chemotherapy cannot be cured and can only alleviate and can only palliative, and can not cure and can only adjuvant therapy and can not cure.

b, chemotherapy cell medication can only kill the differentiated mature cancer cells, can not kill yet undifferentiated and immature stem cells; this time the chemotherapy kills the differentiate mature cancer cells and after some time, those who have not yet matured stem cells gradually mature,and continue to division, proliferation, and divide into two, two for the four clones, in this way it is the geometric progression so that the foci is "wild fire burned, spring breeze and health", goes on the recurrence, metastasis and progresses. (As the following figure)

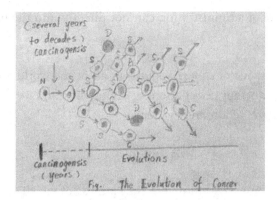

Figure The Cancer Evolution Diagram(several years to several decades)

The picture shows that the principle of chemotherapy does not meet the biological characteristics of cancer cells and biological behavior. N: Normal cells; S:stem cells; T1,2,3: mutated stem cells; 2: stem cells, 4 stem cells: polyploid stem cells; turn: the formation of metastatic cancer stem cells; R: radiation-sensitive stem cells; Resistance: drug-resistant stem cells; D: Dependent-Drug stem cells; ascites: the stem cells adapt to the growth of thousands of cells in the chest and ascites; Dead: a cell where a lethal mutation occurred ; Anti: anti-radiation of the stem cells;

Comment 4: Comment on why the adjuvant chemotherapy after the abdominal solid tumor surgery failed to prevent recurrence, metastasis?

It is because the whole body intravenous chemotherapy cytotoxic medications are injected from the superior vena cava instead of the portal vein, is difficult to reach the portal vein; the vena cava system and portal vein system are generally not connected, this route of administration is unreasonable and unscientific.

Chemotherapy is to kill cancer cells with the drugs. First of all, it must be first clear where the patient's cancer cells are in order to be targeted, clear objectives? Along the line of cancer cell metastasis line it tracks the cancer cells of being transferred in the way.

Where are the cancer cells in the abdominal solid tumor (gastric cancer, colorectal cancer, liver cancer, biliary cancer, pancreatic cancer, abdominal and other malignant tumors? It is mainly in the portal vein system, but in the current global and all of the hospital in China the abdominal solid tumor postoperative adjuvant chemotherapy is given by the elbow vein → superior vena cava → right heart → lungs → left heart → aorta → spray to the body organs. But it can not directly go into the portal vein system because the vena cava system and the portal vein system are generally not connected.

Therefore, in the abdominal malignant tumors (stomach, intestine, liver, gallbladder, pancreas, abdominal and other cancers), after the abdominal surgery the vein route of administration of the adjuvant chemotherapy injected by the elbow vein → venous is unreasonable, is unscientific, does not meet the anatomy and physiological pathology, and does not meet the reality of cancer cell metastasis pathways, because this route of administration can not directly into the presence of cancer cells in the portal vein system.

For half a century, the thousands of cancer patients in all of the world and in China are suffering from the great pain of chemotherapy cells poisoning killing the normal cells of great pain. Clinicians should seriously think, analyze, reflect and evaluate.

How to do?

It should change the route of administration into the pathway of which chemotherapy medication is given inside the target organ vessels so that drugs can directly go into the portal vein, for the solid tumor medication should not be administered by the elbow vein, but should be changed to target organ intravascular administration, the drug targets reaching the target organ foci, which will greatly reduce the dose, improve the efficacy, will certainly reduce or eliminate the toxic side effects of chemotherapy, so that tens of thousands of cancer patients can avoid suffering from the pain and risk of the adverse reactions of chemotherapy and it is for the benefit of patients. To reduce or eliminate the toxic side effects of chemotherapy is bound to greatly reduce the medical costs and will be for the country, for patients to save more medical expenses and help solving the problem of that it is difficult to get medical treatment and the medical cost is expensive, this reform will be tens of thousands of cancer patient benefit.

Comment 5: Comment on there are some important errors in the current chemotherapy

Why did the patient postoperative chemotherapy fail to prevent the recurrence of cancer from the analysis and reflection of the clinical practice of cases?

From the analysis and reflection of the role of chemotherapy drugs in the cancer cell cycle ; from the analysis and reflection of the overall inhibition of chemotherapy to the immune function ; from the analysis and reflection of the drug resistance to chemotherapy it is found that :

①there are still some important errors in the current chemotherapy; the current chemotherapy still exists several major contradictions and needs to be further research and improvement.

It should be updated thinking and update awareness.

After the review, analysis, evaluation and self-reflection of 7 years of experimental experiments and 30 years of specialist outpatient clinics more than 6,000 cases of diagnosis and treatment, it is summed up the success and failure of both positive and negative experience and lessons, thinks of why the traditional therapy did not significantly reduce the death Rate? why did not it control relapse and transfer? What are the questions of the traditional concept of traditional therapy? So I gradually realize that the current cancer traditional therapies may still have some important errors. For example: ① the traditional chemotherapy suppresses the immune function and inhibit the bone marrow hematopoietic function:

It is well known that consist of central immune organs and peripheral immune organs, the former ones are thymus and marrow, the later are spleen and lymph node.

When patients are in chemotherapy, their three immune organs suffer damage (see Fig. 1), which leads to the decrease in immune function. Literature and the experimental results by the author have proved that when cancer emerges, tumors can produce a kind of immunorepressive factor (called factor of inhibiting thymus by cancer temporarily) and make thymus atrophied gradually. At the same time, chemotherapy also inhibits marrow. For the patients with cancer, the inhibition of both thymus and marrow by the chemotherapeutic cytotoxic drug make the function of the entire central immune organs inhibited, which reduces the holistic immune function as one disaster after disaster.

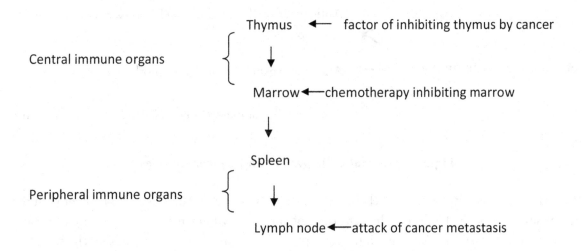

Figure 3. Cancer when the immune organs are damaged

② the conventional intravenous chemotherapy is the intermittent treatment; in the intermittent period cancer can not be treated and intermittent cancer cells continue to proliferate and divide;

③ traditional therapy damage the host, because the chemotherapy cell poison for the "double-edged sword", both kill cancer cells and kill normal cells;

④ traditional therapy goal only focuses on that chemotherapy can kill cancer cells, while ignoring the host itself on cancer resistance and control because the occurrence and development of the tumor depends on the level of host immune function and the biological characteristics of the tumor itself, that is determined by The biological characteristics of tumor cells and the host of the constraints on the impact of the two potential, if it is the balance, cancer is controlled; if the two are imbalance, cancer is progress. Traditional radiotherapy and chemotherapy are to promote the decline in immune function and it may make the two more potential imbalance;

⑤ Traditional therapy neglects the anti-cancer ability of the human body itself, ignores the role of anticancer cells (NK cell population, K cell population, LAK cell population, macrophage population, TK cell population) in the host cancer system and ignores the role of the host of the anti-cancer cytokine system IFN, IL-2, TNF, LT and ignores the role of the host of the tumor suppressor gene and tumor suppressor gene (the human body has oncogenes and tumor suppressor genes, but also cancer metastasis gene and tumor suppressor gene) and ignores the role of the neurohumoral system and endocrine hormone system in the body and ignores the role of anti-cancer agencies and their influencing factors in the human body, as well as its role of the regulation, balance and stabilization of the host mechanism itself and ignores the inherent factors of the human body's anti-cancer activity, Blindly kill cancer cells (Figure 4)

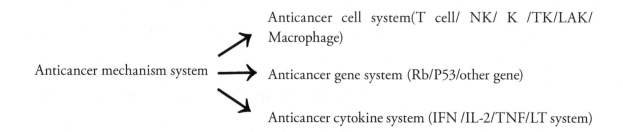

Anticancer mechanism system → Anticancer cell system(T cell/ NK/ K /TK/LAK/ Macrophage)

Anticancer gene system (Rb/P53/other gene)

Anticancer cytokine system (IFN /IL-2/TNF/LT system)

Figure 4 Schematic diagram of anti-cancer agencies

⑥ traditional therapy goal is relatively simple, just kill cancer cells. And it is not consistent with the actual situation of the biological characteristics of cancer now known such as cancer cell invasion behavior; the metastasis is involved in the multiple steps; the incentives factors of the relapse can be the latent months or years and then have recurrence. It has been recognized that antineoplastic agents are not necessarily resistant to metastasis and the anti-metastatic drugs are not necessarily anti-tumor.

If there are the problems as the above-mentioned, we should further study, and we should update our thinking, update our understanding and move forward under the reform and look forward to innovate. Innovation must have the challenge to the traditional ideas and it is not substitute. But it is to overcome the shortcomings and to correct its shortcomings so that it is more perfect. Innovation also has another way and find a new way to overcome cancer. To this end, specially it is put forward the anti-cancer new ideas, new concepts, new principles, new treatment mode; according to the biological characteristics of cancer and the host's immune status and the multi-step, multi-link of metastasis it takes a comprehensive model of comprehensive treatment to be reformed, innovated and developed.

(2) to recognize that the radiotherapy and chemotherapy exist the problems and drawbacks which is difficult to be relied on conquering cancer so that it is put forward the need to launch a general attack. (Abstract, brief introduction)

① Review of the traditional three treatments in the century and historical evaluation

Surgical treatment:

Comment 1 - Surgery is the exact and effective way to treat cancer

Comments 2 - "radical surgery" design need to be further studied and improved

Rating 3 - Surgery is the main treatment for cancer in the future

Radiotherapy:

Comment I- does not attach importance to the patient's protective equipment and facilities

Comments 2 it must pay attention to the prevention and treatment of radiation therapy complications

Comment 3 - Radiotherapy for topical treatment, it can not be anti-metastatic, cancer metastasis for systemic problems, which is a major contradiction.

The key to cancer treatment is how to resist metastasis

Chemotherapy

Comment1: The route of administration of systemic intravenous chemotherapy is not targeted, but the whole body is distributed, and the route of administration is unreasonable, unscientific, Iatrogenic side effects. why? Because through the administration from this route 99.6% of the cytotoxic will kill normal cells, only 0.4% of the dose may kill cancer cells.

Comment 2: The evaluation of the dose of intravenous chemotherapy is to extend the experience and methods of leukemia treatment to solid tumor treatment, the guiding ideology is calculated by the body surface area, which is unwise, unreasonable, will damage Patient, easily lead to iatrogenic side effects, why? It is unreasonable because the solid tumor is confined to an organ and should not be calculated with the body surface area.

Comment 3: Evaluation of the evaluation criteria for the efficacy of systemic intravenous chemotherapy

The current solid tumor evaluation criteria are: a, tumor size; b, remission, remission (CR. PR) - As the name suggests, ease is not cured, just a few weeks of traditional put, chemotherapy goal is relatively simple, just kill cancer cells. And is not consistent with the current understanding of the biological behavior of cancer cells and biological characteristics of the actual situation.

Such as cancer cell invasion behavior; metastasis and multiple steps; relapse incentives, latent months, years and recurrence. It is now recognized that anticancer drugs are not necessarily resistant to metastasis, anti-transfer drugs do not have to kill cancer cells.

Both the above problems, should be further studied, should be updated thinking, change the concept, based on the reform, in the reform forward, innovation. Innovation, there must be a challenge to the traditional concept, to correct its shortcomings, to make it more perfect. Innovation, but also another way to find a new way to overcome cancer.

(2) to recognize the release, chemotherapy problems and drawbacks difficult to rely on the case of cancer, put forward the need to launch a general attack. (Abstract, brief introduction)

① Review of the traditional three treatments in the century and historical evaluation

Surgical treatment:

Comment 1 - Surgery is the exact and effective way to treat cancer

Comments 2 - "radical surgery" design to be further studied and improved

Rating 3 - Surgery is the main treatment for cancer in the future

Radiotherapy:

Comment I- does not attach importance to the patient's protective equipment and facilities

Comments 2 1 must pay attention to the prevention and treatment of radiation therapy complications

Comment 3 - Radiotherapy for topical treatment, it can not be anti-metastatic, cancer metastasis for systemic problems, which is a major contradiction.

The key to cancer treatment is how to resist metastasis

Chemotherapy

Comment 1: The route of administration of systemic intravenous chemotherapy is not targeted, but the whole body is distributed, and the route of administration is unreasonable, unscientific, Iatrogenic side effects. why? Because of this route of administration, 99.6% of the cytotoxic to kill normal cells, only 0.4% of the dose may kill cancer cells.

Comment 2: The evaluation of the body dose of the intravenous chemotherapy of solid body tumor

The calculation of the dose is to extend the treatment of leukemia experience and methods to solid tumor treatment. Its guiding ideology is calculated by the whole body surface area. It is unwise, unreasonable, will damage the patient, easily lead to iatrogenic side effects, why? It is unreasonable because the solid tumor is confined to an organ and should not be calculated with the body surface area.

Comments 3:

The evaluation of Evaluation Criteria for Evaluation of Curative Effect of Chemotherapy in the body solid tumor:

The Current solid tumor efficacy evaluation criteria are: a, tumor size; b, remission,

Relief (CR. PR) - As the name implies, the remission is not cured, Just a few short weeks of improvement. After this short-term improvement, it Will progress, increase, transfer so that the ease is not the purpose of treatment, it can not be cured and can only alleviate, and only short-term relief so that the ease is not the purpose of the patient and should not be the goal of treatment, it is unreasonable.

Comments 4

Why did the abdomen solid tumor fail to prevent recurrence, metastasis after adjuvant chemotherapy? In the Abdominal solid tumors (gastric cancer, cancer, colorectal cancer, menstrual cancer, cholangiocarcinoma, pancreatic cancer, abdominal tumor) the postoperative adjuvant chemotherapy are systemic intravenous chemotherapy, this way from the vena cava can not directly reach the portal vein. Abdominal solid tumor cancer cells mainly are in the portal vein system; the vena cava system and portal vein system is generally not connected. From the superior vena cava it is not easy to reach the portal vein so that this route of administration is unreasonable and does not meet the anatomy.

Comments 5

There are some important errors and shortcomings in current chemotherapy

  a, chemotherapy inhibits the immune function and inhibits the bone marrow hematopoietic function so that the overall immune function declines, and cancer thymus is inhibited, and chemotherapy inhibit bone marrow, as "worse or snow plus frog" which all cause to damage the central immune organs and it further reduce immune surveillance; it is possible to lead that while doing chemotherapy, it has metastasis ; the more chemotherapy and the more metastasis.
  b, the traditional intravenous chemotherapy is the intermittent treatment and during intermittent period cancer can not be treated, and intermittent cancer cells continue to proliferate, split, divided into two, two divided into four, cloning, and thus continue to increase the number of geometric series, Endless, spring and wind ".
  c, chemotherapy only has intravenous infusion of 1-5 days, can kill cancer cells, then no killing effect, and can not once and for all, then cancer cells continue to split, proliferation, will recur, increase, so it Can only alleviate, can not be cured.
  d, chemotherapy target cancer cells, is a one-sided treatment, and ignores the body's own anti-cancer ability, ignores the host anti-cancer system anti-cancer cell system (NK cells, K cells, LAK cells, macrophages), anti-cancer cells Factor gene (1FN-1L2-. ThF, LT and other factors) anti-cancer gene system (Rb gene, P53 gene), ignores the body's anti-cancer mechanism and its influencing factors, ignores the body's own anti-cancer internal factors which are not activated, mobilized, but it only blindly kills cancer cells and it is one-sided treatment view

and it is very unreasonable, it does not meet the biological characteristics of cancer cells and biological behavior.

The goal of the traditional radiotherapy and chemotherapy is relatively simple and is just to kill cancer cells. And it is not consistent with the current understanding of the biological behavior of cancer cells and biological characteristics of the actual situation. For example, cancer cell invasion behavior: metastasis and multiple steps; relapse incentives, latent months, or years and recurrence. It is now recognized that anticancer drugs are not necessarily resistant to metastasis and anti-transfer drugs do not have to kill cancer cells.

Both the above problems should be further studied, should be updated thinking, change the concept, based on the reform, in the reform forward, and courage to innovation.

Innovation must be a challenge to the traditional concept, to correct its shortcomings, to make it more perfect.

Innovation should also find another way and find a new way to overcome cancer.

Such as cancer cell invasion behavior; metastasis and multiple steps; relapse incentives, latent months, years and recurrence. It is now recognized that anticancer drugs are not necessarily resistant to metastasis, anti-transfer drugs do not have to kill cancer cells.

Both the above problems, should be further studied, should be updated thinking, change the concept, based on the reform, in the reform forward, innovation. Innovation, there must be a challenge to the traditional concept, to correct its shortcomings, to make it more perfect. Innovation, but also another way to find a new way to overcome cancer.

3. CHEMOTHERAPY NEEDS TO BE FURTHER RESEARCH AND IMPROVEMENT

- There are some important errors in current chemotherapy
- The main contradiction of traditional chemotherapy

一. Some Wrong Ways in Current Chemotherapy

1. Current chemotherapy emphasizes on only killing cancer cells and neglects to protect or even damage host cells

It is essential to attach importance to the interrelation and the interaction among host cells, tumors and drugs. Here chemotherapy is cytotoxic drug without selectivity, so it can not distinguish tumor cells and the normal with killing them together. The initial target of chemotherapy is to kill cancer cells; however, actually it also kills the proliferative cells of host cells that are damaged as a result. Especially, chemotherapy inhibits the immune system and medullary hemopoietic system of the host cells, which leads to the general decline in immune function. Consequently, that tumors are not monitored by immunity promotes the evolution of tumors. That is the reason why tumors are constringed or relieved temporary, but continue to increase and evolve after a while or even metastasize and relapse during the period of treatment. Therefore, there is one problem about chemotherapy that has not been paid much attention, namely taking no actions to protect host cells and their immune organs and immune function. The strategy of curing cancer is to destroy cancer cells protect autologous functions at the most.

2. Chemotherapy as cytotoxic drug can aggravate the inhibition on central immune organic

It is well known that consist of central immune organs and peripheral immune organs, the former ones are thymus and marrow, the later are spleen and lymph node.

When patients are in chemotherapy, their three immune organs suffer damage, which leads to the decrease in immune function. Literature and the experimental results by the author have proved that when cancer emerges, tumors can produce a kind of immunorepressive factor (called factor of inhibiting thymus by cancer temporarily) and make thymus atrophied gradually. At the same time, chemotherapy also inhibits marrow. For the patients with cancer, the inhibition of both thymus and marrow by the chemotherapeutic cytotoxic drug make the function of the entire central immune organs inhibited, which reduces the holistic immune function as one disaster after disaster.

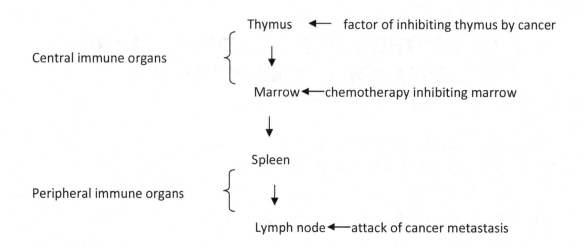

Lymph nodes in peripheral immune organs as well as the areas around the focus, and lymph nodes in the process of metastasis are invaded by cancer metastasis and lost partial function, which lead to further decrease in immune function consequently. It is inevitable that tumors will evolve further, relapse and metastasize with weak immune monitor or even without it.

Due to the decline in the holistic immune function, the anti-infection ability is weakened, so chemotherapy can not continue. There may be serious complications during the process of chemotherapy, such as mycotic superinfection, viral and infectious infection. However, the antibiotics can not control them efficiently. As a result, the patients die of immune function prostration.

3. During chemotherapy general untoward reaction may occur due to the effect of cytotoxic

During chemotherapy, general untoward reaction can bring down immune function, and lead to arrest of bone marrow, hepatic and nephric toxic reaction, gastrointestinal response dysfunction, phalacrosis, etc. However, there is no positive and effective protection currently.

Inhibition of marrow is a usual clinic toxic reaction as marrow is the organ to store hematopoietic stem cells. It is mainly the dynamic effect of antineoplastics to the specific stem cells that chemotherapeutic drugs destroy the specific stem cells in marrow, which can reduce the number of mature and functional blood corpuscles in peripheral blood. The degree of reduction is related to the lifetime of cell components in peripheral blood, for instance, the lifetime of hematid is long, so the number of hematid in the peripheral does not change apparently; while the lifetimes of blood platelet and granular cell groups are shorter with 3 days and 67 hours respectively, so the numbers of peripheral blood platelet and granular cell groups reduce rapidly if the groups of megakaryocytic stem cells and granular cell groups are destroyed. After administering drugs, stem cells increase the time of division to make up for the amount in the process of restoration.

Most antineoplastics can result in the gastrointestinal mucosa reaction by inhibiting gastrointestinal mucosa epithelial cells.

Many kinds of antineoplastics can lead to renal toxic reaction and also affect the excretion of drugs through the kidney. It must be noticed that the damage of renal function can aggravate the general toxic symptoms or worsen the inhibition of marrow. Many kinds of antineoplastics can damage liver in different degree and affect liver function.

Such serious geneal toxic reaction of chemotherapy can lead to nausea, vomit as well as anorexia, even being unable to take food. Consequently, the general anticancer ability declines obviously and the function of anticancer system of host cells is weakened apparently. The anticancer ability of organism and evolution of cancer are locked in a "zero-sum" game, which conduce to the further development of tumors.

4. Theoretic foundation of choosing chemotherapeutic drugs

Choosing chemotherapeutic is based on cell generation cycle and pathology and physiology of cancer, or accords to the principle of pharmacokinetics. The current chemotherapeutic scheme does not always accord with the theory of cell generation cycle. During the period of treatment (3-5d), cytotoxic drugs will inhibit cancer cells. After the treatment, these cancer cells continue to proliferate and divide. Currently, the use of chemotherapeutic drugs differs in different medical institution, in which some use the treatment of 5 days, others are 3 days; some of the used drugs aim at S stage and some are for M_1 stage. No matter the treatment is 3 to 5 days or 5 days, the effective period of cytotoxic drugs on cancer cells is less than 120 hours with cell generation cycle of 50 to 80 hours, so the treatment can only act on one and a half cell generation cycles. However, the proliferating cycle of cell mass continue for years, while the effect of chemotherapeutic drugs can only last from 3 to 5 days, so the effect of killing cancer cells can just happen at the stage of proliferating cycle when the drugs take effect, such as S stage, and then disappear. After the treatment of 3 or 5 days, cancer cells continue to proliferate and divide. As a result, tumors and the metastasized lymph nodes may shrink in volume, but they are likely to augment soon.

5. Failure to take actions to control cancer cells continuously and consolidate the effect at the interval of two times of chemotherapies

The treatment between two times of chemotherapies is blank, and the actions to continuous killing or control on cancer cells are not taken to consolidate the curative effect. What have been done is waiting the restoration of leucocytes and blood platelets to achieve the aim of stand chemotherapy next time. Actually, the treatment at the interval is very important, for cancer cells are out of control and proliferate and divide further positively and potentially at intervals due to the heavy decline in immune function. The more times of chemotherapies and the larger dosage of drugs, the more cytotoxic drugs will be used correspondently, so that the general immune function is worse and worse and the immunity of organism is less and less able to control the proliferation of oncocytes and prevent the metastasis leading to relapse and metastasize after continuous chemotherapies. Therefore, it is necessary to adopt immunological therapy or Chinese traditional medicine for regulating immunity to avoid relapse.

6. Theoretical foundation of postoperative auxiliary chemotherapy, the length of the intervals between two times of chemotherapies and the time of chemotherapy

The arrangements of chemotherapy differ in different locations and medical institutions, among which some use once a month or once every two months, some adopt six times in a row, or continuous four or eight times. The treatment is much blinder, especially postoperative auxiliary chemotherapy. The current arrangement of chemotherapeutic period is that only when leucocyte and blood platelet restore, can the next chemotherapy be taken. In fact, it is more helpless instead of meeting the pathological and physical demands (since the time of restoration is longer for some patients, when cancer cells have been in the process of division and proliferation continuously). What is the aim of auxiliary chemotherapy? How to achieve the aim? Are there any residual cancer cells in the body although the aim of chemotherapy is to kill cancer cells? Where do the cancer cells hide after surgeons, in the local of the surgeon, lymph nodes or in the blood? Taking gastrointestinal surgeon for instance, do the residual cancer cells hide in portal vein blood, or in celiac lymph nodes, or even in the local area of the surgeon? How long can the residual cancer cells lurk after surgeons before devastated by host cells? How to arrange the period of postoperative auxiliary chemotherapy? Knowing the location of cancer cells may be good for controlling the residual cancer cells in the area of surgeons and portal vein.

In a word, the current choice of postoperative auxiliary chemotherapy and the arrangement of chemotherapeutic period are very blind. It is essential to do further clinic research to ensure the indication, contraindication, medication and route of administration as well as a more uniform scheme so as to conclude analysis and evaluate.

7. Blindness of current chemotherapy

It may be helpful for some patients to take on chemotherapy blindly just according to experience, but it is harmful for a considerable number of patients. For instance, if some patient was resistant to this kind of drug, it would be harmful, rather than fruitless, for the cytotoxic drugs of chemotherapy can not act on cancer cells, instead of killing normal histiocyte, especially immunocyte, myeloid cell, which will lead to the prostration of immune function.

Drugsensitive test is a must to verify whether the patient is allergic to the used drugs. Only doing like this can ensure the accuracy of administering drugs. Currently, it is common that clinical administrate of drugs depends on experience blindly. Such blind administrate is potentially dangerous. If the drug is really sensitive to the patient's cancer cells, it will be effective (CR, PR). But if the drug is not sensitive to the cancer cells, it will only kill the normal cells and inhibit the marrow hematopiesis leading to the reduction in leucocyte and blood platelet as well as the decline in immune function without any damage on cancer cells, which will definitely promote the evolution of tumors and result in the prostration of immune function and hematopiesis. The decrease in immune function makes tumors be beyond the immune monitor and develop further, and then promote the relapse and metastasis. Therefore, it is necessary to take on individual drugsensitive test and drug resistant test.

8. Cure of cancer aims to kill tumors, reserve organism and regain health

The cure of cancer should always run through both strengthening health and wiping evil off, in which wiping evil off means inhibiting and killing cancer cells, clearing up lumps; strengthening health means protecting organismal ability to recognize dissidents, exciting the organismal positive factors of anti-cancer and improve the organismal ability to resist cancer. These two are dialectic and united. However, the current treatment on cancer only emphasizes killing cancer cells and ignores the protection of host cells, which damages the immune system and the system of marrow hematopiesis resulting in wiping both evil and health away. If tumors are drug resistant to this chemotherapeutic drug, it is likely to be harmful to health without wiping evil away. The treatment on cancer needs a scientific designed scheme, for cancer results from losing the balance between the organismal immune capacity of anti-cancer and the development of tumors, and from losing immune monitor, which leads to the further development of tumors. So it is necessary to try to restore the balance. Taking teeterboard in a children's playground for instance, tumor and the immunity of host cells represent the two ends of a teeterboard respectively. The comparison of the two parties' power decides the direction of tilt and the final result. Besides, the example of "scale" can be explained in the same way. However, chemotherapy does not emphasize the protection of host cells but promotes the diffuse and evolution of tumors.

9. Standards for the curative effects of chemotherapy should be good quality of life and prolonged lifetime

How to evaluate the curative effect of postoperative auxiliary chemotherapy? As the tumor has been ablated, it is unable to evaluate the effect in terms of its shrink.

Most patients only regard untoward reactions after chemotherapy, like decline in leucocyte and blood platelet, nausea and disgorge, anorexia, hypodynamia and abdominal distention as the curative effects, but they hardly realize that these symptoms are not the effects at all. It is unable to evaluate the postoperative curative effects until now. The current diagnostic methods are still laggard, as when tumors are detected, they have been very serious. Therefore, molecular biology is the only way to solve this problem.

Generally speaking, the standard for curative effects is remission. In terms of remission, the efficiency is defined as the shrink of the tumor, however, the quality of life is not improved and the lifetime is not prolonged, which is not the aim of handling diseases for the patients with cancer.

10. Anti-Carcinomatous drugs used currently can not always resist metastasis and relapse and the drugs for anti- carcinomatous metastasis and anti-cancer should be different

For many cases, postoperative auxiliary can not prevent relapse and metastasis, which relates to the fact that the current anti- carcinomatous drugs are not always able to resist metastasis and relapse besides other various possible factors mentioned above. Drugs for anti-metastasis should be different from anti-carcinomatous drugs as generally anti-cancer drugs have cytotoxicity and aim at killing cancer cells, destroying and inhibiting cell division and proliferation, whereas drugs for resisting metastasis are mainly used to resist the invasion of tumor cells, to antagonize the adherence of cancer cells inside the blood vessels, to inhibit the nascent micrangium and strengthen the organismal immunity to kill cancer cells. Most of anti- carcinomatous metastasis drugs have no cytotoxicity.

Research on anti-cancer drugs has stepped into a new stage. It is confronted with theoretical and technical renovations and the change in the train of thoughts when the field of research on anti-cancer drugs is not restricted to the traditional thoughts based on cytotoxic and the working method of cytotoxic drugs. New methods like inducement of differentiate, regulator of biological reaction, immunoregulation, genetherapy, combination of Chinese and western medicine, etc. have been taken into consideration in succession.

Although chemotherapy has been applied for sixty years, it is not satisfactory that many problems still exist reflected by the statistic, analysis and evaluation of applied information from a large number of clinical suffers. It is pitiful that cancer may metastasize and relapse after or during the process of chemotherapy.

In conclusion, the possible reasons that postoperative auxiliary chemotherapy is unable to prevent relapse and metastasis are, ①chemotherapeutant can promote the decline in immune function and inhibit hematopoiesis of marrow; ②failure to continue aftertreatment at the intervals of chemotherapies; ③chemotherapeutic drugs can not protect host cells; ④lumps may has drug resistance; ⑤chemotherapeutic drugs may be not sensitive; ⑥chemotherapeutic drugs for solid tumor may be not infiltrate into tumors; ⑦the arrangement of chemotherapeutic period is not reasonable; ⑧drugs may not act on the sensitive period of cell proliferation; ⑨it is difficult to restore immune function and hematopoiesis probably.

二,Main Contradictions in Traditional Chemotherapy

So far, the aim of chemotherapy has been still focusing on killing cancer cells. The majority of chemotherapeutic drugs are cytotoxic drugs without selectivity, so both cancer cells and normal ones will be damaged. Besides, chemotherapy has serious untoward reaction, suffers will have intensive feeling and have to give up the treatment at last. In the last ten years, the author has helped nearly ten thousand cancer cases in Wuchang Shuguang Tumorous Clinic, many of whom have tried chemotherapy. They came to anti-carcinomatous clinic for treatment as there were no curative effects after several periods of treatment. It can be implicated that auxiliary treatment does not prevent carcinomatous invasion, relapse and metastasis, and it also can not improve the quality of life and prolong lifetime obviously. Through the feedback of those cases, analysis, evaluation and reflection, the author have recognized that there are the following contradictions in traditional chemotherapy.

1. The contradiction between chemotherapeutic cytotoxic and the damage to host cells

The aim of curing tumor is to eliminate tumors and preserve the organism as well as regain health. However, currently the chemotherapeutic cytotoxic kills both cancer cells and the normal with internecine result of damaging host cells, which is the heavily unreasonable contradiction between cytotoxic and suffers (or host cells). What should be done is to try to eliminate or resist the effect of killing normal cells and to research positively on intelligent anti-carcinomatous drugs with selectivity.

2. The contradiction between succession and discontinuity

It means the contradiction between the continuous divisions of cancer cells and the discontinuous chemotherapeutic period of treatment. The division and proliferation of cancer cells are continuous according to cell cycle, but chemotherapeutic drugs can be used with intervals for they inhibit the hematopoiesis of marrow and the blood corpuscle in the peripheral, which results in the severe contradiction between continuous divisions and proliferation of cancer cells and the discontinuous chemotherapies. Cancer cells divide successively, whereas chemotherapies are of interval, so cancer cells continue to divide during the intervals. Even a large dosage of chemotherapeutic drugs can only kill limited number of cancer cells, but can not destroy the whole. Even the majority of the cancer cells can be killed during the 3 to 5 days with chemotherapeutic drugs, the residual tumorous stem cells will continue to divide, to proliferate, to clone, and then metastasize and relapse when the effects of medicine fade away after several days. Therefore, killing cancer cells simply does not accord with the biological traits and behavior of cancer cells.

3. The contradiction between increase and decrease in immunity

That chemotherapeutic drugs usually can reduce the immunity contradicts the fact that the treatment on cancer should improve the immunity. As chemotherapeutic drugs can weaken the immunity, the longer the period of treatment, the more decrease in immunity, which promotes the decline in immunity, and even leads to lose monitor and the further development of tumors. This unreasonable contradiction between chemotherapy and immunity can weaken the curative effects heavily and even lead to diffuse. Therefore, treatment on tumors must aim at improving immunity and restoring immune monitor so as to stabilize the cancer, to make it and regain health.

4. The contradiction between periods of treatment and curative effects

That chemotherapy can inhibit marrow forces the peripheral leucocytes and blood platelets decline, so it is necessary to design the time of administering with intervals, which means the next time of chemotherapy should be taken on after restoration. Currently the intervals are just for waiting, instead of taking any measure to control cell division. On one hand cancer cells proliferate successively, on the other hand the chemotherapy stops. Due to this contradiction, it is difficult to gain the curative effects though chemotherapy. The more times of chemotherapy, the more serious immune inhibition will be, the more actively cancer cells proliferate during intervals, which results in evolution and metastasis during the process of chemotherapy.

5. The contradiction between the period when drugs act and the cell cycle during the period of administer through intravenous drip

It is only effective when the time of administer meets the sensitive cycle of cancer cells. If not, it is of no effect. Chemotherapeutic administer aims at cell cycles. During the period of administer, the cell cycles of most cancer cells in the crowds are not simultaneous but much different from each other, for instance, administer via intravenous drip from 8 am to 10 am when some of the cancer cells are in S stage, others are in G_1 or M stage. Thus, if the drug aims at S stage, it is effective to the cancer cells in S stage, but the drug given at this period (8 am to 10 am) is of no effect to the cancer cells in other stages, that is to say the sensitivity of chemotherapeutic drugs to cancer cells in different stages are differential. So during the period of administer through intravenous drip, it is effective to some sensitive cancer cells but not to those in insensitive periods.

6. The contradiction between inhibition and protection of marrow

Chemotherapy is cytotoxic and can inhibit the hematopiesis of marrow where hematopoietic stem cells are stored. Inhibition of marrow is a common clinical toxic reaction, which is the kinetic effect of chemotherapeutic drugs on specific stem cells. Chemotherapeutic cytotoxic drugs can damage the specific crowd of stem cells in marrow and will definitely reduce the number of mature and functional blood corpuscles in the peripheral blood. The degree of reduction relates to the lifetime of the cell components in the peripheral blood, for instance, the lifetime of hematid is longer, so the degree of reduction in the amount of blood corpuscles in the peripheral blood and the number of blood corpuscles in the peripheral blood during the treatment do not change obviously. However, the lifetimes of blood platelet and granular leucocytes are shorter with 3 days and 67 hours respectively, so the numbers of peripheral blood platelet and granular leucocytes reduce rapidly if the groups of megakaryocytic stem cells and granular cell groups are destroyed. If the amount of leucocytes and blood platelets decline to a very low level, it is extremely easy to cause subsequent serious infection or haemorrhage. In some cases, using large amount of broadspectrum antibiotic to resist the serious infection may lead to double infection or mycotic ingestion, even endangers the life.

To sum up, in order to solve the contradictions in the current chemotherapy, to ameliorate its disadvantages and make it better, the author thinks that it is necessary to update thoughts and to research on new drugs and new principles to resist cancer and metastasis as well as relapse, except improving chemotherapy further in traditional thoughts, only the changes in the opinions on curing cancer and the creativities and reforms of technologies can bring further development into the treatment of cancer.

4. THE INITIATIVE TO CHANGE THE SOLID BODY TUMOR INTRAVENOUS CHEMOTHERAPY INTO THE TARGET ORGAN INTRAVASCULAR CHEMOTHERAPY

- Advocacy for traditional cancer therapies
- Assessment of problems and disadvantages of solid body tumor intravenous chemotherapy
- To change and perform the Intravascular chemotherapy into the target organ intravenous chemotherapy for solid tumors
- The initiative of specific methods and approaches of target organ intravascular chemotherapy of abdominal solid tumor

The author reformed the systemic intravenous chemotherapy of solid tumor (especially the tumor of liver, gallbladder, pancreas, spleen, kidney, lung, uterus, ovary, abdominal cavity and pelvic cavity) to intravascular chemotherapy in target organ. This is the reformation after we have deeply taken cognizance of its disadvantages. Over the past half a century, millions of cancer patients have had chemotherapy and undertaken the side reaction of chemotherapy once and again after receiving the chemotherapy.

I. Evaluation of Problems and Disadvantages of Systemic Intravenous Chemotherapy for Solid Tumor

(I) Evaluation of the route of administration of systemic intravenous chemotherapy for solid tumor

The route of administration, not the specific targeting administration, distributes the cytotoxic drug in the whole body through the general blood circulation. In this way, it does not have a definite object for administration, but administers drugs in the whole body, resulting in:

1. The diseased cancer lesion area is very small (accounting for very small ratio of the body surface area of the whole body) only can obtain very little cytotoxic drug, resulting in very little action and curative effect.

2.However, the disease-free normal tissue in the whole body is damaged by the reaction of 99.6% of the cytotoxic drug. The normal tissue in the whole body does not need the cytotoxic drug, but it obtains a large number of cytotoxic drugs. However, the cytotoxic anti-cancer drug has relatively toxicity to the tissue with relatively rapid proliferation, such as the toxicity of alimentary canel, hemopoietic system, heart, liver, spleen, lung, kidney, nervous system and endocrine system, in this way, so many patients cannot receive the treatment or have to interrupt the treatment. Killing the tissue with relatively rapid proliferation in the whole body leads to harm to the patients instead of benefits to the patients.

3. The medication of this route of administration, does not have a definite object for administration, but the blind administration, which is non-targeting administration. Without the definite object, it only distributes and administers the drug in the whole body, as a result, the cancer lesion obtains a minute of cytotoxic drug while the area of the tissue in the whole body damaged by the cytotoxic drug is very large, resulting in bad curative effects, large side reaction and many and heavy complication, so the medication is unreasonable and unscientific.

4. With the above-mentioned medication, the cytotoxic drug administered in chemotherapy does not greatly attack the cancer cells, but only attach the cancer cells slightly (0.4%) while the normal tissue is greatly attacked in an all-round way by the cytotoxic drug (99.6%), at the same time, the cancer patient has low immunologic function by nature, now the cytotoxic drug in chemotherapy kills the hematopoietic cells, immunological cells, T lymphocyte, blood cells and blood platelet of the bone marrow again, resulting in further drop of immunologic function, the cytotoxic drug in chemotherapy attacks and kills the hematopoietic cells and immunological cells of the bone marrow once and again, resulting in the future drop of the immunologic function, in this way, one disaster comes after another, some cytotoxic drugs even urge the breakdown of the immunologic function.

(II) Elevation of calculation of dose for systemic intravenous chemotherapy for solid tumor

1. Since the systemic intravenous chemotherapy for solid tumor is not the specific targeting administration, but blindly distributed in the whole body, it necessarily needs much dose of cytotoxic drug; furthermore, it needs the combination of multiple drugs, in this way, it is possible to make the cancer lesion with very small area obtain the dose for remitting and shrinking the cancer lesion. The reason for large dose is that the 99.6% of the dose is absorbed by the whole body while only 0.4% is absorbed by the local cancer lesion. As a result, the relatively larger the dose, the larger and the more obvious the side reaction, resulting in remarkable drop of white blood cells and blood platelets, sometimes it also needs drug for increasing white cells, so it is unreasonable to calculate the dose.

2. At present, the systemic intravenous chemotherapy for solid tumor is the experience and the method obtained from the treatment of leukemia, however, as to the treatment extended to the solid tumor, its guiding ideology is to administer the drug as per the calculation of the body surface area of the whole body, which is unadvisable. Why? Because the leukemic cells are distributed in the general blood circulation system, in the organs and tissues in the whole body, the target to be treated exists in the general blood circulation system, therefore, it is reasonable and advisable to adopt the systemic intravenous chemotherapy and conforms to the targeting treatment. Because the target cells of the leukaemia are distributed in the general blood circulation system, so it is reasonable and advisable. However, since the solid tumor is limited to a certain organ, its target to be treated is mainly a certain

organ suffering from cancer, so it shall adopt the route of intravascular administration in the target organ and specific targeting administration, in this way, it can greatly reduce the dose of cytotoxic drug, as well as greatly reduce and eliminate the side reaction of the cytotoxic drug.

3. The calculation of the dose of systemic intravenous chemotherapy for solid tumor as per the body surface area is not based on therapeutical does by which how many cancer cells can be killed but on the tolerance dose of the organism to the cytotoxic drug. It is unknown whether one chemotherapy and two chemotherapies kill the cancer cells and how many cancer cells are killed by the chemotherapy. It is unknown. Whether there are cancer cells in the body of the patient? And where? It is unknown. Only one chemotherapy is carried out and only one task is accomplished.

(III) Evaluation of curative effect evaluation criterion of systemic intravenous chemotherapy for solid tumor

In a word, the curative effect evaluation criterion of systemic intravenous chemotherapy for solid is mainly embodied in three points: size of tumor, remission and remission time. As to the size of tumor, it is mainly based on CT, MRI or type-B ultrasonic, however, all of the images only reflect the size of occupation. As to the size of occupation, in our opinion, "the big" does not mean "the bad" and "the small" does not mean "the good". In addition, most of the occupations are short-term, the reason has been mentioned above.

2. Remission and remission time. Why the remission is regarded as the curative effect evaluation criterion and why the remission has a certain period? Apparently, the remission is not the objective of treatment or the treatment requirement of the patient or the objective of determination of treatment of the doctor just because the patient pays a certain price after several chemotherapies and only obtains a short-term remission. However, at present, the tumor medicine cannot heal all cancers (namely non-recurrence and non-metastasis) for a long time. Then, to say the latest, remission is better than the failure to remission. It is practical and realistic. Why it only can remit the cancer? Because the cytotoxic drug only harms the cancer cells and destroys their DNA rather than killing all cancer cells, which is only the first order kinetics. In addition, the reaction duration of cytotoxic drug only lasts 24h~48h even 72h after drug injection, after several days, the cancer cells will also be divided, proliferated and cloned in geometric progression, one into two, two into four and four into eight. Since the cytotoxic drug cannot kill the stem cells of the tumor, after administration for chemotherapy, the stem cells of tumor are still divided, proliferated and cloned. So in out opinion, killing the cancer cells does not conform to biological characteristics and behaviors or multi-link and multi-step of the metastasis of cancer cells, it only can regulate and control the cancer cells and prevents their division, proliferation and clone rather than the simple killing.

(IV) Evaluation of side reaction of systemic intravenous chemotherapy for solid tumor

Why the side reaction is so large? Just because this kind of route of administration needs so much dose or has to adopt combined administration. In order to remit and shrink the cancer, it has to determine the tolerance dose of the patient as the dose, in this way, the reaction is necessarily large and the damage is large, the distribution mode of this kind of route of administration leads to large dose or combined administration, otherwise, it is difficult to realize the curative effect criterion of shrinkage, in fact, it is avoidable to administer 99.6% of the cytotoxic drug to the normal tissues, in other words, it is avoidable to reform this route of administration to the specific targeting administration. If it is reformed to intravascular administration in the specific target organ, naturally, the side reaction will become little or be eliminated.

II. We Propose to Reform Systemic Intravenous Chemotherapy for Solid Tumor to Intravascular Chemotherapy in Target Organ

Since the above-mentioned problems are in existence, they shall be further studied. We should continue to improve the traditional curative therapeutic method as per the traditional idea, in the meanwhile, we should update the idea and the understanding, make progress in reforming and have the courage to innovate. Innovation, must challenge the traditional idea instead of replacement, it shall overcome the disadvantages, correct the defects so as to make it more perfect. Innovation, shall open a new path to overcome the cancer. Therefore, we specially propose the new idea, new concept and new principles of anti-cancer as well as new treatment mode and adopt organic integral new treatment mode to reform and innovate the traditional problems based on the biological characteristics and behaviors of cancer as well as the immunologic conditions of the host and the multi-link and multi-step of metastasis.

(I) Necessity, reasonableness and scientificalness of reform the systemic intravenous chemotherapy for solid tumor to intravascular chemotherapy in target organ

1. As above-mentioned, the route of administration of systemic intravenous chemotherapy is not the specific targeting administration but the blind general distribution, which is unreasonable and scientific distribution, so it must be reformed. The cancer lesion is limited to the local of the viscera, so it is necessary to adopt the specific targeting administration with clear target, which is reasonable and scientific. As to the systemic intravenous chemotherapy, since most of the cytotoxic drugs are administered to the general normal tissues, if the drugs are administered to the target organ, it can save the dose administered to the whole body, in this way, the dose can be greatly reduced, thus the side reaction is greatly reduced even eliminated, so the chemotherapy even may have no toxicity.

2. Analyze the source and formation of the side reaction of chemotherapy and probe into the method to eliminate the side reaction. Through review, reflection and analysis, we deeply realize that the source, the blind distribution of the cytotoxic drug in the whole body by the systemic intravenous chemotherapy for solid tumor, is unreasonable. In order to shrink the tumor, it necessarily increases the dose, resulting in unavoidable side reaction.

The increased dose of cytotoxic drug does not entirely react on the cancer lesion, but mainly on the whole body to damage the normal histiocytes while these general normal tissues do not need the cytotoxic drug, however, they get most of the cytotoxic drugs in fact, which is unreasonable. It is necessary to study and reform it.

In view that its source and formation is based on the blindness of the route of administration of systemic intravenous chemotherapy, resulting in increased dose and combined administration and leading to unavoidable side reaction, so the solution is to reform the route of administration.

How to reform the route of administration?

Professor Xu Ze proposes to reform the systemic intravenous chemotherapy for solid tumor (especially the tumor of liver, gallbladder, spleen, pancreas, stomach, intestine, uterus, ovary, pelvic cavity and abdominal cavity) to intravascular chemotherapy in target organ, in this way, the drug is administered to the specific target and then to the cancer lesion of the target organ, necessarily leading in the greatly decreased dose; the reduction of dose of cytotoxic drug necessarily leads to the reduction and elimination of side reaction. The elimination of side reaction of the traditional chemotherapy, makes millions of cancer patients free from the pains and risks of side reaction of chemotherapy and benefits the patients.

Professor Xu Ze holds: the intravascular administration in the specific target organ, reduces the dose, improves the curative effects, eliminates the side reaction, necessarily leading to great reduction of medical charge, saving billions of medical charges and expenditures (in RMB Yuan) for the state and the patients and being advantageous for settling the problems of being difficult and expensive in taking medical treatment.

Over half a century, millions of cancer patients have been deeply damaged by the side reaction of the chemotherapy, therefore, this reform will benefit millions of cancer cells, which is a great pioneering undertaking and an original innovation and promotes the further development of the oncology in the 21st century.

(II) It is necessary to firstly study and make clear where the target is so as to carry out the intravascular chemotherapy in target organ; it is necessary to study and make clear where the cancer cells are so as to kill the cancer cells with cytotoxic drug in chemotherapy? In this way, it can have a definite object.

1. The primary lesion of the solid tumor is in the organ, for example, the stomach cancer lies in the stomach, the liver cancer lies in the liver, the lung cancer lies in the lung, the intestinal cancer lies in intestine, that is to say, the primary cancer lesion lies in the organ, even if it meets with metastasis in the advanced stage, its primary cancer lesion is still in the organ.

2. Where are the cancer cells? The cancer cells of stomach cancer, intestinal cancer, liver cancer, lung cancer and so on are mainly in the portal system and meet with metastasis via the portal system. An example of liver cancer: the main blood supply of liver cancer is from the hepatic artery, the most primary route of the metastasis of liver cancer is the venous system in the liver. The metastasis of liver cancer in liver is the most common metastasis mode, the cancer cells invade the branch of the portal vein, form the cancer embolus in the portal vein, continually extend to the hepatic portal until the left and right branch of the portal vein and its beam are blocked by the cancer embolus, the deciduous cancer cell balls are floating in the portal vein and are spread to the liver through blood.

The hepatic vein wall is thin and receives the blood flowing back from the cancer lesion, so it is easy to be encroached and the cancer embolus is formed in the hepatic vein, sometimes, the embolus can reach to inferior vena cava and to right atrium and then meet with metastasis via the lung.

The liver is one of the organs meeting with metastatic carcinoma most commonly. According to information of pathologic anatomy, among the cases of the patients who die of the malignant tumor, about 40% meet with the liver metastasis and its incidence rate is next only to lymphatic system. The liver metastasis of malignant tumor of gstrointestinal tract is the most common.

The liver receives the dual blood supply from portal vein and hepatic artery, the liver metastasis can come from the portal vein circulation and systemic circulation, that is to say, the cancer cells enters the systemic circulation via pulmonary capilliary station. The blood supply is complicated, about 90%of the blood supply is from the hepatic artery.

3. The administration along the route of hematogenous metastasis of cancer cells for tracking and killing shall follow the flow direction of the tumor vein, the chemotherapy drug follows the flow direction, killing the cancer cells in metastasis with small dose. As to the cancer cells, the cancer cell groups and micro-metastasis cancer embolus in metastasis, it is only necessary to kill $10^{4.5}$ cancer cells with eth cytotoxic drugs for chemotherapy, the rest $10^{4.5}$ cancer cells can be eliminated by the immunological cells and immunological surveillance in the blood circulation of the organism. According to the plan, it is satisfactory for the dose to kill $10^{4.5}$ cancer cells, the dose cannot go so far to kill too many immunological cells. To kill some cancer cells and to protect the immunological cells from being damaged excessively as well, shall be judged with the sign of not affecting the drop of white blood cells and blood platelets. The viscera and organs in the abdomen, such as stomach, rectum, colon, liver, gallbladder, pancreas, uterus and ovary and other tumor-producing vein gather at the portal vein system, therefore, the target organs of tumor at the abdomen shall focus on the portal vein system and hepatic artery.

III. Xu Ze Proposes to Reform the Systemic Intravenous Chemotherapy for Solid Tumor at the Abdomen to the Specific Method and Approach of Intravascular Chemotherapy in Target Organ

(I) Intravascular administration for chemotherapy in target organ

1. Administration via arterial route

> (1) The chemotherapy pump shall be arranged in the hepatic artery;
> (2) Hepatic artery interventional therapy, embolism + chemotherapy;
> (3) Interventional chemotherapy perfusion of bronchial artery;
> (4) Interventional chemotherapy perfusion of internal iliac artery;
> (5) Interventional chemotherapy of arteria pancreatica;
> (6) Interventional chemotherapy perfusion of gastric artery;
> (7) Hepatic artery chemotherapy pump through laparotomy.

2. Administration via portal vein route

    (1) Portal vein chemotherapy pump through laparotomy;

    (2) Omentum venous pump through laparotomy;

    (3) Subcutaneous chemotherapy pump through laparotomy via mesentery vein;

    (4) Subcutaneous deep vein conduit chemotherapy pump: can be used in the treatment of malignant tumor of the intestines and stomach tract.

Surgical interventional chemotherapy for tumor patient has been widely applied, now the subcutaneous chemotherapy pump for drug delivery system is mostly adopted at present and it is a good route of administration for tumor chemotherapy, which can be divided into three classes: venous duct chemotherapy pump; ductus arteriosus chemotherapy pump and celiac duct chemotherapy pump, compared with the peripheral vein chemotherapy and artery interventional chemotherapy, it has a lot of advantages.

3. Administration via target organ at the abdomen

Oral administration: oral administration→ stomach→ vena coronaria of stomach (left vein and right vein of stomach)→ splenic vein→ portal vein, for example, oral administration of Xeloda.

Oral administration: oral administration→ stomach→ lymphatic vessel under gastric mucosa →lymph node around the stomach→ lymph node behind peritoneum→ cisterna chyli→ thoracic duct, for example, oral administration of Brucea emulsion.

Rectal suppository: rectal suppository (a few of chemotherapy drug) → venae intestinales → vein under mesentery → portal vein.

Route of administration for the target organ of lung cancer:

A. vein of antibrachium → superior vena cava → double lungs

B. Portal vein conduit or pump → liver → hepatic vein →lower caval vein → right ventricle → double lungs

C. Oral administration: oral administration → portal vein →liver →lower caval vein → right ventricle → double lungs

(II) Paying attention to arterial interventional administration

An example of liver cancer: since the onset of liver cancer is insidious, when the patient see a doctor, it is mostly in intermediate and advanced stage, followed by other factors such as high combined hepatocirrhosis rate, relatively low surgical removal rate and high recurrence rate after operation, most of the patients need non-operation therapy. At present, among the non-operation therapies with positively curative effects, interventional therapy is most widely used.

Its indication can be used to the liver cancer in different stages and it is better for the liver cancer in early and intermediate stage. These suffering from serious icterrus, voluminous ascites, serious damage to liver function and widespread metastasia shall be abstained from contraindication.

Generally, the first period of treatment of interventional therapy of liver cancer needs 3-4 times, with the interval of 2-3 months. In principle, the next interventional therapy shall be carried out only after the general condition and liver function of the patient are basically recovered over 3 weeks.

Interventional therapy

Since the interventional therapy will damage the normal tissue especially the liver and the immune system of the organism synchronously, the organism needs a certain time for recovery to understand the second interventional therapy, in the interval of interventional therapy, it shall nourish the liver, improve the immunity and adopt the complex treatment. In Shuguang Tumor Clinic of Shugang Tumor Research Institute, in the past 16 years, all the patients of liver cancer receiving the interventional therapy administer XZ-C medicine after operation and they take oral administration of XZ-C$_{1+4+5}$ for protecting the chest, improving the immunity, protecting the bone marrow, enhancing hematopiesis, protecting liver and great curative effects have been made. Most of the patients have been in good condition and have had good appetite, their symptoms have been improved, their survival quality has been improved, and most of them have had an obviously prolonged survival period.

(III) Paying attention to the route of administration of chemotherapy pump in portal vein

It is necessary for the specific targeting administration for target organ to understand where the target organ of the cancer cells is. The tumor-bearing vein of stomach cancer, colon and rectal cancer, gallbladder cancer, pancreas cancer, cancer of pelvic cavity and oophoroma flows into the portal vein system, therefore, the cancer cells, and the ones in metastasis are flowing into the portal vein system, therefore, attention shall be paid to the chemotherapy pump in portal vein for targeting tracking and killing the cancer cells.

Chemotherapy pump in portal vein is remained in the portal vein after exploration of laparotomy or remained in the lower omentum vein after laparotomy; or remained in the drug delivery system in the mesentery under the direct vision of the laparotomy.

Chemotherapy pump embedded in portal vein body, also called implanted drug delivery system or subcutaneous embedded drug delivery system, is a kind of drug subcutaneously embedded for local perfusion, which is used for the guiding chemotherapy of cancer and oriented local perfusion chemotherapy for preventing the recurrence after removal of tumor. The drug can directly enter the target organ through drug pump and conduit, improving the lethality and the curative effects to cancer cells and reducing the side reaction of chemotherapy. It is reported by the literature that when the density of the local chemotherapy drug is increased one time, the lethality to the tumor can be increased 6-12 times. This system can increase several times of the density of the local drug.

At present, this system is widely used for the clinic at home and abroad and great curative effects have been made.

In a word, as above mentioned, the systemic intravenous chemotherapy for solid tumor, only has a few of drug reaching to the cancer lesion while most of the cytotoxic drugs react on the normal histiocyte in the whole body, especially, they are relatively toxic to the tissue with rapid proliferation such as hemopoietic system of bone marrow, immune system and alimentary system and have the side reaction, however, these normal tissue, not needing the cytotoxic drugs, obtains a large number of cytotoxic drugs, which is unreasonable.

As to the chemotherapy through intravascular administration in the target organ, the drug is directly sent to the target organ via the conduit, the cytotoxic drugs obtained by the cancer lesion are all drugs administered, which is reasonable and scientific, greatly reducing the dose for chemotherapy. The specific targeting administration, reduces the does, improves the curative effects, reduces or eliminates the side reaction. In this way, it improves the curative effects, eliminates the reaction, resulting in the reduction of expenses. It is advantages for settling the problems of being difficult and expensive in taking medical treatment. Since it reduces or eliminates the side reaction, necessarily reducing the medical charge and saving billions of medical expenses and expenditures (in RMB Yuan) for the state.

This topic is my third book "new concept of cancer treatment and a new method," the core of the twelfth chapter, this article advocates "on the solid tumor systemic intravenous chemotherapy should be the target organ for intravascular chemotherapy"

Why is this initiative?

Because half a century, the size of the world's hospitals in all countries to buy body tumors are using systemic intravenous chemotherapy, the hospital tumor chemotherapy are busy patients with systemic intravenous chemotherapy, cancer patients are also hospitalized for intravenous chemotherapy, the above Through our in-depth measurement found and commented on the existence of systemic intravenous chemotherapy problems and disadvantages,

In this paper, we put forward this: a review of solid body intravenous chemotherapy route of the drawbacks of the second assessment of solid body tumor intravenous chemotherapy dose calculation; three evaluation of solid tumor systemic intravenous chemotherapy efficacy evaluation criteria ; Four assessment of solid body tumor intravenous chemotherapy side effects. Since the discovery of the existence of the problem, it should try to improve, how to improve, how to reform?

First of all to study the patient's cancer cells where? Through our laboratory for many years of animal experimental research and clinical research found that abdominal surgery, gastrointestinal cancer patients with cancer cells are homogeneous in the portal vein system, the abdomen of various metastases to the liver metastases of cancer cells are also cancer Into the hepatic portal vein or hepatic vein, we found in surgery is also true.

Therefore, we advocate should be reformed for the portal vein system drug pump, change the body of the drug distribution for the target organ administration, the target clear, directly to the chemical drug by the drug pump directly to the portal vein system, direct contact with the presence of portal vein cancer cells The In my nearly 10 years follow-up cases, the portal vein system to set the pump long-term effect is better, in this paper, I put forward specific programs and methods.

The reform of the hospital on the National Academy of Oncology will cause a huge shock and change the current national hospitals of the Department of Chemists doctors, on the daily work is to make the whole body intravenous chemotherapy venous puncture, observation care, if the reform For the portal vein to set the pulp, the soil to be carried out by the surgeon, rather than chemotherapy doctors and nurses involved, involving a series of reforms, changes. For half a century, tens of thousands of solid tumor cancer patients around the world have undergone systemic intravenous chemotherapy, drug body distribution, but so far cancer is still the first death, and can not prevent recurrence and metastasis.

In this paper, this solid tumor intravenous chemotherapy route of the proposed challenge, challenge, criticism and reform, will be possible to correct the change over half a century to the whole body of intravenous chemotherapy to the irrational status quo. (The above are our first in the international, independent innovation, the international leader.)

In the last two centuries, the treatment of malignant tumors has occurred twice leap:

The first time was 1890 Naistad proposed the concept of radical surgery.

The first time in the 1970s, Fish integrated chemotherapy into radical surgery (adjuvant chemotherapy or neoadjuvant chemotherapy).

Since then, the treatment of malignant tumors wandering.

Fis): is the route of systemic intravenous chemotherapy, after half a day, so far failed to reduce the mortality rate also failed to prevent the hair, transfer, mortality is still the first. Now we are on this traditional doctrine, the traditional method of questioning and reforming the idea of innovation, instead of target organ administration, combined with the establishment of xz-c comprehensive treatment concept and xz-c immunomodulation therapy (ie immunotherapy) will be helpful To promote the current situation of the current hovering.

5. INITIATIVES TO STRATEGIES OF IMPROVING CANCER POSTOPERATIVE ADJUVANT CHEMOTHERAPY

- **Why should cancer postoperative adjuvant chemotherapy be performed?**
- **The analysis of reasons why Postoperative chemotherapy did not meet the desired**
- **how to do cancer postoperative adjuvant chemotherapy well**

Since 1990s, in view that the reoccurrence and metastasis rate of cancer after operation was very high, in order to prevent the reoccurrence and metastasis after operation, a series of assistance chemotherapy after operation has been adopted, what's more, the chemotherapy was made before operation (for example, the breast cancer), however, the results had been not so satisfactory. Reoccurrence and metastasis take place in assistant chemotherapy after operation or in the period of treatment or the metastasis takes place synchronously in chemotherapy. It can be seen from so many patients in Wuhan Shuguang Tumor Special Clinic that neither reoccurrence nor metastasis cannot be prevented by the assistant chemotherapy after operation, even in some cases, the intensified chemotherapy promotes the adynamia of immunologic function. All these things should be seriously, calmly, practically and realistically thought and reflected by the clinicians: why the assistant chemotherapy after operation cannot prevent the reoccurrence? Why the assistant chemotherapy after operation cannot prevent the metastasis? Why the assistant chemotherapy after operation on some patients promotes the adynamia of immunologic function? What's the problem and disadvantage of the assistant chemotherapy after operation? What measures should be taken? How to further study and perfect it? How to reform and innovate in the assistant chemotherapy to improve the curative effects?

I. Why to make the assistant chemotherapy after operation on cancer or assistant chemotherapy in peri-operation period?

Currently, the treatment of cancer mainly depends on the operation, however, the reoccurrence and metastasis rate is still relatively high after operation.

1. The potential reason why the local reoccurrence and metastasis after radical operation on cancer takes place may be the following factors viewed from clinic:

(1) Insufficient attention has not been paid to the free-tumor technique, as a result, the operation such as exploration and touch causes the cancer cells on the serosa surface to fall into the intra-abdominal implantation.

(2) The tumor tissue is not thoroughly removed by the operation, as a result, the remained cancer cells are continually proliferating.

(3) The existing metastasis lesion is not found in operation and is not removed, for example, the lymph node in metastasis is not found or is removed incompletely.

(4) As to the clearing of lymph node in operation, traditionally, it adopts the passive separation, in this way, the apocoptic micro-lymphatic vessel may lead to the fluxion, dissemination, residual and transplantation of the cancer cells.

(5) The operation leads to the transplantation of the cancer cells, the cancer cells invading the esophagus, stomach serosa or colon, recta and serosa may easily fall into the abdominal cavity and form the transplantation lesion and the damaged peritoneum in the area of operation may easily meet with transplnation and reoccurrence. The reoccurrence of anastomotic stoma of the colon may be the intracavity exfoliation and transplantation of the enteral cancer cells in the operation.

(6) The metastasis of the lymph node in the patients in the late stage is relatively wide and syzygial, in this way, it is difficult to remove it with operation.

(7) In the operation on gastrointestinal tract cancer, the metastasis of cancer cells in the portal vein takes place, resulting in the metastasis of liver cancer cells after operation. However, it is unseenable in the operation by the naked eyes. For example, when the "radical operation on gastric carcinoma" is made, the cancerous protuberance and the tumid lymph nodes of gastric carcinoma can be seen by us, however, whether the cancer cells exist in the vein and the blood of the portal vein is unknown? How many cancer cells exist? Where do these cancer cells in the vein go? Whether these cancer cells in cluster that can be touched and extruded into the venous blood in operation arrive at the portal vein? Or arrive at the branch of the portal vein in the liver? It is not impossible to touch the cancerous protuberance in exploration and excision of gastric cancerous protuberance and cleaning of lymph node, the operation necessarily makes a large number of cancer cells be extruded and fall down, then they flow into the portal venous blood, resulting in metastasis in liver after operation.

(8) The operation brings about the traumas to the organism, resulting in the inferior immunologic function, in this way, the organism losses the immunological surveillance or is weakened in immunological surveillance, leaving opportunity to the residual cancer cells or the cancer cells in dormancy for reoccurrence and metastasis.

(9) As to the cancer in the progressive stage, the metastasis of cancer cells may take place before operation while these cancer cells in metastasis cannot be seen by the physician in operation. However, it is reported in the pathological section report that the cancer embolus can be seen in the blood capillary and the lymphatic vessel.

Based on the above-mentioned, after the radical operation of the cancer, the residual cancer cells may still exist, resulting in reoccurrence and metastasis of the residual subclinical cancer lesion after operation.

Then, how to make up for the shortage of radical operation with residual cancer cells? Adopt the chemotherapy in peri-operation period to hunt the residual cancer cells in operation with the chemotherapy cytotoxic drug and remove the cancer cells falling off or remained or transplanted in the operation.

However, could the traditional assistant chemotherapy after operation hunt the residual cancer cells in operation? Could it remove the cancer cells falling off, remained or transplanted in operation?

2. Why the current assistant chemotherapy after operation cannot prevent the reoccurrence and metastasis? It shall be reviewed, analyzed and reflected:

(1) The route of administration of assistant chemotherapy after operation shall be further studied and reformed. At present, it mainly adopts the general intravenous chemotherapy after operation, the cytotoxic drug injected is generally distributed, acting on the histiocytes of the viscera in the whole body, in this way, the ones killed are mainly the proliferative cells, immunological cells and bone marrow cells of the normal tissue organs in the whole body. However, the field of operation accounts for a little ratio in the whole body, in this way, the dose obtained is very small, it is difficult to kill the local residual cancer cells or the cancer lesion in the field of operation or the residual cancer lesion of the cancer cells falling off in the operation, therefore, the route of administration shall be reformed.

(2) The assistant chemotherapy after operation is blinded and the drug administered is not subject to the drugsensitive test. Since the drugsensitive test on the cancer histiocytes of patient is not carried out, the drug is administered by experience, so it is unknown whether the drug is sensitive. If the drug administered is insensitive or drug resistant, it is not only fruitless, without any action on the residual cancer cells, but also kills the proliferative cells, the immunological cells and the bone marrow cells of the normal tissues in the whole body, while these normal tissues in the whole body do not need the cytotoxic drug, resulting in the remarkable side effect, damaging the patient and making the patient suffer from the pain of the side effect. Thus, although the chemotherapy has been made for several times, the expected curative effects cannot be realized, in addition, the cytotoxic drug injected intravenously in the wholly body covers the whole body, kills the general immunological cells and the hematopoietic cells of the bone marrow and makes the immunologic functions of the patient further descend. Actually, the cancer patient is inferior in immunologic function, while the radical operation further brings down the immunologic function, plus the assistant chemotherapy of the cytotoxic drug after operation, the immunological function of the patient is further reduced, like one disaster after another, resulting in metastasis while in chemotherapy. Therefore, as for the assistant chemotherapy after operation, if the drugsensitive test is not made and the drug is administered in form of individualization, the chemotherapy would benefit some patients while damage some patients.

(3) Assistant chemotherapy after operation. **Since the tumor is removed and the lymph clearing is made, the drug administration plan and the dosage should differ from the ones for the patients without removal by operation,** the dosage in the assistant chemotherapy period after operation would differ from the one before operation, before removal of the tumor, the dosage is calculated as per the body surface area so as to realize the goal of remission

and shrinkage, however, after the radical operation, the tumor is removed, so it shall target the potentially residual cancer cells or the micro-metastasis in operation instead of the remission and shrinkage, since both targets differs from each other, in order to remit and shrink the tumor of the patient without operation, the drug must have a certain lethality, as a result, the drug administration plans shall be combined and the dosage shall be up to the one the patient can bear, in this way, the curative effect of remission and shrinkage can be realized. Meanwhile, the assistant chemotherapy after operation, depends on radical operation primarily and the chemotherapy secondarily, only targeted for removal of the potentially residual cancer cells or the cancer cells falling off in the operation or the cancer cells in metastasis to make some subsidiary treatment to prevent the reoccurrence and metastasis. Therefore, its drug administration plan and dose shall differ from the former and the dosage of the cytotoxic drug shall be greatly reduced.

(4) What determines the indications and the contraindications of the assistant chemotherapy after operation? At present, the indications of assistant chemotherapy after operation are discordant, for example, do the residual cancer cells exist in the patient after this operation on earth? Where? How many? To what extent? All those things should be taken into account and estimated, however, most of the patients receive the "radical operation on cancer" in the general surgery or the specialized surgery, after operation, they come back to the local hospitals or the tumor clinic, the chemotherapy after operation is the general intravenous chemotherapy, the plans selected differ from each other in each place, each hospital by each physician, namely there is no uniform plan, these physicians or nurses responsible for general intravenous injection for the assistant chemotherapy after operation are not always aware of the patient's condition, pathological analysis, the range and the extent of cancer invasion seen in the operation as well as the estimation of the potential residual cancer lesion in operation, the extent of the radical operation and so on. They should know TNM stage and the immunity chemotherapy and estimate the potential residual cancer cells. Who knows it clearly? Only the operation doctor because he can see the range and extent of the cancer invasion through exploration in operation. Therefore, what determines the selection of chemotherapy or radiotherapy after operation? The operation physician shall determine the indications and the contraindications of the assistant chemotherapy after operation as well as the chemotherapy plan, times, dosage and so on to satisfy the actual conditions of the patient.

(5) How to assess the curative effects of the assistant chemotherapy after operation? At present, there is no uniform understanding or standard. The objective curative effects of the chemotherapy on the solid tumor before removal of the tumor shall be assessed according to the area of tumor and the remission of the tumor recognized in the world. However, since the tumor is removed, it shall be assessed according to the improvement of the symptom and the condition instead of area of tumor. At present, what role does the assistant chemotherapy after operation play? Does it kill the cancer cells? How many? Do the residual cancer cells exist in the patient's body? What is the effect? All these things are kept unknown. However, it is well known that it kills the normal cells, the immunological cells and the hematopoietic cells of the bone marrow because the white blood cells fall down, the blood platelets fall down too, but it is the extent of the side effect rather than the effect. As to the tumor sign, it is difficult

to determine the definite standard at present and it is necessary to make the fundamental study and clinical study.

II. How to Do well in Assistant Chemotherapy after Operation on Cancer or Assistant Chemotherapy in Peri-operation Period?

XU ZE made a suggestion of reforming and developing the assistant chemotherapy after operation on cancer in abdomen (the malignant tumor such as liver cancer, gallbladder cancer, pancreatic cancer, gastric cancer, intestinal cancer and abdominal cancer) as follows:

1. Reform the route of administration and change the general intravenous chemotherapy into the chemotherapy through intravascular administration in target organ. All of the operations on cancer in abdomen, no matter the radical operation or palliative excision, or the operation only for exploration instead of removal, shall adopt the built-in pump in ductus venosus in stomach omentum, or built-in pump in portal vein, or arterial pump, or built-in pump in vein of mesentery as much as possible. Why is the chemotherapy pump built in portal system? Firstly, it is necessary to know where the cancer cells after operation on cancer exist. The administration must be targeted for the cancer cell group and the cancer cells of liver cancer, gallbladder cancer, pancreatic cancer, gastric cancer and intestinal cancer are in the tuberiferous veins, which flow towards the portal vein and gather at the portal vein, then flow towards hepatic vein via sinus hepaticus and into the lungs via the right atrium. Therefore, the portal system adopts the targeted intravascular administration targeted through the chemotherapy pump, so it is the direct target and it is reasonable and scientific. It can make the residual cancer cells prowling in the portal vein after operation directly contact the chemotherapy drug to produce the curative effect.

2. Reform the dosage of administration: since the built-pump in portal vein is directly targeted for the cancer cell group in the blood of the portal vein and the chemotherapy drug needed is greatly reduced by contrast with the dosage of general intravenous administration. Since the drug is administered through the target organ of the portal vein, the dosage can be greatly reduced. Because the radical operation on cancer has been made, the cancerous protuberance has been removed and the next thing to be done is to remove the potentially residual cancer cells, generally, the immunological cells in the human body can remove these cancer cells, however, since the immunologic function of the cancer patient comes down, the assistant chemotherapy after operation is used to assist in removal, so only a small quantity of dosage is needed, it shall strive for killing 10^{5-6} cancer cells without damage to the normal cells as much as possible. The rest 10^{5-6} cancer cells will be removed by the immunological cells of the organism. However, as to the tracking and hunting of the potential cancer cells in metastasis in the portal system, although the targeted administration reduces the dosage greatly, the drug concentration in the portal vein will be greatly increased out of question, resulting in the improvement of the curative effect. **Since the dosage is greatly reduced, it will necessarily reduce even eliminate the side effect of the chemotherapy greatly. The elimination of the side effect of the chemotherapy, will benefit millions of cancer**

patients. **Over the past half century, millions of cancer patients have deeply suffered from the pain of the side effect from the chemotherapy and the radiotherapy all over the world, what's more, the lives of some patients have been endangered. Since the side effect of chemotherapy is eliminated, so many cancer patients are secured. The cancer seriously endangers the health of the human beings and makes the medical expenses rapidly increase as well. The direct expenses for cancer treatment in China are approximately RMB one hundred billion Yuan, bringing a heavy economic burden to the patients even the whole society. Now Professor Xu Ze holds: the intravascular administration in the specific target organ, reduces the dose, improves the curative effects, eliminates the side reaction, necessarily leading to great reduction of medical charge, saving billions of medical charges and expenditures (in RMB Yuan) for the state and the patients and being advantageous for settling the problems of being difficult and expensive in taking medical treatment.**

3. Reform the blindness of the drug administered for assistant chemotherapy after operation. The drug for chemotherapy after operation shall be subject to the drugsensitive test together with the histiocytes of the cancer tissue of the patients for the individualized chemotherapy. All operations on cancer, no matter the radical operations or the palliative operations or the exploratory operations, shall try to obtain the specimen of the cancer tissue, the cancer tissue will be cut up into two halves in aseptic manipulation, one for cultivation of cancer tissue and drugsensitive test and another for pathological section and chemotherapy of immunity group for definite pathological diagnosis.

Why the specimen of cancer tissue is selected for cultivation of cancer cells and the drugsensitive test? Since the detection of sensitivity and drug resistance of tumor chemotherapy is the foundation of "individualized" chemotherapy. To this day, the tumor chemotherapy has stridden forward to the "individualized" chemotherapy. In the past days, the different tumor patients receive the same chemotherapy mode (plan), resulting in blindness inevitably. It is shown by the study that the same kind of tumor with the same tissue, even the same tumor in different stages has the incompletely consistent sensitivity to the chemotherapy drug. Therefore, it is necessary to make the drugsensitive test on the tumor patient to select the sensitive drug. Especially, with the increase of the anti-tumor drug at present, it is more urgent. It is proven by the clinical experience in tumor chemotherapy that the effective rate of drug administered by experience is very low (14%) while it will be increased to 28%-35% if the results measured with the existing drugsensitive test method is used to guide the selection of the drug, which is a great fruit.

The detection of the sensitivity and drug resistance of tumor chemotherapy offers an important basis to the foreseeable chemotherapy to reasonably use the anti-tumor drug to reduce the blindness and improve the pertinence, which would undoubtedly improve the level of tumor chemotherapy greatly.

4. The key is to manage and disposal the pump after operation: the drug pump for portal system is in-built in the operation. After operation, it is necessary to continually adopt the long-term light (trace) nontoxic chemotherapy drug and inject the heparin to prevent the

embolism, prevent the cancer embolus and prevent the cancer cell group. Where are the cancer cells in the peri-operation period? The cancerous protuberance of liver, gallbladder, pancreas, spleen, stomach and intestine will be carried off by the blood separately after flowing into the blood of the portal vein or many cancer cells meet with homoplasmic adhesion or heterogenetic adhesion with other cells to form the cancer cell group, which floats with the blood and forms the cancer embolus in the blood vessel, then the deciduous cancer cell embolus moves along the direction of the blood of the venous system. The cancer cells continually enter the blood circulation and transfer along the normal direction of the blood. Most of the cancer cells entering the blood circulation will be eliminated by the host and only a few of the cancer cells survive. Within several days after operation, a large number of cancer cells flow over into the portal system via tumorigenic vein in virtue of operation technique and exploratory extrusion. The surviving cancer cells are adhered to the endothelial cells of the wall of the target organ and then enter the target organ after passing through the wall and form the minute metastasis lesion. The cancer cells from gstrointestinal tract can flow into the liver along the portal vein and the liver is the end point of the blood of the portal vein, therefore, the cancer of gastrointestinal tract often transfers to the liver, forms the cancer cells of the metastasis lesion of the metastasis liver cancer and invades the central vein via the minute branch of the portal vein. The cancer cells can enter the hepatic vein and then flow back to the right atrium via the lower caval vein, then to the lung via the pulmonary artery and form the metastasis lesion of lung.

It can be often seen that the cancer embolus exists in the portal vein branch in the pathological report or the cancer embolus forms in the portal vein branch in CT or MRI report. The cancer embolus is the main factor in the formation of the metastasis lesion. The cancer cells, the fibrin and the blood platelet constitute the embolus and then it is carried to other parts, passes through the wall and forms the secondary tumor around the blood vessel. The formation of cancer embolus is related to the following factors: ① the inherent adhesion and aggregation of the cancer cells; ② the action of Thrombo-Pletinlike substances; ③ action of blood platelet; ④combined action of fibrin.

It is important to do well in management and application of pump after operation. Someone is inbuilt with chemotherapy pump and does not pay a return visit or use the pump after leaving hospital. After operation, the regular return visit shall be paid and the heparin shall be injected via the pump to prevent the blockade and the cancer embolus. A few of chemotherapy drugs shall be injected to hunt the floating cancer cells remaining in the the blood circulation of portal vein.

The surgeons and the nurses shall be responsible for the arrangement, follow-up survey, registration, filling, consultation answer, statistics and summary of the assistant chemotherapy after operation.

5. Reform the single goal of killing cancer cells into the immunological mediation and control therapy in an all-round way. Abandon the goal of only killing the cancer cells, attach importance to the resistance of the organism, reform it into the immunological

mediation and control therapy in an all-round way and give attention to both of them, thus, the curative effect will be improved. XZ-C medicine shall be orally taken in the period of assistant chemotherapy after operation and after the treatment course of the assistant chemotherapy to carry out the immunological chemotherapy (immunity + chemotherapy) or immunological chemotherapy radiotherapy (immunity + radiotherapy) so as to reform the unilateral therapeutic outlook of singly killing the cancer cells into an all-round therapeutic outlook of killing the cancer cells as well as improving the immunity of the organism.

III. Why the Assistant Chemotherapy after Operation Cannot Achieve the Expectation

In the past 10 years, the assistant chemotherapy after operation has been widely adopted all over the country, however, most of the assistant chemotherapy after operation is made by experience, the treatment plans differ from each other in different hospitals; the chemotherapy drugs selected differ from each other; the same to the departments and doctors in the same hospital due to the difference experience. The days and the interval of chemotherapy drugs administered differ a little from each other in different hospitals in different places: once per month for someone, once per two months for someone, once per week for someone, 4 times continually for someone, 6 times continually for someone and even 8-10 times continually for someone. The treatment courses are arranged with a certain blindness and differ from each other, without uniform or consistent standard. Because most of the hospitals have not made the drugsensitive test, so the "individualized" chemotherapy cannot be made.

At present, the plans for assistant chemotherapy after operation adopted in different places are basically similar to the ordinary chemotherapy plans, however, the goal or target of the ordinary tumor chemotherapy aims at the primary cancer lesion or the metastasis cancer lesion and the goal of treatment is to shrink, eliminate or remit the primary cancerous protuberance or metastasis cancerous protuberance or the tumid lymph node. These solid cancerous protuberances occupy a relatively large area, so, in order to shrink the cancerous protuberance, it is necessary to take the combined chemotherapy drugs with a relatively large quantity, otherwise, it is difficult to shrink the cancerous protuberance.

However, the assistant chemotherapy after operation is entirely different from this because the radical operation removes and cleans down the primary cancerous protuberance and the tumid lymph node around it, in this way, there is no solid cancerous protuberance. Since the cancerous protuberance is removed, the assistant chemotherapy after operation aims at the potentially residual cancer cells after operation, the potentially remnant micro-metastasis cancer cells or the cancer cells in metastasis and it is targeted for the remnant cancer cells or the potentially metastasis cancer cells instead of the solid cancerous protuberance, so the dosage shall be relatively small, without damage to the immunological cells of the host or with a little damage to the host. So how to assess the curative effect of the assistant chemotherapy after operation shall be measured according to the assessment standard including the improvement of immunity, the improvement of the survival quality, the improvement of the symptom, the elevation of the immunity indexes, the descent of the tumor sign and good mental state and appetite instead of the shrinkage of the tumor.

How to do well in assistant chemotherapy after operation? It is held by us that attention shall be paid to the following:

1. As to the patients receiving the radical operation on the cancerous protuberance, the fresh tumor specimen shall be selected for the chemotherapy drug sensitive test so as to individualize the assistant chemotherapy after operation to avoid the blindness of drug administration.

2. How to judge or estimate whether the remnant cancer cells exist in the body after radical operation so as to determine the indication of the assistant chemotherapy after operation, in this way, the immunity indexes and the tumor signs shall be detected.

3. How to judge the curative effect of the assistant chemotherapy after operation? Are the cancer cells killed or not? Since the tumor is removed, the curative effect cannot be judged as per the existence of the tumor of the volume of the tumor. The immunity indexes, the cytokines and the tumor signs shall be detected to judge the possibility of the reoccurrence and metastasis after operation.

4. The drug administered for the assistant chemotherapy after operation shall differ from the one for primary tumor or the metastasis cancer lesion because the goals are different: the former is to eliminate the primary cancer lesion and the latter is to eliminate the residual cancer cells, as a result, the dosage shall be different and it shall be greatly reduced.

5. The patient receiving the radical operation on cancer is very weak in the body condition and inferior in immunologic function, so the assistant chemotherapy after operation must be accompanied with the immunological mediation and control therapy, namely the immunological therapy + chemotherapy, called immunological chemotherapy. As above-mentioned, the elimination of the cancer cells in metastasis or the cancer cells or the cancer cell group in the blood circulation after operation mainly depends on the immunological cells in the organism of the host. It is shown by the experimental study that the immunological cells in the organism can eliminate 10^5 cancer cells, so the dosage for the assistant chemotheray after operation shall not be too large under the precondition of not damaging or slihgtly damaging the immunological cells because it is very important to carry out the immunological mediation and control therapy and improve the immunity of the organism to eliminate the cancer cells in metastasis. We deeply realize that in the past 16 years, Wuhan Shuguang Tumor Special Clinic under Wuhan Research Institute of Anti-cancerometastasis and Anti-reoccurrence has diagnosed so many patients like this, some of them are of valetudinarianism or accompanied with other diseases, resulting in failure to chemotherapy and radiotherapy; some of them fail to the chemotherapy again due to the severe response after 1-2 chemotherapy after operation; some of them refuse the chemotherapy after operation; most of the patients meet with the cancer invading serosa and are accompanied by metastasis of lymph node, so

they take XZ-C medicine for treatment in the new mode of XU ZE new concept of anti-cancerometastasis treatment and orally take XZ-C medicine for a long term, resulting in a relatively good curative effect.

6. Although the assistant chemotherapy after operation has been widely popularized all over the country at present, there are short of the forward-looking, comparable and appreciable reports on the assistant chemotherapy after operation. According to the report on 5-year's follow-up survey of the assistant chemotherapy or radiotherapy after operation on the patients suffering from the stomach cancer by American Stomach Cancer Group, it was reported by Lence (1994, 3, 3, 1390) that the total survival rate was still low in the patients suffering from the stomach cancer even the patients with the cancer removed through operation, therefore, the people hope to improve the prognosis through the assistant chemotherapy and radiotherapy for the patients with low tumor load after operation. It was shown by the results of the assistant treatment with mitomycin and fluorouracil on the first group of the patients in 1976 by British Stomach Cancer Organization that it had no benefit to the patients after operation, for this reason, the study on the assistant treatment of another group of patients had been made.

The forward-looking, random and contrapositive grouping study had been made on 430 patients suffering from the gastric gland cancer in Stage II and III after operation, accompanied with radiotherapy or the combined chemotherapy of mitomycin, adriamycin and fluorouracil (MAF) plan over 5 years, among which 372 patients died, 7 of which died of the surgical complication and 327 of which died of the reoccurrence of tumor. In the random grouping study, 145 cases only adopted the operation therapy; 153 cases accepted the assistant chemotherapy with the rang of irradiation including hilum of spleen and porta hepatic with the dosage of 4500cGy and the increase in dosage of 500cGy in operative field area; another 138 cases accepted the combined chemotherapy (MPA Plan) with mitomycin 4mg/m², adriamycin 30mg/m² and fluorouracil 600 mg/m², intravenously injected, 3 weeks as a cycle, totaling 6 cycles. The total two-year's survival rate of this group of patients was 33% and the total five-year's survival rate was 17% (13%~21%), compared with the patients with the single operation therapy, as to the patients accepting the assistant chemotherapy, the survival rate was not raised: the five-year's survival rate of the patients with single operation therapy was 20% and the one of the patients accepting the operation plus radiotherapy was 19%.

Therefore, operation is still the standard therapeutic method of the stomach cancer and the assistant therapeutic measures shall be restricted within a certain scope of study.

To sum up, it is held by the author: some large hospitals or medical centers in China should make the forward-looking comparable grouping study to obtain a large number of appreciable scientific data in China. At present, the assistant chemotherapy after operation is still restricted within a certain scope of study.

This topic for my monograph "new concept and new way of cancer treatment ". In this book in the international community it is the first time to initiative that cancer surgery after rejuvenation chemotherapy should be reformed and innovated:

This initiative will cause the work of the General Surgery and Chemotherapy Division of China's top three hospitals, the preparation of redeployment, postoperative adjuvant chemotherapy to perioperative adjuvant chemotherapy, the postoperative chemotherapy is the implementation of the surgeon and surgical nurses, that is, the surgeon and surgery nurses conduct the postoperative treatment and follow-up, so that the statistical results of the recent short-term efficacy and long-term efficacy can be understood ; because the surgeon understands the patient's condition, the surgeon should determine whether the need for chemotherapy and chemotherapy or not? This is suitable for the actual condition, improve efficacy. However, chemotherapy can greatly reduce the work of the preparation. This will be a major improvement measures to improve the quality of medical care and improve the level of team therapy.

6. THE OPINION OF IMPROVEMENT AND PERFECTION OF THE TRADITIONAL CHEMOTHERAPY CANCER TREATMENT

- Discussion about the "get" and "lost" after the use of anti-cancer drugs
- The status of tumor chemotherapy is the main reason for further improvement of efficacy
- Suggestions for improving and improving chemotherapy

I. On "gain" and "loss" after taking anti-cancer drugs

The treatment of cancer, no matter in early stage, mid stage or advanced stage, involves the comprehensive multi-discipline treatment.

The operation is a method of local treatment. The surgical oncology scientists hold that the cancer occurs locally at first, then encroaches the peripheral tissues and transfers to other places via lymphatic vessel and blood vessel, as a result, they stress on the local treatment, that is to say, the stress on control over the local growth and diffusion, especially when the cancer meets with metastasis via lymph, the lymph node is cleaned down by operation. For years, although the operative treatment has been improved continually in methodology, the long-term curative effects have not made remarkable progress as yet. The reoccurrence and metastasis after operation seriously threatens the prognosis of the patients, attracting high attention from the medical field, however, there has been no effective prescription up to now.

The radiotherapy is also a method of local treatment, which plays a role in killing off the cells from the local tumor per unit dosage. The radiotherapy effects are mostly affected by the factors including oxygenation of cells, type of tumor and restoration of cells and so on, all these characteristics determine that the radiotherapy is locally inferior to the surgical removal with respect to tumor.

The biological characteristics of cancer are invasion, reoccurrence and metastasis, which are the important reasons why the treatment with operation and radiotherapy fails.

In recent years, some one holds that cancer is a kind of generalized disease, so the generalized treatment should mainly depend on radiotherapy, however, it is a pity, in despite of the emerging new drugs and continually undated therapeutic methods and plans, the radiotherapy effects are not satisfactory. Since the cytotoxic drugs have no selectivity, they kill the cancer cells as well as the normal cells of the host, especially the immunological cells, in addition, they have severe side effects, inhibiting hematopiesis function of the bone marrow and reducing the immunity. Therefore, the traditional radiotherapy does not entirely conform to the well-known actual conditions of the biological behaviors of the cancer at present, for example, the invasion behaviors and metastasis of the cancer cells are of multi-link and multi-step. At present, people have cognized that the anti-tumor drugs do not always prevent the metastasis and reoccurrence.

In 1980s, the tumorous bioremediation emerged, such as immunological therapy, cytokine therapy and gene vaccination therapy. It was proven that some therapies could mediate the immunity of the patients, however, it has not proven that which immunological preparation or method could induce the extinction of tumor.

In the recent 20 years, so many reports on treatment of cancer with traditional Chinese medicine have been made and its outlook has been concerned by the people. Especially, with the further development of the study on medicine and immunology, people have realized that the disorder of the immune system of the organism is closely related to the occurrence and development of tumor and traditional Chinese medicine has its own characteristics and advantages in tumor treatment through mediating the immunologic function of the organism. The immunoregulation of traditional Chinese medicine and development of immunoregulator of traditional Chinese medicine will attract more attention and favor all over the world. With the assistance of operation, radiotherapy and chemotherapy, the traditional Chinese medicine can bring its immunoregulation into full play in the process of treatment and obviously prolong the survival time and improve the survival quality, in this way, the characteristics and advantages of the traditional Chinese medicine are fully embodied, however, it is disadvantageous in unremarkably improving the tumor.

Since the above-mentioned methods have different characteristics in action mechanism and effect with respect to treatment of cancer and different curative effects as well as their own disadvantages, so it is necessary to focus on the advantages and disadvantages of various therapies aiming at the "gain" and the "loss" of the paints, for example, what's the "advantage" and the "disadvantage" after taking the therapy, what's the "gain" and the "loss" of the patients? We should learn from the strong points of one therapy to offset the weakness of the other therapies and combine these therapies organically and reasonably to form the comprehensive therapeutic plans for cancer, only in this way, can the side effects from the drugs be obviously reduced, the survival quality of the patients be improved and the total survival time be prolonged. In the past 16 years, Tumor Specialized Clinic of Shuguang Tumor Research Institute has treated over 12000 cancer patients in mid and advanced stage with XZ-C immunoregulation therapy in practice and most of the patients have achieved the effects of improving the survival quality, stabilizing the lesion, controlling the metastasis, keeping survival with tumor and remarkably prolonging the survival time.

II. Actual conditions of chemotherapy in tumor: main cause affecting further improvement of curative effects of chemotherapy

The total effective rate of treatment with anti-tumor drug in clinic is only 14%, the factors impeding chemotherapy' better curative effects mainly include:

1. Blindness of current chemotherapy. Now it is unknown whether the chemical medicine used in the current therapeutic plan for chemotherapy is sensitive to the cancer cells of the patients just because most of the patients are not subject to the drugsensitive test to cancer cells. If the medicine is used by experience, it has blindness, that is to say, it may be beneficial to some patients while harmful to other patients. Based on the drugsensitive test results, remarkable curative effects have been made in treating the infectious diseases with antibiotics, as enlightens us on reasonably and jointly administrating drug through testing the sensitivity of the cancer cells of the patients to the cytotoxic drugs for chemotherapy so as to replace the blind chemotherapy with "individualized" chemotherapy. It is shown by the data that it can double the effective rate of chemotherapy.

2. **Drug resistance of chemotherapy.** Most of the solid tumor, such as stomach cancer, cancer of large intestine, is lowly sensitive or insensitive to the chemotherapy. Some tumor is remitted after chemotherapy, however, it meets with reoccurrence, resulting in ineffective chemotherapy, indicating that the cancer cells has the drug resistance to the chemotherapy drug. The reasons why the drug resistance appears include many factors such as drug transmission disturbance of solid tumor, cell proliferation, difference in dynamics, immunity and metabolism and so on.

3. Selectivity toxicity of chemotherapy anti-cancer drug. The chemotherapy drug is the cytotoxic drug, killing the cancer cells as well as the normal histiocytes, without selectivity, especially the hemopoietic stem cells of the bone marrow with exuberant proliferation and immunological cells as well as stomach cells and intestinal cells. Compared with the volume of the normal tissue, since the cancerous protuberance only accounts for a minimal proportion, it is possible to "kill one hundred enemies while injuring three thousand soldiers on one's own side". The blindness of chemotherapy and the drug resistance of chemotherapy result in low curative effects, in case that it is expected to improve the curative effects by means of increasing the dosage, increasing the kinds of drugs and shortening the time, the toxic effects will be further aggravated, so the chemotherapy in cancer is still satisfactory in despite of great progress. The drugs shall be selected by testing the sensitivity and drug resistance of the chemotherapy drug so as to have a definite object in view. If the drugsensitive test is made on the chemotherapy patients so as to avoid the damage on the patients from the blind chemotherapy and benefit the chemotherapy patients, the epoch of chemotherapy will be opened up.

III. Suggestion on improving and perfecting the chemotherapy in cancer

Since nitrogen mustard drugs were reported by Gillman and Phillips in 1946 to treat the tumor in hematopiesis function, the chemotherapy has made great progress for 60 years and the great achievements have been made in therapeutics of the malignant tumor, for example, the chemotherapy has cured over 10 kinds of malignant tumor including chorionepithilioma, acute lymphocytic leukemia, Hodgkin disease, seminoma of testis, small-cell carcinoma of the lung and Wilms tumor and so on, and remitted the tumor including breast cancer, children' lymphadenoma, neuroblastoma and osteosarcoman and so on, resulting in prolonged survival time. Thus three principles of treatment including operation, chemotherapy and radiotherapy are established. Since the chemotherapy has made great achievements, especially in the recent 20 years, it has been widely used for various solid tumor, especially in the assistant treatment after operation, so the metastasis and dissemination in some patients has been restrained and improved, giving hope to treatment of solid tumor after operation. However, it is a pity that the reoccurrence and the metastasis happen again after several months and the patients still die of the cancer despite chemotherapy or intensive chemotherapy again. According to the follow-up survey to over 12000 metastasis and reoccurrence patients and the analysis of and experience in treatment summarization in Tumor Specialized Clinic of Shuguang Tumor Research Institute, it is found neither metastasis nor the reoccurrence could not be restrained on thousands of patients receiving the assistant chemotherapy after operation, the survival time and the survival time without cancer are not obviously improved. At present, although the assistant chemotherapy after operation has been made all over the country, there has been no prospective and correlatable scientific data, the assistant chemotherapy after operation is still in study. Of course, there are lots of patients receiving assistant chemotherapy after operation who have been in good condition over 10 years even 20 years, however, due to lack of prospective and correlatable scientific data, what is the comparison result between chemotherapy and non-chemotherapy in the patients after operation? What is the long-term survival rate of the patients not subject to chemotherapy? How to prove the long-term survival results from the chemotherapy after operation? All of these issues shall be further studied. At present, the reports in China lack lots of prospective and correlatable follow-up survey analysis data as well as the prospective and correlatable evaluation data about the assistant chemotherapy after operation just because the case history is kept by the patient instead of the hospital, as a result, the doctors and the hospital cannot make the follow-up survey. Of course, the in-hospital case history is kept for study, however, the in-hospital case history just reflects the short-term curative effects, most of the effects reflected in the in-hospital case history are relatively good because if it is not so good, the patient is not allowed to leave hospital. However, most patients are in good condition temporarily, for example, after the incision heals up, the patient begins to take food again and takes case of itself, the short-term curative effects are good, but it is hardly realized that the cancer cells may be in metastasis and it cannot be tested at present, of course, some tumor markers can be dynamically observed, such as CEA and AFP and so on.

Then, how to make the further study? Start from the existing problems to settle the problems through experiments and clinical study. The treatment of cancer shall be people-oriented and aim at curing the sickness to save the patient.

1. Actively searching, studying and developing intelligent anti-cancer drugs. The main contradictions in chemotherapy have been mentioned above and now we should pay attention to how to study and perfect them. The main issue is: the chemotherapy is the cytotoxic drug, without selectivity, so it cannot selectively distinguish the cancer cells from the normal cells, killing off all of them, resulting in some side effects and contradictions. So we should update the thought and actively study, search and develop the "intelligent anti-cancer drug" that only selectively kills the cancer cells instead of the normal cells of the organism, especially the immunological cells. In June 2004, American Society of Clinical Oncology held the annual meeting in New Orleans, with over 20000 oncologists as the attendants and 3700 papers called. Among these 3700 papers, there were 30 papers greatly affecting the treatment of cancer, of which there were 9 papers discussing the intelligent anti-cancer drugs. The intelligent anti-cancer drugs only affect the specific molecules in the cancer cells. The research findings of intelligent anti-drugs come into the world, indicating the treatment of cancer would shift to the epoch of accurate administration with little side effects from the one of chemotherapy with very great side effects. In research and development of the intelligent anti-cancer drugs, the research and development personnel do not spread these drugs at present. I believe that in the coming future, with the wide use of these drugs, people would feel the great effects from them and the patients would benefit from them. **Among the 48 kinds of anti-cancer drugs with relatively good tumor-inhibiting rate screened by this lab from 200 kinds of natural vegetable drugs, there are 3 kinds of vegetable drugs that can entirely inhibit and kill the cancer cells entirely and has no effects on the cultured epithelial cells or fibrous cells in the culture in vitro experiment on cancer cells, including XZ-C1-A, XZ-C1-B and XZ-C1-C. In the in vivo tumor-inhibition experiment on tumor-bearing animals, their tumor-inhibiting rate is 85%-95%. They are a part of XZ-C1, XZ-C immunoregulation anti-cancer medicine.** This experiment takes chemotherapy drug CTX as the control group and CTX obviously inhibits the immunity and the bone marrow. XZ-C anti-cancer medicine has no effects on bone marrow.

2. Suggestion on immunologic chemotherapy. Namely immunological treatment + chemotherapy. The immunological drugs can be administered in peri-chemotherapy period so as to reduce the side effects from chemotherapy; after chemotherapy, the immunologic treatment should be continued for a period to enhance the curative effects. The immunological treatment is the most reasonable treatment, it is of 0 order kinetics, however, it ① has relatively small acting force, it acts on $10^{5\text{-}6}$ cancer cells strongly; beyond this range, it acts weakly. ②The immunological drug can improve the immunity of the organism and enhance the immunological surveillance in the organism. ③ It can be continually administered or taken orally. Because the cancer cells are continually divided and proliferated, the treatment shall be also continual. XZ-C immunoregulation medicine can protect the hematopiesis function of the bone marrow, protect the thymus, improve the immunity, improve the symptom and raise the life quality; the action is relatively slowly, little but durably. Since the biological characteristics of the cancer cells are the continual division and proliferation, our countermeasures must be also continual.

Chemotherapy and immunological treatment currently adopted should learn from other's strong points to offset one's weakness and be comprehensively applied so as to improve the curative effects. The chemotherapy is of intermittent administration while the immunoregulation treatment is of continual treatment. If both of them assist with each other, the curative effects will be improved undoubtedly. If the cancer patient has inferior immunologic function, the operation on cancer will bring down the immunologic function further. In operation, the cancer cells entering the blood circulation by extrusion increase. How to eliminate or control the cancer cells entering the blood circulation in operation? It is held by us that XZ-C medicine should be added before, in and after operation for immunological treatment. XZ-C$_4$ can protect the thymus and XZ=C$_8$ can protect the bone marrow. In this way, the central immune organ and immunologic function of the host can be protected, the curative effects of the chemotherapy can be strengthened and the side effects of the chemotherapy inhibiting the immunologic function can be reduced, as a result, it will reduce the opportunity of metastasis of cancer cells, therefore, the improvement of immunologic function of the patient in the peri-operation period or in the period of assistant chemotherapy after operation is an important link of comprehensive treatment.

3. Making sensitivity test of chemotherapy drugs and implementing "individualized" immunological chemotherapy. Now the chemotherapy in cancer has stepped into the stage of "individualized" chemotherapy in many hospitals. Previously, the different cancer patients are subject to the same chemotherapy plan, unavoidably resulting in blindness, not conforming to the actual conditions of the patients. It is shown by the study that even though the same kind of tumor with same type of tissue, even the different stages of the same cancer, has different sensitivities to the chemotherapy drugs, therefore, it is necessary to make the drugsensitive test on the individual cancer patients and it is urgent to select the sensitive drugs from various anti-cancer drugs. It is proven by the clinical experience in chemotherapy that the effective rate of administration by experience is very low (14%), if the drug can be selected according to the results measured by drugsensitive test, the effective rate can be raised to 28%-35%.

The effect of chemotherapy in the solid tumor is not as good as the one in malignant tumor in the blood system and the transmission hindrance of drug in the solid tumor is the upmost factor of drug resistance of solid tumor.

It is an important way and one of the current study hotspots to make the sensitive test on chemotherapy drug for tumor and carry out the individualized chemotherapy plan so as to improve the effects of chemotherapy in tumor and reduce the side effects.

Generally, the drugsensitive test on tumor can be made with the method of culture in vitro and culture in vivo, the former includes cell culture method and tissue culture method and the latter refers to the method of culture in vivo in animal. Among the test methods, the method of transplantation in vivo in the nude mice can obtain true and reliable results with respect to drug test or new drug screening, however, the process is long, the operation is complicated and the price is high. The method of cell culture is the most simple, convenient and feasible, however, since the kinetics is not entirely same to the tumor in vivo, the test results often differ from the drug reaction of the tumor in vivo, so it cannot be used to directly guide the administration of the different tumor patients.

Someone makes a study on 3D tissue culture method of tumor, namely Hoffman 3D tissue culture method, which directly uses the clinical samples, avoids the repeated digestion of tumor cells with enzyme or mechanically and features quickness and relatively high success ratio. This method would be helpful to guide the individualized chemotherapy, improve the chemotherapy effects and reduce the drug resistance.

(1) In vitro drugsensitive test: it is very important to establish the reliable anti-cancer in vitro drugsensitive test method so as to help the clinicians select the effective chemotherapy drugs, reasonably design the therapeutic method, improve the curative effects, avoid the side effects from the ineffective drugs and directly screen the new anti-cancer and anti-metastasis drugs with the fresh human tumor samples.

There are so many methods of in vitro sensitive test of anti-cancer drug and they have the common characteristics: simple method, high sensitivity, smaller dose than the in vivo method, quick judgment results, without too many animals; in addition, they also can screen the anti-cancer drugs and most of them are parallel to the in vivo method with respect to the procedures.

(2) in vivo chemotherapy drug sensitive test: at present, as to the chemotherapy drug sensitive test methods, the in vitro method prevails and it has the advantages of quickness, convenience and simple as well as good clinical correlation and good repeatability, however, it also has some disadvantages because it breaks away from the in vivo environment of the tumor and is not consistent with the human tumor in histology and cell kinetics, reducing the coincidence rate of the test results and the clinic.

Various drugs have different concentrations in the body fluid and are affected by the body weight, route of medication, liver and kidney function and so on, in this way, the in vitro method cannot represent the change in drug concentration. Some drugs should be activated and metabolized in vivo before playing a role in anti-cancer, such as CTX; some drugs acting on the cancer cells will bring into play through the immune system. The reaction of the cancer cells to these drugs cannot be tested with in vitro method.

The solid tumor are the spatial structure occupying a certain space. Besides the tumor cells in blood, breast and ascites are directly contact with the drugs, the solid tumor is not so simple. The drugs cannot reach up to the deep part easily; the anoxia caused by ischemia; the uneven blood flow in the tumor; the difference in PH value and osmotic pressure will affect the sensitivity of the solid tumor cells to the chemotherapy drugs.

It is necessary to select the optimal "individualized" joint chemotherapy plan through the drugsensitive test.

7. THE BASIC MODEL AND SPECIFIC PROGRAMS OF ANTI-CANCER METASTASIS

- The basic pattern of anti-cancer metastasis
- The specific treatment plansof anti-cancer metastasis
- Immunotherapy plays an important role in anticancer treatment

Traditional chemotherapy against metastasis mainly aims to kill cancer cells. No matter it is the primary carcinoma, metastatic carcinoma, the postoperative adjuvant chemotherapy preventing reoccurrence and metastasis or when metastasis of lymph nodes is found, intravenous chemotherapy drugs are adopted in all cases. However, because chemotherapy drugs are of no selectivity and kill both cancer cells and normal cells (especially the immunological cells), they act as a double-edged sword. The author holds that various schemes for intravenous chemotherapy are mainly the different combinations of cytotoxic drugs, which are not certainly in line with the multi-link and multi-step biological characteristics of the cancerometastasis process.

I. The basic model of anti-cancerometastasis treatment

Among the innumerable patients in this clinical practice, it is not uncommon to see that some of them are not free from metastasis after the postoperative adjuvant chemotherapy. What is worse is that some of them suffered a simultaneous metastasis in chemotherapy or suffered from the metastasis again after chemotherapy again. All these phenomena make us deeply think about the reason behind the failure to prevent metastasis. Is it the traditional chemotherapy not in line with the biological characteristics of cancerometastasis process? Whether it is necessary to update our knowledge and thinking, or to change our conceptions and treatment model on anti-cancerometastasis? Xu Ze's design concept of anti-cancerometastasis countermeasures is just an innovation of the concepts, thinking, methods and models of the traditional anti-metastasis treatment.

Anti-metastasis drugs tend to interfere or blockade a certain link or step of the metastasis process of cancer cells or the cancer cell clusters so as to inhibit the formation of metastasis focus. Although the chemotherapeutic cytotoxic drugs can kill tumor cells, suspend the growth of primary carcinoma and delay the occurrence time of metastasis, they fail to inhibit the process of invasion and metastasis. At present, the ideal drugs killing the primary carcinoma and inhibiting invasion and metastasis are unavailable. Thus, it is necessary to study the strategy of interdiction, prevention and treatment aiming at the development steps and mechanism of the cancerometastasis summarized as "eight steps and three stages".

The invasion and metastasis of carcinoma is a complicated process of many steps and the metastasis process could be generalized as following: proliferation of primary cancerous protuberance→ the formation and growth of newly born micrangium of tumor→ invading and breaking through basement membrane→ cancer cells breaking away from parent tumor and breaking through basement membrane and then perforating micrangiums or micro lymphatic vessels→ the survival and floating of invading blood in the circulatory system→ formation of small cancer embolus from cancer cells clusters wrapped by blood platelet and delivery to remote target organs together with blood stream→ the detention in the micrangium of target organs→ the attachment or adherence of cancer embolus to the wall of micrangium→ breaking through blood vessels and forming micro metastasis focus→formation of newly born micrangium of tumor as the metastasis focus→ the proliferation of the metastasis focus. If we could find the way to blockade one or several links or steps, it is possible to control metastasis, as is the context in which Xu Ze's new model of anti-cancerometastasis treatment is formed and developed.

II. The specific plan of anti-cancerometastasis treatment

According to biological behaviors of modern oncology on cancerometastasis and theory of reoccurrence and metastasis, this libratory has been always searching for new anti-metastasis drugs among traditional Chinese herbs extracted from natural herbs for years. Through experimental study on of tumor-bearing animal bodies with traditional Chinese medicine as well as the combination of traditional Chinese medicine and western medicine, we interfere, obstruct and intercept all the links of the metastasis, and develop an anti-metastasis scheme and countermeasure with XZ-C medicine, including XZ-C-TG against the formation of micrangium, XZ-C-AS dissolving cancer embolus, XZ-C-MD against invading into and breaking through blood vessels, XZ-C-LM with antigenicity, XZ-C-Ind against PGE2; VA and XZ-C-CA as calcium channel blocking drugs against invasion, XZ-C-GB against adherence, XZ-C-TIMP against the resistance to drugs, XZ-C$_1$ inhibiting cancer cells rather than normal cells; XZ-C$_4$ protecting thymus and improving immunity; XZ-C$_8$ protecting bone marrow and improving hematogenesis function and Emulsion of Brucea Javanica into lymph nodes. The comprehensive measures of the above-mentioned treatment schemes have achieved sound curative effects in the clinical practice by our anti-cancer cooperative group.

Because cancerometastasis is a complicated process of multi-step and multi-link, it is necessary to adopt the comprehensive measures in an all-round way to treat the cancerometastasis instead of a certain drug or measure. Thus aiming at the steps of metastasis, we scientifically design and adopt different treatment schemes and countermeasures shown in the following table. Those treatment schemes and countermeasures aiming at the steps of metastasis are to achieve the same goal of anti-metastasis.

The new model of anti-cancerometastasis treatment of Xu Ze's new concept
(treatment schemes and countermeasures for the steps of canceromestasis)

Metastasis step	Treatment countermeasures	XZ-C medicine and its role
Proliferation of primary cancerous	Operation, chemotherapy	$XZ-C_1$ inhibiting cancer cells
		$XZ-C_4$ protecting thymus and improving immunity
		$XZ-C_8$ protecting bone marrow and improving hematogenesis function
Growth of newly born micrangium of tumor	Inhibiting the formation of micrangium	XZ-C-TG against formation of micrangium
		XZ-C-CA against adherence
Invasion into basement membrane	Anti-adhesion, anti-kinesalgia and inhibiting the activity of hydrolase	XZ-C-K(LWF) against adhesion
		Ind against PGE2
		XZ-C-MD against kinesalgia
Breaking through blood vessels or lymphatic vessels	Anti-adhesion, anti-kinesalgia and inhibiting the activity of hydrolase	XZ-C-MD against invasion into blood vessels
		XZ-C-K (LWF)
		$XZ-C_{1+4}$ mediating immunity
In the blood of circulatory system	Inhibiting the aggregation and coagulation of blood platelet. Biological response modification (BRM)	XZ-C-N (CZR) against the aggregation of blood platelet
		XZ-C-LM
		XZ-C-ASP dissolving cancer embolus
		$XZ-C_{1+4}$ mediating immunity
The formation of cancer embolus	Promoting blood circulation and removing stasis and resisting thrombus	XZ-C-K (NSR) against cancer embolus
		XZ-C-N (CZR) against aggregation of blood platelet
The breaking out of cancer embolus from blood vessels	Resisting adhesion, kinesalgia, and the activity of hydrolase	XZ-C-MD against the breaking out of cancer embolus
The formation of metastasis focus	Operation, radiotherapy, chemotherapy	$XZ-C_{1+4}$ mediating immunity
		XZ-C-TG inhibiting the growth of blood vessels
The metastasis of lymph nodes	Liposoluble drugs	The Emulsion of Brucea Javanica as the carrier of lipa entering into the lymph nodes

The correlative factors of the invasion of cancer cells are adherence, enzymatic secretion and kinesalgia. The inhibition of adhesion, kinesalgia and enzymatic secretion is also helpful to inhibit the exfoliation of cancer cells from parent tumor, its break into matrix and the formation of the newly born blood vessels of the tumor besides its contribution to prevent the invasion of primary carcinoma. For years the researches on inhibitors inhibiting the growth of newly born blood vessels are seen in reports. Meanwhile, it is also discovered in the tumor-bearing animal experiment screening the anti-cancerometastasis drugs by this libratory that traditional Chinese medicine TG is of sound inhibiting effects on newly born blood vessels. Tumor cells are in weakest condition to resist the host environment when entering into the blood of the circulatory system and can be easily eliminated by the immunological cells of the host. It is proved by some literature that a vast majority of cancer cells entering into the circulatory system are killed by immunological cells and only a number of approximately 0.01% thereof could survive and possibly become the focus of metastasis. Except the mechanical damage factors, the cancer cells in blood stream are mainly eliminated by the damaging effects of the immunological function of the hosts against tumor cells. Tumor-bearing patients usually suffer low immunological function inhibited by tumor and chemotherapy. Therefore, it is necessary to adopt immunotherapy, biotherapy and biological response modification and traditional Chinese medicine for immunological mediation to protect the function of immune organs so as to improve the immunity of the host. It is found that XZ-C medicine can protect bone marrow and improve hemogenesis function, protect hemogenesis function of bone marrow as well as stem cells, improve immunologic function and inhibit the metastasis of tumor. According to the clinical application on the innumerable patients in the clinic of Anti-cancer Cooperative Group of Traditional Chinese Medicine Combined with Western Medicine over ten years, XZ-C medicine against cancer and metastasis has achieved significant curative effects.

III. The important role of immunotherapy in anti-cancerometastasis treatment

Among all the current therapeutic methods, operation and radiotherapy are both local therapy while chemotherapy, immunotherapy, biological therapy, therapy with traditional Chinese medicine are systematic therapy. At present, the chemotherapy mainly targets the focus of primary cancer or metastasis focus and the criterion to judge the curative effects is to alleviate and shrink the tumor. In order to fulfill of the above criterion, a significant dose of chemotherapeutic cytotoxic drugs are in need to shrink the lump. Additionally in view of the cell cycle, medicines are necessarily combined in order to achieve a certain level of lethality. If it is a 1cm×1cm^2 lump, it would contain a number of 10^{12} cancer cells and this, requires a considerable dose of chemotherapeutic drugs to shrink it into half. However, it only needs a slight dose if cancer cells are eliminated in the process of metastasis by chemotherapy, because the amount of cancer cells in metastasis process only accounts to 10^7 to 10^8 and most of them could be eliminated. The problem happens as a large amount of immunological cells in blood circulation are destroyed by chemotherapeutic cytotoxic drugs whereas the anti-metastasis mainly depends on the system against cancer cells of the organism itself. Thus it would be a great loss to patients. Chemotherapy could only be conducted with intermission during which time a large amount of cancer cells and immunological cells would be both eliminated. However there still exist a handful of escaped cancer cells during this period which continually split and proliferate or are even more active. More than that, the destroyed immunological cells, decreased immunity and weakened immune surveillance would also lead or contribute to the development and metastasis of cancer cells.

Therefore, the chemotherapeutic drugs should not be overdosed in the anti-metastasis treatment and should not impair a large amount of immunological cells. Meanwhile, chemotherapy should be accompanied by Immunotherapy, Biotherapy, Biological Response Modification (BRM), XZ-C medicine and tonic traditional Chinese medicine so as to give play to each other's advantages and make up each other's imperfections. Because a properly protected and activated immune system of the body could eliminate 10^6 cancer cells and additional chemotherapeutic drugs could destroy most cancer cells in the process of metastasis, it is possible to hold up and cut off the metastasis path and put the diffusion and metastasis under further control.

Xu Ze's new concept of anti-metastasis treatment promotes the application of immunochemotherapy, namely the combination of immunotherapy and chemotherapy. To be specific, immune drugs would be used in the peri-chemotheraputic period, in other words, at the week before the chemotherapy to be implemented, and would not be ceased in the chemotherapy period unless in case of serious chemotherapy response. The immunotherapy will continue for 6 to 9 months after chemotherapy and during intermission for the maintenance of a certain level of immunity and the consolidation of the curative effects. All these above are proved to be reasonable. For 16 years the Dawn Specialist Out-patient of our anti-metastasis laboratory uses XZ-C anti-cancer traditional Chinese medicine for immunological mediation to coordinate chemotherapy, which usually causes less chemotherapy response. Most of the postoperative in our out-patients suffer the liver, gallbladder, pancreas, stomach, intestine, lung and breast cancer. Some suffer a multi-part lymphatic metastasis after radical operations but then meet with serious response after chemotherapy thus come to our out-patient for treatment. Some fail the exploratory operation and some are under palliative operations. Therefore, the author, through combining the small-dosed chemotherapy with XZ-C medicine, usually finds less response and hemogram variation. Because of different conditions of the patients and the absence of comparability, it is impossible to conduct the comparative observation of perspective random allocation. Therefore, the perspective clinical study is conducted by comparatively observing the curative effects of the immunotherapy group and the chemotherapy group with immune indexes (IFN, IL-2 and TNF), the level of tumor marker, the quality of life and the survival time as the evaluative criteria of the two groups.

The immune drugs used in the above-mentioned immunochemotherapy shall increase the immunity indexes of the body. Actually not all traditional Chinese medicine that support healthy energy and eliminate evil are able to improve immunity because some are of bidirectional regulating function, which would improve immunity at a certain dosage range but lower immunity at another dosage range. For example, the glossy privet fruit could significantly increase the spleen and thymus indexes; the bupleurum roots lead to the atrophy of the mice thymus; and the liquid made from the pilose antlers of a young stag could improve the weight of the spleen and thymus of the mice if it is poured into their stomach. Additionally, barrenwort polysaccharide would lead to the atrophy of the thymus but a long-term oral administration turns to increase the weight of thymus. $XZ-C_{1+4+8}$ medicine is proved to be able to increase cytokines like IFN, IL-2, TNF etc and to decrease the level of tumor markers of many terms by many animal experiments and long-term clinical observation. To be specific, $XZ-C_4$ could protect bone marrow and thymus and improve hematopoiesis functions and immunity thus raises the overall immune level. The test by cultivating cancer cells in vitro reveals that the series of XZ-C1 medicine, including $XZ-C_1$-A, $XZ-C_1$-B and $XZ-C_1$-C, are the three pharmaceutics that 100% kill cancer cells, 100% cause no harm to normal cells and achieve an 85% to 95% tumor-inhibiting rate in tumor-inhibiting experiments on the body of tumor-bearing animals.

Cyclophosphane (CTX) as the control group only achieves a tumor-inhibiting rate of 45% and also significantly decreases the immunity.

The removal of focus of primary cancer and metastasis focus depends on local surgical removal or radiation exposure. The focus of primary cancer should be removed by surgical removal if possible and in case of impossibility, it would be helpful to turn to interventional therapy, radiotherapy, radio frequency, focused ultrasound or the injection of absolute ethyl alcohol so as to control the local focus.

The metastasis of tumor is an essential expression of malignancy. The reason why cancer treatment is failed is that the treatment isn't proper and the immunity of the patients isn't sufficiently strong to kill all the cancer cells. Literatures show that a marginally small tumor (1 to 8g) could release millions or even thousand millions of cancer cells in 24 hours into blood. However, a vast majority of these cancel cells would be eliminated by the human body's immune system and only 1% of them are possibly able to survive and evolve into metastasis tumor. The test data of our libratory reveals that the immunity of mice is capable of killing 100,000 cancer cells. The amount could be increased to more than 1,000,000 if XZ-C$_1$ medicine is used. The question is what destroys them? It is the immunological cells of the body itself. Thus Xu Ze's new concept holds that the immunological cells of body should be protected and not be damaged by any treatments. It is necessary to find ways to protect and activate the immunological function of the host. It would be beneficial for the patients if the immunotherapy and a small-dosed chemotherapy are combined as immunochemotherapy, learning from each other's strong points and offsetting each other's weakness.

8. THE NEW MODELS AND NEW METHODS OF CANCER TREATMENT

- Strengthen immunotherapy, to improve adverse reactions to chemotherapy
- Change intermittent treatment for continuous treatment
- change the damage to the host into protecting the host
- change the potential of the tumor and the host, and strive imbalance into the balance
- change from damaging the central immune organs into protecting the central immune organs
- change the injury therapy into non-injury therapy

I. Strengthening of immunological therapy and improving side effects from chemotherapy

1. Side effects of traditional chemotherapy: when chemotherapy is made on cancer, it usually inhibits immunologic function and hematopoiesis function of the bone marrow, descends WBC and PLT and damages liver and kidney function as well as gastroenteric function, leading to the side effects such as nausea, emesis, abdominal distension, anorexia and so on.

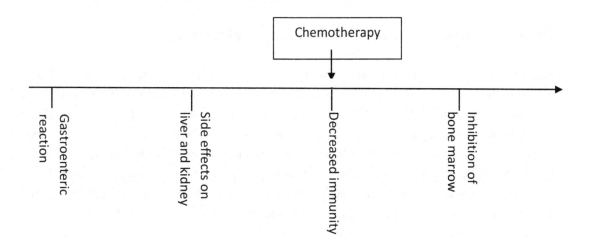

Fig. 1 Side effects of traditional chemotherapy

273

2. The countermeasures of Xu Ze's new concept: the method to improve the side effects of chemotherapy is to strengthen the supporting therapy and take effective measures to protect the host. Among the traditional Chinese medicine for immunological mediation, XZ-C$_4$ can protect thymus thus and improve immunity; XZ-C$_8$ can protect hematopoiesis function of the bone marrow and generate more stem cells; XZ-C medicine for immunity mediation can strengthen physical strength of cancerous patients. See Fig. 2.

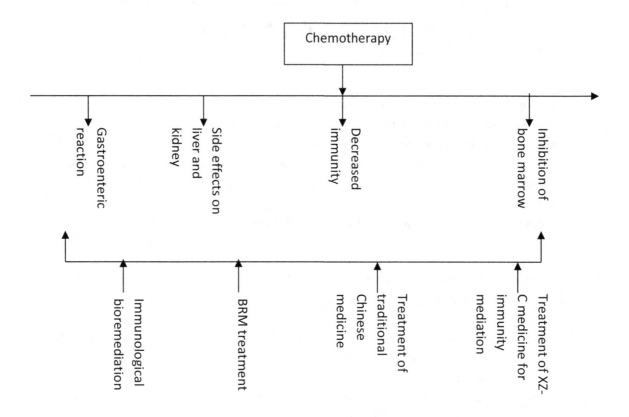

Fig. 2 Countermeasures for side effects of chemotherapy

II. Changing intermittent treatment into continual treatment

1. Traditional intravenous chemotherapy is an intermittent therapy, that is to say, after the drug for chemotherapy is applied for 3-5 days, it is necessary to apply the chemotherapeutic drug for the second course of treatment when WBC and PLT return to normal after 3-4 weeks. The drug for chemotherapy shall not be continually applied during the intermission between the first and the second course of treatment, whereas the cancel cells are still continually and uninterruptedly proliferated and divided in the intermission and increase at the speed of geometrical progression. In addition, because of the inhibition of immunologic function caused by chemotherapeutic drug, the cancel cells escape from or are free of the immunological surveillance, their proliferation and division are quickened during the intermission between these two courses, in other words, the longer the course of treatment of chemotherapeutic drug, the more the combined drug and the more the dose, the more serious of the attack against immunity of the human body, resulting in lack of immunological surveillance, and even resulting in reoccurrence and metastasis in chemotherapy, and shrinkage of tumor firstly before

continual enlargement later (see Fig. 3). These cases occur commonly, how to treat them? It is held by us that the following model should be adopted for a continuous immunological therapy in the intermission between two courses of treatment.

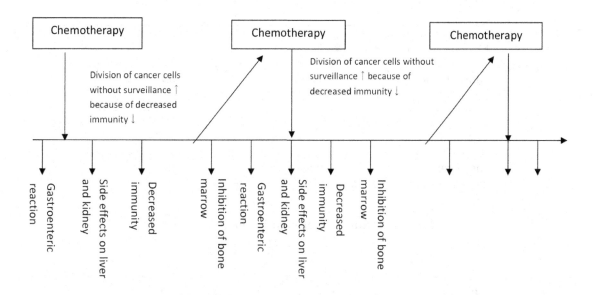

Fig.3 Easy reoccurrence of tumor without treatment in the intermission

2. Xu Ze's new concept and model of cancer treatment is a continuous treatment. It adopts traditional Chinese medicine for immunological mediation, namely $XZ-C_1 + XZ-C_4$, or BRM for treatment during the intermission. $XZ-C_1$ was screened through the experimental study on tumor-bearing animals over 7 years and has been proven by a sixteen-year clinical verification that it has only inhibited the cancel cells rather than normal ones and that it can benefit spleen and stomach. $XZ-C_4$ can protect thymus from atrophy, prevent immunity from decreasing and make it better. Continual treatment in the intermittence with XZ-C medicine can control proliferation of caner cells and also protect the function of immune organs such as thymus.

The combination of chemotherapeutic drug and XZ-C medicine can decrease teh side effects from chemotherapy and strengthen chemotherapy effects against the loss of immunological surveillance as well meanwhile. See Fig. 4.

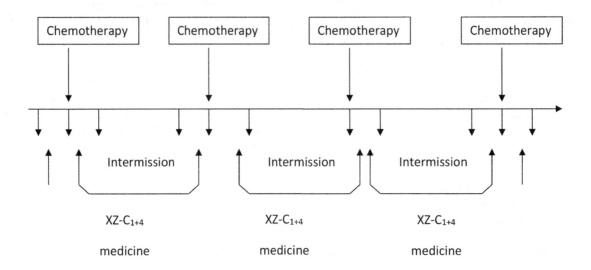

Fig. 4 Continual treatment in the intermission

III. Therapy of protecting the host instead of damaging the host

1. Traditional chemotherapy tends to damage the hosts: chemotherapeutic drugs are the x drugs and function as a double-edged sword, killing both cancer cells and normal ones for the lack of selectivity, inhibiting bone marrow and decreasing peripheral WBC and PLT. See Fig. 5.

2. Xu Ze' new concept and model of cancer treatment tends to protect the hosts: the new-type anticancer drugs only inhibit cancer cells, have no effects on normal cells, protect thymus, improve immunity and protect bone marrow. Among XZ-C medicine, $XZ-C_1$ only inhibits the cancel cells and have no effects on normal cells; $XZ-C_4$ protects thymus from atrophy and improves immunity; $XZ-C_8$ protects bone marrow and produces blood, all of which have been screened through the experiments on tumor-bearing animals over 7 years and have been proven by the clinical data of nearly 10000 cases in the cooperative anti-cancer clinic over 10 years. See Fig. 6.

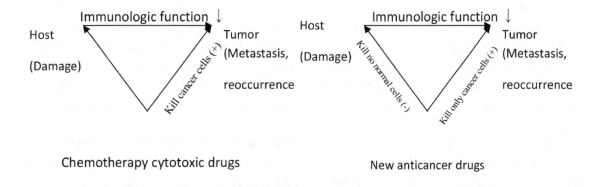

Fig. 5 Effects of traditional chemotherapy　　**Fig. 6 Effects of Xu Ze's new model of cancer treatment**

IV. Rebalancing the unbalance between the host and tumor

It has been proven by the abovementioned findings from the experimental study that the positive relationship exists between the occurrence and development of tumor and the structure and immunologic function of immune organs of the host such as thymus and marrow. Enlightened by the seesaws in children's park and the weighing scale in the laboratory, the author took a tumble: if immunologic function was too inferior, tumor would grow up, meanwhile, when the former was improved to a certain level, then the later would be controlled in a stable or improvement condition (Fig. 7). However, the fluctuation of the level depends on further experimental observation and test.

Thus, the occurrence and development of tumor depends on the relationship between immunologic function of the host and the intrinsic biological characteristics of tumor. Similarly, the invasion and metastasis of cancer also rests with the relationship, namely, carcinoma would be put under control in case of the balance between biological characteristics of tumor cells and impacts of the host on the inhibition factors; otherwise, the cancer would grow up.

Traditional radiotherapy and chemotherapy are inclined to weakening immunologic function and lead to a worse unbalance between both of them.

Xu Ze's new model of cancer treatment aims to improve the immunity of patients as much as possible, level off the decreased *immunity* (Fig. 8) and thus inhibit tumor growth and strengthen immunological surveillance.

Immune system is the one composed of immune organs, immunological cell and molecules executing immunologic function, mainly including central lymphatic tissue, peripheral lymphatic tissue and immunological cells. Central lymphatic tissue, the home to immune cells for their occurrence, differentiation and maturation, includes thymus and bone marrow. Peripheral lymphatic tissue includes lymph nodes, spleens and stomachs, in which T cells and B cells settle and these cells make their immune response after the identification of foreign antigen.

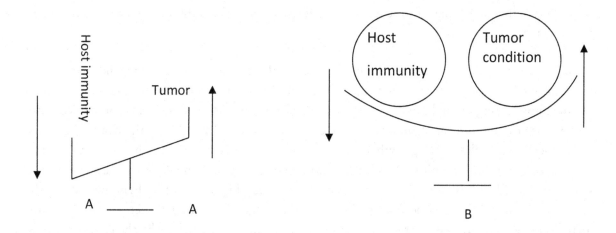

Fig. 7 Schematics of "seesaw" and "weighing scale"
A. tumor grows up in unbalance; B. stabled improvement conditions in balance

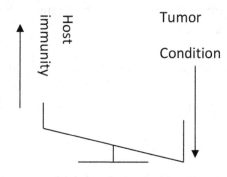

Fig. 8 Improved immunity and controlled tumor

V. Protecting central immune organs instead of damaging it

1. Traditional chemotherapy inhibits immunologic function: when cancer happens, thymus has been inhibited by "cancer-inhibiting thymic factor" and atrophied. Meanwhile, chemotherapy inhibits immunity and bone marrow, damages hemopoietic system and finally lead to the adynamia of the central immune organs as a whole.

In case of cancerometastasis, a large number of cancer cells are swarming into lymph nodes and destroy their immunologic function. As to the spleen, it could inhibit or destroy cancer cells intruding in the spleen along the blood and provide nowhere for the existence of free cancer cells due to its intrinsic structures and functions. Thus there is generally no primary or secondary malignant tumor in the spleen. However, it is shown by the experiments that the immunologic function of the spleen to tumor is bidirectional, namely, it effectively inhibits tumor in the early stage of cancer but fails in the late stage.

2. Xu Ze's new model of cancer treatment can protect thymus and bone marrow and prevent the immunologic function of the host from damage. According to anatomic experiments on more than 2,000 tumor-bearing animal models, it was found that the growth of tumor is accompanied with the thymus atrophy in form of simultaneously direct proportion. In addition, the death of mice is also proportional to the tumor growth and thymus atrophy. Conclusively, it is necessary to protect thymus and improve immunity. As well as that, in studying the reason why cancer leads to death on thousands of late tumor-bearing animal models, it is found by us that the thymuses apparently atrophied among all grouped dead animals in the final stage of carcinoma, their central immune organ met with atrophy and malfunction. It may be one important reason why the cancer patients died of cancer. It is a common fact that most cancer patients die of cancer in clinic. But further careful analysis and profound consideration would reveal the close relationship between infection bleeding, the failure of organ function and adynamia of immunologic function, which enlightens us to try to prevent or inhibit the thymus atrophy of tumor-bearing animal models in the late stage of tumor. We just aim to find the way to prevent or alleviate thymus atrophy, no matter what measure is taken. After a long-term experimental research, it is found by us that XZ-C$_4$ and XZ-C$_8$ screened from the natural herbs, the former can protect thymus and improve immunologic function and the later can protect bone marrow and produce the blood.

XZ-C$_4$ can protect thymus from atrophy and increase lymphocyte and T cells.

XZ-C$_8$ can protect hematopoiesis function of the bone marrow, rebuild erythrocyte and leucocyte system and correct anemia.

VI. Non-damage therapy instead of damage therapy

1. For half a century, the traditional anti-cancer therapies have been always the operation, the radiotherapy and the chemotherapy, the first two are the local therapy and the last one is the systematic therapy, all of which would damage the patients to a certain extent. To be specific, operations would attack the ability of the patients to resist disease at a certain level and also cause an implantation, dissemination or residue of exfoliated and free cancer cells, thus resulting in reoccurrence or metastasis after operation. Radiotherapy would cause radioactive inflammatory pathological changes. Chemotherapy has great systemic side effects on the human body. Although currently the traditional therapies have been gradually improved as regional selective local therapy with intubation or catheter on target organs, which aims to increase local concentration and narrow down the damage range of cytotoxic drug, the whole body would still under the effects of medicine disseminated systemically and be subject to obviously toxic effects such as decreased immunity, inhibition of bone marrow, gastroenteric reaction, hair shedding, renal and hepatic injuries and so on. In addition, radioactive rays and chemotherapeutic drugs are two carcinogenic factors despite

of the ability of radiotherapy and chemotherapy to kill cancer cells, thus they would be obviously harmful to the patients.

2. The characteristics of the effects of the new non-damage therapy and Xu Ze's new model of cancer treatment: so many new therapies such as biotherapy, immunotherapy, differentiation and induction therapy, gene therapy, Chinese medicine treatment, combined therapy of traditional Chinese and western medicine and so on, have been emerging in the past 10 years, most of which devote to improving immunity, protecting the host, simulating and inducing the anticancer cell clusters within the anticancer system of the host (including NK cell clusters, K cell clusters, LAK cell clusters, macrophage cell clusters and TK cell clusters) as well as the factor system of anticancer cells (including IFN, IL-2, TNF, LT), regulating and controlling neurohumor system and endocrine system, strengthening the immunologic function and antineoplastic ability of the host and maintaining a balance and sustainability for the host. Z-C medicine was screened from natural herbs on tumor-bearing experimental animals, got a remarkable curative effect by a ten-year follow-up clinical verification with data of approximate 10,000 clinical cases and categorized as non-damage medicine, which could actually constitutes a non damage therapy.

The effects of burgeoning non-damage therapy could be summarized as follows: ① directly improve the anti-tumor ability of the host; ② indirectly improve the anti-cancer ability of the host by diminishing inhibition mechanism; ③ improve the resistance power of the host against oncotherapy; ④ enhance the immunogenicity of tumors.

No matter the traditional therapy or the new concept therapy, operation is the preferred method to treat solid tumor. Radical surgery to resect tumor is the currently best therapeutic method in the range of indication. In 1960s, the author resected huge abdominal tumor more than 6kg for 4 patients, one of which was a female patient, aged 50, with a hysteroma over 18kg. Such a huge solid tumor can't be removed by chemotherapy, immunity, traditional Chinese medicine or BRM. The strategy for treatment of cancerous protuberance is to adopt different methods to eliminate the number of cancer cells to a certain order of magnitude (Someone fixes the order of magnitude at 10^6 mice cells or corresponding 3.5×10^9 human cells and describes it as a spherical nodule with a diameter of 1.5cm) and remediate the human body under this condition. $Z-C_{1+4}$ are verified by the experiments from this laboratory that they could put 10^5 cancer cells under control. Thus if XZ-C medicine is applied in adjuvant therapy after the tumors resection surgery of patients, the body resistance could be strengthened so as to eliminate pathogenic factors and diminish reoccurrence and metastasis.

9. "THREE STEPS" OF ANTI-CANCER METASTASIS THERAPY

- The metastasis step should be understood so that the goal of treatment is more specific
- Try to break each step by step
- Three major strategies of anti-cancer treatment (trilogy)

[Abstract]

Objectives: Probing into the detailed strategies of therapy of carcinoma metastasis.

Methods: Deeply analyzing "Eight Steps" and "Three Stages" of carcinoma metastasis and trying to destroy the metastasis steps respectively.

Results: Putting forward the three countermeasures for therapy of carcinoma metastasis, namely "Three-Steps" through analysis.

Conclusions: The space allocation of XU ZE Three Steps of Therapy of Carcinoma Metastasis is in blood circulation and its time allocation is in three different stages. XU ZE Three Steps of Therapy of Carcinoma Metastasis attach importance to the immunity of the host and improvement of immune surveillance of the immunological cells in blood circulation on the cancer cells in the routing of metastasis.

[Keywords]: Anti carcinoma metastasis; three steps; immune surveillance

1. The metastasis step should be understood so that the goal of treatment is more specific

As to how to make clearer the extremely complicated dynamic and continuous biological process of carcinoma metastasis with multi-step and multi-element, through repeated thinking and carefully analysis, we summed up and put forward Eight Steps of Metastasis of Cancer Cells in the aforesaid. Based on Eight Steps, we tried to make clearer and more particular of the concept of extremely complicated dynamic and continuous biological process of carcinoma metastasis with multi-step and multi-element with respect to understanding. In order to take scientific measures to obstruct and intercept each metastasis step and destroy it one by one, it is necessary to make clear the concept of each step in the metastasis process. Only when the target of each step is made clear, can the prevention and cure countermeasures be carried out, researched and probed into.

In the above, we have mentioned "Three Stages" of carcinoma metastasis and illuminated it in details. The reason why "Three Stage" is put forward is that one of the keys to therapy of cancer is to anti metastasis, however, at present, the understanding of the concept of metastasis is still ambiguous and it is not clear and particular. People only understand the severity of the harm of the metastasis to the patients, however, it lacks of effective prevention and therapeutic countermeasures with clear concept and detailed profile. In order to take scientific measures to obstruct and intercept each metastasis step, based on the Eight Steps, Three Stages and the molecular mechanism of carcinoma metastasis, we try to establish the preventive and therapeutic countermeasures for each stage and called it Xu Ze Three Steps of Therapy of Carcinoma Metastasis.

2. Try to break each step by step

The basic process of carcinoma metastasis is: the cancer cell falling from the primary tumor---degrading the basement membrance---migrating into blood capillary and small vein---survived cancer cell adhering to endothelial cell of blood capillary or basement membrance under the exposed endothelium---passing through wall---growing up in the remote target organ and forming the metastatic carcinoma, which is an extremely complicated, dynamic and continuous biological process, composed of several relatively independent but interlocked steps. In each step, a series of molecular biological events will happen between cancer cells, and between the cancer cells and the host cells, finishing the whole metastatic process and finally forming the metastatic carcinoma.

That is to say, it is necessary for the cancer cells to be subject to and finish the whole metastatic process before forming the metastatic carcinoma. any failure of each step will result in the stop of the whole metastatic process, which presents that if we take measures to destroy the metastatic steps one by one and carry out the strategy and tactics of obstruction and interception of the cancer cells in the routing of the metastasis, it is certainly possible to break or intercept the metastatic routing and intercept and kill the cancer cells in the routing of metastasis.

Xu Ze New Concept and Mode of Therapy of Carcinoma and Carcinoma Metastasis are to try to intercept one or several steps or links of the above-mentioned metastatic process so as to control the metastasis.

In order to realize the above-mentioned objectives, what measures shall be taken by us for anti metastasis? With which theory? Which technology and which drug? In which step or in which stage and link to intercept the cancer cells in the routing of the metastasis?

3. Three Steps of Therapy of Carcinoma Metastasis or three major strategies of anti-cancer treatment (trilogy)

1. First step of anti carcinomatous metastasis: in this stage, the metastatic process of cancer cells is as follows: cancer cells falling from the primary carcinoma---adhering to the stroma outside the cells---degrading ECM to open up a road for cancer cells---carrying out cell movement via the adherence of degraded stroma or the degraded stroma for adherence---then arriving at the external wall---degrading basement membrane of blood vessel---doing Amoeba movement, firstly stretching out the pseudopodium---then passing through the wall.

Prevention and cure countermeasures: this stage is the intervention and repression countermeasure before the cancer cell falls from the primary carcinoma and enters the blood vessel. In this stage, the therapeutic "targets" are mainly anti-adherence, anti-degradation, anti-movement and anti cancer cell attack. The therapeutic goal is to prevent the cancer cells from entering the blood vessel so as to realize the goal of "turning the enemy back at the border".

2. Second step of anti carcinomatous metastasis: in this stage, the metastasis process of cancer cell: it will pass through the wall and enter the blood circulation. The cancer cell will be interweaved in various blood cell components including blood plasma and blood or will be adhered to cancer cell group together with homo-cancer cell, or will be adhered to slight cancer embolus together with the alloplasm such as blood platelet and white blood cell and float in venous system→turn back to the right ventricle→circulate→enter pulmonary vein→turn back to left ventricle together with the venous blood, some cancer cells can stay in the pulmonary microcirculation blood vessel (forming the pulmonary metastasis lesion), some will enter the pulmonary vein→turn back to the left ventricle via the pulmonary microcirculation. The cancer cell, interweaved in the blood, enters the aorta and then jets into the small artery of the parenchymatous viscera and then enters the microcirculation of each organ (especially the parenchymatous organ, such as liver, kidney, brain and porotic substance of bone through the impact force and vertex flow and pump flow of the heart valve blood. Most of the cancer cells in the circulation will be damaged and killed by the immunological cells in the circulation or the strong blood impact force and shearing force, the tiny minority of the survived cancer cells form the micro-cancer embolus, adhering to the endothelial cell of the micrangium, degrading the basement membrane and passing through the blood vessel.

In this stage, the cancer cell will contact various immunological cells in floating in the blood circulation and cannot survive possibly due to being captured and phagocytized by various immunological cells in the blood. Few survived cancer cells will be adhered to the endothelial cell of the blood vessel due to escaping from the monitoring of the immunity in the blood circulation.

Prevention and cure countermeasures: in this stage, the "target" of therapy of carcinoma metastasis is to protect and enhance the immunologic function of various immunological cells in the blood circulation, activate the immunological cytokine and resist adherence (homogenous adherence of cancer cells and cancer cells, alloplasmatic adherence of cancer cells with blood platelet and so on), resist movement, resist aggregation of blood platelet, resist high coagulation and resist cancer embolus.

Therapeutic goal: activating the immunological cell, protecting function of thymus organization, improving immunity, protecting the bone marrow and producing the blood and promoting the cancer cells floating in the blood circulation to be captured, phagocytized, surrounded and annihilated and intercepted by the immunological cell group.

The second step is the main battlefield to kill off the cancer cells floating in the blood circulation as well as the main countermeasures to interfere and repress the carcinoma metastasis.

3. Third Step of anti carcinomatous metastasis: the metastasis process of the cancer cell in this stage: the cancer cell escapes the monitoring of the immunological cell in blood circulation and the annihilation of the immunological cell, passes through the wall and anchors itself in the organs with agreeable local microenvironment for settlement, in this way, the new blood capillary of tumor forms and then it gradually forms the metastatic carcinoma.

Prevention and cure countermeasures: the interference and repression countermeasures, mainly aiming at improving the histogenic immunity of the local microenvironment and regulating the local microenvironment to make it adverse to the survival and nidation and repress the angiogenesis factor and the new angiogenesis.

To sum up, space allocation of Xu Ze Three Steps of Therapy of Carcinoma Metastasis is in the blood circulation and the time allocation is in three different stages. It attaches importance to improvement of the host immunity. It can be summed up and concluded as Table 1

Table 1 Xu Ze Three Steps of Therapy of Carcinoma Metastasis

Metastasis stage of cancer cell	Metastasis process	Prevention and cure countermeasures
The stage before the cancer cell intrudes the circulation First step of anti metastasis	Separating the cancer cell from the primary cancer→degrading ECM→adherence and de-adherence→movement→before entering the blood vessel.	● anti-adherence ● anti-degradation ● anti-movement anti stroma metal protease
Transportation stage of cancer cell in blood circulation Second step of anti-metastasis	The cancer cell group and micro cancer embolus float in the blood circulation and are damaged due to being phagocytized and captured by the immunological cell and be subject to the shearing force of the blood.	● enhancing and activating various immunological cells in circulation, improving the immunologic function as the main battlefield of killing off the cancer cells in the routing of the metastasis

The stage in which Cancer cell escapes the blood circulation and anchors "target" organ Third step of anti metastasis

After cancer cell escapes from the blood vessel, it anchors the organ for nidation, forms the new blood vessel and forms the metastatic lesion.

● anti-adherence
● anti-aggregation of blood platelet
● anti cancer embolus
● TG
● Inhibiting angiogenesis factor
● Inhibiting angiogenesis
● Improving immunological regulation
● Improving the immunity of local microenvironment.

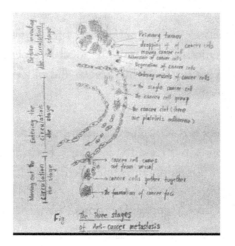

Fig the three stages of Anti-cancer metastasis

The metastatic lesion is not the terminal. When the metastatic lesion grows up to a certain size, it has the cancer cells separated, intruded and transferred, in this way, it will become a new original place of the cancer cell metastasis. At this moment, the primary lesion and metaststic lesion will become the original place of the ablation and metastasis of the cancer cells via blood metastasis. Therefore, the more and larger the metastatic carcinoma is, the more the cancer cells in the blood circulation are. The number of the immunological cells in the blood circulation of the body of the patient is far insufficient for controlling a large number of cancer cells falling from the carcinoma lesion and entering the blood circulation. The immunologic function of the organism will be severely unbalanced, even the immunologic function will break down, resulting in the hematogenous dissemination. At this time, the organism of the patient will meet with the functional crisis of the immunologic cells. As to how to perfect and deal with this situation, there are only two methods, one is foreign aid and another is endogeny. The foreign aid is the transplantation of stem cell and the endogeny is bioremediation, immunological therapy, genetherapy, molecular biological therapy, treatment by Chinese herbs, Z-C immunologic regulation therapy by Chinese herbs and BRM therapy.

10. REVIEW AND ANALYSIS OF CLINICAL CASES OF POSTOPERATIVE ADJUVANT CHEMOTHERAPY FOR CARCINOMA

- The cases of which cancer postoperative adjuvant chemotherapy failed to prevent recurrence
- The cases of which cancer postoperative adjuvant chemotherapy failed to prevent metastasis
- The cases of which chemotherapy promotes immune failure

In view of the recurrent relapse and metastasis after surgical radical operation, therefore, postoperative adjuvant chemotherapy has been prevailing universally after the 1980s. While cancer experts have different perspectives whether postoperative adjuvant chemotherapy has arrested relapse, or whether it has prevented metastasis. Specific research report has not yet appeared. According to a group of case reports for five-year follow-up results of postoperative adjuvant chemotherapy or radiation patients by British Stomach Cancer Group, this cancer group adopted mitomycin and fluorouracil to provide adjuvant treatment for the first group patients in 1976. But the result showed that this treatment didn't benefit the postoperative patients. Therefore British Stomach Cancer Group carried out adjuvant treatment research for another group of patients again.

British Stomach Cancer Group adopted prospective, randomized, controlled grouping research for 436 sdenocarcinoma of stomach patients, whose postoperative staging was phase II to phase III. The 436 postoperative patients were respectively treated by radiation or combined chemotherapy of mitomycin, adriamycin and fluorouracil treatment (MAF). During five-year follow-up, 372 patients died, in which 45 patients died from surgical complications and 327 patients died from tumor relapse. In this randomized grouping research, 145 patients adopted surgical operation. 153 patients accepted adjuvant radiation, and the range of irradiation included hilus lienis and porta hepatis region, also the radiation dose was 4500cGy. Another 138 patients accepted combined chemotherapy (MAF Treatment). Mitomycin was 4mg/m^2; adriamycin was 30 mg/m^2; fluorouracil was 600 mg/m^2. The three drugs were all intravenous injections, and the treatment cycle was 8 cycles, which three weeks were one cycle. Overall two-year survival rate of this group was 33% (31%~35%), and five-year survival rate was 17% (13%~21%). Compared with the survival rate of patients only adopting surgical operation, the survival rate of patients accepting adjuvant treatment had no increase. The five-year survival rate of patients only adopting surgical operation was 20%, rate of surgery and radiation was 12%, and rate of surgery and chemotherapy was 19%.

Thus, surgical operation remains to be the standard treatment for sdenocarcinoma of stomach. The adjuvant treatment measure should be limited within certain field of research.

The writer of this book sorts, analyzes, evaluates and rethinks the following part of the cases (cases with personal inquiry of medical history, medical examination, diagnosis and treat, complete observation) with nearly ten-year personal clinical diagnosis and treatment.

I. Failure Cases of Postoperative Adjuvant Chemotherapy to Arrest Relapse

Case 1 Patient Wei ××, female, fifty, Changsha Hunan, engineer, patient history number: 3300653

Diagnosis: Cystosarcoma phylloides of left breast had serious malignant change and relapse. In July 1996, the patient was found the enlargement of lump in her left breast. The puncture of the lump diagnosed that the lump was fibroma. In October 1996, the left breast was removed. Pathological examination: cystosarcoma phylloides of left breast, level II. Since December 19, 1996, the patient began to accept VAD treatment for chemotherapy and get chemotherapy once every three weeks. The second chemotherapy was on January 16, 1997. Constantly, the third chemotherapy was on February 24, 1997; and then the fourth chemotherapy on March 6, 1997; the fifth chemotherapy on April 8, 1997; the sixth chemotherapy on April 29, 1997. On July 2, 1997, type-B ultrasonic examined that there was a 15mm×12mm sized lump in the similar 9 o'clock position of the right breast. Considering the relapse and metastasis, the patient came to the anti-cancer coordination group (Hubei Group) for outpatient treatment, adopting traditional Chinese and western medicine combination treatment.

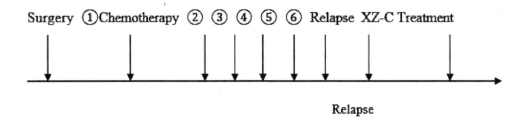

Analysis: This patient had one-year postoperative chemotherapies continuously, defining once every month and five days one time. The treatment was standard systematic chemotherapy. But after stopping chemotherapy for two months, the tumor appeared local relapse. That explained that the chemotherapy failed to arrest relapse. It was speculated that chemotherapy might cause the continuing decline of patient's immunity functions beyond retrieval. The tumor lost the immunoregulation and made rest tumor cells set into the cell cycle. Then the tumor was induced. It prompted that long-time continuous chemotherapy must attach importance to protect the host and confront side effects of chemotherapy drugs to avoid the damage for the host. Although chemotherapy killed off tumor cells, it damaged the body at the same time.

Case 2 Patient Yang ××, female, fifty-four, cadre, Honghu, patient history number: 7201432

Stomach cancer relapsed after surgery. The pain of superior venter had continued for one year. The result of stomachoscopy was stomach cancer. On August 26, 1997, the patient accepted radical operation for stomach cancer. The radical operation was $_2$B1 type. There was a 8mm×5mm sized lump in the lateral side of the lesser curvature of stomach, which caused the pyloric obstruction and enlargement of lymph nodes on the side of the arteria coeliaca. The patient began to accept postoperative chemotherapy after a month. MMC and 5-Fu were seven days one time and the intervals between two times were three weeks. There were total six times in September, October, November, December 1997 and January, February 1998. After that no other treatments were adopted. In January 1999, the patient appeared swallow obstruction and emesis. On February 24, 1999, the patient accepted the stomachoscopy. Front and back of gastric remnant which closed to anastomotic stoma swelled and developed pathological changes. There were mucosal erosion and ulcer. Stomach cancer patient had the postoperative relapse. On March 4, 1999, the patient came to the anti-cancer coordination group (Hubei Group) for XZ-C$_{1+4+2}$ treatment.

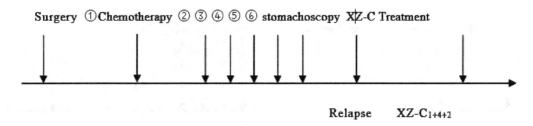

Analysis: This patient had six-time postoperative chemotherapies, defining once every month and seven days one time. The sixth chemotherapy was in February 1998. Until January 1999, the patient appeared swallow obstruction. The result of stomachoscopy was the postoperative relapse of stomach cancer. In this case, the patient had six-time postoperative chemotherapies continuously. It prompted that postoperative adjuvant chemotherapy failed to arrest relapse.

Case 3 Patient Li ××, male, forty-two, Shanxi, cadre, patient history number: 7201427

On November 18, 1997, the patient was found left-liver space occupying lesion through CT in 161 Hospital. On December 2, 1997, the patient accepted the left-liver lateral lobectomy. After 20 days, the patient began to accept postoperative chemotherapy. The chemotherapy drugs were 10mg/dl with intravenous injection and 20mg of hydroxycamptothecine with intravenous injection every other day in two weeks. A course was 15 days. And then the patient needed to repeat the last course after resting 15 days. Before chemotherapy, SGPT was 77μ. After chemotherapy, SGPT was 500μ. In the operation, chemotherapeutic drugs above the chemotherapy pump of portal vein (no chemotherapy pump in the artery) were injected into the organism through the pump. Before the operation, AFP was 200μ. After the operation, AFP was 200μ. In April 1998, the patient accepted the third chemotherapy in the hospital. Chemotherapeutic drugs were injected through the pump. The chemotherapy adopted the high dose pulse therapy, using 6mg of MMC, 200mg of carboplatin and 750mg of 5-Fu. Before chemotherapy, AFP was 180μ. After chemotherapy, AFP was 302μ. On May 19, 1998, the patient accepted the fourth chemotherapy, using the chemotherapy pump as the third time. On June 30, 1998, the patient accepted the fifth chemotherapy with pump. When the AFP was 219μ, it should be detected every other day. On July 28, 1998, the patient accepted the sixth chemotherapy, adopting the high dose pulse therapy through the pump. The reexamination showed that AFP>363. In early August 1998, the examination found that there was a 4cm sized lump under the incision of abdominal wall. On August 27, 1998, the lump was removed in tumor hospital. On September 29, 1998, the patient accepted the seventh chemotherapy with pump. After chemotherapy, the reexamination of type-B ultrasonic, CT and intrahepatic widespread metastasis showed that there were many ball shadows and metastases. In December 1998, the patient accepted hepatic artery embolism and pulmonary intervention in the general hospital of a military region. The examinations found that there were lumps equivalent to the size of an adult fist and infant's head in epigastrium and right abdomen. The lumps were stiff. On March 1, 1999, the patient came to the anti-cancer coordination group (Hubei Group) for outpatient treatment, adopting traditional Chinese and western medicine combination treatment and XZ-C$_{1+4+5}$ series treatment.

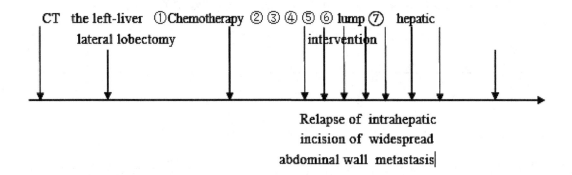

Analysis: This patient suffered from cancer of the liver. After the left-liver lateral lobectomy, the patient had seven-time postoperative chemotherapies continuously, defining once every month. The seventh chemotherapy showed the intrahepatic widespread metastasis and pulmonary metastasis. It prompted that postoperative adjuvant chemotherapy failed to arrest relapse and prevent metastasis.

Case 4 Patient Xiang ××, male, forty-three, cadre, Chongyang, patient history number: 6801345

In June 1994, the disease of this patient was treated as gastroenteritis. Until December, the X-ray examination in city hospital showed that the patient suffered from intestinal obstruction. In early January 1995, the emergency operation explored the disease as a transverse colon tumor. Then the tumor was removed, adopting the end to end anastomosis. Pathological examination showed that the tumor was a malignant tumor. In February, March, April, May, June, July 1995, the patient had six-time postoperative chemotherapies continuously, defining five days one time. In January 1996, the colonic neoplasm of anastomotic stoma was found. The patient accepted the radical excision. At the end of December 1997, the tumor of anastomotic stoma was found again. On March 31, 1998, the patient accepted the palliative excision. In September 1998, another 5.6cm×4.6cm sized lump equivalent to the size of an adult fist was found between stomach and caput pancreatic. On November 24, 1998, the patient underwent an operation again to remove the lump. Those lesser tubercles, such as the omentum, were difficult to be removed completely. And the operation could only remove big ones. In 1996, the patient once accepted four-time postoperative chemotherapies in Tumor Department, defining five days one time. And the patient also took Doxifluridine orally for two months. In April, May 1998, the patient accepted twice chemotherapies. And as well, the patient took two courses of traditional Chinese medicine dispensed by Wang Zhenguo of Shenyang. But the course didn't work. Then the patient took one course of Shijiazhuang Chinese medicine. The course also didn't work. On November 13, 1998, the patient came to the anti-cancer coordination group for outpatient treatment, adopting traditional Chinese and western medicine combination treatment, XZ-C$_{1+4}$ treatment and XZ-C$_2$ treatment. In November 1999, the patient accepted the reexamination, which showed the stable condition.

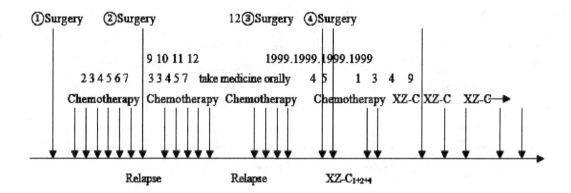

Analysis: This patient underwent the colon cancer operation of removing the tumor. After that, the patient had six-time postoperative chemotherapies continuously, defining once every month and five days one time. Five months later, the colonic neoplasm of anastomotic stoma relapsed and was removed by surgery. During the one year after operation, the patient proceeded with postoperative chemotherapies monthly and continuously. The tumor of anastomotic stoma relapsed and was removed again. The patient proceeded with postoperative chemotherapies. This case prompted that chemotherapy failed to arrest relapse and prevent metastasis. In November 1998, the patient came to the outpatient department for traditional Chinese and western medicine combination treatment, and also took traditional Chinese medicine of XZ-C$_{1+4+2}$ immunoregulation series chronically and continuously. After taking medicine orally, the patient's condition was improved. In November 1999, the patient accepted the reexamination, which showed the stable condition.

Case 5 Patient Li ××, male, fifty, cadre, Hanchuan, patient history number: 5701131
Diagnosis: Rectum cancer relapsed after surgery.

In December 1994, the patient underwent a radical operation for rectum cancer. The operation was Dixon type. The length of rectum cancer lesion was 12cm. The patient had six-time postoperative chemotherapies continuously, defining once every month and seven days one time. The condition was good after operation. On April 30, 1998, the patient accepted the colonoscopy examination. There was a lump at the area of rectum, having 10cm distances to the anus. The 3cm×3cm sized lump had a rugged surface and swelled towards the intracavity. The biopsy of four living tissues showed that the cell had became allotypic gland cell. On June 25, 1998, the patient suffered from the incomplete intestinal obstruction. Then on July 9, 1998, the patient underwent the Hartmann operation and partial cystectomy. The surgery proved it the recurrent rectum cancer, which had involved the bladder. The patient had five-time postoperative radiotherapies for pelvic cavity with accumulated dose of 5000CGY (from October 12, 1998 to November 13, 1998). The patient also had postoperative chemotherapies for one month. The chemotherapy drugs were 5-Fu and calcium leucovorin (five days, once a day). Since the proctoscopy examined the relapse of rectum cancer in May 1998, the patient came to the anti-cancer coordination group for the traditional Chinese medicine treatment of XZ-C immunoregulation series, which was adopted to control the relapse and metastasis. On November 28, 1999, the patient accepted the reexamination. After taking the medicine orally, the patient regained a high spirit, a good appetite and enough physical strength, which showed the stable condition. The patient continued to live normally without any discomfort.

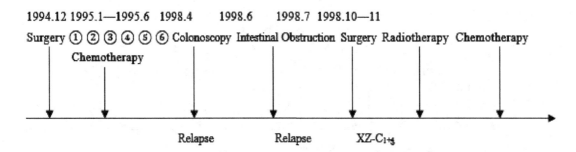

Analysis: After a radical operation for rectum cancer, the patient had six-time postoperative chemotherapies continuously, defining once every month and seven days one time. Two years later, rectum cancer appeared the local recurrence and widespread metastasis. Then the patient continued to accept the chemotherapy, but the rectum cancer relapsed again. It prompted that postoperative adjuvant chemotherapy failed to arrest relapse and prevent metastasis. After the relapse in April 1998, the patient came to the anti-cancer coordination outpatient department for the traditional Chinese medicine treatment of XZ-C$_{1+4}$ immunoregulation series. After taking the medicine orally, the patient's condition was stable and improving. The patient had been persisting in taking the XZ-C medicine for over one year and was being in good health.

Case 6 Patient Luo ××, female, housewife, Gongan county, patient history number: 521020

In September 1994, the patient found a lump in the left breast. The local hospital scanned the lump as a fibroma. In September 1995, because of the enlargement of the lump (5cm×5cm×3cm), the patient underwent a radical operation for breast cancer in the district hospital. Pathology: infiltrating ductal cancer of right breast, ER (+), P.R (+), removal of one subclavicular lymph node and two axillary fusional lymph nodes. After the operation, the patient accepted chemotherapies with CMF treatment for one week. On December 6, 1995, the patient accepted chemotherapies with CAF treatment for one week. On December 26, 1995, the patient accepted chemotherapies with CAF treatment for one week again. From February 5, 1996 to March 30, the patient accepted radiotherapies. In August 1996, the patient continued to accept two courses of chemotherapies, defining three weeks of one course. In September 1997, a

lump was found in the right axilla. There were tubercles under the prethoracic skin again. The breast cancer appeared relapse and metastasis. Then the patient came to the anti-cancer coordination outpatient department for the traditional Chinese medicine treatment of XZ-C immunoregulation series. On January 4, 1998, the patient began to take XZ-C medicine during the outpatient treatment. After taking 45-day medicine, the patient's condition kept stable. In October 1998, the patient accepted the reexamination in the outpatient department, which showed the stable condition. There was a tubercle equivalent to the size of the little finger in the top part of right axilla. Above this tubercle, there was another tubercle equivalent to the size of a rice grain. But it had no more growth.

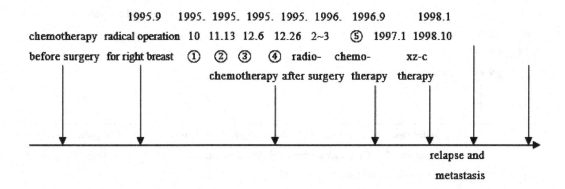

Analysis: The patient suffered from the breast cancer. Before the surgery, the patient accepted one-week chemotherapies. After the surgery, the patient accepted postoperative chemotherapies, defining once every month and one-week one time. But the treatment failed to prevent metastasis, diffusion and progression. In January 1998, the patient came to the outpatient department and took 10-month traditional Chinese medicine of immunoregulation. The patient's condition was stable. The breast cancer had no more progress. The general condition was improving.

Case 7 Patient Yang ××, female, fifty, Hankou, technical cadre, patient history number: 54001079

Diagnosis: Rectal adenocarcinoma relapsed after surgery.

In June 1996, the patient was diagnosed with rectum cancer for diarrhea. On July 11, 1996, the patient underwent a radical low anterior resection operation for rectum cancer. In the operation, the tumor located under the reflection, which was 5cm×4cm and invaded the muscular layer. The lymph node under the mesentery developed obvious enlargement. The patient recovered well from the operation. Nine days after the operation, the patient accepted chemotherapies of 5-Fu and MMC series. After leaving hospital, the patient took Mifulong orally. On October 4, 1996, the patient accepted chemotherapies in a tumor hospital and then left it. From August 17, 1996 to October 5, the patient accepted three courses of chemotherapies with ELF treatment. From January 14, 1997 to February 3, the patient accepted the third chemotherapies in a tumor hospital of MMC and 5-Fu series. After the chemotherapy, the patient began the attack of diarrhea more than ten times every day. From May 1997 to July 1997, the patient took Mifulong orally. On February 4, 1998, the patient had a return visit for the rectal examination. In the area of the anastomotic stoma, the tubercle could be touched. The rectum cancer relapsed. The patient accepted eight chemotherapies again and 21 radiotherapies. Then the patient had hematuria and diarrhea. It showed that the patient suffered from the radioactive cystitis and radioactive rectitis.

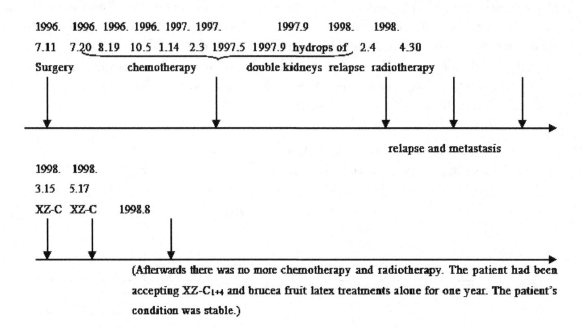

Analysis: This case was the rectal adenocarcinoma. After the radical operation, the patient accepted chemotherapies continuously. On February 4, 1998, the rectum cancer relapsed in the area of the anastomotic stoma. The patient had accepted continuous and multiple chemotherapies, involving intravenous chemotherapies and oral chemotherapy drugs. But it failed to arrest the relapse of rectum cancer in the area of the anastomotic stoma. After finding the relapse, the patient accepted radiotherapies and chemotherapies continuously again. These treatments also evoked the radioactive cystitis and other complicating diseases. The treatments failed to prevent the progression of recurrent cancer.

On March 15, 1998, the patient came to the anti-cancer coordination group for outpatient treatment, simply adopting the traditional Chinese medicine of XZ-C immunoregulation series and brucea fruit latex for enema. After taking the medicine, the patient's general condition was getting better. And the spirit and appetite were improving. The patient had chronically been taking the traditional Chinese medicine of XZ-C immunoregulation series for eighteen months. The condition of illness was stable. The tumor had been controlled, and it was stable with no more progression. The patient's condition was getting better markedly.

Case 8 Patient Xu ××, female, fifty-six, Macheng, patient history number: 7401472
Diagnosis: Lymph nodes of the left ventral groove metastasized. The adenocarcinoma of anal canal relapsed.

For the blood-stained stool, three blood examinations showed that the patient suffered from the cancer of anus. On February 25, 1997, the patient underwent a Miles-type radical operation for cancer of anal canal. The appendages of ambo-uterus were removed. Lymph nodes of the left perineum and ventral groove were cleaned. The patient had six-time postoperative chemotherapies. The first chemotherapy was on May 24, 1997 with MMC+5-Fu treatment. The second chemotherapy was on July 2, 1997. The third chemotherapy was on August 13, 1997. The fourth chemotherapy was on September 17, 1997. The fifth chemotherapy was on February 8, 1998. The sixth chemotherapy was on November 15, 1998. Since September 1997, the patient began to have the feeling of swell, distention, burn and urodynia in the area of anus. On April 14, 1999, the detected value of CEA was 5.8mg/ml. On April 16, 1999, the patient came to the anti-cancer coordination group for the traditional Chinese medicine treatment of immunoregulation. The patient had the feeling of swell, ache and tenderness in the area of anus. There was a very high chance that exfoliated survival cancer cells had relapsed.

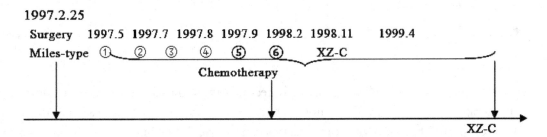

Analysis: After the Miles-type radical operation for cancer of anal canal, the patient accepted chemotherapies of six courses continuously. In September 1997, the patient began to have the feeling of ache and tenderness in the area of anus. And the feeling of pain became doubly intense. It was obvious that exfoliated survival cancer cells were proliferating and relapsing. The poisonous drugs for cancers cells in continuous chemotherapies failed to totally destroy these exfoliated survival cancer cells. Thus, these cancer cells revived again, proliferating and relapsing in partial place.

Case 9 Patient Xiong ××, male, forty-two, worker, Wuhan, patient history number: 6501291
Diagnosis: Rectum cancer relapsed after surgery.

In March 1998, for the blood-stained stool, the disease of this patient was treated as "hemorrhoid". In May 1998, the proctoscop biopsy examination showed that the patient suffered from rectum cancer. On May 29, 1998, the patient underwent a Miles-type radical operation for rectum cancer. The postoperative plug was poorly differentiated rectum cancer. The cancer cells had invaded to the full-thickness of intestinal wall, involving the adipose tissue around the rectum. The lymph nodes around the rectum also had metastases (16/17). The patient accepted the postoperative chemotherapies. The first chemotherapy was in June 1998, adopting the MMC+5-Fu treatment for five days. In July 1998, the patient accepted chemotherapies for twelve days (pelvic cavity, front and back of abdomen) with twenty-four times. And then the second chemotherapy was in September 1998, adopting the MMC+5-Fu treatment for six days. The third chemotherapy was in November 1999, adopting the same drugs as the second chemotherapy for five days. On November 2, 1998, the patient accepted the reexamination of type-B ultrasonic. There was no abnormality in the pelvic cavity. In February 1999, the patient began to feel pain in the area of anus. The examination of type-B ultrasonic still showed no abnormality. In March, the CT examination showed that there was a lump in the deep part of pelvic cavity (the area of anus). On March 15, 1999, the patient accepted the radiotherapies of pelvic cavity for fifteen days. In the following five days, the patient had the chemotherapies. And then the patient proceeded with radiotherapies for six times. During the radiotherapies and chemotherapies, the patient was treated by XZ-C4 to fight against the toxic side effect and protect the chest and marrow for hematopoiesis and immunization. There was no untoward effect in the whole process. Since November 1998, the patient had been using the XZ-C series for the traditional Chinese medicine treatment of immunoregulation. The condition of the illness was stable and getting better.

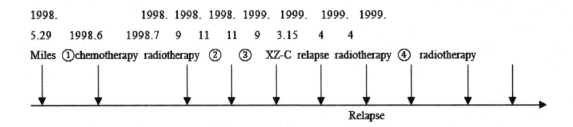

Analysis: After the Miles-type radical operation for rectum cancer, the patient accepted chemotherapies and radiotherapies continuously. Three months later, the CT examination showed that there was a lump in the deep part of pelvic cavity. The patient began to have the feeling of ache in the area of anus. The rectum cancer relapsed in partial place. It prompted that postoperative continuous chemotherapy failed to prevent the local recurrence.

Case 10 Patient Zhang ××, female, forty-four, married, Hankou, patient history number: 7101407

Diagnosis: Infiltrating ductal cancer of right breast relapsed after surgery.

In October 1997, the patient underwent the radical operation of mastocarcinoma for breast cancer (above 5m²). Twenty days later, the patient accepted intravenous chemotherapies for eight days with CMF treatment. In December after leaving hospital, the patient accepted radiotherapies for twenty-five times. After that, the patient accepted the chemotherapies again. In February, March, April, May and June 1998, the patient accepted chemotherapies for six times, defining once every month. In April 1998, at the lower end of the incision, a tubercle about the size of a bean could be touched. Since then, the skin tubercles grew more and more. Now eczematoid lesion was diffusing around the skin incision, and the cancer cells had been metastasizing through the whole body. There was a cauliflower-shaped ulcer (3cm×3cm) in the middle part of incisional scar. On February 3, 1999, the patient came to the anti-cancer coordination group for outpatient treatment, adopting the traditional Chinese medicine treatment of XZ-C immunoregulation series and brucea fruit latex treatment. The condition of the illness was stable.

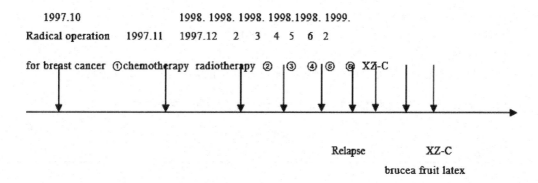

1997.10   1998. 1998. 1998. 1998.1998. 1999.

Radical operation   1997.11   1997.12   2   3   4   5   6   2

for breast cancer ①chemotherapy radiotherapy ② ③ ④ ⑤ ⑥ XZ-C

Relapse   XZ-C

brucea fruit latex

Analysis: After the operation for breast cancer, the patient accepted chemotherapies and radiotherapies continuously. Six months after the operation, when the patient was accepting chemotherapies, the cancer relapsed in partial places and the cancer cells metastasized through the whole body. It prompted that postoperative continuous radiotherapies and chemotherapies failed to prevent relapse and metastasis.

Case 11 Patient Yang ××, female, forty-three, accountant, Henan Luoshan, patient history number: 521024

There was red mucus in the stool for one month. Then on December 23, 1997, the patient accepted the fibercoloscope examination. There was an irregularly shaped new growth (3cm×5cm) at the ascending colon of the blinding end, which had 100cm to the fibercoloscope. The surface of the new growth was rugged and anabrotic. The pathological test proved it villoglandular adenocarcinoma. On December 30, 1997, the patient underwent the radical operation for colon cancer to remove the right hemicolon. In the operation, it could be found that there was a 4cm×4cm sized lump in the juncture between the blind gut and the ascending colon. The lymph nodes of the mesocolic root enlarged. The cancer cells had no metastases to the liver. Pathological test showed that villoglandular adenocarcinoma (part of mucinous adenocarcinoma) had invaded to the full-thickness of intestinal wall. Twenty-two lymph nodes had no metastases. The patient accepted postoperative chemotherapies for six times, defining once every month. The first chemotherapy was on November 26, 1998, continuing for eight days with FAP and hydroxycamptothecine. The second time started from February 12, 1998. A month later, the third time proceeded. The fourth time was on April 25, 1998 with FP treatment. The fifth time was on May 27, 1998. And the sixth time was on June 27, 1998. The chemotherapy continued for eight days. The patient had mild side effects. The white blood cell count (WBC) was 2100. On January 4, 1999, the patient accepted chemotherapies for ten days with MMC and hydroxycamptothecine. From February 1, 1999 to February 10, the patient accepted the tenth chemotherapy. In April 1999, the fibercoloscope reexamination showed the anastomosis ulcer of the colon. And the cancer relapsed in the anastomotic stoma. Then the patient came to the anti-cancer coordination group for outpatient treatment, adopting traditional Chinese and western medicine combination treatment, i.e. XZ-C$_{1+4}$ and brucea fruit latex. The condition of the illness was stable and getting better.

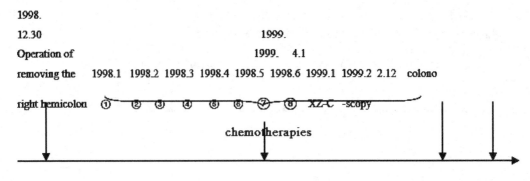

Analysis: After the radical excision for adenocarcinoma of ascending colon, the patient accepted chemotherapies for eight courses, defining one course of one month and eight days of one course. After the eighth course, the fibercoloscope reexamination showed the recurrence of anastomotic stoma. It prompted that postoperative continuous chemotherapies with eight lengthy courses still failed to prevent relapse.

Case 12 Patient Fu ××, male, twenty-four, demobilized soldier, Henan, Hu Aibin. patient history number: 8201626

Diagnosis: The carcinoma of colon relapsed after surgery.

Medical History: In February 1996, the abdominal pain was falsely diagnosed as appendicitis. Then the patient underwent the operation of removing the appendix. Pathological examination of appendicitis showed no inflammation. After the operation, the patient still felt pain in the abdominal region with recurrent paroxysmal pain. And it was treated as the spasmolysis of intestinal adhesion. Until December 1996, the patient underwent the operation of abdominal laparotomy in 153 Hospital of Zhengzhou because of intestinal obstruction. The operation showed that there was a tumor in the right hemicolon. Then the patient underwent the radical excision for right hemicolon. The pathological report was as follows. The patient suffered from the carcinoma of colon. Half month after the operation, the patient began to accept chemotherapies. The first chemotherapy started from January 1997 and continued for five days with the intravenous injection (iv). And the chemotherapy drugs were 5-Fu+cis-platinum+MMC. The second chemotherapy was in March 1997. The third time was in May. The forth time was in August. The fifth time was in October. The sixth time was in December 1997. In the following year, the patient accepted the chemotherapy every three months. The seventh time was in March 1998. The eighth time was in June 1998. The ninth time was in September 1998. The tenth time was in December 1998. (In 1997, there was one time every two months with a total of six times. In 1998, there was one time every three months with a total of four times.) The eleventh time was in October 1999. In January 1999, the patient began to feel pain and constantly pain in the lumbosacral portion. In August 1999, the patient began to feel pain in the abdominal region and have the abdominal tympania. And there was mucus in the stool. On November 14, 1999, the patient came to the anti-cancer coordination outpatient department for XZ-C$_{1+3+4}$ treatment. On November 15, 1999, the patient underwent a colonoscopy in the general hospital of Chinese People's Liberation Army (301 hospital). The examination showed that there was a recurrent tumor in the region, having 10cm to 30cm distances to the anus. Pathological examination showed that this tumor was the anaplastic adenocarcinoma.

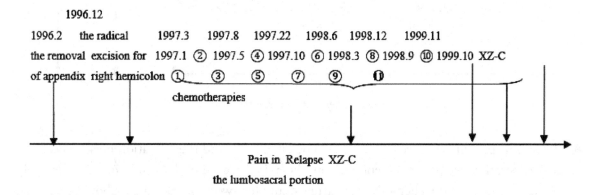

Analysis: This patient suffered from the carcinoma of colon. After undergoing the radical excision for right hemicolon, the patient accepted chemotherapies for eleven times continuously, defining two courses of one month in the first year after the operation and one course of three months in the second year after the operation. Until the tenth chemotherapy, the patient began to feel pain in the abdominal region. Retroperitoneal metastases appeared. The left colorectal cancer relapsed. Relapse and metastasis appeared while the chemotherapies were continuing. It prompted that postoperative adjuvant chemotherapy failed to arrest relapse and prevent metastasis.

II. Failure Cases of Postoperative Adjuvant Chemotherapy to Prevent Metastasis

Case 1 Patient, Xu ××, male, fifty-two, peasant, Xinzhou, patient history number: 6901374
Diagnosis: The hepatic metastases happened after the operation of carcinoma of anal canal.

The patient suffered from the carcinoma of anal canal. On September 23, 1997, the patient underwent the Miles-type radical operation. The tumor had 2cm from the anus, having the size of 3cm×3cm×2cm. The pathology was squamous cell carcinoma of anal canal. The patient accepted the postoperative chemotherapies once a month. There were five days per month for intravenous injection with carboplatin+5-Fu in October and November 1997. There were also five days per month for intravenous injection with MMC+5-Fu in December 1997, January 1998, February 1998 and March 1998. In April and May 1998, the patient switched to the oral route of Ftorafur-207 tablets. In June 1998, the type-B ultrasonic showed no abnormality. But on January 8, 1999, the type-B ultrasonic showed that there were multiple occupying nidi in the liver. The biggest nidus had the size of 8.2cm×8.6cm, diagnosed as intrahepatic metastases and retroperitoneal lymphatic metastases. There were several lymph nodes with the size of 2.1cm×0.5cm.

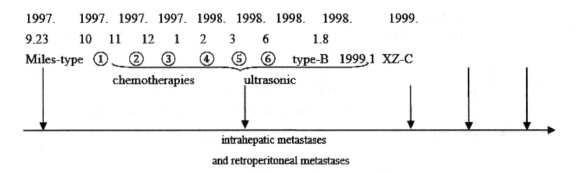

1997.	1997.	1997.	1997.	1998.	1998.	1998.	1998.		1999.
9.23	10	11	12	1	2	3	6		1.8

Miles-type ① ② ③ ④ ⑤ ⑥ type-B 1999.1 XZ-C

chemotherapies   ultrasonic

intrahepatic metastases
and retroperitoneal metastases

Analysis: This patient underwent the Miles-type operation. And the operation means was right. After the operation, the patient accepted chemotherapies once a month for six times continuously. Then the patient took the chemotherapy drugs orally for two months. The carboplatin, MMC and 5-Fu failed to prevent carcinomatous metastases. The tumor was the carcinoma of anal canal. But the first metastasis was hepatic metastasis. It prompted that continuous and systematical chemotherapies after the operation still failed to prevent hepatic metastases.

Case 2 Patient Yu ××, male, fifty-seven, worker, Nanchang, patient history number: 6901366

On October 22, 1995, the patient underwent the Miles-type radical operation for rectum cancer in a central hospital of Nanchang. After operation, the patient accepted the first chemotherapy was on December 5, 1995 with intravenous injection of 1000mg of 5-Fu once a day (d_1, d_2, d_3, d_4) and intravenous injection of 6mg of MMC (d_1). The second time was on February 2, 1996 with the same FM treatment as the first time. The third time was on March 18, 1996 with the same treatment. The fourth time was on May 24, 1996. The fifth time was on August 14, 1996. The sixth time was on September 14, 1996. All of the chemotherapies adopted the FM treatment. After the chemotherapies, the patient underwent the CT examination. On December 28, 1998, the report showed three points: ①fatty liver and metastatic liver cancer, ②colorectal cancer metastasis, ③polycystic kidney and calculus of kidney. On December 25, 1998, the type-B ultrasonic found the space occupying lesion of liver.

On December 30, 1998, the patient came to the anti-cancer coordination group for outpatient treatment with XZ-C$_{4+5+3}$. The examination showed that a lump in the form of bar could be touched in the right liver and the lump was hard. On January 20, 1999, the type-B ultrasonic in a central hospital of Nanchang found several tumors of unequal size about 4cm×2.1cm, 2.2cm×1.8cm and 2.0cm×1.7cm in the liver. There was a metastatic liver cancer with the size of 3.0cm×2.9cm in the right liver. On February 20, 1999, after taking the XZ-C$_{1+4}$, the patient's condition was stable and the patient regained a high spirit, a good appetite. The liver was functioning normally. The patient could walk on the street as a normal people. The symptom had an obvious improvement.

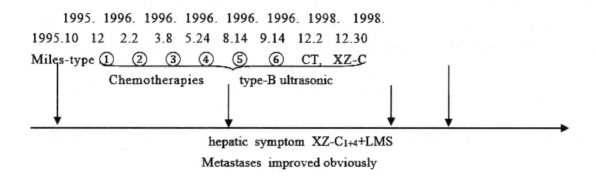

hepatic symptom XZ-C$_{1+4}$+LMS

Metastases improved obviously

Analysis: After the radical operation of rectum cancer, the patient accepted continuous chemotherapies for six courses. One year later, the hepatic metastases happened. It prompted that systematical chemotherapies failed to prevent metastases.

Case 3 Patient Guo ××, male, thirty-six, teacher, Wuhan, patient history number: 7201425

In October 1996, the patient suffered from gastric bleeding. Then the stomachoscopy showed that the patient suffered from the stomach cancer. The patient underwent the total gastrectomy in a general hospital. Two months after the operation, the chemotherapies started. The patient accepted once every two months, defining ten days of one time. The chemotherapy drugs were MMC and 5Fu with intravenous injection. This course lasted for one year (six times). In the second year, the patient accepted once every half year. The chemotherapies in 1998 were carried out once every three or four months. In September 1998, the patient accepted one time. Every time before the chemotherapy, the patient needed to undergo the examination of type-B ultrasonic. If the type-B ultrasonic showed that there was a problem, the type-B ultrasonic would be switched to CT. The patient underwent the CT examinations for five times successively, and the CT was strengthened. After the last chemotherapy in September 1998, CT showed that the cancer cells were metastasizing to liver and retroperitoneum. Then the patient underwent the photon knife (X-knife) treatment for one time and the interventional chemotherapy for hepatic vessels embolism. In October 1998, the sclera of the patient turned yellow. The CT showed that the nubbly lump of caput pancreatic was oppressing the bile duct. Then the patient underwent the radiotherapies continuously for three times in October, November 1998 and January 1999. The doses at a time were 4000 dela. The patient had an intense reaction with bad physiques and vomiting, and couldn't feed at all. The patient couldn't undergo it and stopped the treatment. On February 28, 1999, the patient came to the outpatient department of anti-cancer coordination group for traditional Chinese and western medicine combination treatment. At that time, the patient had been bedridden. The patient was not able to take in any food for the repeated nausea and vomiting. After taking the XZ-C drugs, the patient was getting better.

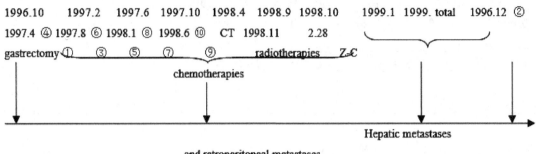

Analysis: After the total gastrectomy, the patient underwent the continuous chemotherapies and radiotherapies for a long time. After the last chemotherapy in September 1998, the CT reexamination showed the hepatic metastases and retroperitoneal metastases. It prompted that continuous and long-term treatments still failed to prevent metastases, even resulting in the failure of immunologic system and threatening the patient's life.

Case 4 Patient Cao ××, male, thirty-five, married, peasant, Hanchuan, patient history number: 470928

Diagnosis: The hepatic metastases happened after the operation of stomach cancer.

On June 28, 1996, the pre-operative diagnosis in the People's Hospital of Hanchuan certified it as the ulcer of gastric angles. The property of the illness was yet to be investigated. The patient underwent the massive resection of the stomach and the resection of great epiploon. The operation was B1-type anastomosis. The postoperative pathological report showed it the sdenocarcinoma of stomach. The cancer cells had invaded the full-thickness of stomach wall with lymphatic metastases of lesser curvature side (4/4). The lymph nodes of greater curvature side had reactive hyperplasia. The patient underwent the postoperative chemotherapies for four times in July, August, September and October 1996, defining once a month and three days every time. The chemotherapy drugs were 5-F and MMC. In September 1997, after the half month of swelling pain in right upper abdomen, the type-B ultrasonic and CT prompted that there were several low-density shadows in the right and left lobe of liver. Those were metastatic hepatic tumors and could be touched below the right costal margin of 3cm with pressing tender. On September 30, 1997, the patient underwent the interventional chemotherapy for hepatic artery. On October 5, 1997, the patient came to the anti-cancer coordination outpatient department, adopting the Z-C series for the traditional Chinese medicine treatment of immunoregulation. After taking the medicine orally, the patient regained a high spirit, a good appetite and enough physical strength. The lump below the right costal margin became soft and narrowing.

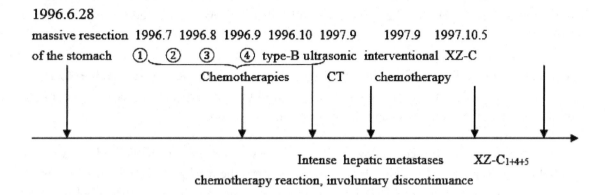

Analysis: After the operation of stomach cancer, the patient underwent the continuous chemotherapies for four times, defining once a month and three days every time. One year after the last chemotherapy, the CT reexamination showed that there were several metastatic lesions in the right and left lobe of liver. It prompted that postoperative adjuvant chemotherapies still failed to prevent metastases.

Case 5 Patient Li ××, male, fifty-five, Huangshi, second-grade actor, patient history number: 2700530

Diagnosis: The cancer cells metastasized to pancreas after the operation of stomach cancer.

In October 1995, the patient suffered from the epigastric discomfort. In November, the stomachoscopy in Huangshi Hospital diagnosed it as the stomach cancer. On November 27, 1995, the patient underwent the massive resection of the stomach. After the operation, the patient accepted five courses of chemotherapies with one course per month. In early May 1996, the last course ended. On June 4, 1996, the CT reexamination showed the space occupying lesion of pancreas. The patient began to have the abdominal distension and bad appetite. Then the patient came to the anti-cancer coordination group for outpatient treatment, adopting the $XZ-C_{1+4+2}$ series for the traditional Chinese medicine treatment of immunoregulation. After taking the medicine orally, the patient regained a high spirit, a good appetite.

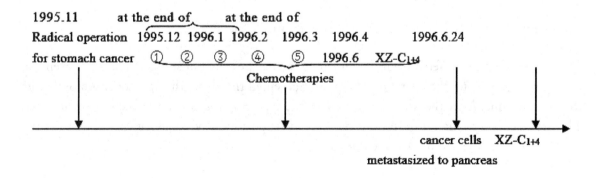

Analysis: After the radical operation of stomach cancer, the patient accepted five courses of chemotherapies with one course per month. After the five courses, the patient underwent the CT reexamination, finding the space occupying lesion of pancreas and metastatic carcinoma of pancreas. It prompted that postoperative chemotherapies still failed to prevent postoperative carcinomatous metastases.

Case 6 Patient Li ××, female, forty-five, Guangshui, teacher, patient history number: 6701324
Diagnosis: The stomach cancer relapsed and metastasized to ovary after the operation. The middle and down section of choledochus had solid space occupying lesions.

In April 1998, the stomachoscopy showed that there was a new growth in the body of stomach with bulb ulcer. On April 20, 1998, the patient underwent the total gastrectomy and lienectomy. Esophagus and empty intestine were connected by the end-to-side anastomosis. The pathological test showed that the patient suffered from the mucinous adenocarcinoma of stomach. The cancer cells had invaded the full-thickness of stomach wall with lymphatic metastases of lesser curvature side. On May 13, 1998, the patient accepted the first chemotherapy, adopting 1000mg of 5-Fu with five-day intravenous injections. On the first day the chemotherapy drugs were added with 10mg of Mitomycin. On June 3, 1998, the patient accepted the second chemotherapy with 10mg of Mitomycin. The third time was on July 1, 1998. The fourth time was on July 29, 1998. The fifth time was on September 9, 1998. The reexamination found the relapse. On December 24, 1998, the type-B ultrasonic showed the cancer of biliary duct and ovarian metastasis. On December 26, 1998, the patient came to the anti-cancer coordination group for outpatient treatment, adopting the XZ-C series for the traditional Chinese medicine treatment of immunoregulation. After taking the medicine orally, the symptom was improving, and the condition of the illness was getting better.

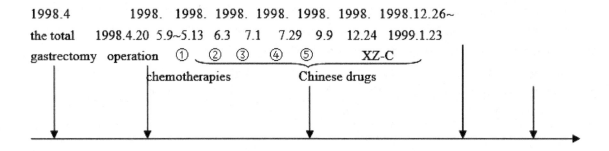

Type-B ultrasonic: relapse of cancer of biliary duct, ovarian metastasis.

Analysis: This patient suffered from the mucinous adenocarcinoma of stomach and underwent the total gastrectomy. After the operation, the patient accepted the chemotherapies once a month with five days per time. After the fifth chemotherapy, the type-B ultrasonic found the relapse of cancer of biliary duct and ovarian metastasis. It prompted that postoperative adjuvant chemotherapies still failed to arrest relapse and prevent metastasis.

Case 7 Patient Li ××, female, thirty-seven, worker, Yingcheng, patient history number: 7401473
Diagnosis: The rectum cancer cells metastasized to ovary after the operation.

Since 1997, the stool had been being with the blood. In June 1998, the colonoscopy showed it as the rectum cancer. On July 9, 1998, the patient underwent the anterior resection of the rectum (Dixon-type, anastomat). There were six-time postoperative chemotherapies. The first time was on July 27, 1998 with carboplatin and 5-Fu. The second time was on September 6, 1998. The third time was on October 2, 1998. The fourth time was on November 19, 1998. The fifth time was on December 25, 1998. The sixth time was on January 31, 1999.

On April 16, 1999, the patient came to the anti-cancer coordination group for outpatient treatment with the XZ-C series. In May 1999, the CT examination showed the rectum cancer cells metastasized to bilateral ovaries.

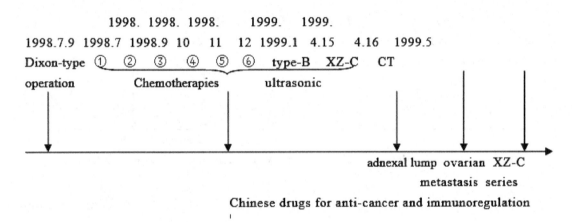

Chinese drugs for anti-cancer and immunoregulation

Analysis: After the operation of rectum cancer, the patient accepted continuous chemotherapies for six courses. Three months after the last course, the type-B ultrasonic and CT found that rectum cancer cells metastasized to bilateral ovaries. It prompted that such continuous and long-term chemotherapies still failed to prevent metastases.

III. Cases of Chemotherapy Accelerating the Failure of Immunologic Function

Case 1 Patient, Xu ××, male, forty-two, cadre, Wuhan, patient history number: 420836
Diagnosis: Lung cancer of right middle lobe

In February 1997, fluoroscopy of chest showed no abnormity. Because of the home decorating, the patient had contacted the marble powder bed for about one month. Then this patient began to have a complaint of the chest. On June 1, 1997, X-ray chest film showed the atelectasis of right lung. On June 13, 1997, the CT reported the lung cancer of median lobe and metastases of hilar lymph nodes. The examination of bronchofiberscope showed that each bronchus of the right side became narrower. The brushing biopsy showed it as the adenocarcinoma cell. Right now, the patient had no cough and emptysis. There was a lymph node about the size of fingertip in the right neck region. On June 13, 1997, the patient underwent the interventional therapy for one time. Because of the intense reaction, there was no more interventional therapy. On July 25, 1997, the patient began to accept chemotherapies for two times. The first time adopted the intravenous injection with a large dose of Adriamycin, Cyclophosphane, Cis-platinum and Xierke. On August 9, the white blood cell count (WBC) was 1100. Then the patient accepted the blood transfusion, adding with injections of interleukin-2, tumor necrosis factor and interferon. The second time was on August 20. The chemotherapy drugs were same as the first time with intravenous injection. On September 10, X-ray chest film showed no obvious pathological change. On September 11, the patient left the hospital. On October 10, 1997, Emission Computed Tomography (ECT) showed widespread metastatic tumor of bone of the whole body. On October 13, 1997, X-ray chest film showed the lung cancer of double lungs. The lesions increased significantly as compared with the past. After undergoing the reinforced chemotherapies of two courses, the lesions of double lungs spread. The cancer cells quickly metastasized to skeletons of the whole body. The immunologic function broke down. By the end of October 1997, the patient died from the failure of immunologic function.

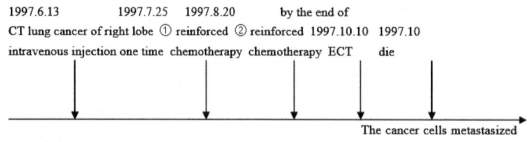

Analysis: This patient suffered from lung cancer of right middle lobe. The left lung had carcinomatous metastasis. So the patient couldn't accept the operation. Since July 1997, the patient accepted the reinforced chemotherapies of two courses with four kinds of drugs. The patient began to vomit and couldn't feed at all. After the treatment, the immunologic function of the patient broke down. Emission Computed Tomography (ECT) showed that there were several dozen osseous metastases in the whole body. It prompted: ① the reinforced chemotherapies failed to prevent metastases. ② the reinforced chemotherapies severely suppressed the immunity, which led to the severe failure of immunologic function. The host lost the immune surveillance. The cancer cells immediately spread to the whole body. The osseous metastases resulted in the failure of immunologic function and shortened this patient's life.

Case 2 Patient Feng ××, female, fifty-one, Xiangfan, doctor, patient history number: 4900972
Diagnosis: After the operation of the breast cancer, the cancer cells metastasized to bones, liver and brain.

In February 1995, the patient underwent the modified radical mastectomy for the lump in the right breast. The patient suffered from the metastatic carcinoma of axillary lymph nodes (3/6). Pathology: infiltrating ductal cancer became partly hard. On February 19, 1995, the patient accepted the chemotherapy with the drugs of Adriamycin and Cyclophosphamide. On April 28, 1995, the patient transferred to Wuhan for eleven cycles of chemotherapies with CMF treatment. On May 21, 1996, the CMF treatment was switched to Xierke treatment in the eleventh cycle. The arrest of bone marrow became obvious. The white blood cell count (WBC) dropped to 300! Transfusion of 20g of leucocytes eventually made it come back to the normal value. The doctor gave express order that the patient couldn't accept the treatment after leaving hospital. On June 4, 1996, the Ct reexamination found metastatic carcinoma of the ninth rib. Then the patient accepted the radiotherapies without any chemotherapy. On July 7, 1997, the type-B ultrasonic found the metastatic carcinoma of liver. There was a tumor about the size of 3.2cm×3.9cm in the right anterior lobe of liver. The MRI and CT examinations diagnosed it falsely as radioactive hepatic lesion. On July 17, 1997, the angiography proved it as the metastatic carcinoma of liver. On July 28, 1997, the patient underwent the resection of the right anterior lobe of liver. And the patient was inserted a catheter into the hepatic artery for implantation of the drug pump. The chemotherapy drugs of epirubicin, cis-platinum and 5-Fu had been pumped successively for four times. On November 10, 1997, the type-B ultrasonic found that there were a metastatic carcinoma about the size of 3.4cm×3.3cm in the right lobe of liver and another metastatic carcinoma about the size of 1.7cm×1.9cm in the right anterior lobe of liver. The patient couldn't undergo the surgery, radiotherapy or chemotherapy any more. That was because none of the three treatments could prevent metastasis and extension. On November 16, 1997, the patient came to the anti-cancer coordination group for outpatient treatment, adopting the XZ-C series for the traditional Chinese medicine complex treatment of immunoregulation. After taking the medicine, the patient regained a high spirit, a good appetite. The general condition was improving. On March 17, 1998, MRI showed that there were multiple occupying nidi inside the calvarium. The cancer cells were metastasizing to the brain. Then the patient accepted the reinforced chemotherapies. After a course of reinforced chemotherapies, the patient gradually faded away.

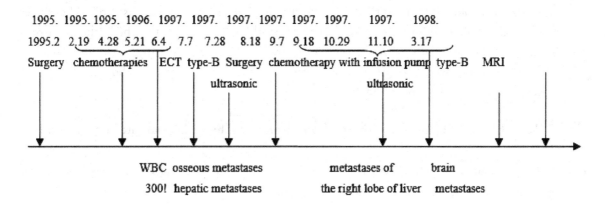

Analysis: (1) After the operation of breast cancer, the patient accepted the continuous chemotherapies, starting with short-course chemotherapies and proceeding with the eleven courses of chemotherapies. And then, the patient was injected with the chemotherapy drugs by the infusion pump. Although the patient continuously accepted the chemotherapies and other treatments without a stop, the cancer still ignored those treatments, slowly and gradually making the distant metastases through the whole body. Why did so many treatments fail to stop metastases and extensions? What kind of role and status did those chemotherapy anti-cancer drugs play and have in this case? The chemotherapies didn't produce the due effect, because after the chemotherapy the cancer cells immediately metastasized to bones, liver.

(2) The chemotherapy suppressed the immunologic function and marrow hematopoietic function. The question was whether the suppression would promote osseous metastases. The reinforced chemotherapies of this case once made WBC reduce to 300. The body's immunological function suffered the severe suppression. The cancer cells lost the immune surveillance and would inevitably have the further multiplications, extensions and metastases.

(3) Why were the chemotherapies of this case useless? The question was whether the chemotherapy drugs had the drug tolerance. If having the tolerance, the chemotherapy drugs of more than one year were totally useless. The drugs didn't produce the due effect on cancer cells. On the contrary, the normal cells of visceral organs in the patient's body, especially the cells of immune organ (Marrow was the central immune organ), ceaselessly suffered form the damage. Then the ability of the body resistance and immunological function severely fell off. It promoted multiplications, extensions and metastases of cancer cells. The chemotherapy not only failed to achieve the therapeutic effect, but also conversely had the adverse effect on attacking the ability of the body resistance and promoting the metastases and multiplications of the cancer cells.

(4) Why were the continuous chemotherapies of this case useless? The question was whether the selected joint chemotherapy drugs were not sensitive to the cancer cells of this patient. (The anti-cancer drugs couldn't accept drug sensitive test as the antibiotic. Thus the drugs were selected according to the experience with certain blindness.) When doctors couldn't get the curative effect, they would increase the dose, intensify the chemotherapy or switch to use the better chemotherapy drugs. In this way, it would produce the more severe immunological suppression, result the failure of immunological function and lead to the further multiplications of the cancer cells, which the cancer cells would present the multiplication like the geometrical logarithm. But the chemotherapy drugs couldn't increase exponentially with the toxic side effect. Thus the increasing speed and quantity of chemotherapy drugs would never be able to catch up those of cancer cells. So the continuous chemotherapies still failed to control metastases and extensions.

Case 3 Patient Lu xx, female, forty-three, shop employee, Changsha, patient history number: 4300857

Diagnosis: The patient suffered from the carcinoma simplex of left breast. The cancer cells had metastasized to the back bone, pelvis and liver.

Medical History: (Omission).

1996. 1996. 1996. 1996. 1996. 1996. 1996. 1996. 1996. 1996. 1997. 1997. 1997. 1997. 1997. 1997. 1997.

7.15 7.22 7.29 8.30 9.9 9.16 9.23 10.2 11.14 12 1 3.19 4.16 4.23 6.12 7.21 7.23

Chemotherapies Surgery   Chemotherapies   XZ-C

osseous metastases osseous hepatic metastases

destruction of lumbar multiple metastases

308

Analysis: This patient accepted the preoperative and postoperative chemotherapies continuously and chronically. After the operation, the patient accepted the chemotherapy once a month, defining five days every time. During the five months after the operation, there were over forty times of radiotherapies and eight times of chemotherapies. The patient underwent continuous multiple CT scans and ceaselessly continuous chemotherapies. But after eight months the cancerous protuberance widely metastasized and spread to skeletons of the whole body. Every time the patient accepted the radiotherapy or chemotherapy, she had to suffer the suppression, bone marrow suppression and the attack to the organisms of the body. The long-term and continuous chemotherapies were essentially the chronic and continuous attack to the immunologic function. The immunologic function of organisms and marrow hematopoietic function suffered such long-term and continuous damage that they couldn't restore the functions. Losing the immune surveillance, the cancer cells were bound to invade and metastasize widely to all of the visceral organs in the whole body.

The real effect of this case was that the treatment killed off tumor cells but damaged the body. It didn't turn out as it should be. In fact, the treatments failed to prevent carcinomatous metastases, essentially damage the function of immunologic and defensive system of the host, attack the ability of the body resistance and promote the invasion and dissemination of cancer cells.

Six months after the operation, metastatic carcinoma of bone appeared. Eight months after the operation, metastatic carcinoma of liver appeared. The radiotherapy and chemotherapy failed to prevent the progression of this disease. How to evaluate the therapeutic effectiveness that the radiotherapy and chemotherapy had on the patient? What kind of role and status did those treatments play and have?

Case 4 Patient Chen ××, male, Thirty-four, counterman, Wuhan, patient history number: 430849

This patient had suffered from the repetitious and irritative dry cough without phlegm for three years. Then this disease was treated as bronchitis. In January 1997, X-ray film of the chest showed large compact shadows in the right upper lung. CT examination reported that there was a compact shadow about the size of 6cm×9cm in the right upper lung. And there was another sarcoidosis behind it about the size of 1.2cm×1.5cm. The sarcoidosis was the central type and had multiple metastases in the lung. On January 11, 1997, the patient underwent the exploratory thoracotomy. In the operation, it could be easily seen that the nidi had widely infiltrated and couldn't be cut off. The tissue slice showed it as the poorly differentiated adenocarcinoma in the right upper lung. Then the chest was closed. In February, March, April and May 1997, the patient accepted postoperative chemotherapies with the drugs of DDP and ADM for one course a month. On July 14, 1997, scanning reexamination showed the enlargement of lump in the right lung. Because the patient suffered from the headache for one week and felt dizzy. The CT scanning of brain showed the brain metastases. Then on July 22, 1997 and July 27, the patient successively underwent the r-scalpel operation for two times. The headache was eased and then disappeared. And on July 13, 1977, the patient came to the anti-cancer coordination group for outpatient treatment, adopting the drugs of XZ-C series. After taking the medicine, the condition of illness was stable. The patient regained a high spirit, a good appetite. The headache and vomit disappeared. The patient walked and talked as the normal people. Three months (one course) after taking the Wuhan Chinese herbal anticancer medicine of XZ-C series, the condition of illness had an obvious improvement. The patient had a rosy cheek, regained the physical strength and walked as the normal people. There was no cough or any kind of discomfort. The breathing sound of right lung faded out. Afterwards the patient accepted the chemotherapy in another hospital, continuously increasing the dose for reinforced chemotherapies. The white blood cell count (WBC) dropped to 300, which was an extremely low value. The immunologic function crocked up.

Analysis: This patient underwent the exploratory thoracotomy for the cancer of right lung. The nidi couldn't be cut off. Then the patient accepted the continuous reinforced chemotherapies. The cancer cells metastasized to the brain. After the r-scalpel operation, the headache disappeared and obtained satisfactory effects. With the immunoregulation treatment of XZ-C series, the general conditions of this patient were getting better obviously and the symptoms improved. But the continuous reinforced chemotherapies resulted in the failure of immunologic function.

11. REVIEW AND PROSPECT OF SURGICAL TREATMENT OF TUMORS

- The achievement of surgical resection of the tumor in the 20th century
- 21st century surgical goal should be prevention and treatment research for cancer recurrence and metastasis after surgery radical resection
- The design of tumor radical surgery should be further studied and perfected
- The molecular biology basic research and clinical basic research of metastasis should be strengthened after the radical resection
- To prevent cancer recurrence and metastasis should be done from the surgery

Surgical operation is a definite and effective cure for malignant tumor therapy. Even though today's cancer treatment has developed to the multi-discipline and multimodality treatment, surgical operation is still one of the most central and common means for malignant tumor therapy, and makes itself an integral part of multi-discipline and multimodality treatment.

In the 18th century, therapists held that the early cancer was a local disease, which could be cured by surgical treatment. In 1881, Bill-roth first carried out the surgical removal of tumor — subtotal gastrectomy. In 1890, Halsted actualized the radical resection of breast. He first elucidated the principle of en bloc resection, which meant resections of lymphatic vessel and lymph node in the chosen zone of primary tumor. This resection laid a good foundation for most modern surgical operations of tumors. The surgical technique of tumor resection has been developing along with surgery. After the middle of the 20th century, it gradually developed into an independent subject — tumor surgery. Since the 1950s, due to the improvement and development of surgical technique, preoperative (postoperative) care and operative supporting measures, such as blood transfusion, anesthesia, aseptic technique and antibiotics, the surgical risk, complications and fatality rate have reduced greatly; the range of tumor surgical technique tends to expand; a series of super radical operations arise, such as expansive radical mastectomy. But many years' practice proves that expanding the range of surgical resection cannot improve the survival time without tumor and total survival time of most tumors, such as lung cancer, liver cancer and pancreatic cancer.

Since the 1970s, people's understanding of tumor biology has changed a lot. At present, people hold that most tumors are not local diseases and may have been systemic diseases since the clinical examination. The hematogenous spread is common. When finally diagnosed, many patients may have suffered from micro-metastases. Whether obvious metastases have happened since the clinical examination, depends upon biological characteristics of tumor cells and interactions between tumors and hosts. Neither the more extensive regional surgery nor the share of surgery and radiotherapy can affect metastases.

1. Great Achievements in Surgical Removal of Tumor in 20th Century

In the 20th century, great achievements mainly focus on researching various methods of tumor surgical resections, operation procedures, preoperative (postoperative) care and cleaning range of lymph nodes; studying, understanding and getting familiar with regional anatomy and pathophysiology of bearing cancer organs, such as resection technique and organ reconstruction technique of liver cancer, pancreatic cancer, stomach cancer, esophageal cancer, colorectal cancer, lung cancer, breast cancer, cervical cancer, brain cancer and so on; taking measures to raise resection rate, reduce complications, lower operative mortality rate and improve perioperative care. In terms of esophageal cancer surgery, how to raise the resection rate? How to reduce anastomotic leakage? How to improve Esophagogastrostomy upon (down) Aortic Arch? How to carry out the cervical anastomosis? How to improve anastomose technique, such as scarf-type anastomosis? And in the case of liver cancer, how to perform regular or irregular hepatectomy? How to conduct (expanding) lobectomy of liver? How to carry out combined segmentum hepatis resection, second resection of intrahepatic recurrent cancer after resection, and liver cancer resection of special regions? How to retain residual liver functions? For the breast cancer, how to perform radical or super radical operation? Then how to conduct conservative operation procedures? In the case of stomach cancer, how to carry out D2 and D3 operations? How many groups of lymph nodes are needed to clear? For the operation procedure of rectal cancer, select Mile or Dixon procedure? Retain anus or not? Use anastomat or not? In terms of pancreatic cancer, select Whipple or Child procedure? How to conduct anastomose procedure of gall bladder and bowel? How to perform the resection of hepatic hilar cholangiocarcinoma? For the lung cancer, how to carry out the resection of pulmonary segments, lung lobes or the whole lung? In conclusion, researches are about how to resect the tumor en bloc and completely? How to increase operative resection rate? How to reduce or avoid complications? How to lower operative mortality rate? And how to help patients recover? By the 1990s, cancer resections of esophagus, stomach, bowel, liver, gall bladder, pancreas, lung, mammary gland and thyroid gland fully pass the test. All the operative routine techniques are already mature. Operative mortality rates have dropped to a very low level. Operations are basically safe. Many cancer radical operations have been widely diffused among county hospitals and basic hospitals. But how to prevent recurrence and metastasis has not yet generally attracted people's attention.

In some large hospitals, doctors have perceived that though operations are performed very thoroughly and canonically, postoperative recurrence and metastasis in the short (long) term still puzzle some specialists. Then in the 1990s, some experts have followed suit, announcing the study that disposes cast-off cells caused by operative wound. Chen Junqing in Shenyang has spent over ten years on researching and processing cast-off cells of stomach cancer, finally making brilliant achievements. The study conducted by South Hospital, which heats, washes and processes cast-off cells after the operation of rectum cancer, has got satisfactory efficacy. Yang Chuanyong at Tongji Hospital has always been devoting himself to exploring the pharmacokinetics of intraperitoneal chemotherapy of hepatic portal venous blood. At present, the technique of surgical excision of the tumor is basically successful, which is an honorable achievement in the 20th century. But these difficulties that cancer patients suffer from postoperative recurrences and metastases with no good countermeasure, and frequently come back to the clinic for further consultation, still bother vast numbers of medical workers.

2. The Objectives of Surgery in 21st Century Should Be the Study on Prevention and Control of Recurrence and Metastasis after Radical Operation of Carcinoma

In 1985, the writer himself made follow-up to more than 3,000 patients who had accepted surgical radical excisions of tumors. The results show that 2~3 years after the operation, most patients suffer from recurrences or metastases. While some patients even bear it after six months, less than a year or just over one year. These patients do not always come back to the previous surgery physician for further consultation but go to Tumor Hospital or Tumor Department for medical treatment. Once recurrences appear, however, only a few patients can accept the second operation. But most patients cannot receive effective therapies and soon pass away. It has made the writer more aware that though the operation at that time was successful and standard, the long-term follow-up result is dissatisfactory. That is, the late result is a failure (Certainly tens of patients can survive for 10, 20 or 30 years after the operation, but it is only a very few cases.). Therefore, the study must be done to prevent postoperative recurrence and metastasis. Follow-up results present an important problem that postoperative recurrence or metastasis is the key factor for long-term postoperative effectiveness. While researching method and measure of preventing postoperative recurrence or metastasis plays the key role in improving long-term effectiveness and lengthening survival time. Therefore, the clinical fundamental research must be done for preventing cancer recurrence and metastasis. If no breakthrough in the field of fundamental research, it will be hard to improve clinical effectiveness. Then the writer as well as his colleagues has established the Institute of Experimental Surgery, where they have carried out experimental tumor research, implemented transplantation of cancer cells to animals, constructed tumor animals' models. They have also developed a series of experimental tumor researches: ① Explore mechanism and rule of cancer recurrence and metastasis; ② Probe into the relationship between tumor and immunity, and that between tumor and immune organ; ③ Research into the method of arresting progressive atrophy of immune organs with the growth of tumor and the way of immunologic reconstitution; ④ Seek effective measures to adjust and control cancer invasion, recurrence and metastasis; ⑤ Conduct inhibition rates experiments of tumor-bearing animals to respectively filter 200 literature-approved traditional Chinese medicines which are commonly used for anti-cancer; ⑥ Carry out experimental researches to seek new drugs from natural drugs with resistances to cancer, recurrence and metastasis.

The writer has gone through a complete review of almost 54-year practical cases of clinical treatment and also made the follow-up. Then he analyzes and rethinks the lessons of success and failure, from which he comes to understand a truth. That is, conquering cancer needs to break with the conventional ideas and update the thought; conduct investigations, researches and analyses with patients; carry out self-reflection and self-evaluation. Renew ideas, innovate methods, look for an opening in urgent problems of tumor researches and weak links of modern medicine. The writer has also realized that techniques of surgical resections of tumors in the 20th century have made brilliant achievements. The next researching objective and task of surgeons are not only to have further studies on seeking for greater perfection of radical operation, but also to prevent postoperative recurrence and metastasis. Experiments and clinical researches on preventing recurrence and metastasis after cancer radical operation should be done to further improve postoperative long-term effectiveness. Because the operation is just a regional treatment, if the tumor is limited in a certain visceral organ, the surgical effect may be very good; but if the tumor is not just limited in this visceral organ but has invaded the serosa outside the organ, no matter how thorough the operation is, the possibility of recurrence and metastasis is still in existence. Especially for stomach cancer and rectum cancer, though lymph nodes are cleared completely, many cancer cells still remain in venous blood vessels. A lot of research materials have identified that clearance of lymph nodes is only to prevent lymphatic metastasis but that is just one side. The involved lymph nodes should be cleared, but excising lymph nodes cannot prevent hematogenous metastasis. Therefore, hepatic metastases rates in the short/long term are both high after operations of stomach cancer and intestinal cancer. At present, surgical excision of the tumor as well as regional lymphatic vessels and lymph nodes cannot prevent hematogenous metastasis and spread, implantation and dissemination of cast-off cells. Consequently, the next objective of tumor surgeons' research work should focus on experiments and clinical researches for preventing cancer recurrence and metastasis after radical operation. That is, in the early 20th century, researchers should make great achievements on studies of preventing cancer recurrence and metastasis. If postoperative recurrence and metastasis cannot be solved, short/long-term effectiveness of surgical cancer treatment will fail to get satisfactory result.

3. Design of Surgical Radical Operation of Tumor to be Further Studied and Perfected

Since recurrence and metastasis happens after the radical operation, it is necessary to analyze whether the radical operation itself has connection with postoperative recurrence and metastasis, and carry out retrospective analysis and reflection. Among the present radical operations, some have been used for over 100 years, such as the radical operation of breast cancer. Over a century, thousands of cancer patients have accepted different kinds of radical operations, the majority of which have got satisfied short-term effectiveness. But long-term recurrence and metastasis rates are still very high. As the name implies, "radical cure" means thorough or eradicating treatment; but if it is "radical operation", why the purpose of radical cure fails to achieve and the recurrence still happens? Now that lymph nodes have been cleared, why the metastasis still appears? The question is whether those recurrences and metastases are due to cast-off cells left by operation or operative techniques, related to procedure design, concept foundation of operative design or not entirely consistent with the present known Biological characteristics and biological behaviors of cancer cells. The present radical operation refers to the en bloc resection of primary tumor and regional lymph nodes. Logically, it is not the radical cure, and cannot approach the purpose of radical cure. That is because the malignant tumor has four routes of metastasis, which are lymphatic channel metastasis, hematogenous metastasis, implantation metastasis and direct spreading. While the surgical operation just completely clears lymph nodes and radically cures the route of lymphatic channel metastasis, it has no specific technical measure to prevent hematogenous metastasis, and also do nothing to bring forward definite and effective countermeasures to implantation of cast-off cancer cells as well as implantation and dissemination of chest and peritoneal cavity. Lymph nodes having been thoroughly cleared off cannot prevent hematogenous metastasis, and moreover, only the clearance of lymph nodes can't prevent peritoneal implantation and dissemination of peritoneal cavity by cast-off cancer cells, either. Surgical operation belongs to a regional treatment. Experts in tumor surgery hold that cancer develops in a local area of the body, invades the surrounding tissues and metastasizes to other areas through lymphatic vessels, etc. Accordingly, the main point of treatment is often put on the local area, controlling local growth and diffusion, especially lymph nodes metastasis, such as the clearance of lymph nodes. For years surgical treatment has been updating on the operation method and type, but its long-term effectiveness — 5-year survival rate still has no obvious improvement. The postoperative recurrence and metastasis seriously threaten patients' postoperative survival. Therefore, the present radical operation is just a relative one, which is on a quote. Young doctors should know that the present type design still has weak links, which need the further experimental and clinical studies to explore new techniques and methods to definitely and effectively prevent routes of metastases. Accordingly, in recent years the writer's laboratory has always been doing experimental exploration in this respect, such as experimental study of free-tumor technique in radical operation (Fig. 1), free-tumor technique study in radical operation of cancer-bearing animal models, counting of intraoperative cast-off cancer cells as well as detection and counting of cancer cells in venous angioma, experimental observation of dyeing tracking of gastric lymph nodes. Preventing postoperative cancer metastasis and recurrence must be started from the radical operation.

In order to study why cancer cells can dissociate and cast off from the tumor body, cast-off cancer cells still have the vitality and can implant to other areas, the writer's laboratory use electronic microscope to observe and study cancer cells' ultrastructural organization of cancer-bearing animal models (Fig. 2, 3).

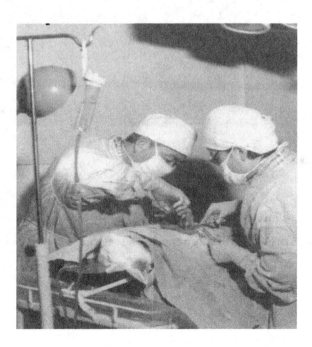

Fig. 1 Experimental study of free-tumor technique in radical operation

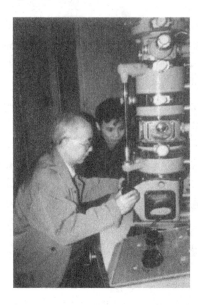
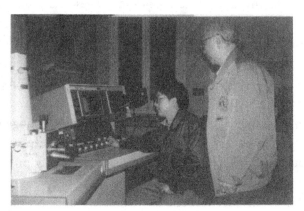

Fig. 2 Observation of ultrastructural organization of experimental model's cancer cells with electronic microscope

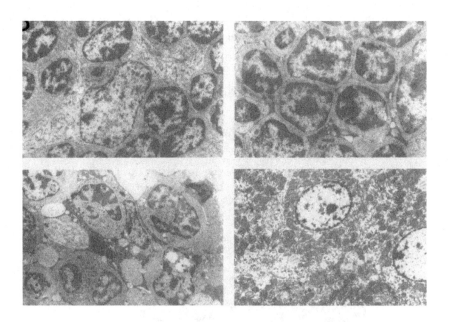

Fig. 3 Ultrastructural organization of hepatic cancer cells of cancer-bearing mouse H$_{22}$

4. Strengthening Fundamental and Clinical Study on Molecular Biology of Radical Operation of Recurrence and Metastasis after Operation

Inhibiting angiogenesis factors to induce the formation of blood vessels and preventing endothelial cells to construct new blood vessels are both new ways to explore preventions from recurrence and metastasis. In the experimental study of inhibiting actions of ethyl acetate extractives (TG) of traditional Chinese medicine — Common Threewingnut Root with different dosages on new blood vessels of transplanted tumor of mice peritoneum, the writer's laboratory observe influences of TG on the form and number of new-born micro-vessels in and around transplanted tumor of mice peritoneum, and on the diameter and flow rate of tumor arterioles and venules. They have made the preliminary confirmation that TG has certain inhibiting actions on new-born blood vessels of metastatic carcinoma focus and has been taken on clinical trials.

Study of preventing postoperative recurrence and metastasis of cancers must base on establishing animal models of recurrence and metastasis, and also proceed on levels of Molecular Biology and Gene. In the past decade and more, due to the rapid development of Molecular Biology, experts have found that the generation, progress, invasion, metastasis and recurrence of tumor are all in connection with cancer genes, cancer suppressor genes, metastatic genes and suppressor metastatic genes. To research related genes and seek control methods to prevent recurrence and metastasis as well as clinical measures of preventing recurrence, such as biological therapy, gene therapy, biological reaction control agent therapy, may be an important research aim in the future. In the 21st century, gene therapy will provide new efficient way for tumor therapy, and Molecular Biological Immunology will also stimulate the development of tumor therapy.

5. Prevention of Recurrence and Metastasis after Operation Should Be Established in Operation

(1) Surgical techniques of cancer surgery

Free-tumor technique is vitally important, which should prevent operation techniques from causing or actuating hematogenous metastasis of cancer cells.

Surgical principles of general surgery also applies to tumor surgery, such as operation techniques of aseptic operation, sufficient exposedness of operative location, the least intraoperative damage of normal tissues for the early-stage healing, etc. In addition, tumor surgery should take note of preventing the dissemination of cancer cells in the operation, in which the free-tumor technique is vitally important.

Ever since the end of the nineteenth century, people have realized that operation techniques may cause or actuate the dissemination of cancer cells. Therefore, the free-tumor technique of tumor surgery has been attracting more and more attention in recent years. For instance, intraoperative procedures of preserved skin, extrusion and anatomy can directly lead to the dissemination of tumor cells, stimulate formations of tumor embolism and metastasis which are near to or far away from blood vessels and lymphatic vessel. And tumor cells cast off and pollute surgical wounds, which results in local implantation recurrence, etc. Along with the development of Cell Pathology and inspection technology of tumor cells in blood stream, the phenomenon of tumor dissemination has been confirmed in clinical trials and animal experiments. For example, active cancer cells and cancer tissue masses can be found in vessel douche and surgical wounds douche of tumor operative specimen; cancer cells can be easier found in the output venous blood flow of tumor during the operation. Therefore, it is important that in the operation surgeons should first ligate and cut off output vena of tumor.

It should be noted in surgical operation that all the techniques are favorable toward preventing cancer cells' metastases. Do not stimulate or increase chances of cancer cells' metastases to cause iatrogenic metastasis and dissemination. For the surgical resection of tumor, all the operations must stress and observe free-tumor concept and technique, no matter big or small. Surgeons should give equal emphasis on free-tumor concept and aseptic concept, free-tumor technique and aseptic technique. The free-tumor technique is even stricter than aseptic technique. The surgical knife, scissors, needle and thread in the surgical operation, even every procedure is possible to cause metastasis of cancer cells. Such a possibility may increase with excessive extrusion, needle punching through the skin, knife cutting and other negative operative procedures by surgeons on tumor body or tissues. At present, applied molecular biology or immunohistochemistry method has proved that the operation technique itself can cause iatrogenic implantations, diffusions and metastases of cancer cells. Cancer cells can be found in surrounding blood circulations when many patients are undergoing the surgical operation; or cancer cells convert from the preoperative negative result to the postoperative positive result. The above evidences indicate that operation techniques are possible to induce the diffusion of cancer cells. It also suggests that some patients' postoperative recurrence and metastasis may be caused by improper operation techniques, such as the incision implantation.

Therefore, preventing postoperative recurrence and metastasis must start out from all the techniques in the surgical operation.

The route and type of tumor dissemination vary according to different pathologic types of tumor. Whether or not the metastasis can come into being is also related to the body's immune state. Consequently during the therapeutic process, the modern tumor surgeons should both prevent tumor dissemination and be careful to maintain the body's resistibility or immunity.

(2) Prevention from the dissemination of cancer cells

It is well-known but always overlooked that tumor's localized examination and operation techniques should be gentle and skillful to prevent the dissemination of cancer cells. Therefore, the following points should be noted: ① Preoperative tumor palpation should be gentle, and the number of times ought to be minimized. ② Preserved skin for operation should be gentle and skillful, or more cancer cells will invade small veins by the over friction. ③ operation techniques should be gentle and skillful, incision must be sufficient to expose, dissect and resect. Avoid pressing the tumor. ④ Adopt sharp dissection (dissecting knife or scissor); Strictly avoid blunt dissection to reduce dissemination. ⑤ Deal with the output vein before the artery. ⑥ Dispose the farther lymph nodes before the nearby lymph nodes to resect them wholly with the tumor.

(3) Prevention from the implantation of cancer cells

Cast-off cancer cells easily implant and grow on the traumatic tissue wounds, so: ① Use the gauze pad to protect cutting shoulder and wound surface. ② if the tumor is unwittingly incised or cracks, it should be covered and bound up with gauze pads. Replace timely polluted gloves and surgical instruments. ③ Adequate excision extent, involving enough normal tissues around the pathological changes. ④ Avoid the blood out-flowing from polluted wounds when anatomizing tissues near the tumor. Therefore, when two blood vessel forceps are used to clamp blood vessels, they should stick close to each other. Ligate immediately after being cut off. Replace timely gauze pads that are contaminated with blood.

Postoperative local recurrence (cover about 10%) of colon and rectum cancers often occurs in anastomotic stoma, incision of abdominal wall or outside of intestinal wall. This kind of recurrence is usually caused by the implantation of cancer cells. In recent years, a strip of cloth is used to ligate intestinal canals belonging to the upper and lower segment of tumor before the excision of intestinal loop, in order to stop cast-off cancer cells from continuing to diffuse along the intestinal cavity in the surgical operation. Use 1:500 corrosive sublimate or fluorouracil solution to douche intestinal cavities of both ends before the anastomosis, which can obviously improve the long-term effectiveness and may be relevant to the before-mentioned reduction of recurrence.

After all, to review significant achievements of 20-century techniques of surgical tumor excision; to preview glary prospects of 21-century tumor surgery study of prevention from recurrence and metastasis. In the coming period, the highlight of anti-cancer work should be anti-invasion, anti-metastasis and anti-recurrence. Anti-recurrence is the key of operative effectiveness; and anti-metastasis is the core question of cancer treatment. Cancer invasion and metastasis depend on specific potentials of two factors: biological characteristics of tumor cell itself and the host's influence on its restraining factors. To keep a balance is to control; to lose a balance is to progress.

The initiative of the following reforms and development were made for traditional therapies

In the last two centuries the treatment of malignant tumors appeared twice leap

↓

The first time was in 1989 that Halsted proposed the concept of radical surgery

↓

The second was in the 1970s that Fish integrated chemotherapy into the radical surgery (adjuvant chemotherapy or neoadjuvant chemotherapy)

↓

Since then the treatment of malignant tumors was wandering and the malignant tumor death is still the first

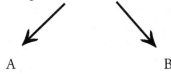

A   B

(**A and B** are the following parts):

A,

Radical surgery
↓
Expand radical surgery or radical surgery
↓
Improved radical surgery
↓
Professor Xu Ze proposed the following four points of reform and development proposals:

•The design of radical resection should be further studied and perfected

•It is extremely important to propose tumor-free surgery

•Surgery should prevent the spread of cancer cells

•Surgery should prevent shedding of cancer cells

B, Chemotherapy is integrated with radical surgery (adjuvant chemotherapy or neoadjuvant chemotherapy)

↓

The target of Radiotherapy and chemotherapy is to kill cancer cells; while it is killing proliferation cells, it is killing immune cells

↓

And it failed to improve the efficacy and it caused the toxic side effects and reduce immune function

↓

Professor Xu Ze proposed the following six points of reform and development proposals:

- It is pointed out that healing should be done by regulation rather than by single killing
- It should also aim at the host and cancer cells and establish a comprehensive view of treatment
- It is Indicating that chemotherapy should be further studied and improved and it should be immunochemotherapy
- The route of administration On the solid tumor systemic intravenous chemotherapy should be questioned
- Advocacy of changing the solid tumor systemic intravenous chemotherapy into the target organ intravascular chemotherapy
- Advice of changing the cancer postoperative adjuvant chemotherapy into Omentum vein catheter pump chemotherapy

VOLUME VIII

The Research of XZ-C immune regulation and control anticancer medications-------The series of the scientific achievement and the innovation the scientific and technology

CONTENTS VOLUME VIII

Preface

Immunomodulatory drug looks promising

No matter how complex the mechanism behind cancer, immune suppression is a key cancer progression. Removal of immunosuppressive factors and restoration of recognition system cells to cancer cells can effectively resist cancer. More and more evidence shows that by regulating the body's immune system, it is possible to achieve the purpose of controlling cancer. Many researchers in the field are currently excited by activating the body's anti-tumor immune system to treat cancer. The next major breakthrough in cancer is likely to come from this.

In order to investigate cancer etiology, pathogenesis, pathophysiology, we conducted a series of animal studies, the experimental results from the analysis, access to new discoveries and new revelation: thymus atrophy and immune dysfunction is one of the cause of cancer and pathogenesis, therefore Ze (Xu Ze) professor proposed causes of cancer at international conferences, one of the mechanisms that may be thymus atrophy, central immune sensory dysfunction, immune dysfunction, decreased immune surveillance and immune escape ability.

As a result of experimental studies real laboratory findings: in cancer-bearing mice thymus showed progressive atrophy, central immune sensory dysfunction, decreased immune function, immune surveillance decrease so that its treatment principle must be to prevent atrophy of the thymus, to promote thymic hyperplasia and protect bone marrow function improve immune surveillance, which provides an experimental evidence and theoretical basis for the immune regulation treatment of cancer.

Based on the above revelation about cancer etiology, pathogenesis of experimental results, is put forward a new concept and new methods of xz immunomodulatory therapy. After 16 years of oncology clinics in more than 12,000 cases, clinical validation of Advanced cancer patients, confirming that protection of thymus and increase immune function treatment principle is reasonable, the efficacy is satisfactory. Application of immune regulation medicine has achieved good results, improving the quality of life and prolong the survival.

Professor Xu Ze immune regulation law is that XZ-C(XU ZE-China) first proposed in 2006 in his monograph << new concepts and new methods of treatment of cancer metastasis>> which he believes under normal circumstances the body's defenses and cancer are in a dynamic equilibrium and the cancer is caused by the dynamic balance disorders. If the state has adjusted to normal levels, it can control cancer growth and make it subside.

As we all know, the incidence of cancer development and prognosis, depending on the comparison of two factors, namely, the biological characteristics of cancer cells and the host defense against the body's own cancer-dimensional constraint cells, such as the balance between these two, the cancer can be controlled, if the two of those are imbalances, then the cancer develops.

Under normal circumstances, the host organism itself has a certain capacity constraints against cancer cells, but in cancer patients, these constraints are subject to different levels of defense suppression and damage, leading to the loss of the immune surveillance of cancer cells, immune escape occurred so as to lead to the further development of cancer cells and metastasis.

Through Basic experimental study of investigated the recurrence and metastasis mechanism by more than four years, and after three years of the inherent natural medicine herbal experiment in vivo anti-tumor cancer-bearing mice, herbs selected from a group of traditional Chinese medicine which have better inhibition rate are composed of anti-cancer immune regulation medications $XZ-C_{1-10}$..

1. OVERVIEW

XZ-C immunomodulatory anticancer medications are the selected 48 kinds of anti-tumor Chinese herbal medication with the better inhibitory rate from traditional Chinese herbal medication in the tumor-bearing mice experiments. After made up into the composition of the compound, and then tested in the inhibiting tumor experiments in cancer-bearing mice, the compound inhibitory rate is much greater than single herbs. $XZ-C_1$, $XZ-C_4$ are consisted of 28 Chinese herbal medications, of which $XZ-_{C1-A}$, $XZ-C_{1-B}$ can 100% inhibit cancer and 100% don't kill normal cells with righting and firming the body, improve the role of the body's immune function. From our experiments XZ-C pharmacodynamics study the results show: they has a good inhibitory rate on Ehrlich ascites carcinoma, S_{182}, H_{22} hepatocellular carcinoma; there are obvious synergy and toxicity attenuation; the experiments also demonstrated that XZ-C immune regulation traditional Chinese medications have significantly improved immune function.

After the acute toxicity test in mice, there is no obvious toxicity and no significant side effects for the long-term oral clinical taking (2--6 years). XZ-C can significantly reduce the toxicity of chemotherapy while the oral immune regulation medications are used with chemotherapy. The oral XZ-C drugs can increase the white blood cells; the hemoglobin increases during the Chemotherapy Intermittent periods. The advanced cancer patients mostly have weakness, fatigue, loss of appetite. After taking XZ-C immunomodulatory anticancer medications 4-8-12 weeks, the patients have more significantly improved on the appetite and sleeping and have the relieved pain and gradually recuperate.

(1) Among the 4,277 carcinoma patients in medium and advanced stage who took Z-C medicine with the return visit over 3 months, the case history had the specific observation record of the curative effect, see Table 1. It improved the quality of life of the patients in an all-round way, see Table 2.

Table 1 General information about 4,277 patients suffering from recurrence and metastasis

		Hepatic carcinoma	Carcinoma of lung	Gastric carcinoma	Esophagus cardia carcinoma	Rectum carcinoma of anal canal	Carcinoma of colon	Breast carcinoma	adenocarcinoma of pancreas
No. of cases		1 021	752	668	624	328	442	368	74
Male: female		4:1	4.4:1	2.25:1	3.1:1	1:1	2.1:1	Female	3.2:1
Focus	Primary	694 (68.6%)	699 (93.9%)						
	Metastasis	327 (31.2%)	53 (6.1%)						

Xu Ze; Xu Jie; Bin Wu

		Metastatic lung (2) From the stomach (31.2%)	Metastasis of supraclavicular lymph nodes (11.6%)	Metastatic lever (23.8%) Lung metastasis (3%)	Upper metastasis of compact bone (13.1%)	Reoccurrence rate (14.8%)	Metastatic lever (16.0%)	Metastasis of supraclavicular lymph nodes (17.5%)	Metastatic lever (11.7%)
Usual metastasis part in this group		From esophagus cardia (19.5%) From recta (31.2%)	Brain metastasis (3.1%) Bone metastasis (4.6%)	Metastasis of peritoneum (29.1%) Upper metastasis of compact bone (6.1%)	Metastatic lever (8.3%)	Metastatic lever (7.0%)	Metastasis of peritoneum (6.0%)	Metastasis of axillary lymph nodes (15.0%) Bone metastasis (5.0%)	Rear metastasis of peritoneum (39.1%)
Age	high invasion (year) %	30~39 (76.2)	50~69 (71.6)	40~49 (73.4)	40~69 (80.4)	40~49 (75.2)	30~69 (88.0)	40~59 (65.9)	40~59 (70.0)
	Oldest (year) %	11	20	17	30	27	27	29	34
	Youngest (year) %	86	80	77	77	78	76	80	68

Table 2 Observation of curative effect on 4 277 patients: fully improving the quality of life of the carcinoma patients in medium and advanced stage

Improvement	Vigor	Appetite	Reinforcement of physical force	Improvement in generalized case	Increase of body weight	Improvement of sleep	The restriction of improvement activity and capability released activity	self servicing normal walking	Resumption of work Engaged in light work
No. of cases (%)	4071	3986	2450	479	2938	1005	1038	3220	479
	95.2	93.2	57.3	11.2	68.7	23.5	24.3	75.3	11.2

In this group, all of them were the patients in medium and advanced stage. After taking the medicine, their symptoms were improved to different extents with the effective rate of 93.2%. With respect to the improvement of the quality of life (as per Karnofsky Performance Status), it rose to 80 scores on average after administration from 50 on average before administration; the patients in this group met with the different metastasis and dysfunction of the organs about Stage III. It was reported by the previous statistic information that the mesoposition survival time of this kind of patients was about 6 months. The longest time among this group of the cases reached up to 11 years; another patient suffering from hepatic carcinoma had taken Z-C medicine for ten years and a half; two patients suffering from hepatic carcinoma met with frequency encountered carcinomatous lesion in the left and right liver and it entirely subsided through secondary CT reexamination after the patient took Z-C medicine for half a year and the state of the disease had been stable over half a year. One patient suffering from double-kidney carcinoma met with the widespread metastasis of abdominal cavity after removal of one kidney, after taking Z-C medicine, he was entirely recovered and began to work again. 3 patients suffering from carcinoma of lung, with the lung not removed through explaraton, had taken

Z-C medicine over three years and a half. 2 patients suffering from gastric remnant carcinoma had taken Z-C medicine for 8 years. 3 patients suffering from reoccurrence of rectal carcinoma had taken Z-C medicine for 3 years. 1 patient suffering from metastatic liver and rib of the mastocarcinoma had taken Z-C medicine for 8 years. 1 patient suffering from the recurrent bladder carcinoma after operation of renal carcinoma had not met with the carcinoma for 9 years and a half after taking Z-C medicine. All of these patients were the ones in the medium and advanced stage that could not be operated once more or treated with radiotherapy or chemotherapy. They only took Z-C medicine without other medicines for treatment. Up to today, they are reexamined and get the medicine at the out-patient department every month. Through taking the medicine for a long time, the state of the disease is controlled in the stable state to make the organism and the tumor in balanced state for a relatively long time and get a relatively good survival with tumor, in this way, the symptoms of the patients are improved, the quality of life is improved and the survival time is prolonged.

(2) As to 84 patients suffering from solid tumor and 56 patients suffering from enlargement of upper lymph node of metastatic compact bone, after taking Z-C series medicines orally and applying Z-C3 anti-cancer apocatastasis paste, they met with good curative effects, see table 3.

Table 3 Changes of 84 patients suffering from solid tumor and 56 patients suffering from metastatic mode after applying Z-C paste externally

	Solid tumor				Enlargement of upper lymph node of metastatic compact bone			
	Disappearance	Shrinkage 1/2	Softening	No change	Disappearance	Shrinkage 1/2	Softening	No change
No. of cases (%)	12 14.2	28 33.3	32 38.0	12 14.2	12 21.4	22 39.2	14 25.0	8 14.2
Total effective rate (%)	85.7				85.7			

(3) 298 patients suffering from carcinoma pain obtained the obvious pain alleviation effects after taking Z-C medicine orally and applying Z-C anti-cancer apocatastasis paste externally, see Table 1-4.

Clinical menifetation	Pain			
	Light alleviation	Obvious alleviation	Disappearance	Avoidance
No of cases (%)	52 17.3	139 46.8	93 31.2	14 4.7
Total effective rate (%)	95.3			

3. IMMUNE PHARMACOLOGY OF XZ-C IMMUNE REGULATION CONTROL MEDICATION

Compared with western medication immunity pharmacology, the traditional Chinese medication pharmacology has own characteristics and advantages which the long-term clinical experience of Chinese medication has accumulated a large number of prescriptions regulating body's immune function, especially the beneficial Chinese medications generally have dynamic regulation of the immune benefits.

Whether the single herb medication or prescription will have a variety of active ingredients, and unlike the western medication(synthetic drugs) it is a matter of a single structure. The roles of Chinese medications have many aspects, in addition to the regulation of immune function, which has a certain role on the whole system function.

The main role of XZ-C immune regulation and control medications regulates the cellular immune response which regulate all of the cell-mediated, including various cytokines or lymphokines. The immune function of XZ-C medication has the major role on stem cells immunity, such as the thymus, gonads and lymphatic systems and T, B cells and various cytokines.

China ancient medication has the concept of that righteousness isn't false and evil doesn't come into which constitutes an integral part of traditional Chinese medication theory. Its essence is to maintain the balance of the overall function and to enhance resistance to disease. Its main role is to enhance immune function, in fact, the tonics medication is based on immune pharmacology. Immunity pharmacology is an emerging interdisciplinary and serves as a bridge contact between pharmacology and immunology. XZ-C immune control regulation medication has obvious immune function, as an effective immune enhancers, this area should be vigorously developed to get a new type of immune accelerator, making them become reliable, efficient and safe drugs. The various Chinese herbs in XZ-C4 has substantially immune enhancer effects. In animal experiments XZ-C4 has been proven to significantly promote thymus function. The main role of Chinese medication immunomodulator is to regulate cellular immune and various cell-mediated immune response, including cytokines or lymphokines.

4. THE PHARMACOLOGICAL RESEARCH OF XZ-C IMMUNE REGULATION ANTICANCER CHINESE MEDICATIONS

1. To sum anticancer pharmacology and experimental cancer-bearing animal solid tumors in vivo anti-tumor experiments, XZ-C drugs have significant anti-tumor effects. The inhibition rate of antitumor activity $XZ-C_1$ medication was 58% in the first six weeks; the inhibition rate of $XZ-C4$ was 70% in the first six weeks; the inhibition rate of cyclophosphamide amine (CTX) was 49% in the first 6 weeks in liver cancer H_{22} bearing mice. Life span in $XZ-C_1$ was 9.8% which indicates XZ-C drug has a good anti-cancer effect.

2. XZ-C drug has synergistic effect of attenuating the toxicity from chemotherapy drugs, as said anti-cancer pharmacology above, $XZ-C4$ has been shown to have better function to reduce the toxicity from chemotherapy.

3. XZ-C anti-cancer medication protects immune hematopoietic function. Chemotherapy drugs such as MMC or CTX cause bone marrow hematopoietic system suppression such as WBC↓, PLT↓, and then served $XZ-C4$ for 4 weeks Hb, WBC, PLT were improved significantly in cancer-bearing mice.

4. XZ-C immunomodulatory anticancer medication has a role in protecting the immune organs and improving human immune function.

CTX caused leukopenia, reduced immune function and kidney damaged on pathologic slices ; after taking $XZ-C4$, it can significantly improve immune function and can recover white blood cells and red blood cells in H_{22} cancer-bearing mice. There is no thymic atrophy but a little hypertrophy, lymphocytes intensive, increased epithelial reticular cells in XZ-C treatment group.

5. THE RESEARCH ON CYTOKINE INDUCTION FACTORS OF XZ-C ANTICANCER IMMUNE REGULATION AND CONTROL MEDICATION

1. XZ-C4 induces endogenous cytokines

(1). Through the experiments: XZ-C4 has many immune strengthening functions and has closely relationship to the induced endogenous cytokines

(2). XZ-C4 can recover the reduction of the white blood cells, granulation cells and platelets.

(3). XZ-C4 can have the direct function on GM-CSF production from granulation cell (GM) through IL-1β, also increase TNF, IFN etc all of kind of the cell factors, which are possible the indirect function.

(4). XZ-C4 can increase the Th1 cell factors, which were decrease in the cancer patients. There are the curative effects on the anemia and the white blood cells decrease due to the chemotherapy.

(5). The experiment analysis showed that XZ-C4 not only protects the bone marrow function, but also has direct function on the tumor cell division.

In brief, XZ-C4 can induce the tumor division and natural death through the autocrine which produce all of kind of factors. The autocrine is the secretory things from the host to affect the host's function. XZ-C4 probably will become the induction therapy to the tumor division in the future.

2. XZ-C4 inhibiting cancer development and metastasis

The malignant development is defined as tumor cells accepting invasion and metastasis characters during the proliferation. Cancer research need to have good repeated animal models. Then the good repeated animal model was made from the mice fibrosis cancernoma QR-32. QR-32 cannot proliferate after inoculation in the skin, and will completely disappear; there were no metastasis lump after injecting into the vein. However, if QR-32 was injected with Gelatin sponge together under the skin in the mice, QR-32 will become the proliferating tumor cells QRSP.XuZe XuJie Bin Wu• 140 •

In vitro culturing QRSP and then transfer into another mice, even if there is no foreign thing, the tumors will grow such as the lung metastasis will happen after injection in the vein.

XZ-C4 was used in the animal models to search the effects of the tumor development. To divide this animal models into two steps: the process from QR-32 to QRSP(early progress) and from the QRSP to tumor(later progress). After using XZ-C4, the tumor development will be inhibited in these two models, especially the former will be inhibited significantly. And this has relationship with the dose of the medication.

On the survival experiment the animal models of the inoculation of the QR-32 AND Gelatin sponge died during 65 days, however in XZ-C group the mice survival rate for 150 days was 30%. XZ-C4 can increase the immune effects and reduce the side effects of other anticancer medication.

This research proved that XZ-C4 has inhibition of the cancer progression function and inhibit cancer invasion and metastasis.

6. THE TOXICOLOGY STUDIES OF XZ-C IMMUNOMODULATORY ANTICANCER MEDICATION

$XZ-C_1$ can be long-term use. Acute toxicity experiments showed that: 100 times the adult dose to mice fed (10g / kg) were observed at 24, 48, 72, 96 hours in 30 purebred mice without a death. The median lethal dose (LD50) is difficult to make and is a quite secure prescription.

According to WHO "cancer medicine and acute toxin Classification Standard" assessment patients with different measurement, different forms of treatment, changes in the peripheral blood, liver and kidney function in order to understand its toxicity and adverse circumstances, XZ-C medication was oral taken in more than 6000 cases, continuous medication at less 3 months, some for years. The patients have no abnormal phenomenon before and after treatment and blood tests such as WBC, RBC, Hb, PLT are checked and the results are improvement. In order to control cancers the patients with advanced cancer in our specialty clinics took XZ-C for a long-term such as using $XZ-C_{1+4}$ 10 or more years and the patient didn't have metastasis and non-proliferation, the disease condition is stable, and lived with cancer. Adhere to long-term medication XZ-C medication can stabilize condition, inhibit cancer proliferation, improve the quality of life and prolong their lives, did not show toxicity, we insist on a longer-term experience serving XZ-C medicine and can help prevent the patients from short and long term recurrence and metastasis after radical surgery.

7. THE ACTIVE INGREDIENT OF XZ-C ANTICANCER IMMUNE CONTROL AND REGULATION MEDICATIONS

$XZ-C_{1+4}$ is a compound consisting of 28 Chinese herbs. The extraction work of total effective ingredient compound is extremely difficult, the technology is complex and it was exceedingly difficult to extract the active ingredient compound. Active ingredients of a single herb can be extracted. Thus, XZ- C series drugs except XZ- C_1 outside is boiling agent, and the rest are used every herb of fine powder or capsules in order to remain independent of each herb's active ingredients which can play its antitumor effects. The powders are mixed fine powder and the active ingredient can remain independent of each drug; however, after the drug is boiled, the chemical element changes so as to inevitably change the active ingredient of the drug and make it difficult to know the active ingredients after boiling.

But overall the active ingredients of various medications in the prescription are:

1.Alkaloids

2. Glycosides: saponins and glycosides

Each herb in the prescription has anti-tumor active ingredient, for example prescription Ganoderma lucidum, its anti-tumor component A is Ganoderma lucidum polysaccharides, antitumor effect is: with a hypodermic method, graft inoculation 7 days of S_{180} ascites carcinoma on mouse right groin, at a dose 20% mg / kg 10 days the inhibition rate is 95.6-98.5%. The inhibition rate of treatment of leukopenia was 84.6%, the treatment of leukopenia, recent efficiency 84.6% and total WBC increases 1028 / mm3. Anti-tumor component B is Fumaric acid. Its anti-tumor effect: with Gavage 60mg / kg 10 days in S180 cancer mice, then weighed tumors: the inhibition rate was 37.1% -38.6% and the body weight of mice did not decline.

Another example is the prescription FRUCTUS LIGUSTRI LUCIDI, its anti-tumor components of ursolic acid (Ursolic acid). Its anti-tumor effect on liver cancer cells in vitro with a very significant inhibition rate, can prolong life Ehrlich ascites carcinoma in mice. Pharmacological experiments show its flooding agent capable of inhibiting certain animals transplanted tumor growth. This product contains oleanolic acid with enhancing immune function, recovering peripheral leukocyte, enhancing phagocytes in reticuloendothelial cells, recovers white blood cells of the reduction induced by radiation or chemotherapy, strengthens cardiac functions and diuretic function and protects liver function.

Another example is the prescription of Sophora, its anti-tumor component A: Sophocarpine. Its anti-tumor effect: In vitro experiments showed that Sophocarpine have a direct killing effect on Ehrlich ascites tumor cells: the inhibition rate was 30 to 60% on mice transplanted U_{14} or S_{180}. There is clinical application effect. Sophora antitumor component B is Oxymatrine. Its anti-tumor effects: for S_{180} mice there is significant activity, 500ug and 250 ug per day administration, a total of five days, in treatment groups, respectively tumor weight was 26.1% and 57.9%.

3. Another example is the prescription of bamboo ginseng, its anti-tumor component A, as β-Elemene. Its anti-tumor effects: on the EAC, ARS etc two kinds of ascites cancer there is significant anti-graft tumor effect; also it has effect on YAS and S180 ascites. Its anti-tumor components: ginseng total polysaccharides. Its anti-tumor effects of animal experiments show: total ginseng polysaccharides has a stimulating effect on immune function for Ehrlich ascites cancer in mice at 400- 800mg / kg with significant cancer inhibition. Ginseng polysaccharide on many tumor cells doesn't have directly killing effect and its anti-tumor effect may be due to the adjustment of the body's immune function so that cancer-bearing host enhanced antitumor capacity. Its anti-tumor component C is Ginsenoside which has inhibition for S180 cancer cells which its tumor weight inhibition rate was 36.4% in 120mg / kg 7d. Ginsenosides may act directly on cancer cells to inhibit cancer cell growth; also available through effects on metabolism and regulation of immunity so that the body's resistance to disease increased and tumor growth was inhibited. Ginseng extract can inhibit Marine tumor, sarcoma S_{180} and lung cancer T_{55}.

8. THE PRINCIPLES OF XZ-C PRESCRIPTION

XZ-C1,XZ-C4 of XZ-C immunomodulatory anticancer medications are compound as a powder, or capsules, the compound is a mixture rather than multi-flavored powder, so each herb's active ingredients, pharmacological effects are alone Each herb can be individually separated.

XZ-C compound is completely different with traditional Chinese medicine. After A, B, C, D compound are boiled, the component is completely changed, like eating, "pot", the original pharmacological effect of every taste was widowed after boiling together, and the original pharmacological effect of each flavor was lost after boiled, and after cooking it is difficult to know what the pharmacological effects and what the active ingredient is. It is very difficult and very complex technology to extract the active ingredient after boiling the compound. Our XZ-C drugs are completely different, not boiling, every individual taste is grinded into fine level, and then mixed in different amounts (cannot afford a compound effect), the pharmacological effects of each herb and its active ingredient completely do not change while retaining all herbs and pharmacological effects of the active ingredient. This is the reform and innovation for traditional Chinese medicine formulations.

Why use compound rather than single herb? Because the role of power is not enough, more herbs together have stronger effects such as A = a + b + c + d.. then there must be A> a, A> a + b, A> a + b + c, etc., such as the inhibition rate of its single flavor was 20%, another flavor was 30%, and then another 31%, which totally the inhibition rate of this mixed serving may be 20 + 30 + 31 which may reach 81%. To improve the immune system, such as one flavor is 19%, the second flavor is 40%, the third flavor is 24%, then the mixed one together may be 83%. Holding constant every individual taste is the most important; each herb play its independent role in anti-cancer and increasing the role of immunity function.

Furthermore, XZ-C prescription principles also are followed the biological characteristics of cancer and cancer metastasis multi-link, multi-step characteristics so over the years we achieved remarkable results on anti-recurrence and anti-metastasis for the patients with long-term XZ-C immunomodulatory medications. Many patients with advanced cancer are inoperable and also should not have radiation and chemotherapy; however after long-term taking XZ-C immune regulation medication can achieve stable condition, control metastasis, improve quality of life and significantly prolong survival time. Every herb in XZ-C immunomodulatory anticancer medication was selected by two step in solid tumor-bearing mice in vivo anti-tumor screening: the first step is screening a single flavor for the better inhibition rate, and the second step is to select prescription which there are three indicators: 1). it has a good anti-tumor effect; 2).without damage the normal cells of the body 3).increase immune function. If it has a high inhibition rate, but reduced immunity, it will not be chosen. In "new concept and new methods of cancer treatment," recently published a book written specifically for 16 years in our laboratory experiments work in cancer research confirmed cancer development and recurrence, metastasis and host immune organ function and immunity have certainly clear relationship. The medication which protects the immune organs and enhances immunity function are more important than the medication which inhibit or kill cancer drugs. XZ-C anti-tumor immune regulation medicine through experimental research and clinical validation observations show that:

1. There is significant anti-tumor effect, a higher inhibition rate;
2. Better improve the body's immune function, it can be cancer mouse experiments showed incomplete atrophy of the thymus and improve immune function;
3. Protect the hematopoietic system of the role of the chemotherapy drugs inhibit the outer periphery of the bone marrow after the white blood cells, platelets, red blood cells have been significantly improved;
4. Have a good effect for advanced cancer patients. Can significantly change the patient's appetite, sleep, physical and mental state, can significantly improve symptoms, improve quality of life;
5. Have a role in reducing the toxicity in advanced cancer patients with chemotherapy drugs. Its efficacy is superior to the treatment of chemotherapy drugs;
6. In animal experiments there is no toxic side effects. In clinics for 16 years on 16000 patients, especially in many cases of advanced cancer patients the medication were used for a long-term 3--5 years, and some patients even served 8--10 years, it showed no toxic side effects. If the patients have long-term medication adherence, their spirit, appetite, physical strength are good, significantly prolonged survival.

9. THE MOLECULAR LEVEL IMMUNE FUNCTION OF XZ-C IMMUNOMODULATOR ANTI-CANCER MEDICINE

With more and deeper researches on traditional Chinese medication, it has been proved that many kinds of traditional Chinese medications can regulate and control the production and biological activity of cytokine and other immune molecules, which is meaningful to explain the immunological mechanism of XZ-C immunologic regulation and control anti-carcinoma medication from the level of molecule.

I. Protecting Immune Organs and Increasing the Weight of Thymus and Spleen

1. XZ-C-T (EBM): Using its 15g/kg and 30g/kg extracting solution (equivalent to 1g original medicine) along with 12.5mg/kg, 25mg/kg ferulic acid suspension to feed the mice for seven days in a raw can increase the weight of thymus and spleen obviously, especially the effects of the group with high dose are more apparent. Intraperitoneal injection of EBM polysaccharide can also alleviate thymus and spleen atrophy obviously caused by prednisolone.

2. XZ-C-O (PMT): Extract PM-2, feed the mice with 6g/kg PMT decoction for successive seven days which can increase the weight of thymus and celiac lymph nodes and antagonize the reduction in the weight of immune organs caused by prednisolone. Drenching the mouse of 15 months old with 6g/kg decoction (with the concentration of 0.5g/ml) for 14 days can increase the weight and volume of thymus, thicken the cortex and raise cellular density apparently. The combined use of PM and astragalus root can promote non-lymphocyte hyperplasia and benefit the micro environment of thymus.

3. XZ-C-W (SCB): SCB polysaccharide can gain weight of thymus and spleen of a normal mouse. Lavage with it enables cyclophosphane to control the gain in the weight of thymus and spleen.

4. XZ-C-M (LLA): Drench a mouse with LLA decoction for seven days resulting in increasing the weight of thymus and spleen.

5. XZ-C-L: For a 15-month old mouse, its thymus degenerates obviously. Astragalus injectio can enlarge the thymus significantly. The cortex under microscope is thickened and the cellular density increase obviously.

II. Effects on Proliferation, Differentiation and Hematopiesis of Marrow Cells

1. XZ-C-O (PMT): Extract PM-2
2. XZ-C-Q (LBP): (1)Effects on the proliferation of hematopoietic stem cell (CFU-S) of a normal mouse: inject PM-2 with the dose of 500mg/kg ×3d or 10mg/kgx3d LBP into the experimental mice respectively by venoclysis and kill them in the ninth day. It can be found that the number of spleen CFU-S in the group with administration increases obviously. The number of CFU-S in group PM-2 is 21% higher than that of the control group and it is 36% in the group with LBP;(2)Effects on colony forming unit of granulocytes and macrophages (CFU-GM): the experimental results indicate that LBP with the dose of 5~30mg/kg×3d can increase the number of CFU-GM and PM-2 can also strengthen the effect of CFU-GM with the effective dose of 12.5~50mg/kg×3d. In the early stage of cultivation, most CFU-GMs are units of granulocytes and then units of macrophages increase gradually. In the anaphase units of macrophages take over the dominance.

   From the above experiment, it can be found that PM-2 and LBP can promote hematopiesis of normal mice obviously. The experiment proves that during the process of restoring hematopiesis damaged by CTX, PM-2 and LBP stimulate the proliferation of granulocytes at first, and then marrow karyocytes multiply; at last these two promote the restoration of peripheral granulocytes.

3. XZ-C-D (TSPG):Ginsenoside, which is the active principle of ginseng to promote hematopiesis, can bring the recovery of erythrocyte in peripheral blood, haemoglobin and myeloid cell of thighbone in the mice of marrow-inhibited type, increase the index of myeloid cellular division and stimulate the proliferation of myeloid hematopoietic cell in vitro so as to make it into cell cycle with active proliferation (S+G_2/M stage). TSPG can promote the proliferation and differentiation of polyenergetic hematopoietic cells and induce the formation of hemopoietic growth factor (HGF).

4. XZ-C-H (RCL):Steamed Chinese Foxglove can promote the recovery of erythrocyte and haemoglobin for animals with blood deficiency and accelerate the proliferation and differentiation of myeloid hematopoietic cell (CFU-S) with the effect of predominance and hematosis significantly. Peritoneal injection of rehmannia polysaccharides for successive six days can promote the proliferation and differentiation of myeloid hematopoietic cells and progenitor cells as well as increasing the number of leucocytes in peripheral blood.

5. XZ-C-J (ASD):ASD polysaccharide has no effects on erythrocytes and leucocytes of normal mice, but for those damaged by radiation, injection of ASD polysaccharide can influence the proliferation and differentiation of both polyenergetic hematopoietic stem cells (CPU-S) and hemopoietic progenitor cells. But its decoction has no obvious effects.

6. XZ-C-E (PEW):Poria cocos (micromolecule chemical compound extracted from Tuckahoe polysaccharide) is the active principle that can strengthen the production of colony stimulating factor (CSF) and improve the level of leucocytes in peripheral blood inside the mouse's body.

It can also prevent the decline in leucocytes caused by cyclophosphamide and accelerate the recovery with the effects better than sodium ferulic which is used to increase leucocytes.

7. XZ-C-Y (PAR): Its polysaccharide can obviously resist the decline in leucocytes caused by cyclophosphamide and increase the number of myeloid cells to promote the proliferation of myeloid induced by CSF as well as the recovery and reconstitution of hematopiesis for the mice irradiated by X ray. It can also increase the number of hematopoietic stem cells and myeloid cells along with leucocytes.

III. Enhancing Immunologic Function of T Cells

The active principles of XZ-C traditional Chinese medicine and their effects are following.

1. XZ-C-L (AMB): It can raise the percentage of lymphocytes in peripheral blood obviously. The LBP in small dose (5~10mg/kg) can cause the proliferation of lymphocytes, indicating that LBP can promote the proliferation of T cells apparently. 50mg/(kg·d)×7d is the best dose in that it will have no effects if lower than the level and it will bring the effects down if higher than the level. Oral administration of LBP can raise the conversion rate of lymphocytes for the sufferers who are weak and with fewer leucocytes.

2. XZ-C4: It can regulate immune system and active T cells of aggregated lymphatic follicles, as well as stimulate the secretion of hemopoietic growth factor in T cells. Among the crude drugs of XZ-C4, the extract from the hot water of atractylodes lancea rhizome can obviously stimulate the cells of aggregated lymphatic follicles, which is regarded as the base of XZ-C4 immunoloregulation.

IV. Activating and Enhancing NK Cell Activity

Natural killer cell, NK cell is another kind of killer cell in lymphocytes for human beings and mice, which needs neither antigenic stimulation, nor the participation of antibodies to kill some cells. It plays an important role in immunity, especially in the function of immune surveillance as NK cell is the first line of defense against tumors and has broad spectrum anti-tumor effects.

NK cell is broad-spectrum and able to kill sygeneous, homogenous and heterogenous tumor cells with special effects on lymjphoma and leucocytes.

NK cell is an important kind of cells for immunoloregulation, which can regulate T cells, B cells and stem cells, etc. It can also regulate immunity by releasing cytokines like IFN-α, IFN-γ, IL-2, TNF, etc.

The active principles in XZ-C traditional Chinese medicine and their effects are following.

1. XZ-C-X (SDS): Divaricate Saposhniovia Root can strengthen the activity of NK cells of experimental mice. When combined with IL-2, it can make the activity of NK cell higher,

indicating that its polysaccharide can give a hand to IL-2 to activate NK cells and improve the activity. LBP can strengthen T cell mediated immune reaction and the activity of NK cells for normal mice and those dealt by cyclophosphamide. Peritoneal injection of LBP can improve the proliferation of spleen T lymphocytes and strengthen the lethality of CTL increasing the specific lethal rate from 33% to 67%.

2. XZ-C-G (GUF):Glycyrrhizin can induce the production of IFN in the blood of animals and human beings and strengthen NK cell activity at the same time. Clinical tests made by Abe show that after intravenous injection of 80mg GL, the raise of NK cell activity reaches 75% among 21 sufferers. Peritoneal injection of 0.5mg/kg GL on mice can strengthen the activity of NK cells in liver.

3. XZ-C-L (AMB): Its bath fluid can promote NK cell activity of mice both in vivo and in vitro, and can also induce IFN-γ to deal with effector cells under the certain concentration of 0.1mg/ml. Cordyceps sinensis extract can strengthen NK cells activity of the mouse both in vivo and in vitro. Fluids with the concentrations of 0.5g/kg, 1g/kg and 5g/kg can strengthen NK cell activity of mice.

V. Effects on LAK Cell Activity

Lymphokine activated killer cell, namely LAK cell can be induced by IL-2 cytokine. LAK cells can kill the solid tumors that are both sensitive and insensitive to NK cells with broad anti-tumor effects.

The active principles in XZ-C anti-carcinoma traditional Chinese medicine and their effects are following:

1. XZ-C-L (AMB): Its polysaccharide can strengthen LAK cell activity within a certain range of dose with 0.01mg/ml being the most effective, which is three times better than the damage effects of LAK cells. The concentrations of both higher and lower than this level can not achieve the effects.

2. XZ-C-U (PUF):It can significantly strengthen the spleen LAK cell activity of killing tumor cells and improve the activity of erythrocyte C3b liquid. PUF and IL-2 are synergistic that can be used as regulator for biological reaction in tumor biological therapy based on LAK/Ril-2.

3. XZ-C-V:ABB polysaccharide can also raise LAK cell activity for the mouse and inhibit tumors remarkably. Its anti-tumorous mechanism relates to its strengthening immunity and changing cell membrane features.

VI. Effects on Iterleukin-2 (IL-2)

The active principles in XZ-C anti-carcinoma traditional Chinese medicine and their effects are following:

1. XZ-C-T:EBM polysaccharide can enhance obviously the production of IL-2 for human beings when the concentration is 100ug/ml. At higher concentration (2500ug/ml and 5000ug/ml), it will lead to inhibition. Hypodermic injection of barrenwort polysaccharide for seven days in a row can significantly improve the ability of thymus and spleen of the mouse induced by ConA to produce IL-2.

2. XZ-C-Y:PAR polysaccharide has strong immune activity and is able to promote the production of IL-2. For the mouse bearing S-180 tumor, it can raise the ability of spleen cells to produce IL-2 obviously。

3. XZ-C-D: Ginseng polysaccharide has great promotion on IL-2 induced by peripheral monocytes for both healthy people and sufferers with kidney troubles. The effects are relevant to the dose positively.

VII. Function of Inducing Interferon and Promoting Inducement of Interferon

IFN are broad-spectrum in resisting tumors and can regulate immunity. It can also inhibit the proliferation of tumor cells and activate NK cells and CTL to kill tumor cells. Meanwhile, IFN can cooperate with TNF, IL-1 and IL-2 to enforce anti-tumorous ability.

The active principles in XZ-C anti-carcinoma traditional Chinese medicine and their effects are following:

1. XZ-C-Z: 250mg/kg or 500mg/kg CVQ polysaccharide can improve significantly the level of IFN-γ produced by mouse spleen cells.

2. XZ-C-D: Ginsenoside (GS) and panaxitriol ginsenoside (PTGS) can induce whole blood cells and monocytes of human beings to produce IFN-αand IFN-γ. It can also recover the low level of IFN-γand IL-2 to the normal. The IFN potency of ASH polysaccharide on S-180 cell line of acute lymphoblastic leukemia and S7811 cell line of acute myelomonocytic leukemia produced after acanthopanax polysaccharide stimulation is 5~10 times more than that of normal control group.

3. X-C-E

Hydroxymethyl Poria cocos mushroom polysaccharide has many kinds of physical activity like immunoloregulation, promoting to induce IPN, resisting virus indirectly and alleviating adverse reaction resulting from radiation. Do IFN inducement dynamic experiment on S-180leukaemia cell line by using 50mg/ml Hydroxymethyl Poria cocos mushroom polysaccharide. The results indicate that its potency to induce interferon at all stages is better than that of normal inducement.

1. X-C-G (GL): It can induce IFN activity. Make peritoneal injection of 330mg/ kg GL on mice. IFN activity reaches the peak after 20 hours.

VIII. Function of Promoting and Increasing Colony Stimulating Factor

Colony stimulation factor, namely CSF is a kind of glucoprotein with low molecular weight that can stimulate the proliferation and differentiation of marrow hematopoietic stem cells as well as other mature blood cells. Cells that can produce CSF include mononuclear macrophages, T cells, endothelial cells and desmocytes. CSF not only take part in the proliferation and differentiation of hematopoietic stem cells and regulating mature cells, but also play an important role in anti- tumorous immunity of host cells.

The active principles in X-C anti-carcinoma traditional Chinese medicine and their effects are following:

1. X-C-Q:PAR polysaccharide is able to promote to produce CSF by spleen cells of experimental mice. 100~500ug/ml PAP-II can encourage spleen cells to produce CSF depending on the dose and time with the fittest dose of 100ug/ml and best time of 5d. Moreover, lentinan can also increase the amount of CSF.
2. X-C-Q:Injection of LBP can facilitate the secretion of CSF by mouse spleen T cells and improve the activity of CSF in serum.
3. X-C-T:EBM icariin can promote the proliferation of mouse spleen lymphocytes induced by ConA and bring CSF activity.

IX. Function of Promoting TNF

Tumor necrosis factor, namely TNF is a kind of cytokine that can kill tumor cells directly. Its main effect is to kill or inhibit tumor cells, which can kill some tumor cells or inhibit the proliferation both in vivo and in vitro.

The active principles in XZ-C anti-carcinoma traditional Chinese medicine and their effects are following:

1. X-C-Y (PEP):It can induce the production of TNF, so as PEP-1. Inject 80~160mg/kg PEP-1, once every four days. Collect peritoneal macrophages (PM), add 10ug LPS into culture medium to cultivate PM. Take the supernatant to determine TNF and IL-1. It can be found that PEP-1 can parallelly increase the auxiliary production of TNF and IL-1. The time of TNF inducement reaches the peak on the 8th day after the second intraperitoneal injection. Compared with the known startup potion BCG, the inducement of TNF has no difference.
2. X-C-E:Carboxymethyl-pachymaran (CMP) is the principle essential component distilled from traditional Chinese medicine Tuckahoe. It can not only strengthen the ability of mouse spleen to create IL-2 and macrophages and promote the activity of T cells, B cells, NK cells and LAK cells; but also encourage the production of TNF. The experiment proves that CMP is an effective potion to promote and induce cytokines.
3. X-C-V: ABB polysaccharide can promote the production of TNF-b in mouse cells induced by ConA. It can also induce the synthesis of peritoneal macrophages and secrete 20ug/ml

TNF-αachyranthes bidentata polysaccharides. The time of TNF-α to reach its peak is 2-6 hours after effects. Peritoneal injection of 100mg/kg achyranthes bidentata polysaccharides can accelerate the production of TNF-α, whose intensity of effects is comparable to that of BCG.

X. The Effects on Cell Adhesion Molecule by Z-C immune regulator and control medications

Most adhesion molecules are glycoproteid and are distributed on cellular surface and extracellular matrix. Adhesion molecules take effect in the corresponding form of ligand-acceptor, resulting in the adhesion between cells, or between cell and stroma, or the adhesion of cell-stroma-cell. These molecules take part in a set of physical pathologic processes, like cellular conduction and activation of information, cellular stretch and movement, formation of thrombus as well as tumor metastasis, etc. Intercellular adhesion molecule-1, namely ICAM-1 is one kind of adhesion molecules in the super family of immune globulins.

Z-C immune regulator and control anticancer medications have effects on ICAM-1

The effect of an active ingredient in XZ-C traditional Chinese anti-carcinoma medication :

Corn stigma or hair, Hobtemariam has proved that alcohol extract from corn stigma has significant inhibition on the adhesion of endothelial cells to inhibit effectively the expression of ICAM-1 and the adhesive activity with TNF, LPS as agents.

10. THE ANTITUMOR COMPOSITION OF Z-C IMMUNE REGULATION AND CONTROL ANTI - CANCER TRADITIONAL CHINESE MEDICATIONS: STRUCTURE; THE EXISTING SITE : THE ANTICANCER ACTION

(1).Z-C1 - A ApL

Anti-tumor components: agrimonniin
Effective parts: the whole plant for the plants.

Anti-tumor effect: Okucla other scholars isolated out agrimonniin from ApL grass which has proven to be the main component. Before and after inoculation MM2 breast cancer cells, 10mg /kg of this product is given by ip, the results were all tumor are rejected. No matter how it was given by P.O. or I.P., it can prolong survival time in tumor-bearing animals. Agrimonniin can inhibit MH 134 liver cancer and sarcoma Meth-A cellulose growth. With or without calf serum medium, MM2 breast cancer cells and agrimonniin together for 2h, then for 48h at 37 humidified CO2 incubator, and found time without calf serum, agrimonnii on breast cancer cells showed MM2 strong cytotoxicity, and its IC50 is 2.66ug / ml, but adding fetal calf serum in the culture medium, then weakened to around 4% of the original, namely an IC50 of 62.5% ug / ml, after intraperitoneal injection of agrimonniin 4d, the absorption of H3- thymine on MM2 breast cancer and MH134 hepatoma cells was obviously inhibited.

These results indicate that agrimonniin is a potent anti-tumor acid and its anti-tumor effect may be due to the drug action on tumor cells and enhance the immune re ApL grass produces 1: 1, PH6.5 (1g crude drug / ml) solution by water extraction method to inhibit $_{S180,}$ cervix U_{14}, brain tumors B_{22}, Ehrlich EAC, melanoma B_{10}, rats W_{256} cancer. The results show that for more than transplanted tumors better inhibition, the inhibition rates were between 36.2 -6.59%, P<0.05, there is a significant difference.

ApL grass water extract has a strong inhibitory effect on human JTC-26 canein vitro and inhibition rate reaches 100% and meanwhile it promotes the growth 100%. While 30mg / kg ApL grass phenol was injected daily in intraperitoneal cavity, it has a significant therapeutic effect on rat sarcoma S_{37} and cervical cancer U_{14}. The inhibition rates on tumor growth were 47.0% and 38.7%. The inhibition was 47.4% on sarcoma S_{180} mice with 0.625g / day and was 52.6% on liver cancer.

Fluid extracted from liver cancer ascites was diluted with sterile physiological water 1-2x10⁷/ml, then inoculated into mice, each mouse by intraperitoneal injection 0.2ml, the next day were randomly divided into treatment group and control group 30mg / ApL grass phenol was injected in intraperitoneal cavity once daily for 7 days, saline was injected in control group, then observed 30 days to calculate life span. Results: the mean survival day was 26.2 disabilities 0.9 in 24 animals treatment group; the average rival was 17.5 + 1.3day in control group. Life span prolonged above 49.6%. ApL grass phenol has significantly prolong life in animal liver cancer ascites carcinoma.

Z-Cl - B SLT

Anti-tumor components: p-SoIamarine
Structure:

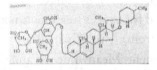

Effective parts: the SLT whole plant.

Anti-tumor effect: the whole plant has anti-tumor effect, in many countries for a long time as a folk medicine to cure cancer, p-Solamarine its active ingredient, at 30mg / kg on S_{180} mice the tumor weight from control group 1285 mg reduced to 274mg, the Inhibition rate was 78.6%.

The whole plant has anti-cancer effects on human lung cancer.

The studies have reported recently, extracted from the SLT anti-tumor active ingredient o health foods, it has given anti-tumor effect and almost no toxicity. SLT also contain solanine Australia which has inhibitory activity on S_{180} mice.

Recently it has been reported: an effective anti-tumor ingredient was extracted from SLT through water or an organic solvent or a mixture of water capacitive solvent, then be made into oral or parenteral medication: the oral dose serving as 1g /d; the parenteral drug as 60mg / d. The drug can inhibit a variety of tumors, such as S_{180} neck cancer with its low toxicity. Murakami Kotaro etc isolated two different body sugar from SLT, each with some anti-tumor effect.

SIT can inhibit S_{180}, cervical cancer U_{14} and Ehrlich ascites carcinoma. In vitro the product of hot water extract can has inhibition rate 100% on human cervical cancer JTC-26 system. And there was no effect on normal cells; in vivo experiments on mice S_{180} inhibition rate was 14.57%. This product contains an effective anti-cancer ingredient β -bitter solanine which significantly inhibited mice S_{180} and W256 mouse cancer.

Z-C1-C SNL

Antitumor Ingredient A: Vitamin A
Structure:

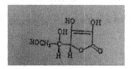

Existing parts: the whole plant for an amount of 9666 IU%.

Anti-tumor effects: vitamin A(Va) has anti-tumor activity. Wald had conducted a survey in 1975-1979, indicating Va having anti-tumor effect in vivo; Bontwell found that Va can stop cell membrane mucopolysaccharides aggregate effect induced by tumor promoters and block the receptor which bindstumor promoters. A new method for cancer treatment: normal sugar plus LETS (large cells are transferred outside sensitive protein from), two of which are affected Va material synthesis, which shows Va is important in cancer treatment. Meanwhile, Va and their derivatives can reverse cancerous cells inducedv by chemical carcinogens, viruses, and ionizing radiation.

Antitumor Component B: Vitamin C(Vc)
Structure:

Existing parts: the whole plant for the plant, its content is 20mg%

Anti-tumor effects: Vc is antioxidants in anti-tumor effects in blocking nitrite and primary amine to synthesize carcinogenicity compounds in vivo. Cameron will use 10g / day Vc to hundred cancer patients from long-term, 42 times of higher efficacy than control group and has better effect in gastrointestinal cancer. Murata use Vc high-dose to treat cervical cancer and its effect is 5.7 times higher than the effect of small doses. Malistratos induced sarcoma growth with benzo, then treat them with lots of Vc. Vc inhibited sarcoma growth and occurrence. For bladder cancer and skin cancer, it has the preventive effect. In epidemiology cancer occurrence is also related with the intake of Vc.

Vc with various anticancer drugs in combination can increase the efficacy of the drug. As with Vincristine (VCR) it has a synergistic effect and V + CCNu have higher treatment efficacy than single CCNu in leukemia. The survival time extencle: twice, but also alleviate the condition of patients with advanced cancer. Cisplatin anticancer drugs, because of its toxicity and the larger application subject to certain restrictions, if Vc their combination, can reduce toxicity. New Jersey now Englehard company Hollis developed a cisplatin and Vc mixture composition which has better efficacy.

The whole plant contains Solasonine and solanine which also have activity against S_{180} sarcoma. Nigrum extract of dried green fruit of total alkali Solanum nigrum can inhibit animals transplanted tumor system by 40- 50%. In tissue culture 50-500mcg/ml 24h total alkali Solanum nigrum inhibit meningioma cells growth. Alkali component isolated from total alkali Solanum nigrum has the strongest antitumor activity and there are significant cytotoxicity. 10mcg / ml 15h concentration causes cells to collapse. A total extract also has inhibition effect on mice ascites sarcoma S_{180}. Solamine also be used as hematopoietic system stimulant, increasing leukocyte. barbata and comfrey it was used to treat malignant mole and the result is good. With surgery, chemotherapy, radiation it was used to treat uterine choriocarcinoma, -_in cancer, liver cancer and had effectiveness.

This product can inhibit cervical cancer U_{14} and S_{180}, Ehrlich ascites carcinoma and -hosarcoma, Ehrlich ascites carcinoma, L_{615} lymphatic leukemia, S_{180}, gastric cancer cells and leukemia in mice, etc

SNL has anti-cancer effect on nuclear division. Extract of SNL has inhibition rate of -50% on animal transplanted tumor. In tissue culture 50-50Oug/ ml 24 hr total SNL can inhibit brain tumor cell growth.

Z-C-D PGS
Anti-tumor components A: β-Elemene
Structure:

Existing parts: the root of the volatile oil and flowers of about 10%.

Anti-tumor effects: The product has significant anti-tumor effect on ECA and ARS etc transplanted animal ascites and S_{180} ascites.

Anti-tumor component B: PGS total polysaccharides:

Anti-tumor effects: animal experiments show: PGS total polysaccharides have a stimulating effect on immune function. It inhibit mice transplanted tumor S_{180} to a certain extent and significantly inhibited Ehrlich ascites tumor cells in mice at 400-800mg / kg. PGS polysaccharide doesn't directly kill many tumor cells; its anti-tumor effect may be due to the adjustment of the body's immune function so that =or-bearing hosts enhance antitumor capacity. There are also reports: PGS total - polysaccharide is administered at 460.620mg / kg / d in S_{180} abdomen the inhibition of tumor weight was76.81% (P <0 001.).

Another report, PGS total polysaccharides have some anti-tumor activity, its system may be induced tumor necrosis factor: PGS total polysaccharides on normal mice d tumor-bearing mice can enhance immune function and activation, PGS total polysaccharides also inhibit cancer cell growth.

Anti-tumor components C: PGS saponin Ginsenoside
Formula formula :

Anti-tumor effects:

On mouse sarcoma S_{180} it had significant inhibition at 120mg / kg/d x7 and the inhibition rate of its tumor weight was 60.48%; on Ehrlich ascites carcinoma (ECS) at a dose of I00mg / kg / d x70, its inhibition rate was 36.40%; on S_{180} at a dose of 100 mg / kg / dx10 its inhibition rate was 41-61% (P <0.05); large doses on U_{14} also have some anti-tumor effect.

With chemotherapy drugs CXT used in conjunction, it can enhance the anti-tumor effects of chemotherapy drugs.

Its anti-tumor effect is more complex; one, it can act directly with the cancer cell- -that the cancer cell growth was inhibited or be reversal. Second, it can also regulate the body metabolism and the immune function to resist diseases so that the tumor growth was inhibited. National and international clinical trials have proved: it has therapeutic effect on gastric cancer, not only reduces tumor; but also increases appetite, improves immunity and prolongs patients' survival time.

PGS soap component as a human anti-tumor agents, adapt to a wide range, almost no side effects. The application ranges: gastric cancer, colorectal cancer, breast cancer, uterine cancer, mouth, esophagus, gallbladder cancer, kidney cancer, lung cancer, brain cancer, liver cancer, skin cancer, etc., are valid for almost all tumors. The mode of administration: it can be taken orally at 100-300mg/day x2-3 doses. It can also used 1-10% of hydrophilic or hydrophobic ointment topically.

Korea Atomic Energy Research Institute Nguyen and other reports: Application -- carcinogens in laboratory animals treated, serving long red ginseng can reduce the incidence of cancer and inhibit tumor growth. Small Tajima and other reports: cultured hepatoma cell PGS soap can change the cancer cell structures indicating PGS can induce cancer cells to be reversed. Hiroko Abe and other reports: PGS saponin induced reversal to hepatic cancer cells. Li xianggao believes: PGS soap can inhibit 3-O- methyl glucose through the cell membrane and overflow on liver cancer cells so presumably the inhibition of membrane transporters of PGS saponin may non-specific.

In addition to the relevant ginseng root soap antitumor activity studies, ginseng flower total inhibition has also been reported: Yuyongli and other scholars studied, the effect of a total ginseng flower soap on NKC-IFN-IL-2 regulatory network and inhibition of tumor Effect. The results showed that: PGS total promote natural killer activity in vitro mouse spleen, and in the presence of Con-A induces the production of Y-IFN and IL-2, indicating the total soap flower PGS has regulation -KC-IFN-IL-2 network to regulate the immune function by this adjustment extensive network.

Liang Zhongpei etc applied PGS to study how dimethyl buttery yellow sugar induced rat liver cancer. The results showed that: PGS can increase the percentage of ANAE e lymphocyte cells, reduce the incidence of liver cancer, the tumor is smaller, a degree of differentiation of cancer cells, the longitudinal fibers hyperplasia and cute infiltration around tumor tissue, indicating that PGS should be able to promote immune function so that it has prevention or control action to the chemical carcinogen-induced liver cancer.

Ginseng inhibits variety of experimental animals. Ginseng had reduced tumor incidence nor growth inhibition after rats and mice were fed with ginseng long-term for aflatoxin-induced rat lung adenomas, urethane-induced lung cancer in mice. Its main anti-tumor ingredient is Ginseng saponin of which ginseng saponin Rg3 can - inhibit tumor formation of new organs, inhibit tumor recurrence, proliferation and metastasis in mouse melanoma and S_{180} tumor. The inhibition rate was 60% and on a variety of animal and human tumor lung metastasis, liver metastasis the inhibition ached 60% -70%. Ginseng saponin Rg3 is promising as anti-metastatic drugs.

Z-C-E PCW

Antitumor points A, Adenine
Structure:

The presence of areas: plant sclerotia.

Anti-tumor effect: for the prevention and treatment of various leukopenia, particularly caused by chemotherapy, radiotherapy and benzene poisoning. Its phosphate stimulates - blood cell hyperplasia. It was found that Leukocyte recovered about 2-4 weeks after administration. It can extend the time of chemotherapy and prevent the occurrence of leukopenia if used before chemotherapy or simultaneously.

Anti tumor B: Pachyman
Structural formula:[13-D-Glcp- (1.-3) a 13-D.-Glcp- (1 - 3)] n

Antitumor effects: Studies have shown that: new Pachymaran: in 1970 Chihara etc slightly transform pachyman structure into pachymaran of removing the side chain β (1--6) with significant anti-tumor activity, but the poor water-soluble activity.

Carboxymethyl Pachymaran was synthesized by Hamuro etc. in 1971 with pachymaran carboxymethylation which has significant anti-tumor activity in animal experimeriments.

Hamuro, J and other experiments proved: new biological Pachymaran of pachyman such as CM-pachymaran and HM-pachyman 2-4, have significant anti-tumor actin activity of its agents and routes of administration have a great relationship and the appropriate route of administration of the optimal dose must be selected.

About pachyman antitumor mechanism of action and its derivatives, it has also reported: think no direct cytotoxicity; however through the host's intermediary it played anti-tumor roles which enhance the body's immune system.

Chaoqiaoli etc. observed inhibition of carboxymethyl Pachymaran mouse lung metastasis of inbred uterine cancer U_{615}. The results show that the non-transfer 64% tumor control group were 94%; metastasis inhibition rate of 75.68%, significantly higher than the control group, the experimental group tumor weight, inhibition rate was 23.58%, the above results suggest that: indeed carboxymethyl Pachymaran has some anticancer activity.

Data reported also: carboxymethyl tuckahoe polysaccharide is a good immune enham: and apply the treatment of various tumors.

Patent No. 4339435 reports: A Poria sclerotium obtained cultured mycelium, tilt-the mycelium of the water or that the water-soluble organic solvent such as ethanol extraction, to obtain an anti-cancer medicament "A-1", it is not only very good anti-cancer activity and no toxicity, 92% inhibition of the S_{180}, this anti-cancer substance accounted for 24.2% cultured mycelia. Xu Jin et al reported that a group of fat-soluble organic tetracyclic three, collectively known as Poria factors was isolated from Pachyman and significantly inhibited Ehrlich ascites carcinoma, S_{180} metastasis of Lewis lung carcinoma in mice. When administered with Cyclic amines and phosphorus, there is a certain synergy and it proved Poria increases immune function.

In 1986 Japanese scholars Jinshan isolated a water-soluble anti-tumor polysacchariL called Pachymaran H11 from cultured mycelia of Poria, accounting for about 0.69c dry mycelium. With 4mg / kg injection JCR / TCL mice subcutaneously x10 days S_{180} the inhibition rate was 94%, this report shows that there have been polysaccharide which has anti-cancer activity with no structural transformation in Poria.

There are also reports, after Poria cocos contained β- polyester (β-pachyman) was treated and approached to obtain Poria cocos glycan complex (abbreviated UP), it had a significant anti-tumor effect and the inhibition rate was 57%. It can extend tumor-mice survival time, improve the spleen index, and it has a direct effect on cancer cells.

Wu Bo and other scholars also conducted experiments to observe PPS's anti-tumor effect and mechanism on mouse S_{180} cells and human leukemia cells K5G2. It was that PPS has a strong suppression effect and discusses its anti-tumor mechanism of S_{180} cell membrane composition. The results showed that after PPS contacts with cells 24h, the membrane phospholipid content decreased and cell membrane sialic content increased, but the membrane cholesterol content, membrane fluidity membrane fatty acid composition is not affected. When PPS membrane put together with S_{180} under appropriate conditions, it was found that PPS interference of membrane of inositol phospholipid metabolism is critical step. Changes related to PPS antititumor mechanism and biochemical characteristics also have some reports. PPS significantly inhibited DNA synthesis in mouse L_{1210} cells with irreversible inhibition increased with the dose.

Poria has anticancer drug synergistic effect : on mitomycin and using inhibitory (mouse sarcoma S_{180}) was 38.9% (5-Fu alone 38.6%) ; in mouse leukemia L1210 cyclophosphamide alone amines life extension of 70%, combined with phosphorus domide was 168.1%.

PPS and thymus-related anti-tumor effect. Polysaccharides can nonspecifically stimulate the reticuloendothelial system function and enhance the host of cancer-specific antigen immunity to resist the effects of cancer.

Pachymaran with Poria known significant anti-tumor effect, can inhibit the growth solid tumors, extend survival time in mice S_{180} and Ehrlich ascites carcinoma. Pachymaran has distinct anticancer roles on cultured mouse sarcoma S180 cells and human chronic myelogenous leukemia K562 cell. Antitumor mechanism includes two aspects of increased immune system and direct cytokine roles. Antitumor mechanism y be suppressed by inhibiting tumor cell nuclear DNA synthesis and enhance production of tumor necrosis factor (TNF) from macrophage and the ability to enhance or cell killing effect.

Intraperitoneal injection of polysaccharides (PPS) 5-200mg / kg continuous 100, above 10mg, it inhibited S_{180} significantly. On S180 sarcoma in mice and Ehrlich ascites cinoma (EAC) orally taken 8d, it can enhance tumor necrosis factor (TNF) levels and significantly increase natural killer (NK) cell activity.

It significantly inhibited lung metastasis from U_{14} after mice were fed carboxymeth-. tuckahoe polysaccharide (250mg / kg/d) 25d. The mouse sarcoma S_{180} cells were seeded in ICR / JCL mice subcutaneously, 24 hours later 5mg / kg polysaccharides once daily once 10 days injected intraperitoneally. The results showed that inhibition rate was 95%.

Carboxymethyl Pachymaran strongly inhibited U_{14} in mice. Using 500mg / kg, 100mg / kg, 50mg / kg, the result of inhibition rate was 75.5%. 92.7% 78.7%, respectively, which 100 mg / kg dose was the best. Intraperitoneal injection carboxymethyl tuckah polysaccharide 100mg / kg/ d 10d extended lifetime was 23.49% compared with control in Ehrlich ascites carcinoma. It reduced the amount of ascites 7%, reduced total number of cancer cells 139.20%. PPS can inhibit DNA synthesis in Ehrlich ascites tumor cells. The inhibition role of PPS is related to the dose which using 100 / 50mg / kg, 5mg / kg 3 the results of tumor inhibition rates were 92.3%, 96.1%, 53.4%.

Z-C1-G GuF

Anti-tumor components A: Glycyrrhiza acid
Structure:

Existing parts: wooden grass roots, rhizomes.

Antitumor effects: The product can produce morphological changes on rat hepatoma and Ehrlich ascites carcinoma (EAC) cells and inhibit subcutaneous Yoshida sarcoma. Licorice as raw material soluble Monoaniniornum glycyrrhetate, namely licorice acid amine, can inhibit Ehrlich ascites carcinoma and muscle tumor. Meanwhile, licorice acid amine has some detoxification for certain toxic of anti-cancer drugs. Natural products such as having a certain anti-tumor effect: Caniptotliecine causes toxic reactions and limits the use of drugs, but a licorice acid amine can lower camptothecin toxicity by not reducing its efficacy and having a certain synergy. On animal experiments: the number of white blood cells caused by camptothecin, Glycyrrhizinate amine has protective effect.

This product is hot-water extract on human cervical cancer cells JTC-26 and inhibition rate is 70%- 90%.

Anti-tumor component B: Gycyrrhetinic aicd
Struture:

Existing parts: the herbal roots, rhizomes.

Antitumor effects: glycyrrhetinic acid inhibited transplanted Oberling-Guerin myeloma on rat. Its sodium salt has been inhibition on the growth of mouse Ehrhlich ascites carcinoma and sarcoma -45, even orally.

Anti-tumor components: Liguirtin
Structure:

Existing parts: the root herbal.

Antitumor effects: The product can inhibit morphological changes and also have anti-rumor effect on rat hepatoma and Ehrlich ascites carcinoma cells and rat mammary tumor. It has the preventive effect on rat stomach cancer, can reduce the incidence of rastric cancer. In addition, grass sweetener has inhibited aflatoxin B1-induced hepatic precancerous lesion.

Z-C-K LwF

Antitumor points: (Tetrainethylpyrazine, TTMP)

Anti-tumor effects: TTMP can inhibit TXA2 synthetase activity. Li Xue Tang et al reported: TTMP administered once has a certain anti-metastatic effect on hepatoma cell metastasis. Jin Rong and other reports: TTMP anti-tumor effect and its mechanism, the experimental results show that: TTMP at 20mg/d x 18d could significantly inhibit the artificial lung metastasis in B16-F10 melanoma and TTMP can enhance normal and tumor-bearing spleen NK cell activity in isotope incorporation assay in mice and antagonized cyclophosphamide inhibition of NK cell activity. TTMP anti-metastatic effect may be related to reduce plasma TXB content and to enhance NK cell activity.

Some academics have also been reported: isolated from this plant gland (Adenine), its pharmacological activity has been confirmed that stimulate white blood cell proliferation, prevent fine thrombocytopenia, particularly for leukopenia caused by radiotherapy or chemotherapy. TTMP has a certain anti-metastatic effect on liver cancer cells.

Z-C-L AMB

Anti-tumor component B: p-Sitosterol
Structure:

Existing parts: The root of the plant.

Anti-tumor effects: p-Sitosterol has an edge activity for lymphocytic leukemia P134; has effect on mouse adenocarcinoma 715, which inhibition rate of tumor weight (TWI) was> 58%; it has effects on Lewis lung carcinoma,its TWI was > 58%; for the rat carcinoma Wacker cancer 256 its TWI was > 58%.

Reports: AMB roots have in a certain amount of polysaccharide; AMB polysaccharide contains 1.34-2.04% and there are several polysaccharides. It has broad biological activity and has anti-tumor effect in vivo, but does not directly kill cancer cell in vitro which means that AMB polysaccharide works by enhancing immune function.

AMB can improve human and mouse plasma cAMP levels, can inhibit tumor growth, and make tumor cells even reversed; can promote animal leukocytosis; can recover leukopenia induced by chemotherapy or radiotherapy; can promote immune function and inhibit tumor cell killing effect. The inhibition rate of its water extract was 41.7% in vivo experiments on mice sarcoma -180. The alcohol extract AMB is currently used clinically as an anticancer drug righting.

ZhouShuYin reported: the results of AMB polysaccharide show in vivo experiments: APS 2.5mg/kg, 5mg/kg, 10mg/kg, 20mg/kg significantly inhibited on transplanted tumor S_{180} liver cancer; in vitro results showed that: APS and interleukin-2 can significantly improve the compatibility of applied rate LAK cell killing target cell P851 and Yae cells. Its anti-tumor mechanism is related to increasing immune function.

In vivo the inhibition rate of AMB hot extract was 41.7% on mice sarcoma S180; was 12.25% on human lung adenocarcinoma SPC-A- 1. The inhibition index Iodized oil was induced with MCA human-mouse lung which the injection group with MCA was 16.28%, the control group was 51.52% cancer, the difference is very significant. MCA can inhibit DNA synthesis in human ovarian cancer cells. When the concentration increases, the inhibition will strengthen and the duration of action of the drug will prolong and inhibition of DNA synthesis of cancer cells also will be enhanced. MCA polysaccharides have synergies on T lymphocyte activation at malignant ascites.

Z-G-M LIA

Fight tumor components: Ursolic acid
Structure:

Exist parts: the leaves of the plant.

Anti-tumor effect: it has a very significant inhibition rate on cancer cells in vitro culture and can prolong the life on Hershey ascites carcinoma mice.

Pharmacological experiments show that: the goods flooding agent can inhibit certain animals transplanted tumor growth; it can increase immune function; it can recover leukopenia induced by chemotherapy and radiotherapy. There are also reported thr the active ingredient in this product is Oleanic acid.

Z-C-N CzR

Anti-tumor component A: Turmeric alcohol Curcumol
Structure:

Exist parts: roots for the plants.

Anti-tumor effects: Curcumol has anti-tumor effect. At 75mg/kg the inhibition rate -Nis 53.47-61 .96% on mice sarcoma S37; at 75ug/kg the inhibition rate was 45.1-77.13% on mice cervical cancer U14; the inhibition rate was 65.8- 78.9% at the same doses on EAC. There is better effect on treating cervical cancer.

Antitumor Component B: Turmeric dione /Curdione
Structure:

Exist parts: roots for the plants.

Antitumor effects: turmeric significantly inhibited mouse sarcoma 37, U_{14} and neck cancer and mouse Ehrlich ascites carcinoma and can make cancer cells degeneration end necrosis. After this product is processed in Ehrlich ascites carcinoma it can be successfully immunized mice to obtain initiative. The clinical results indicate that cervical cancer has a good effect.

There are also reports: In its same plant Curcuma wenyujin Y.H. Chen etc isolated β-elemene which has anti-cancer activity. The research proved that β-elemene could significantly prolong the survival time on Ehrlich ascites carcinoma and ascites reticulocyte cell sarcoma in mice and has strong killing effect on liver cancer cells in vitro. It also reduced nucleic acid content on EAC, especially in RNA content decreased more significantly. On leukocyte and bone marrow nucleated cells and Immune test: β-elemene has relatively small toxicity.

100% 0.3-0.5ml of Curdione has a good effect and the inhibition rate reached over 50% when it was injected to mice abdominal in S_{180}.

Z-C-Q LBP

Antitumor components:. Lycium burbarum Polysaccharides LBP Structure: The main components are arabinose, glucose, galactose, mannose, xylose, rhamnose and other components. Exist parts: to have come from the fruit.

Anti-tumor effect: Wangbekung etc proved: LBP enhanced immune function on normal mouse cells. At 10mg / kg it can improve the immune function and have inhibitory effect on S180 tumor-bearing mice, and synergistic anti-tumor effect with chemotherapy cyclophosphamide. There are also reports: LBP has a certain influence on the immune function. Lu Changxing and other reports: LBP showed significant radiosensitization with radiotherapy.

In addition, its roots and skins have Betaine, which also have anti-cancer function: with D-isoascorbic together it can inhibit mitosis in vitro on sarcoma 37, Ehrlich cancer and lymphoid leukemia L1210 which is stronger than alone medication. LB P contained (3- sitosterol, ascorbic acid, etc. which has anti-tumor effect.

There are also reports: LBP and interleukin-2 have the regulation effect on two anti-tumor LAK activity.

Z-C-R

Panax pseudo-Wall, var.notoginseng Hooet Tseng
Anti-tumor components: Notoginsenoside R1
Effective parts: that the roots of plants.

Antitumor effects: 180 μg/ml 5 days Panax saponin R can induce 68% HL-60 cell differentiation which proved Panax saponin R1 is a strong inducer of HL-6 0 cell lines and can induce HL-60 neutrophil cell differentiation. H-TdR incorporation assay results show: notoginsenoside R1 can induce differentiation of HL-60 cells while it affects DNA and RNA synthesis. There are also reports: during Cr release assay with soap studied Panax test it induced mouse spleen activity against tumor; have a strong anti-tumor effect with ConA / PHA together. Further experiments showed that soap Panax has no stimulation on proliferation of splenocytes, but changes the level of intracellular CAMP in spleen cells.

Z-C-Z1

Corioius versicolor Quel.

Anti-tumor components: Polysocohaitibe-piptide

Structure: a, R (1-4) dextran as main chain of Polysaccharide with 15% protein and kinds of amino acids

The presence of site: mycelium body

Antitumor effects: target cells: human gastric cancer cell lines (SGC79O1); hum:- lung adenocarcinoma fine lines (SPC); human monocytic leukemia cell line (SLY human skin cell lymphoma cell lines (MEI)

In vitro inhibitory test of PSK Application the results showed that: PSK has moderate inhibition of proliferation at a concentration dose 1000ug / ml on human lung adenocarcinoma cell line (SPC). The Japanese scholars shared PSK (Kiestin) has effects on sarcoma 180, liver AH-13, AH-7974, AH-66F, leukemia P388 in vivo by intravenous, intraperitoneal, subcutaneous, or oral administration and has almost no toxicity. Its mechanism is to improve the immune function through "host agency" role.

Li Jian and other scholars in the report: versicolor extract has no inhibition on ascites hepatoma on subcutaneously transplanted mouse while it has significant effects on the subcutaneous mouse ascites sarcoma S_{180}.

In clinical the extracellular polysaccharide PSK is used on primary liver cancer and alone n improve the clinical symptoms and prolong life, anticancer drugs; in combination with antitumor drugs it also reduces the toxic side effects of antitumor drugs. Japanese vood has developed into proteoglycan "PSK" anti-cancer drugs.

Lentinus edodes Sing
Anti-component A: Lentinan

Structure: The structure of p-D- (1 3) glucan backbone, C-6 has two fulcrum of every D- glucosyl, connecting p-D- (1 6) and p-D- (13) glucose branched-chain, also containing small amounts p-D- (16) branches.

Existing parts: its fruiting bodies.

Anti-tumor effects: Lentinan has some anti-tumor effect and improve the body's immune function. At a dose of 0.2, 1, 5, 25mg /kg, the daily cavity injection for consecutive 10 days, the inhibition rates were 78, 95.1, 97.5 and 73% on S180. It can Increase their compatibility of anti-tumor effect with chemotherapy drugs.

Lentinan can induce DNA synthesis and immune globulin and interferon-inducible, and non-specific cell-mediated cytotoxic effect in human peripheral mononuclear cells (PMNC, mainly lymphocytes); can enhance the cytotoxic response of NK cells of NK cell activity is very low and even absent in Leukemia patients; the general immune enhancer treatment increases the risk of cancer of the white blood cells. Lentinan can Increase the activity of NK cells. It induced β-IFN which has stronger anti-cancer effect than α and β -IFN, can enhance the phagocytic activity of white blood cells in patients with hormone production. At the same time, it can prevent patients with cancer from bacteria and viruses infection.

Shiio T et al reported: LNT and chemotherapeutic agents together can inhibit tumor metastasis in mice which the effect is the best when it is administrated after the surgery. Fachet T et al found Lentinan and their preparations A/ph(A/ph B10) F1hybrid mice A/ph, MC, S1 fibrosarcoma have significant anti-tumor alivity; however, Lentinan does not directly affect tumor growth in vitro. Shiio T et al also studied the inhibitory effect of Lentinan on cancer lung metastasis; intravenous Lentinan can inhibit Lewis system cancer (3LL), melanoma (B6) and fiber sarcoma (ML-CS-1) transfer.

11. THE EXCLUSIVE RESEARCH AND DEVELOPMENT PRODUCTS: A SERIES OF PRODUCTS OF Z-C IMMUNE REGULATION OF ANTI-CANCER CHINESE MEDICATION (INTRODUCTION)

Exclusive research and development of products: XZ-C immunomodulatory anticancer medicine products (Profile)

Independently developed XZ-C (XU ZE China) series of anti-cancer immune regulation medicine preparation, from experimental research to clinical validation, in animal experiments on the basis of success in clinical practice, clinical experience over the years a large number of clinical cases verification, a significant effect. The results are self-invention, the Department of independent innovation and intellectual property rights.

The research of Looking from traditional Chinese medications, and screening anti-cancer, anti-metastatic new drug:

The purpose is to screen out non-resistance, non-toxic side effects, a high selectivity, long-term oral anti-cancer, anti-metastatic and anti-recurrent cancer drug. It is well known now for the world's anti-cancer agent does inhibit proliferation of cancer cells, but it only kill cancer cells but also kill normal cells, especially the bone marrow of immune cells, a host of serious damage, because of chemotherapy cytotoxic and non-selectivity. And traditional chemotherapy can suppress the immune function and inhibit bone marrow function. Traditional intravenous chemotherapy treatment is interrupted, the cancer cells cannot be treated during the gap period which cancer cells continued proliferation and division. Although chemotherapy drugs can inhibit the proliferation of cancer cells, but because of its toxic side effects when cancer has not yet been eliminated, administration had to stop. After treatment, cancer cell proliferation up again, and began to have resistance. When resistance, this dose would not work so as to increase the amount executioner. However, if the dose is increased, it may endanger the lives of patients. If the chemotherapy drug resistance has been given, then the cancer is not only ineffective; Contrary to killing only patient's normal cells so cancer cells resistance to cancer drugs and toxics of cancer drugs on the host side effects is a long vexing problem. And we are looking for new drugs, the purpose is to avoid these drawbacks.

According to the theory of cell cycle, anticancer agents must be able to continue long applications so that cancer foci can bath in anti-cancer agents long lasting time, and is available without stopping to prevent their cell division and to prevent recurrence and metastasis. Must be long years, have been conducting long-term, it is best to long-term oral drugs to control existing foci and prevent nascent cancer cells to form. Due to large toxicity the currently used anticancer medication cannot long continuous use, but only short cycle applications. Existing anticancer medication has suppressed immune function, bone marrow suppression, suppression thymus, bone marrow suppression side effects. The formation and development of cancer is due to the patient's immune system to reduce lost immune surveillance, therefore, all anticancer medications should be increased immunization, protection immune organs, immune suppression and should not use drugs.

To this end, we conducted the following experiment laboratory screening of new anti-cancer research from the traditional Chinese medicine, anti-metastatic drugs:

(A) The method of cancer cells in vitro, the experimental study of Chinese herbal medicine suppressor screening rates:

In vitro screening tests: The cancer cells in vitro was observed for sore drugs directly damage cells.

Screening in vitro culture of cancer cells in vitro tests respectively allowing raw and crude drugs of crude product (500ug / ml) to be used and to observe whether there is inhibition of cancer cells, we believe that 200 kinds of traditional Chinese medicine herbs have anticancer function performed one by one in vitro screening tests. And under the same conditions with a normal fiber cell culture to test the toxicity of these cells, and then compared.

(B) Building cancer-bearing animal model for the screening of Chinese herbs for cancer-bearing animal experimental tumor suppressor rate

Suppressor in vivo screening test, each batch experiments with mice 240, divided into 8 groups, each group 30, the first group was the control group 7, group 8 with 5-Fu or CTX control group, the whole group of small mice was inoculated with EA C or S 180 or H22 cancer cells. After inoculation 24h, each rat oral feeding crude product of crude drug powder, long-term feeding the screened the herbs, observed survival, toxicity, computing prolong survival rate calculated suppression sores.

So, we conducted experimental study for four consecutive years, and has conducted a 3-year incidence of tumor-bearing mice and transfer mechanism, the experimental study of the mechanism of relapse, and experimental studies to explore how cancer causing death of the host each year with more than 1,000 tumor-bearing animals model, made a total of nearly four years, 6000 tumor-bearing animal models, mice each were carried out after the death of the liver, spleen, lung, thymus, kidney pathological anatomy, a total of 20,000 times slice to explore to find out whether There may be slight carcinogenic pathogens, with microcirculation microscope 100 tumor-bearing mice were tumor microvessels bell establish and microcirculation.

Through experimental study we first found in China a medicine to inhibit tumor angiogenesis TG had a significant effect, more than 80 cases have been used in clinical treatment of patients Hang metastasis being observed.

Results: In our laboratory animal experiments screened 200 kinds of Chinese herbs and screened48 kinds of certain and excellent herbs with inhibition of cancer cell proliferation, inhibition rate of more than 75 to 90%. But there are some of commonly used Chinese medicine which consider to have the anticancer roles, after animal in vitro and in vivo inhibition rate anti-cancer screening, showed really no effect, or little effect which 152 kinds of medications having no anti-cancer effect had removed from the phase-out of animal experiments.

Screening out of this real 48 kinds of traditional Chinese medications with having good tumor suppression rates, and then optimized the combination and repeated tumor suppression rate experiments in vivo, and finally developed immunomodulatory anticancer Chinese medication XU ZE China1-10 with Chinese own characteristics China (ZC $_{1-10}$).

Z-C$_1$ could inhibit cancer cells, but does not affect normal cells; Z-C$_4$ specially can increase thymus function, can promote proliferation, increased immunity; Z-C$_1$ can protect bone marrow function and to product more blood.

Clinical validation: Based on the success of animal experiments, clinical validation was conducted. Namely the establishment of oncology clinics and Western medicine combined with anti-cancer, anti-metastasis, recurrence Research Group, retained patient medical records, to establish a regular follow-up observation system to observe the long-term effect · face from experimental research to clinical evidence, the discovery of new clinical validation process issue, went back to the laboratory for basical research, then the results of a new experiment for clinical validation. Thus, a clinical experiment again and again clinical experiment, all experimental studies must be clinically proven in a large number of patients observed 3--5 years, or even clinical observation of 8 to 10 years, according to evidence-based medicine, and can have long-term follow-up assessment information, verified indeed have a good long-term efficacy, the efficacy of the standard is: a good quality of life, longer survival. XZ-C sectional immune regulation anti-cancer medicine made after a lot of applications in advanced cancer patients verification, and achieved remarkable results. XZ-C sectional immune regulation anti-cancer medicine can improve the quality of life of patients with advanced cancer, enhance immune function, increase the body's anticancer abilities, increased appetite and significantly prolong survival.

(C) XZ-C immunomodulatory anticancer Chinese medication Mechanism of Action

With the deepening of traditional Chinese medicine research, it is known to produce a lot of traditional Chinese medicine and biological activity of cytokines and other immune molecules having a regulatory role, this time to clarify XZ-C from the molecular level immunomodulatory anticancer Chinese medication immunological mechanisms very important.

1. XZ-C immunomodulatory anticancer Chinese medication can protect immune organs, increasing the weight of the spleen and chest pay attention.
2. XZ-C immunomodulatory anticancer Chinese medication for hematopoietic function of bone marrow cell proliferation and significant role in promoting.
3. XZ-C immunomodulatory anticancer Chinese medication on T cell immune function enhancement effect on T cells significantly promote proliferation.
4. XZ-C immunomodulatory anticancer Chinese medication for human IL-2 production has significantly enhanced role.
5. XZ-C immunomodulatory anticancer Chinese medication activation of NK cell activity and enhance the role, NK cells with a broad spectrum of anticancer effect, can anti-xenograft tumor cells.
6. XZ-C immunomodulatory anticancer Chinese medication for LAK cell activity can enhance the effect, LAK cells are capable of killing of NK cell sensitive and non-sensitive solid tumor cells, with broad-spectrum anti-tumor effect.
7. XZ-C immunomodulatory anticancer Chinese medication to induce interferon and pro-inducing effect, IFN has a broad-spectrum anti-tumor effect Wo immunomodulatory effects, IFN can inhibit tumor cell proliferation, IFN can activate the skin to kill cancer cells and OIL cells.
8. XZ-C immunomodulatory anticancer Chinese medication for colony stimulating factor can promote credit enhancement, CSF not only involved in hematopoietic cell proliferation, differentiation, and in a host of anti-tumor immunity plays an important role
9. XZ-C immunomodulatory anticancer Chinese medication can promote tumor necrosis factor (TNF) role, TNF is a class can directly cause tumor cell death factor, its main biological role is to kill or inhibit tumor cells.

D. Bilogical response modification(BRM), traditional chinese anticancer medicine similar to BRM and tumor treatment

1. Biological reaction modification (BRM) explores the new field of the tumor biological therapy. Currently BRM as the fourth methods of the tumor treatment gets widely attention in the world.

Oldham in 1982 built BRM theory. Based this in 1984 he advanced the fourth modality of cancer treatment-----biological therapy again. According to this, in the normal condition, there is the dynamic equilibrium between the tumor and the body. The development of the tumors, and even invasion and metastasis, completely is caused by the loss of this equilibrium. If this unbland situation is adjusted to the normal level, the tumor growth can be controlled and will disappear.

The anticancer mechanism of BRM in details as the following:

1.) Improve the host defence abilities or decrease the immune inhabitation of the tumors to the host to reach the immune response to the tumors.

2.) Look for the biological active things in natural or gene combination to enhance the host defense abilities.

3.) Reduce the host response induced by the tumor cells

4.) Promote the tumors to division and mature to become the normal cells

5.) Reduce the side effects of the chemotherapy and redio therapy and enhance The host toleration.

2. XZ-C immune regulation anticancer medicine have the functions and curative effects similar to BRM

After four years experimental research and 16 years clinical research which are the drugs similar to BRM selected from traditional Chinese medicine.

XZ-C is the drugs that XU ZE in China professor selected from two hundreds of the anticancer herbs after the experiments. At first the culturing tumor were done. The in vitro was done One by one to select and asberve the direct damage to tumor cells in the culture setting and the control groups of the rate of the anticancer are the chemotherapyxxxx and the normal culture tube cells. The results are to select the a series of the medicine of the anti-cancer proliferation, then made the animal modes which 200 drugs were used on one by one. These experiments of the analysis and evaluation are steps by steps, scientific, practical and strict, etc. The results proved that48 of them have the excellent tumor inhibition effects, however the rest 152 of the tumors anticancer medicine are all common old anticancer medicine which proved no anticancer or less inhibition of the tumors in the animal models during these medicine selection experiments.

The medicine which the author selected on the tumor animal models and had excellent anticancer rat XZ-C can improve immune function, protection of the central immune organs such as thymus and, improving the cell-mediated immune functions, protecting the thymus function, protect the bone morrow function, increase the red blood cells and white blood cells number, active the immune factors, improve the immune surveilence in the blood ect.

XZ-C the main anticancer pharmacology function si anticancer and increase of the immune function. The above XZ-C has the following function as :

1.) Activing the host immune system to promote the host immune function to reach the immune respond to the tumors.

2.) Activing the host immune factors of the anticancer systems to strengthen the host immune function and improve the immunce surviellence of the host immune systems.

3.) Protecting the thymus and bone marrow, improve the immune system, and stimulate the bone marrow function to reduce the inhibition of the bone marrow and increase the white blood cell and red blood cells etc.

4.) Reduction of the side effects of the chemotherapy and radioactive therapy to increase the tolerance of the hosts.

5.) Increaseing thymus weight and stop the shrinkle of thymus because when the tumor develop thymus goes on shrinkles.

As the above statement, the basic mechanism of XZ-C is similar to BRM and the clinical application is similar to those of the BRM.

(A) XZ-C1 "Smart grams cancer"

The main components are eight Chinese herbs.

Anticancer pharmacology

1. Detoxification, increasing blood circulation, righting, dispelling evil without injury, strong inhibition of cancer cells and inhibition of cancer cell metastasis without inhibition of normal cells.
2. In anti-cancer in vivo tests in mice, they have inhibitory activity in the mice Ehrlich ascites tumor cells which there had been significant differences in the control group.
3. Can prolong survival of mice bearing cancer, increased the survival rate of 26.92%.
4. The main prescription drugs Z-C1-A and Z-C1-B has a stable and significant anticancer effects, 100% inhibition of cancer cells, cancer cell mitotic reduced and degenerated and necrosed seriously and epithelial cells or fibroblasts is no impact in the administration group. XZ-C1-D extract have inhibitory activity on human cervical cancer cells, on mouse sarcoma s180 inhibition rate was 98.9%, several other ingredients also have a strong anticancer effect.
5. Z-C1 Herbs inhibition effect on Mice bearing H22 hepatoma tumor: z-c1 drug inhibition rate was 40 percent in the second week, the first four weeks was 45%, the first six weeks of 58%; in the control group CTX medication first two weeks inhibition rate was 45%, the first four weeks inhibition rate was 45%, 49% for the first six weeks.
6. Z-C1 medicine influence on survival in mice bearing H22: life-prolonging rate was 85% in z-c1 group; life extension was 9.8% in CTX control group ; in Z-C1 group Thymus did not shrink; however thymus shrank in Control group.

Clinical application

1. Indications: esophageal cancer, stomach cancer, colorectal cancer, lung cancer, breast cancer, liver pain, bile duct cancer, pancreatic cancer, thyroid cancer, nasopharyngeal cancer, brain tumors, renal cancer, bladder cancer, ovarian cancer, cervical cancer, various sarcoma and a variety of metastasis, recurrent cancer.
2. Usage: after taking z- c1 continuously 1 - 3 months, the patients felt better. This medication can be taken for long-term and can be taken one dose every other day after three years; can be taken two doses weekly after 5 years to retain immune function and cytokine long-term stable at a certain level.

Toxicity Test

ZX-C1 can be used for long-term. The acute toxicity test showed that when adult mice was fed a dose 104 times (10g / Kg body weight), respectively, in 24, 48, 72, 96 hours of observation, 30 purebred mice didn't die. The median lethal dose (LD5O) didn't have any number so that it is a rather safe prescriptions.

In the oncology clinic it has been used for many years and some patients have taken more than three to five years and more than 8 to 10 years in order to maintain immunity and to stop recurrence. It can be taken for long-term and it is quite safe oral cancer.

(B) XZ-C2

Ingredients: 9 kinds of anticancer herbs

Anticancer pharmacology

1. Animal experiments show that it can prolong L7212 mouse (mouse leukemia) survival, well-behaved compared to the control group, there were statistically significant.
2. Can improve inhibition rate in the L7212 in mice
3. Z-C1-A and Z-C2-B on mouse sarcoma (s180) has a strong inhibitory effect.

Application

Indications: leukemia, upper gastrointestinal cancer, tongue, larynx, nasopharynx cancer, cervical cancer, bone metastasis, esophagus cancer or gastric ulcer anastomotic recurrence narrow (no longer surgery). It has general effect on Acute leukemia lymph and has obvious efficiency of each of the other type of leukemia. It has a more significant effect on Bone metastasis

Usage: one capsule Qid generally or two capsules tid

Leukemia 3 capsules tid after meal and seven days for a course.

(C) XZ-C3 topical pain Patch

Prescription Content: kaempferol, turmeric, etc. 14 flavors

Anticancer pharmacology

1. Detoxification, anti-inflammatory pain, qi Sanjie pain;
2. Increasing the blood circulation, reducing swelling and pain, played a total of detoxification, swelling and analgesic effect, while the most prominent role in cancer treatment is to stop pain.
3. For point application, applicator than simply pain, can better play the efficacy and achieve rapid pain relief purposes.

Clinical application

Indications: liver cancer, lung cancer pain, back pain from pancreatic cancer, bone pain, neck and supraclavicular lymph nodes metastasis.

Usage: A total of research and go take honey, mix, stir into a paste backup, lung disease spreads in milk root point (nipple straight down 5, 6 ribs), liver cancer spreads on the door hole (milk midline 6-7 rib room), treated and covered with gauze and tape securely, severe pain 6h for a second, lesser pain, 12h replacement of 1: continuous use to relieve pain or disappeared.

Experience: Treatment of 84 cases of liver cancer, lung cancer pain patients, have analgesic effect, general medicine three times, will receive different levels of pain relief, 3 to 7 days after a significant analgesic effect, some basical pain.

(D) ZX-C4 anticancer medication of protecting thymus and increasing immune function (5g / bag)

Ingredients: including 12 valuable herbs
Anticancer pharmacology

1. To promote lymphocyte transformation, enhancing immune function, increased white blood cells, inhibit cancer cell, Warming blood.
2. Ehrlich ascites tumor cells transplanted into the abdominal cavity of mice, one day after transplantation and 7 Days 2 times for chemotherapy drugs in mice, while serving z -c4 (2g / kg) per day is significantly enhanced the effectiveness of chemotherapy drugs effect.
3. To suppress leukopenia and weight loss induced by chemotherapy medicinal MMC MMC
4. While serving Z-C4, it was found to inhibit cancer cells in terms of improving the effect of intravenously injected anticancer chemotherapy drugs than simply using more than three times in cancer-bearing mice.
5. Chemotherapy drugs for cancer-bearing mice can damage special thymus, spleen and other immune organs, but after adding the service z-C4, thymus, spleen and other organs completely don't shrink, showed z-C4 have effects on the immune organ protective nature function.
6. ZX-C4 extract in Ehrlich ascites disease mouse prolonged the mice life span of up to 167.1%, the average survival time of mice in the control group 15.2 days, and z-c4 administration group is 25.4 days, while reticuloendothelial system function in mice showed significantly higher.
7. Z-C4 allows the chemotherapy drugs cisplatin quickly to mitigate its effects, can enhance the effectiveness of cisplatin. z-C4 can be 100% inhibition of cisplatin toxicity chloroplatinic day conventional dose amount that is human can be. z-c4 not resist cisplatin Chen Hang crazy. z-C4 can protect the kidney, the renal damage cis-platinum chlorine hardly occurs. Z-C4 has highly promising anticancer drug.
8. Z-C4 patients after cancer surgery have a significant effect, gastrointestinal, liver, pancreas and other ulcer disease after radical: all manifestations of physical decline, decreased immunity, fatigue, burnout, loss of appetite and anemia, after 1 a 2 weeks from the beginning can be oral or tube feeding, oral Z-C4 granules, 7.5 g daily, before meals three times a blunt, 12 weeks, during which can be chemotherapy or immune therapy.

9. Z-C4 medicine antitumor effect in mice bearing hepatoma H22: z-C4 first two weeks of medication inhibition rate was 55%, the first four weeks inhibition rate was 68%, the first six weeks inhibition rate was 70% the control group, CTX (cyclophosphamide Yu amine) Week 2 inhibitory drugs was 45%: the first four weeks inhibition rate of 49%.

10. z-C4 medicine for liver cancer H22 bearing mice survival, z-C4 group extend survival rate 200%, CTX group life span was 9.8%.

11. Z-C4 can significantly improve immune function, can increase white blood cells and red blood cells, liver and kidney function had no effect on the liver, kidney slices without damage. CTX cause leukopenia, reduced immune function, kidney sections have kidney damage.

12. Z-C4 treated group Thymus do not shrink and slightly hypertrophy, CTX thymus control group significantly shrink. Z-C4 on mouse sarcoma (S180) has a strong inhibitory effect.

Clinical Application:

Indications: various types of cancer, sarcoma, a variety of advanced cancer, metastasis, recurrence of cancer, radiotherapy, chemotherapy, post-operative patients. It can be applied all kinds of cancer, especially dizziness, weakness, fatigue, lazy words, less gas, spontaneous sweating, heart palpitations, insomnia, blood deficiency were more applicable.

Z-C4 medicine was used before surgery and after starting the medication and medication every four weeks to do a clinical and laboratory tests, for 20 weeks. Test items: conscious and objective symptoms, body weight, total protein and albumin, total cholesterol, dielectric, ALT AST blood and platelets, lymphocytes, T cells and B cells, r globulin, urinary protein.

Treatment Results: ① increase in the number of lymphocytes, inhibit the role of leukopenia; ② no impact on liver function; ③ protect the kidney function, kidney damage is not so; ④ can significantly reduce the chemotherapy and radiotherapy-induced rash, stomatitis etc; ⑤ postoperative, after chemotherapy, effective physical recovery after radiotherapy, can increase appetite, improve the general malaise and weight gain.

ZX-C4 reduce side effects of radiotherapy and chemotherapy and improve the overall state of the patient after surgery. It is a very valuable rehabilitation medication.

Experience: Modern medicine for the treatment of advanced cancer presents a variety of methods, but there are still some problems, it is still not convinced that the combined use of chemotherapy for advanced disease if certain effective drugs. Even if effective, but it also brings serious side effects, may be considered modern medical treatment for cancer is to kill cancer cells, is offensive, while the Chinese places to enhance the body's own functions to draw even tone pull eliminate cancer. To this end, it should find a way to reduce or eliminate symptoms, improve or treat the disease with few side effects, the treatment can prolong life, and Z-C4 being has the features and advantages.

Through experiments ZX-C4 has the role of enhanced anticancer effect ; promote B cell mitosis role; the catch into the effects of radiation damage hematopoietic system recovery; the promotion of the role of phagocytic cells; thymus increased protective immunity, protection of bone marrow Blood role.

Toxicity Test

Z-C4 can be used long-term. Acute toxicity experiments showed that the median lethal dose (LD50) can not do, is safe and herbs, has been used in the specialist clinic for many years, some patients long-term use three to five years, or even take 8-10 years to maintain immunity, prevent cancer recurrence and metastasis. This anticancer and antimetasatasis medication can be taken by oral for long-term oral and is quite safe.

(5) The following XZ-C various immunomodulatory anticancer medicine series and the experimental and clinical contents are too many and too long so that here only gave names and profiles were omitted.

1. XZ-C5:for liver cancer
2. XZ-C6: for bladder cancer
3. XZ-C7: for Lung cancer
4. XZ-C 8: protect bone marrow and increase blood, attenuated toxics of radiotherapy and chemotherapy
5. XZ-C9:pancreas cancer, prostate cancer.
6. XZ-C10: for brain tumor

All of above of a variety of cancer anticancer, antimetastasis, recurrent research Chinese medicine are based on the experimental study and applied by specialist in outpatient clinics more than 20 years and achieved good results.

Our research Chinese medications for cancer complications in out-patient center of cancer treatment:

1. Anticancer eliminate water soup for pleural effusion and ascites
2. Drop yellow soup for liver cirrhosis and jaundice
3. Anticancer soup after surgery for postoperative recovery
4. Starvation soup for cancer loss of appetite
5. Through Quiet soup for anastomotic stenosis
6. Adhesiolysis soup for adhesions after surgery for cancer

Above all research product formulations. Observation by cancer specialist clinic over the years this big boy patient, have achieved good results, reduce patient suffering, improve the survival quality first, extended survival.

Table 9-1 Summary table of the main pharmacological effects of Z-C immune regulation anticancer Chinese herbal medicine (anti-cancer and increasing immune)

	Increased white blood cells	Enhanced phagocytosis	Enhance cellular immune	Enhance humoral immune	Enhanced hematopoietic function	Improve gastrointestinal function	Enhance the weight of the thymus	Promote bone marrow cell proliferation	Enhanced T cell function	Enhanced NK cell activity	Enhanced LAK cell activity	Enhanced IL-2 activity levels	Enhance the level of interferon IFN activity	Enhanced TNF activity levels	Enhanced CSF colony stimulating factor	Antagonistic WCBYC ↓	Inhibition of platelet coagulation and antithrombosis	Antitumor	Anti-metastasis	Antiviral	Anti-cirrhosis	Liver protection	Eliminate free radicals	Protein synthesis	Anti-HIV	
Z-C-A-APL																		+	+							
Z-C-B-SLT																		+	+							
Z-C-C-SNL																		+	+							
Z-C-D-PGS	+	+	+	+	+	+	6	+	+	+	+		+	+	+	+		9	+	+	+		+	+		20
Z-C-E-PCW		+	+				2	+	+			+	+	+	+	+		7	+	+	+					12
Z-C-F-AMK		+	+	+	+	+	5			+		+			+			3	+	+		+				11
Z-C-G-GUF		+	+	+		+	4			+		+				+		3	+	+		+		+		11
Z-C-H-RGL	+		+	+			3		+	+		+	+		+			5	+			+				10
Z-C-I-PLP	+	+	+	+	+	+	6	+	+							+		3	+	+					+	12
Z-C-J-ASD	+	+	+	+	+		5	+	+	+		+	+	+	+	+		8	+			+				15
Z-C-KLWF		+	+				2							+		+		2	+	+						5
Z-C-L-AMB	+	+	+	+	+		5	+	+	+	+	+	+					7	+		+			+		5
Z-C-M LLA	+	+	+	+			4	+		+								2	+					+		5
Z-C-N-CZR		+					1							+		+		2	+	+						5
Z-C-O-PMT	+	+	+	+	+	+	6	+	+	+					+			4	+	+	+	+	+	+		16
Z-C-P-STG							0											0	+							1
Z-C-Q-LBP	+	+	+	+	+		5		+	+	+	+		+	+	+		8	+				4			16
Z-C-R-NSR		+					1	+		+					+			3	+	+	+	+				8
Z-C-S-GLK	+	+	+	+	+		5			+		+	+			+		6	+					+	+	16
Z-C-T-EDM	+	+	+	+	+		5	+		+		+	+		+	+		6	+	+			+			14
Z-C-U-PUF		+	+	+			3		+	+	+							3	+			+				8
Z-C-V-ABB							1		+	+	+			+				4	+							6
Z-C-W-SCB	+						1		+							+		2	+				+	+		5
Z-C-X-SDS							0		+	+	+							3	+							4
Z-C-Y-PAR							0		+	+	+		+	+				5	+							6
Z-C-Z-CVQ							0					+						1	+							2

12. STUDY ON ACTION MECHANISM OF XZ-C TRADITIONAL CHINESE ANTI-CARCINOMA MEDICINE FOR IMMUNOLOGIC REGULATION AND CONTROL

With more and deeper researches on traditional Chinese medicine, it has been proved that many kinds of traditional Chinese medicine can regulate and control the production and biological activity of cytokine and other immune molecules, which is meaningful to explain the immunological mechanism of XZ-C traditional Chinese anti-carcinoma medicine for immunologic regulation and control from the level of molecule.

I. Protecting Immune Organs and Increasing the Weight of Thymus and Spleen

That XZ-C traditional Chinese medicine can protect immune organs resulting from the following active principles.

1. XZ-C-T (EBM):

    Using its 15g/kg and 30g/kg extracting solution (equivalent to 1g original medicine) along with 12.5mg/kg, 25mg/kg ferulic acid suspension to feed the mice for seven days in a raw can increase the weight of thymus and spleen obviously, especially the effects of the group with high dose are more apparent. Intraperitoneal injection of EBM polysaccharide can also alleviate thymus and spleen atrophy obviously caused by perdnisolone.

2. XZ-C-O (PMT)

    Extract PM-2, feed the mice with 6g/(kg·d) PMT decoction for successive seven days which can increase the weight of thymus and celiac lymph nodes and antagonize the reduction in the weight of immune organs caused by perdnisolone. Drenching the mouse of 15 months old with 6g/kg decoction (with the concentration of 0.5g/ml) for 14 days can increase the weight and volume of thymus, thicken the cortex and raise cellular density apparently. The combined use of PM and astragalus root can promote non-lymphocyte hyperplasia and benefit the micro environment of thymus.

3. XZ-C-W (SCB)

SCB polysaccharide can gain weight of thymus and spleen of a normal mouse. Lavage with it enables cyclophosphane to control the gain in the weight of thymus and spleen.

4. XZ-C-M (LLA)

Drench a mouse with LLA decoction for seven days resulting in increasing the weight of thymus and spleen.

5. XZ-C-L

For a 15-month old mouse, its thymus degenerates obviously. Astragalus injectio can enlarge the thymus significantly. The cortex under microscope is thickened and the cellular density increase obviously.

II. Effects on Proliferation, Differentiation and Hematopiesis of Marrow Cells

The following active principles of XZ-C traditional Chinese medicine have effects on hematopiesis of marrow cells.

1. XZ-C-Q (LBP) extracts (PM-2)

(1)Effects on the proliferation of hematopoietic stem cell (CFU-S) of a normal mouse: inject PM-2 with the dose of 500mg/(kg·d)×3d or 10mg/(kg·d)×3d LBP into the experimental mice respectively by venoclysis and kill them in the ninth day. It can be found that the number of spleen CFU-S in the group with administration increases obviously. The number of CFU-S in group PM-2 is 21% higher than that of the control group and it is 36% in the group with LBP.

(2)Effects on colony forming unit of granulocytes and macrophages (CFU-GM): the experimental results indicate that LBP with the dose of 5~30mg/(kg·d)×3d can increase the number of CFU-GM and PM-2 can also strengthen the effect of CFU-GM with the effective dose of 12.5~50mg/(kg·d)×3d. In the early stage of cultivation, most CFU-GMs are units of granulocytes and then units of macrophages increase gradually. In the anaphase units of macrophages take over the dominance.

From the above experiment, it can be found that PM-2 and LBP can promote hematopiesis of normal mice obviously. The experiment proves that during the process of restoring hematopiesis damaged by cyclophosphamide, PM-2 and LBP stimulate the proliferation of granulocytes at first, and then marrow karyocytes multiply; at last these two promote the restoration of peripheral granulocytes.

2. XZ-C-D (TSPG)

Ginsenoside, which is the active principle of ginseng to promote hematopiesis, can bring the recovery of erythrocyte in peripheral blood, haemoglobin and myeloid cell of thighbone in the mice of marrow-inhibited type, increase the index of myeloid cellular division and stimulate the proliferation of myeloid hematopoietic cell in vitro so as to make it into cell cycle with active proliferation (S+G$_2$/M stage). TSPG can promote the proliferation and differentiation of polyenergetic hematopoietic cells and induce the formation of hemopoietic growth factor (HGF).

3. XZ-C-H (RCL)

Steamed Chinese Foxglove can promote the recovery of erythrocyte and haemoglobin for animals with blood deficiency and accelerate the proliferation and differentiation of myeloid hematopoietic cell (CFU-S) with the effect of predominance and hematosis significantly. Peritoneal injection of rehmannia polysaccharides for successive six days can promote the proliferation and differentiation of myeloid hematopoietic cells and progenitor cells as well as increasing the number of leucocytes in peripheral blood.

4. XZ-C-J (ASD)

ASD polysaccharide has no effects on erythrocytes and leucocytes of normal mice, but for those damaged by radiation, injection of ASD polysaccharide can influence the proliferation and differentiation of both polyenergetic hematopoietic stem cells (CPU-S) and hemopoietic progenitor cells. But its decoction has no obvious effects.

5. XZ-C-E (PEW)

Poria cocos (micromolecule chemical compound extracted from Tuckahoe polysaccharide) is the active principle that can strengthen the production of colony stimulating factor (CSF) and improve the level of leucocytes in peripheral blood inside the mouse's body. It can also prevent the decline in leucocytes caused by cyclophosphamide and accelerate the recovery with the effects better than sodium ferulic which is used to increase leucocytes.

6. XZ-C-Y (PAR)

Its polysaccharide can obviously resist the decline in leucocytes caused by cyclophosphamide and increase the number of myeloid cells to promote the proliferation of myeloid induced by CSF as well as the recovery and reconstitution of hematopiesis for the mice irradiated by X ray. It can also increase the number of hematopoietic stem cells and myeloid cells along with leucocytes.

III. Enhancing Immunologic Function of T Cells

The active principles of XZ-C traditional Chinese medicine and their effects are following.

1. XZ-C-L (AMB)

   It can raise the percentage of lymphocytes in peripheral blood obviously. The LBP in small dose (5~10mg/kg) can cause the proliferation of lymphocytes, indicating that LBP can promote the proliferation of T cells apparently. 50mg/(kg·d)×7d is the best dose in that it will have no effects if lower than the level and it will bring the effects down if higher than the level. Oral administration of LBP can raise the conversion rate of lymphocytes for the sufferers who are weak and with fewer leucocytes.

2. XZ-C$_4$

   It can regulate immune system and active T cells of aggregated lymphatic follicles, as well as stimulate the secretion of hemopoietic growth factor in T cells. Among the crude drugs of XZ-C$_4$, the extract from the hot water of atractylodes lancea rhizome can obviously stimulate the cells of aggregated lymphatic follicles, which is regarded as the base of XZ-C$_4$ immunoloregulation.

IV. Activating and Enhancing NK Cell Activity

Natural killer cell, NK cell is another kind of killer cell in lymphocytes for human beings and mice, which needs neither antigenic stimulation, nor the participation of antibodies to kill some cells. It plays an important role in immunity, especially in the function of immune surveillance as NK cell is the first line of defense against tumors and has broad spectrum anti-tumor effects.

NK cell is broad-spectrum and able to kill sygeneous, homogenous and heterogenous tumor cells with special effects on lymjphoma and leucocytes.

NK cell is an important kind of cells for immunoloregulation, which can regulate T cells, B cells and stem cells, etc. It can also regulate immunity by releasing cytokines like IFN-α, IFN-γ, IL-2, TNF, etc.

The active principles in XZ-C traditional Chinese medicine and their effects are following.

1. XZ-C-X (SDS)

   Divaricate Saposhniovia Root can strengthen the activity of NK cells of experimental mice. When combined with IL-2, it can make the activity of NK cell higher, indicating that its polysaccharide can give a hand to IL-2 to activate NK cells and improve the activity.

LBP can strengthen T cell mediated immune reaction and the activity of NK cells for normal mice and those dealt by cyclophosphamide. Peritoneal injection of LBP can improve the proliferation of spleen T lymphocytes and strengthen the lethality of CTL increasing the specific lethal rate from 33% to 67%.

2. XZ-C-G (GUF)

Glycyrrhizin can induce the production of IFN in the blood of animals and human beings and strengthen NK cell activity at the same time. Clinical tests made by Abe show that after intravenous injection of 80mg GL, the raise of NK cell activity reaches 75% among 21 sufferers. Peritoneal injection of 0.5mg/kg GL on mice can strengthen the activity of NK cells in liver.

3. XZ-C-L (AMB)

Its bath fluid can promote NK cell activity of mice both in vivo and in vitro, and can also induce IFN-γ to deal with effector cells under the certain concentration of 0.1mg/ml. Cordyceps sinensis extract can strengthen NK cells activity of the mouse both in vivo and in vitro. Fluids with the concentrations of 0.5g/kg, 1g/kg and 5g/kg can strengthen NK cell activity of mice.

V. Effects on LAK Cell Activity

Lymphokine activated killer cell, namely LAK cell can be induced by IL-2 cytokine. LAK cells can kill the solid tumors that are both sensitive and insensitive to NK cells with broad anti-tumor effects.

The active principles in XZ-C anti-carcinoma traditional Chinese medicine and their effects are following.

1. XZ-C-L (AMB)

Its polysaccharide can strengthen LAK cell activity within a certain range of dose with 0.01mg/ml being the most effective, which is three times better than the damage effects of LAK cells. The concentrations of both higher and lower than this level can not achieve the effects.

2. XZ-C-U (PUF)

It can significantly strengthen the spleen LAK cell activity of killing tumor cells and improve the activity of erythrocyte C3b liquid. PUF and IL-2 are synergistic that can be used as regulator for biological reaction in tumor biological therapy based on LAK/Ril-2.

3. XZ-C-V

ABB polysaccharide can also raise LAK cell activity for the mouse and inhibit tumors remarkably. Its anti-tumorous mechanism relates to its strengthening immunity and changing cell membrane features.

VI. Effects on Iterleukin-2 (IL-2)

The active principles in XZ-C anti-carcinoma traditional Chinese medicine and their effects are following.

1. XZ-C-T

   EBM polysaccharide can enhance obviously the production of IL-2 for human beings when the concentration is 100ug/ml. At higher concentration (2500ug/ml and 5000ug/ml), it will lead to inhibition. Hypodermic injection of barrenwort polysaccharide for seven days in a row can significantly improve the ability of thymus and spleen of the mouse induced by ConA to produce IL-2.

2. XZ-C-Y

   PAR polysaccharide has strong immune activity and is able to promote the production of IL-2. For the mouse bearing S-180 tumor, it can raise the ability of spleen cells to produce IL-2 obviously。

3. XZ-C-D

   Ginseng polysaccharide has great promotion on IL-2 induced by peripheral monocytes for both healthy people and sufferers with kidney troubles. The effects are relevant to the dose positively.

VII. Function of Inducing Interferon and Promoting Inducement of Interferon

IFN are broad-spectrum in resisting tumors and can regulate immunity. It can also inhibit the proliferation of tumor cells and activate NK cells and CTL to kill tumor cells. Meanwhile, IFN can cooperate with TNF, IL-1 and IL-2 to enforce anti-tumorous ability.

The active principles in XZ-C anti-carcinoma traditional Chinese medicine and their effects are following.

1. XZ-C-Z

   250mg/kg or 500mg/kg CVQ polysaccharide can improve significantly the level of IFN-γ produced by mouse spleen cells.

2. XZ-C-D

Ginsenoside (GS) and panaxitriol ginsenoside (PTGS) can induce whole blood cells and monocytes of human beings to produce IFN-αand IFN-γ. It can also recover the low level of IFN-γand IL-2 to the normal.

The IFN potency of ASH polysaccharide on S-180 cell line of acute lymphoblastic leukemia and S_{7811} cell line of acute myelomonocytic leukemia produced after acanthopanax polysaccharide stimulation is 5~10 times more than that of normal control group.

3. XZ-C-E

Hydroxymethyl Poria cocos mushroom polysaccharide has many kinds of physical activity like immunoloregulation, promoting to induce IPN, resisting virus indirectly and alleviating adverse reaction resulting from radiation. Do IFN inducement dynamic experiment on S-180leukaemia cell line by using 50mg/ml Hydroxymethyl Poria cocos mushroom polysaccharide. The results indicate that its potency to induce interferon at all stages is better than that of normal inducement.

4. XZ-C-G (GL)

It can induce IFN activity. Make peritoneal injection of 330mg/kg GL on mice. IFN activity reaches the peak after 20 hours.

VIII. Function of Promoting and Increasing Colony Stimulating Factor

Colony stimulation factor, namely CSF is a kind of glucoprotein with low molecular weight that can stimulate the proliferation and differentiation of marrow hematopoietic stem cells as well as other mature blood cells. Cells that can produce CSF include mononuclear macrophages, T cells, endothelial cells and desmocytes. CSF not only take part in the proliferation and differentiation of hematopoietic stem cells and regulating mature cells, but also play an important role in anti- tumorous immunity of host cells.

The active principles in XZ-C anti-carcinoma traditional Chinese medicine and their effects are following.

1. XZ-C-Q

PAR polysaccharide is able to promote to produce CSF by spleen cells of experimental mice. 100~500ug/ml PAP-II can encourage spleen cells to produce CSF depending on the dose and time with the fittest dose of 100ug/ml and best time of 5d. Moreover, lentinan can also increase the amount of CSF.

2. XZ-C-Q

   Injection of LBP can facilitate the secretion of CSF by mouse spleen T cells and improve the activity of CSF in serum.

3. XZ-C-T

   EBM icariin can promote the proliferation of mouse spleen lymphocytes induced by ConA and bring CSF activity.

IX. Function of Promoting TNF

Tumor necrosis factor, namely TNF is a kind of cytokine that can kill tumor cells directly. Its main effect is to kill or inhibit tumor cells, which can kill some tumor cells or inhibit the proliferation both in vivo and in vitro.

The active principles in XZ-C anti-carcinoma traditional Chinese medicine and their effects are following.

1. XZ-C-Y (PEP)

   It can induce the production of TNF, so as PEP-1. Inject 80~160mg/kg PEP-1, once every four days. Collect peritoneal macrophages (PM), add 10ug LPS into culture medium to cultivate PM. Take the supernatant to determine TNF and IL-1. It can be found that PEP-1 can parallelly increase the auxiliary production of TNF and IL-1. The time of TNF inducement reaches the peak on the 8th day after the second intraperitoneal injection. Compared with the known startup potion BCG, the inducement of TNF has no difference.

2. XZ-C-E

   Carboxymethyl-pachymaran (CMP) is the principle essential component distilled from traditional Chinese medicine Tuckahoe. It can not only strengthen the ability of mouse spleen to create IL-2 and macrophages and promote the activity of T cells, B cells, NK cells and LAK cells; but also encourage the production of TNF. The experiment proves that CMP is an effective potion to promote and induce cytokines.]

3. XZ-C-V

   ABB polysaccharide can promote the production of TNF-b in mouse cells induced by ConA. It can also induce the synthesis of peritoneal macrophages and secrete 20ug/ml TNF-αachyranthes bidentata polysaccharides. The time of TNF-α to reach its peak is 2~6 hours after effects. Peritoneal injection of 100mg/kg achyranthes bidentata polysaccharides can accelerate the production of TNF-α, whose intensity of effects is comparable to that of BCG.

X. The effects on Cell Adhesion Molecule

Most adhesion molecules are glycoproteid and are distributed on cellular surface and extracellular matrix. Adhesion molecules take effect in the corresponding form of ligand-acceptor, resulting in the adhesion between cells, or between cell and stroma, or the adhesion of cell-stroma-cell. These molecules take part in a set of physical pathologic processes, like cellular conduction and activation of information, cellular stretch and movement, formation of thrombus as well as tumor metastasis, etc. Intercellular adhesion molecule-1, namely ICAM-1 is one kind of adhesion molecules in the super family of immune globulins.

The effect of corn stigma as an active principle in XZ-C traditional Chinese anti-carcinoma medicine: Hobtemariam has proved that alcohol extract from corn stigma has significant inhibition on the adhesion of endothelial cells to inhibit effectively the expression of ICAM-1 and the adhesive activity with TNF, LPS as agents.

13. THE SURVEY OF STUDY ON XZ-C IMMUNOLOGIC REGULATION AND CONTROL MEDICATION

I. The Experimental Study

In 1985, the writer made system follow-up statistics to more than 3,000 patients who had accepted cancer operations of chest and abdomen performed by the writer himself. The results show that 2-3 years after the operation, most patients suffer from relapses or metastases. To reduce the relapse rate and increase the curative rate, the clinical fundamental research is a must. If there is no breakthrough of fundamental research, the clinical effect is hard to improve.

Current anti-cancer drugs are cell toxicants that kill both cancer cells and normal cells. The untoward reaction is intense. Now a kind of anti-cancer drug is extracted from traditional Chinese medicine, such as vinblastine, which is extracted from vinca rosea as alkaloid, has been used as anti-cancer drugs for clinical practice. But it will also kill normal cells. So the untoward reaction is intense too. While we hope that anti-cancer drugs have fewer untoward reactions, may be taken by mouth and can build up patient's strength and resistance. Then scientific research is being designed. The plan is to adopt animal experiments of tumor-inhibition in tumor-bearing mice, and from natural drugs to find new anti-cancer drugs, anti-metastasis and anti-relapse drugs, traditional Chinese medicine that only inhibit cancer cells but not normal cells, and new drugs that can adjust the regulation and control relation between host and tumor.

According to cell proliferation cycle theory, anti-cancer drugs must maintain long-term application and make cancer nidi chronically and continuously immerse in drugs. Only in this way can the cell division be inhibited and relapse and metastasis be prevented. Drugs have to be used for a long term, which is the only way to control existing cancer nidi and prevent the formation of nascent cancer cells. But current used anti-cancer drugs induce intense untoward reaction, and therefore they cannot be used chronically and continuously but only be applied as per the treatment course for a minor cycle. All the current anti-cancer drugs have a series of untoward reactions, such as suppressions of immunologic function, bone marrow hematopoietic function and thymus gland, etc. the formation and development of cancer is due to the loss of immune monitoring caused by the reduction of patient's immunity. Therefore, all the anti-cancer drugs must improve immunity and protect immune organs, but should not suppress immunity.

To this end, our laboratory has carried on the following experimental studies for screening of new anti-cancer and anti-metastasis drugs from traditional Chinese medicine.

1. Adopt the method of cancer cells cultured in vitro to carry on the screening experimental study of tumor inhibition rate of traditional Chinese medicine

Screening test in vitro: adopt the method of tumor cells cultured in vitro; observe drugs' direct damage to tumor cells.

1. Method

1.) Preparation of crude drugs' agentia: dry crude drugs; add sixty times of water; heat and extract filtering liquid; decompress filtering liquid; distill it to dryness; form coarse dust; then it can be applied.

2.) Screening test in culture dish: 1×10^5/ml cells of Ehrlich ascites tumor (FAC), or fleshy tumor 180 (S-180), or ascites liver cancer (H_{22}), or carcinoma of uterine cervix, fetal calf serum 10%, coarse crude drugs 500μg/ml, based on the above proportion to inject 20ml solution in culture dish of 10cm×15cm. Place it at 37 centi- degree for a given time. Then compare the quantity of surviving cells with those of control group. Measure suppression ratio of cell proliferation caused by cytotoxicity.

3.) Drug screening: put crude drugs respectively into test tubes that used for culturing human cancer cells. Observe them whether crude drugs have inhibiting action on cancer cells. For 200 kinds of anti-cancer traditional Chinese medicines identified by traditional Chinese doctors, the writer carries on the in vitro screening test in sequence. Also under the same condition, use those medicines to carry on fibrocytes culture of normal person. Measure this medicine's cytotoxicity to fibrocytes, and then compare it with that of control group.

2. The Experimental Result after animal screening tests by the writer in laboratory, 48 kinds of crude drugs (totally 200) certainly have and even hold sovereign inhibiting action on cancer cells proliferation. Tumor inhibition rate is above 90%. But some commonly used traditional Chinese medicines, which are generally considered to have anti-cancer effects, are verified by experiments to have no or little anti-cancer effects. The suppression ratio of another 50 kinds of traditional Chinese medicines is below 30%, such as Chinese clematis, selfheal, earth worm, akebia stem, cortex lycii, rosa multiflora and so on.

2. Make animal model, carry on the experimental study of tumor inhibition rate of traditional Chinese medicine in cancer-bearing animals

1. The screening test of tumor-inhibition in vivo tumor-bearing animal model:

Each batch of experiment needs 240 Kunming mice, divided into 8 groups. Each group has 30 mice. For the first, second, third, fourth, fifth and sixth experimental group, each group chooses one kind of traditional Chinese medicine. The seventh group is set as the blank control group. The eighth group selects fluorouracil or cyclophosphamide as control group. All the mice are inoculated with 1×10^7/ml EAC or S-180 or H_{22} cancer cells through right front axillary subcutaneous injection. After three days, green gram-sized subcutaneous tumor nidi grow. 24 hours after inoculation, each mouse is fed orally with coarse dust of crude drugs, as per the weight 1000mg/kg. The feeding time is once a day for eight weeks. Mice's weights and sizes of tumor nidi need to be measured daily. After eight weeks, 20 mice of each group are executed. Measure their weights of body, tumor, liver, spleen, lung, thymus gland and other organs. Make pathological section to observe tissue condition and know metastatic condition. Another 10 tumor-bearing experimental mice are chronically fed with the screening traditional Chinese medicine. Observe the surviving time and untoward reaction. Calculate prolonged survival rate and tumor inhibition rate. Each batch (i.e. screen each kinds of traditional Chinese medicine) of experimental cycle is three months. Each batch of experiments can simultaneously screen and study six kinds of traditional Chinese medicines or prescriptions. One group of experiments can simultaneously get screening results of six kinds of traditional Chinese medicines.

This research institute can test three experimental groups over the corresponding period. Three master or doctor postgraduates manage one experimental group. In this way can tumor inhibition experiments with eighteen single traditional Chinese medicines or prescriptions be simultaneously studied. In this year, 72 kinds of single traditional Chinese medicines screening experiments which are used for in vivo tumor-inhibition of tumor-bearing mice can be carried on and completed. Thus the writer has continuously carried on four-year experimental studies and another three-year study on pathogenesis and metastatic compound mechanism of tumor-bearing mice and exploration of reasons that why cancerous protuberance can cause the death of host. 1000 tumor-bearing animal models are used every year. A total of about 6,000 tumor-bearing animal models have been done during four years. Each experimental mouse is performed with pathological anatomy on liver, spleen, lung, thymus gland and kidney after death. More than twenty thousand pathological sections have been accomplished to explore and seek cancerogenic micro-pathogens. Use microscopes to observe tumor micrangium establishing and microcirculation condition of 100 tumor-bearing mice. Through experimental studies, the writer firstly finds in China that traditional Chinese medicine TG has obvious effects on suppressing the formation of tumor micrangium. Now this medicine has been used for clinical anti-metastasis treatments on over 200 patients. Curative effects are being observed.

2. Discussion

(1) Through experimental studies, put forward new thought, new knowledge, new concept and new strategy for resisting against cancer: over a period of seven years; over 6,000 tumor-bearing animal models; in vivo tumor-inhibition experiments for anti-cancer, anti-metastasis and anti-relapse in sequence with 200 kinds of natural traditional Chinese medicines; have cognizance of train of thought, knowledge and experience to renew concept, thought, traditional principle and method for traditional anti-cancer work.

Use tumor-bearing animal models to carry on scientific, objective and strict experimental screening, analysis and evaluation on 200 kinds of traditional Chinese medicines in sequence with so called anti-cancer curative effects by Chinese Medicine Literature. Results show that only 48 kinds of medicines have better anti-cancer effects. Although another 152 kinds of medicines are the commonly used anti-cancer medicines by veteran practioner of TCM, they have been verified by this group of experimental screenings to have no anti-cancer effects or little tumor inhibition rate. These 200 kinds of traditional Chinese medicines used for experimental screening are chosen from over ten books with TCM anti-cancer famous prescriptions. They are also common medicines with anti-cancer effects described in

Journal of Traditional Chinese Medicine and literature reports. While the experimental study results prove that 152 kinds of medicines have no tumor inhibition rate or low anti-cancer effects. The reason might be that Chinese Medicine Literature has no distinction between lump, abdominal mass of Chinese medicine and cancer of modern medicine. 48 kinds of medicines in this group, which are screened through animal experiments, really have better tumor inhibition rate. Through optimization grouping and repeated trials, different medicines are composed to XZ-C$_{1-10}$ immunoregulation anti-cancer Chinese materia medica preparation. It has been verified clinically for sixteen years. Over 12,000 cancer patients have used this preparation and obtained better curative effects.

Through experimental screening study results of this group, we have realized that TCM prescriptions are gained from prolonged experience. The prescription matches symptoms of disease and is the synthesis composed with various kinds of crude drugs. As seen from Chinese Medicine Literature, symptoms of abdominal mass and accumulation seem similar to those of cancer. Traditional Chinese medicines are used to treat abdominal mass. Sometimes symptoms can be improved, but not all abdominal mass are cancers. In general, TCM has no effect on cancer. So we should adopt modern scientific methods to verify, observe and reevaluate cancer resistance and carcinogenicity of various crude drugs in prescriptions of traditional Chinese medicine, and avoid unscientific parts of traditional Chinese medicine and pharmacology.

In medicine screening experiments, it's found that single crude drugs have worse tumor-inhibition effects than optimization grouping compound of many kinds of crude drugs. The reason may be that single crude drugs can only suppress tumor proliferation. While optimization grouping compound of many kinds of crude drugs not only can suppress tumor proliferation of tumor-bearing mice, but also can build up strength, improve immunity, promote to produce cancer-inhibition cytokines and protect normal cells.

Since 1992, over seven-year scientific experiments, different medicines are screened and composed to XZ-C$_{1-10}$ immunoregulation anti-cancer Chinese materia medica preparation. This medicine owns curative effects on anti-cancer, supporting healthy energy to eliminate evils, clearing away heat and toxic materials and activating blood circulation to dissipate blood stasis.

From experimental study to clinical verification, and then from clinic to experiment again, the writer has organized to set up the joint breakthrough research coordination group for cancer prevention and resistance. This coordination group has experimental study base and verification base of clinical application. The former is in medical college and medical university laboratory; the latter is in clinical medical department of nationwide coordination group for cancer prevention and resistance studies combined with traditional Chinese and western medicine. From experimental study to clinical verification means the clinical application on the basis of successful experimental study. Then new problems are found during the clinical application, which need fundamental experimental studies. Afterwards new experimental results are applied to clinical verification. Experiments → clinic → experiments once more → clinic once more, recurrent ascent continuously; through eight-year clinical practical experiences, knowledge also continues to improve. Summation, analysis, reflection and evaluation ascend to theory, putting forward new knowledge, new concept, new thought, new strategy and new therapeutic route and scheme.

Breakthrough research experience of coordination group includes: ① Choose the way that professors, experts and postgraduates of universities and colleges coordinate to carry on scientific researches and joint breakthrough; advocate large-scale coordination of scientific researches; give prominence to concentrate scientific research and technology strength of all parties; enrich anti-cancer strength. ② Cancer prevention and resistance should make use of nation-wide advantages; give full play to the advantage of traditional Chinese medicine; conform to actual conditions in China. ③ Fundamental studies are important, but application and development research are more important. It should be observed that fundamental research → applied research →development research. Emphases are application and curative effects. Focus on increasing life quality of cancer patients, improving symptoms and prolonging survival time. ④ Restore the conservation of outpatient records (since 1976, Hubei province cancels conservation system of outpatient records and sends them to patients.); fill in full and detailed outpatient records. Therefore, full information of clinical verification is obtained to be convenient for analysis, statistics and follow-up survey (Generally, 80%~90% patients accept outpatient service, 10%~20% patients receive hospital treatment. At present hospital records are reserved to analyze and study clinical data. That 80%~90% patients accept outpatient service leads to the inexistence of outpatient records. Analysis, statistics and follow-up survey of patients' curative effects in out-patient department, and follow-up statistics of scientific researches may become impossible. Hospital records can only observe short-term curative effects; while the conservation of outpatient records can observe long-term curative effects.) Restoring and reserving outpatient records data is favorable toward outpatient clinical research to improve medical quality.

(2) Experimental work of finding new anti-cancer drugs, anti-metastasis and anti-relapse drugs from natural drugs: it's aimed at screening new anti-cancer drugs with non-tolerance, no untoward effect and high selectivity that can chronically be taken by mouth. As known to all, although current anti-cancer drugs can suppress cancer cells proliferation, due to their severe untoward effect, while using many patients have to stop administration. Afterwards cancer cells proliferate again and begin to have drug tolerance. Such as the famous anti-cancer drug formyli sarcolysine quinine, as seen from ongoing cancer cells tissue cultures, drug tolerance is up to 20,000 times. Before the appearance of drug tolerance, the dosage is usually only several milligrams. While when drug tolerance is produced, such dosage cannot meet the demand. Then it is necessary to increase the dosage. But when its dosage increases to ten times, it will cause the death of patient. Therefore, drug tolerance of cancer cells on anti-cancer drug and untoward effect of anti-cancer drug on host are long-standing problems that puzzle tumor treatment researchers. Our purpose of finding new drugs is to avoid those disadvantages and screen anti-cancer drugs with non-tolerance, no untoward effect and high selectivity that best can chronically be taken by mouth. Western anti-cancer drugs have single ingredient. Micro dosage is effective, but it will suppress normal cells. Its toxic reaction is quite strong. Some current anti-cancer drugs are extracted from traditional Chinese medicine, such as vincristine, camptothecin and colchicine; these alkaloids are similar to traditional anti-cancer drugs, i.e. micro drug is effective, but toxicity is very high.

The question is whether anti-cancer traditional Chinese medicine, which can suppress the growth of cancer cells but not kill normal cells, can be extracted from TCM. Through several years' experimental screening, the writer finally finds such kind of TCM with rather ideal anti-cancer effects. Usually when the dosage reaches 500µg/ml, it has inhibiting action on cancer cells. The writer also finds XZ-C$_1$ and XZ-C$_4$ drugs that can 100% suppress cancer cells and never kill normal cells. XZ-C$_1$, XZ-C$_4$ and XZ-C$_8$ also can improve the immunologic function of host, which is a superior feature of anti-cancer TCM.

As seen XZ-C series of TCM, its anti-cancer effect changes as the change of dosage. When the dosage is 250µg/ml, it can only suppress 60% cancer cells; when the dosage is 125µg/ml, suppression ratio is zero. Micro A-type drugs will be effective, such as vinblastine, berberine in Chinese goldthread, and myrobalan fruit in alkaloid, etc. But they can also suppress normal cell proliferation, which is same to traditional anti-cancer drugs. B-type drugs are other anti-cancer TCM. Only high concentration is effective. That is, micro dosage has no inhibiting action on cancer cells. Effect is directly proportional to dosage. If the dosage is larger, curative effects will be better, such as XZ-C$_{1A}$ and XZ-C$_{1B}$.

3. Verification of clinical effects over the past ten years, the writer has applied experimental crude drugs to clinical medicine. XZ-C series drugs have distinctive clinical effects. That is, a certain period after the administration of B-type drugs, cancer cells neither proliferate nor shrink, while the patient begins to restore vigorous energy. Several months later, the physical strength recovers gradually. The tumor starts to shrink slowly. That is probably not toxic effect on cancer cells, but the result of creating a circumstance that is adverse to cancer cells proliferation in organisms. The long-term administration has no toxic cumulative effect on normal cells. Many patients have taken XZ-C$_1$ and XZ-C$_4$ drugs for 3-5 years, there is still no relapse, metastasis and untoward effect. The long-term plentiful administration can obtain unexpected good results.

Different types of XZ-C preparation match with various kinds of cancers, such as cancer of alimentary canal, lung cancer and cancer of uterus, etc. Compound prescriptions must be made from symptoms. Only in this way can good results be obtained.

Different from traditional medicinal broth, what the writer chooses is the mixture with every kind of single crude drug through 100 mesh screening. These crude drugs are composed as compound prescription, which is not the decoction of combined preparation, but is the mixed preparation. This kind of mixture can preserve pharmacological characteristics of each crude drug. Prolonged use of this drug will not produce the untoward effect. Probing into the application way of crude drugs is quite significant.

In actual clinical medicine, will the prolonged use cause any problems? Patients can be divided into two kinds of cases: one type of patients take considerable amount of drugs with no abnormalities. The curative effects appear slowly. Many patients have taken XZ-C$_4$ drugs for 3-5 years. They have high spirits and good appetites. Physical strength recovers better; body condition strengthens; state of an illness is stable; patient's condition is good. The daily clinical dosage is about 20g of coarse drugs, in which the basic remedy is anti-cancer drugs, accounting for about 10% (equal to 40g crude drugs). It is considerably different from the dosage of traditional Chinese medicine.

When will curative effects present after taking medicine? Usually 1-3 months reach peak. Therefore if patients can survive for more than six months, then about 90% patients' symptoms can be improved remarkably; 50% patients' cancer proliferation will stop; about 80% patients' survival time is lengthened.

The completely significant thing is that XZ-C$_{1-4}$ crude drugs preparations have favorable abirritation. Medium and advanced stages of liver cancer and cancer of pancreas both produce severe pain. Patients who have used this kind of crude drugs preparation for over one month hardly feel any pain. They even don't have to be injected with analgesic drugs. This is extremely amazing.

Extracts of single crude drugs and compounded crude drugs almost produce the same curative effect. But when decocted with traditional compound prescription, extracts of single crude drugs are less effective. Presumably this is caused by the existence of interaction among drugs. In terms of cancer treatment, the better choice is compounded medicinal preparations.

Please note that some crude drugs can also promote the reproduction of cancer cells but suppress normal cells' growth, especially mineral drugs and animal drugs. Such as pallas pit viper, hairy antler and others, even the microdosis can promote above reactions. The centipede can damage renal tubules.

Akihiko Sato says that cancer resistance of natural drugs can be divided into three categories. The first category is that ingredients of natural drugs have the effect on killing cancer cells, such as vinblastine. The second one is that polysaccharides of some drugs (e.g. purple ganoderma lucidum and evodia rutaecarpa), due to the action on enhancing immunologic function, is very popular as immunotherapy. While there is a limit that polysaccharides almost have no effect on progressive stage and advanced stage of cancer. But because of fewer untoward effects, they can be used as favorable adjuvanticity drugs. The third one is B-type anti-cancer drugs, whose active mechanism is not yet clear. When B-type drug is in high concentration, it can suppress the proliferation of cancer cells but not normal cells. Also it has fewer untoward effects and can be taken for a lone time. But it can neither kill cancer cells nor promote immunologic function. The B-type anti-cancer drug is considered as a kind of new drug.

In nearly a decade, because the writer had the heart issues he rarely goes out and doesn't attend the meeting out of town and other places so that sitting down to do the research work solidly on the detail animal experiment and clinical validation and got many results. With the intensive study, the writer has contacted with a large number of patients monthly, and collected much information that is not recorded in books and literature. And the writer has an intimate knowledge of many patients' epidemiology, clinical symptom, evolution of physical sign and analysis, evaluation and reflection on progress. The writer was sitting down to do a series of the basic research animal experimental work with the Master degree students and the experimental researchers.

14. EXPERIMENTAL STUDY AND OBSERVATION OF ITS CLINICAL CURATIVE EFFECTS ON TREATMENT OF MALIGNANT TUMORE WITH XZ-C TRADITIONAL CHINESE ANTI-CANCER IMMUNOLOGIC REGULATION AND CONTROL MEDICATIONS

In order to look for the traditional herb medicine with actually curative effect and without toxication and adverse reaction, this surgical tumor research institute has screened 200 kinds of Chinese herbal medicines with so-called anticancer reaction recorded on Chinese herbal medicine books for tumor-inhibition reaction on the solid carcinoma in the tumor-bearing animal models one by one in the past 4 years. Through long-term in-vivo tumor-inhibiting animal experiments, we have screened 48 kinds of Chinese herbal medicines with relatively good tumor-inhibition rate that can prolong the survival time, protect the immune organ and obviously improve the immunologic function. According to the clinical conditions, the anticancer medicines screened are combined into 2 compounds including $Z-C_1$ and $Z-C_4$ with better anti-cancer reaction than each single medicine. In the original screening, we carried out the tumor-inhibiting animal experiment for each single medicine and now we further carry out the experimental study on these two groups of compounds for the tumor-inhibiting reaction in the solid tumor of the tumor-bearing rats.

1. Experimental Study on Animal

1). Materials and Method

1.) Experimental animal: 260 Kunming clon white rats, half of male and female respectively, weight:21±2g, 8~10 weeks.

2.) Cell strains and inoculation: hepatic carcinoma H_{22} cell strains, the fresh tumor bodies from the rats with tumor were prepared into the single cell suspended liquid, after dyeing and counting of the cancer cells ($1x\ 10^6$/ml), 0.2ml normal saline of cancer cell was subject to subcutaneous vaccination at the front axilla at the right side of each rat.

3.) Drugs and experimental group: the traditional herb medicines $Z-C_1$ and $Z-C_4$ were entirely developed and prepared by Hubei Branch of China Anti-cancer Research Cooperation of Chinese Traditional Medicine and Western Medicine, the former was a compound and the latter was a medicinal powder. The chemotherapy control medicine used by the chemotherapy group was cyclophosphane (CTX).

Experimental group: the animals with H_{22} cancer cell transplanted were divided into four groups randomly: ① traditional herb medicine Z-C_1 group (90 rats). The rats were subject to gastriclavage once every day after 24h of transplantation of cancer cells, 0.8ml per rat every time, equivalent to 1.4mg of the dried medicinal herbs. ②Traditional herb medicine Z-C_4 group (90 rats), as to the dose and gastriclavage method, ditto. ③Chemotherapy group (50 rats), from the next day after transplantation of cancer cells, they were subject to gastriclavage with CTX50mg/kg weight every other day. ④Control group (30 rats), they were subject to gastriclavage with normal saline every day from the next day after transplantation of the cancer cells, 0.8ml/rat.

4.) Observation of indexes: measure the weight of the rats every 3d, measure the diameter of the tumor with vernier caliper, measure the immunologic function and blood picture. Half of each group as Group A, subject to tumor-bearing experiment, regular killing of the rats in batches, separation of tumor and weighing of the tumor and then calculation of tumor-inhabiting rate. The tumor was subject to the pathological section and a few of the specimens were subject to the observation of ultra-structural organization. The rest half of each group as Group B. The tumor-bearing experimental rats were drenched for a long time until they met with natural death. Then the tumor was separated and weighed, the long-term inhibition rate and life elongation rate of the tumor was calculated.

2). Experimental result

1.) The tumor-inhibition effect of Z-C Medicine on Rats bearing hepatic carcinoma H_{22}: in the second week after administration of Z-C_1, the tumor-inhibition rate was 40% and the one in the fourth week was 45% and 58% in the sixth week. The tumor-inhibition rate after administration of Z-C_4 was 55%, 68% in the fourth week and 70% in the sixth week. (P<0.01) the tumor-inhibiting rate after administration of CTX was 45% in the second week, 45% in the fourth week and 49% in the sixth week (See Fig. 1 and 2).

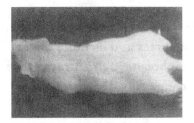

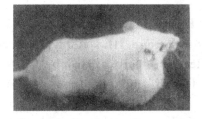

Figure 1 Z-C1, C4 treatment group
30d after inoculation of hepatoma H22

Figure 2 Control group
30d after inoculation of hepatoma H22

2.) The effect of Z-C medicine on the survival time of the rats bearing hepatic carcinoma H_{22}: the average survival time of Z-C_1, Z-C_4 and CTX was longer than the one of the normal saline control group (P<0.01); Z-C medicine played a role in obviously prolonging the survival time. Through comparison with the control group, the life elongation rate of Z-C_1 group was 85%, the one of Z-C_4 group was 200% and the one of CTX group was 9.8%. The rats in Z-C$_1$ and CTX in Group B met with death in 75d. 6 rats bearing carcinoma in Z-C$_4$ survived after seven months.

3.) Both Z-C$_1$ and Z-C$_4$ medicine improved the immunologic function and Z-C$_4$ obviously improved the immunologic function, increased the white blood cells and red blood cells, without any effect on the hepatic function and kidney function and without damage to the hepatic and kidney section. CTX decreased the white blood cells and reduced the immunologic function with the renal damage to the kidney section. The thymus in the control group was obviously atrophic (Fig. 1-4) while the one of Z-C$_1$ and Z-C$_2$ therapy group was not atrophic but a little hypertrophic (Fig.1-3).

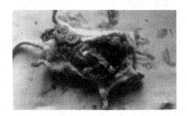

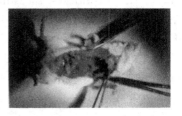

Figure 3 Z-C4 group
30d after inoculation of hepatoma
H22 thymus hypertrophy

Figure 4 Control
30d after inoculation of liver cancer
H22 marked atrophy of thymus

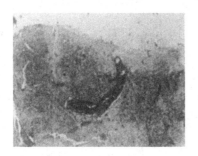

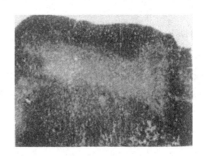

Figure 5 thymic tumor-bearing
control group, HE × 100 lymphocytes
decreased cortical atrophy, Cortex
form a lymphocyte empty band

Figure 6 Z-C4 treated thymus HE × 100
thymic cortex and medulla thickening,
lymphocyte high, intravascular
congestion degree intensive

Pathological section of thymus in the control group: the cortex of the thymus was atrophic, the cells were discrete and the blood vessel met with sludge (Fig. 1-5). The pathological section of the thymus in Z-C$_4$ therapy group displayed that the cortical area of the thymus built up, the lymphocyte was dense, the epithelium reticulocyte increased and the thymus corpuscles increased (Fig. 1-6).

2. Observation on Clinic Application

1. Clinical information

(1) Hubei Branch of China Anti-cancer Research Cooperation of Chinese Traditional Medicine and Western Medicine, Anti Carcinoma Metastasis and Recurrence Research Office and Shuguang Tumor Specialized Outpatient Department had treated 4, 698 carcinoma patients in Stage III and IV or in metastasis and recurrence with Z-C medicine combined with western medicine from 1994 to Nov. 2002, among which there were 3, 051 men patients and 1,647 women patients. The youngest one was 11 years old and the oldest one was 86 years old, the high invasion age was 40~69 years. All groups of the patients were entirely subject to the diagnosis of pathological histology or definitive diagnosis with ultrasonic B, CT and MRI iconography. According to the staging standard of UICC, all the cases were entirely the patients in medium and advanced stage over Stage III. In this group, there were 1,021 hepatic carcinoma patients, among which there were 694 primary lesion hepatic carcinoma patients and 327 metastatic hepatic carcinoma patients; there were 752 patients suffering from carcinoma of lung, among which there were 699 patients suffering from the primary carcinoma of lung and 53 patients suffering from the metastatic carcinoma of lung; there were 668 gastric carcinoma patients, 624 patients suffering from esophagus cardia carcinoma, 328 patients suffering from rectum carcinoma of anal canal, 442 patients suffering from carcinoma of colon, 368 patients suffering from breast carcinoma, 74 patients suffering from adenocarcinoma of pancreas, 30 patients suffering from carcinoma of bile duct, 43 patients suffering from retroperitoneal tumor, 38 patients suffering from oophoroma, 9 patients suffering from cervical carcinoma, 11 patients suffering from cerebroma, 34 patients suffering from thyroid carcinoma, 38 patients suffering from nasopharyngeal carcinoma, 9 patients suffering from melanoma, 27 patients suffering from kidney carcinoma, 48 patients suffering from carcinoma of urinary bladder, 13 patients suffering from leukemia, 47 patients suffering from metastasis of supraclavicular lymph nodes, 35 patients suffering various fleshy tumors and 39 patients suffering from other malignancies.

(2) Medicine and medication: the treatment aims to support healthy energy to eliminate evils, soften and resolve the hard mass and supplement qi and blood. $Z-C_1$ is the compound, 150ml to be taken on the daily basis, $Z-C_4$ is powder, 10g to be taken on the daily basis. According to the analysis and differentiation of the diseases, anti-cancer powder shall be taken orally and the anti-cancer apocatastasis paste shall be applied externally for the solid tumor or the metastatic tumor. In case of being in pain, anti-cancer aponic paste shall be applied externally. Icterus removal soup or dropsy removal soup shall be taken orally for the patients suffering from icterrus and the ascites.

(3) Therapeutic evaluation: it pays attention to the short-term curative effect and iconography indexes as well as the survival time of long-term curative effect, quality of life and immunologic indexes. Attention shall be paid to the changes in subjective signs in administration of drugs. It will be effective when the subjective signs are improved and last over one month; otherwise, it will be ineffective. As to the quality of life (Karnofsky Performance Status), it will be

effective when it is improved and lasts over one month, otherwise, it will be ineffective. As to the evaluation standard of the curative effect of solid tumor, it can be divided into four levels according to the changes in size of tumor: Level I: disappearance of tumor; Level II: tumor reduces 1/2; Level III: softening of tumor; Level IV: no change or enlargement of level tumor.

2. Curative results

(1) The symptom was improved, the quality of life was improved, the survival time was prolonged: among the 4,277 carcinoma patients in medium and advanced stage who took Z-C medicine with the return visit over 3 months, the case history had the specific observation record of the curative effect, see Table 1-1. It improved the quality of life of the patients in an all-round way, see Table 1-2.

Table 1-1 General information about 4,277 patients suffering from recurrence and metastasis

		Hepatic carcinoma	Carcinoma of lung	Gastric carcinoma	Esophagus cardia carcinoma	Rectum carcinoma of anal canal	Carcinoma of colon	Breast carcinoma	adenocarcinoma of pancreas
No. of cases		1 021	752	668	624	328	442	368	74
Male: female		4:1	4.4:1	2.25:1	3.1:1	1:1	2.1:1	Female	3.2:1
Focus	Primary	694 (68.6%)	699 (93.9%)						
	Metastasis	327 (31.2%)	53 (6.1%)						
Usual metastasis part in this group		Metastatic lung (2) From the stomach (31.2%)	Metastasis of supraclavicular lymph nodes (11.6%)	Metastatic lever (23.8%) Lung metastasis (3%)	Upper metastasis of compact bone (13.1%)	Reoccurrence rate (14.8%)	Metastatic lever (16.0%)	Metastasis of supraclavicular lymph nodes (17.5%)	Metastatic lever (11.7%)
		From esophagus cardia (19.5%) From recta (31.2%)	Brain metastasis (3.1%) Bone metastasis (4.6%)	Metastasis of peritoneum (29.1%) Upper metastasis of compact bone (6.1%)	Metastatic lever (8.3%)	Metastatic lever (7.0%)	Metastasis of peritoneum (6.0%)	Metastasis of axillary lymph nodes (15.0%) Bone metastasis (5.0%)	Rear metastasis of peritoneum (39.1%)
Age	high invasion (year) %	30~39 (76.2)	50~69 (71.6)	40~49 (73.4)	40~69 (80.4)	40~49 (75.2)	30~69 (88.0)	40~59 (65.9)	40~59 (70.0)
	Oldest (year) %	11	20	17	30	27	27	29	34
	Youngest (year) %	86	80	77	77	78	76	80	68

Table 1-2 Observation of curative effect on 4 277 patients: fully improving the quality of life of the carcinoma patients in medium and advanced stage

Improvement	Vigor	Appetite	Reinforcement of physical force	Improvement in generalized case	Increase of body weight	Improvement of sleep	The restriction of improvement activity and capability released activity	self servicing normal walking	Resumption of work Engaged in light work
No. of cases (%)	4071	3986	2450	479	2938	1005	1038	3220	479
	95.2	93.2	57.3	11.2	68.7	23.5	24.3	75.3	11.2

In this group, all of them were the patients in medium and advanced stage. After taking the medicine, their symptoms were improved to different extents with the effective rate of 93.2%. With respect to the improvement of the quality of life (as per Karnofsky Performance Status), it rose to 80 scores on average after administration from 50 on average before administration; the patients in this group met with the different metastasis and dysfunction of the organs about Stage III. It was reported by the previous statistic information that the mesoposition survival time of this kind of patients was about 6 months. The longest time among this group of the cases reached up to 11 years; another patient suffering from hepatic carcinoma had taken Z-C medicine for ten years and a half; two patients suffering from hepatic carcinoma met with frequency encountered carcinomatous lesion in the left and right liver and it entirely subsided through secondary CT reexamination after the patient took Z-C medicine for half a year and the state of the disease had been stable over half a year. One patient suffering from double-kidney carcinoma met with the widespread metastasis of abdominal cavity after removal of one kidney, after taking Z-C medicine, he was entirely recovered and began to work again. 3 patients suffering from carcinoma of lung, with the lung not removed through explaraton, had taken Z-C medicine over three years and a half. 2 patients suffering from gastric remnant carcinoma had taken Z-C medicine for 8 years. 3 patients suffering from reoccurrence of rectal carcinoma had taken Z-C medicine for 3 years. 1 patient suffering from metastatic liver and rib of the mastocarcinoma had taken Z-C medicine for 8 years. 1 patient suffering from the recurrent bladder carcinoma after operation of renal carcinoma had not met with the carcinoma for 9 years and a half after taking Z-C medicine. All of these patients were the ones in the medium and advanced stage that could not be operated once more or treated with radiotherapy or chemotherapy. They only took Z-C medicine without other medicines for treatment. Up to today, they are reexamined and get the medicine at the out-patient department every month. Through taking the medicine for a long time, the state of the disease is controlled in the stable state to make the organism and the tumor in balanced state for a relatively long time and get a relatively good survival with tumor, in this way, the symptoms of the patients are improved, the quality of life is improved and the survival time is prolonged.

(2) As to 84 patients suffering from solid tumor and 56 patients suffering from enlargement of upper lymph node of metastatic compact bone, after taking Z-C series medicines orally and applying Z-C3 anti-cancer apocatastasis paste, they met with good curative effects, see table 1-3.

Table 1-3 Changes of 84 patients suffering from solid tumor and 56 patients suffering from metastatic mode after applying Z-C paste externally

	Solid tumor				Enlargement of upper lymph node of metastatic compact bone			
	Disappearance	Shrinkage 1/2	Softening	No change	Disappearance	Shrinkage 1/2	Softening	No change
No. of cases (%)	12 14.2	28 33.3	32 38.0	12 14.2	12 21.4	22 39.2	14 25.0	8 14.2
Total effective rate (%)	85.7				85.7			

(3) 298 patients suffering from carcinoma pain obtained the obvious pain alleviation effects after taking Z-C medicine orally and applying Z-C anti-cancer apocatastasis paste externally, see Table 1-4.

Clinical menifetation	Pain			
	Light alleviation	Obvious alleviation	Disappearance	Avoidance
No of cases (%)	52 17.3	139 46.8	93 31.2	14 4.7
Total effective rate (%)	95.3			

3. Discussion about Z-C Medicine Experiment and Clinic Curative Effect

1.) Tumor-inhibition effect of $Z-C_{1-4}$ Medicine on hepatic carcinoma H_{22} rats bearing tumor

It was found that after the medicine was taken to H_{22} tumor-bearing rats for two weeks, four weeks and six weeks, the tumor inhibition rate increased with the prolongation of the administration time, the tumor inhibition rate of $Z-C_4$ in the 6th week reached up to 70%. Through two repeated experiments in succession, the results were stable, which indicated that the tumor-inhibition effect of Chinese herb medicine was slow and it would increase gradually, that is to say, the tumor-inhibition effect was of positive correlation to the accumulated dosage of Chinese herb medicine.

The effect on the survival time of hepatic carcinoma H_{22} tumor-bearing rats from $Z-C_1$ and $Z-C_4$ medicine: it was proven by the experimental results that $Z-C_1$ and $Z-C_4$ medicine could obviously prolong the survival time of the tumor-bearing rats, especially $Z-C_4$, it could prolong the survival time as long as 200%, more than that, $Z-C_4$ could remarkably improve the immunologic function of the organism, protect the immune organ and the bone marrow, alleviate the toxic action and side effect of the radiotherapy and chemotherapy medicines.

Furthermore, no toxic action or side effect had been found in the past 12 months after the rats took the medicine. The above-mentioned experimental study offered the beneficial basis to the clinical application.

2.) Clinical curative effect

Based on the experimental study, it had been applied to various clinical carcinomas, most of the patients were the ones over Stage III and IV, namely: the ones suffering from the cancer of late stage that could not be removed with exploratory operation; the ones with the exploratory operation without operation indication; the ones meeting with metastasis or reoccurrence in short term or long term after operation of the carcinoma; the ones suffering from hepatic metastasis, lung metastasis or brain metastasis in late stage or the ones accompanied with carcinoma hydrops and hydrops abdominis; the ones suffering from various carcinomas conservative removal operation with the exploratory operation only for the anastomosis of intestines and stomach or colostomy but not for removal and the ones not suitable for the operation, chemotherapy and radiotherapy and so on. Through over 10 years' clinical application and systematic observation, $Z\text{-}C_1$ and $Z\text{-}C_4$ medicine had obtained remarkable curative effect and no toxic action and side effect had been found after long-term administration. It had been proven by the clinical observation that $Z\text{-}C_1$ and $Z\text{-}C_4$ medicine could improve the survival quality of the carcinoma patients in medium and late stage in an all-round way, improve the whole immunity, control the hyperplasia of the cancer cells, consolidate and enhance the long-term curative effect. The oral-taken and external-applied Z-C medicine had good curative effect in softening and shrinking body surface metastatic tumor. With the assistance of intervention or treatment with cannula spray pump for medicine, it could protect liver, kidney and bone marrow hemopoietic system and the immune organ and improve the immune function.

3.) Good pain alleviation effect of Z-C anti-cancer pain alleviation paste

Pain is the relatively remarkable and painful symptom of the carcinoma patients in late stage, the common pain reliever had no remarkable effect on carcinoma pain, the stupefacient pain reliever had the addiction and dependence, Z-C anti-cancer pain alleviation paste had strong pain alleviation effect with a long maintenance time. It was proven through 298 cases of clinical verification that the effective rate was 78.0%, the total effective rate was 95.3%, after repeated application, there were no toxic action or side effect, without addiction. The paid alleviation effect was stable and it was an effective therapeutic method for the carcinoma patients to get rid of the pain and improve the quality of life.

Through experimental research and clinical validation, our experience is: Chinese medicine with Chinese characteristics has its unique advantage in cancer treatment, such as a strong overall concept, conditioning prominent role, mild side effects, can relieve pain, relieve symptoms, and significantly improved quality of life of patients, can mobilize the body's immune function and overall disease resistance, improve the therapeutic effect.

4. The research on cytokine induction factors of XZ-C anticancer immune regulation and control medications

1). XZ-C$_4$ induces endogenous cytokines

(1). Through the experiments: XZ-C$_4$ has many immune strengthening functions and has closely relationship to the induced endogenous cytokines

(2) XZ-C$_4$ can recover the reduction of the white blood cells, granulation cells and platelets.

(3) XZ-C$_4$ can have the direct function on GM-CSF production from granulation cell (GM) through IL-1β, also increase TNF, IFN etc all of kind of the cell factors, which are possible the indirect function.

(4). XZ-C$_4$ can increase the Th1 cell factors, which were decrease in the cancer patients. There are the curative effects on the anemia and the white blood cells decrease due to the chemotherapy.

(5). The experiment analysis showed that XZ-C$_4$ not only protects the bone marrow function, but also has direct function on the tumor cell division.

In brief, XZ-C$_4$ can induce the tumor division and natural death through the autocrine which produce all of kind of factors. The autocrine is the secretory things from the host to affect the host's function. XZ-C$_4$ probably will become the induction therapy to the tumor division in the future.

2). XZ-C$_4$ inhibiting cancer development and metastasis

The malignant development is defined as tumor cells accepting invasion and metastasis characters during the proliferation. Cancer research need to have good repeated animal models. Then the good repeated animal model was made from the mice fibrosis cancernoma QR-32. QR-32 cannot proliferate after inoculation in the skin, and will completely disappear; there were no metastasis lump after injecting into the vein. However, if QR-32 was injected with Gelatin sponge together under the skin in the mice, QR-32 will become the proliferating tumor cells QRSP.

In vitro culturing QRSP and then transfer into another mice, even if there is no foreign thing, the tumors will grow such as the lung metastasis will happen after injection in the vein.

XZ-C$_4$ was used in the animal models to search the effects of the tumor development. To divide this animal models into two steps: the process from QR-32 to QRSP(early progress) and from the QRSP to tumor(later progress). After using XZ-C$_4$, the tumor development will be inhibited in these two models, especially the former will be inhibited significantly. And this has relationship with the dose of the medication.

On the survival experiment the animal models of the inoculation of the QR-32 AND Gelatin sponge died during 65 days, however in XZ-C group the mice survival rate for 150 days was 30%. XZ-C$_4$ can increase the immune effects and reduce the side effects of other anticancer medication.

This research proved that XZ-C$_4$ has inhibition of the cancer progression function and inhibit cancer invasion and metastasis.

3). Z-C1+Z-C4 anti-cancer immune regulation medication

Z-C1+Z-C4 anti-cancer immune regulation medication has the following characteristics:

- An overall improvement in the quality of life of patients with advanced cancer
- Protect Thymus and increase immune function and nurse bone morrow and blood and increase immune function
- Enhance physical fitness, reduce pain and improve physical strength
- Enhance therapeutic effect and reduce the side effects of chemotherapy.

The characteristic of Z-C immune regulation and control anti-cancer medications

A, Chemotherapy

- It causes the side effect of Gastrointestinal system
- It cause the immune function decrease in the whole body
- It caused that Bone marrow is inhibited

B, Z-C1 and Z-C8 therapy

- Increase the immune function in the whole body
- Protect Thymus and Spleen

Increase appetite ; reduce the pain; improve the life quality; enhance fitness and improve physical strength

5. Z-C Medication is the Modern Production of Traditional Herb Medication

Z-C medicine was neither the experiential prescription nor the prescription made by the famous doctor of traditional Chinese medicine, but 48 kinds of traditional herb medicines screened from 200 kinds of common Chinese herbal medicines with so-called anticancer reaction after the animal screening test in batches and vitro screening and screening of tumor-inhibition rate in the tumor-bearing animal body one by one through over 4000 tumor-bearing animal models in the past 7 years with the modern medical method, experimental tumor study method and modern pharmacody and drug effect study method.

The substantial foundation of the traditional prescriptions that bring its unique curative effect into play in clinic was its chemical compositions. The changes in quality and quantity of the chemical compositions would directly affect the curative effect of the prescription in clinic. Therefore, it is necessary to study the changes in quality and quantity of the chemical compositions in the prescription and find out the main effective compositions in the prescription. Z-C medicine basically finds out its effect of medicine, action, molecular weight and constitutional formula and makes the study on the traditional prescription on a new step.

The prescription of Z-C medicine is the innovation and reform of the traditional herbal prescriptions, it is not the bonded solutions through mixing and boiling, but the granular concentration or powder of the medical compounds. The dried medicinal herbs in the medical compound still remain its original compositions without any change in pharmacological action, molecular weight and constitutional formula. It is made with modern scientific method but not through chemical combination, in this way, the original compositions and functions are remained for assessing and affirming the action and curative effect of the medical compounds.

15. BILOGICAL RESPONSE MODIFICATION(BRM), TRADITIONAL CHINESE ANTICANCER MEDICATIONS SIMILAR TO BRM AND TUMOR TREATMENT

Biological reaction modification (BRM) explores the new field of the tumor biological therapy. Currently BRM as the fourth methods of the tumor treatment gets widely attention in the world.

1. The theory of biological reaction modification(BRM)

Oldham in 1982 built BRM theory. Based this in 1984 he advanced the fourth modality of cancer treatment-----biological therapy again. According to this, in the normal condition, there is the dynamic equilibrium between the tumor and the body. The development of the tumors, and even invasion and metastasis, completely is caused by the loss of this equilibrium. If this unbland situation is adjusted to the normal level, the tumor growth can be controlled and will disappear. The anticancer mechanism of BRM in detail as the following:

a. Improve the host defence abilities or decrease the immune inhabitation of the tumors to the host to reach the immune response to the tumors.
b. Look for the biological active things in natural or gene combination to enhance the host defense abilities.
c. Reduce the host response induced by the tumor cells
d. Promote the tumors to division and mature to become the normal cells
e. Reduce the side effects of the chemotherapy and redio therapy and enhance

The host toleration.

The biological therapy is to adjust this biological reaction through from the outside of the body to add,induct or active the cell toxicities biological active factor or cells in. The biological theapy is different from the previous three therapy models such as surgery, radioactive and chemotherapy, to directly attack the target of the tumors.the biological reaction systems inside the host bodys. The therapy ranges of BRM is beyond the traditional immune therapy concepts, which the equilium between the body and the tumors is not limit to the immune reaction, but involved in all kinds of the regulation genes and cell factors related to the tumor proliferations.

The tumor biological therapy mainly includes :1). The injection of the immune active cells2).The production /application of the cytokines and cell factors

3).Specific autoimmune including the application of the tumor cells groups xxxx, monoantibody and its crossing-thingsxxx.

The cytokines and liquid factors in the host immune system is in subtle control. If the balance of them was lost, the body response or the answer abilities will be affected significantly so that BRM can recover this unbalance condtion to the normal equilianume to reach the goal of treating the tumors.

BRM is a group of medicine which can adjust the host body immune function, recovering the immune function from the inhibition conditions, the function mechanism of which are active the immune function systems. Which are mainly from the microbiology agents and the plants, the former is the drugs as the immune strengthener and immune active agents and immune regulator, now the new name is the BRM.

Recurrently there are some BRM-similar medicine from the traditional Chinese medicine, which have excellent results.

2.The classifications of BMR

1). Cytokines: is the production from the immune effective cells and related cells, which are the cell-mediated proteins with the important biological activities. The types of their biological activities as the following:

   a. Interleukin 2, IL-2 is the molecules between the immune cells and active the T cells, Bcells proliferatin, and active the NK cells ect Killer cells
   b. IFN has three types of IFN-A,B, which are groups of glycoproteins.
   c. CSF is the factor which stimulated the blood stem cells growth an division into GM-CSF, M-CSF and G-CSF.
   d. TNF.

2). The immune active cells: so far there are four immune cells which are used to the tumor therapy:

   a. LAK
   b. TIL
   c.PWH-LAK and OKT3-LAK: The PBL or TIL from pwh, okt can stimulated LAK proliferation activity.
   d.CD8 CTL which can recognized the MHCI tumor groups has the strong activities which killed the tumor cells.

3).The vaccines of the tumor molecules: currently the main research on the tumor vaccination is the unique vaccine of antitumor monoantibodys, which can produce the anticancer response after imitating the antigen stimulation.

4). The natural medicine with BRM function: XZ-C have BRM function.

3. The function mechanism of BRM

BRM has the effects on the regulation of the host immmun response to the timor and killing the tumor s. The mechinsum are the following five aspects:

a. Directly regulating the growth and division of the tumors
b. Increasing the sensitivities of the tumors to the anticancer mechnisum in the body to benefit of killing the tumor cells.
c. Acting on the tumor vessels and affects the tumor's nutrition, blood supply so as to lead the death of the tumors and not damage the normal tissues
d. Stimulating the immune response to host antitumors
e. Stimulating the production of the blood to improve the inhibited bone marrow function to increase the tolerance of the the damage from the tumor therapy.

BRM can improve the body immune response and can strengthen the body immune surveillance to the tumors. The patients with the smallest size have good response to the BRM. BRM have very good effects on the early patients or the remaining tumor after surgery, or the tiny tumors and the xxxxx of the tumor cells.

BRM is one of the combination therapy methods to treat the malignant tumors, which some scientists said that immune therap just treat the 105 tumor cells such if the tumor cells formed clearly, the RRM functions will be limit the tumors to growth.

Even if the immune therapy have great development and attacted the whole world attentions, the mature degree of the tumor immune therapy is still in controevent., Currntly this is a worth research and there are some questions as the following:

1.) It is difficult to have effects to the big tumors, only as the supply therapy to the therapy of the operation, chem. And radivation
2.) Because the tumor antigen is specific, it is very difficult to produce the specific antibody.

Some researches showed that the antitumor therapy doesn't need absolute specificity, therefore, even if the tumors don't have the specific antigen, the immune therapy of the tumors is still acceptable. The concentration of the tumor relative antigens in the malignant tumor cells is higher than the normal cells, which this difference can make it possible for these antigens to become the effective attacked target. In addition, because the patients with cancer almost have the decreases of the immune function, and the increase of the immune inhibition factors, and the decrease of IL-2,TNF, and IFN ect, therefore, it is necessary to increase the immune function.

Because of the immune function decrease in the tumor patients, during the therap it should try to improve the immune function in the patients with the tumors. Because of the increaser of the immune inhibiting factors in the tumor patients, it should be treated to black ; because of the decrease of the IL-2, TNF and IFN etc, it should try to stimulate the production of these factors.

In order to improve the effects of the immune therapy, it is necessary to investigate how to get the best combinating forms of these therapies with the current therapy.

4. The research survey on the XZ-C traditional Chinese anticancer medications for the immune regulation control similar to BRM

XZ-C immune regulation anticancer medicine have the functions and curative effects similar to BRM after four years experimental research and 16 years clinical research which are the drugs similar to BRM selected from traditional Chinese medicine.

XZ-C is the durgs that XU ZE in China professor selected from two hundreds of the anticancer herbs after the experiments. At first the culturing tumor were done. The in vitro was done One by one to select and asberve the direct damage to tumor cells in the culture setting and the control groups of the rate of the anticancer are the chemotherapyxxxx and the normal culture tube cells. The results are to select the a series of the medicine of the anti-cancer proliferation, then made the animal modes which 200 drugs were used on one by one. These experiments of the analysis and evaluation are steps by steps, scientific, practical and strict, etc. The results proved that48 of them have the excellent tumor inhibition effects, however the rest 152 of the tumors anticancer medicine are all common old anticancer medicine which proved no anticancer or less inhibition of the tumors in the animal models during these medicine selection experiments.

In the process of the experiments, the main work were conducted on the tumor animal models: one medicine was experienced on one group to observe them about three months and then selected 48 of the effective anticancer medicine, then combination of two or three medicine to do experiment on these animal models so that the single medicine has less effects than the multiple compound effects, which seems that the single medicine has the inhibition only on the tumor cell proliferation, however the multiple combination not inhibition to the tumor proliferation, but have the immune regulation control function of the body regulation, strengthen the energy, improvement of the immune system, promoting the production of the inhibiting cell factors, protecting the normal cells and promoting the anticancer factors etc.

Based on the author's experiments during four years of the single traditional medicine selection in the animal models, then the combination of the experiment, then set up again XZ-C 1-10 recepes of anticancer, antimetastasis and antireccurrency and last conducted the clinical verification. From 1992 the wide clinical tests were set up. After 16 years of the tumor specialty in outpatient centers there were

12000 cases of the tumor patients who were test and showed the excellent effects which their medical condition are stable, improved in there symptoms, the life quality improvement and the survival rates prolong. The medical condition in many metastasis patients were stable and didn't spread. Some of the patients with the number decrease of the white blood cells couldn't have chmetherapy and radicative therapy, however after taking these medicine, there were no metastasis and have excellent effects.

5. The function and curative effect of the XZ-C traditional Chinese anticancer medicine for the immune regulation control similar to BRM

BRM is in 1982 first was described by Oldham, which meaning is that the reaction to foreign attack or response ability is through the BRM.

The cell-mediated and antibody mediated immune response is in the subtle control situation. In the unbalance situation the host response or the response ability will be significantly affected. The application of the BRM regulator can recover the normal equilitiun from the loss of the equilitium to reach the goal of the disease prevention.

BRM explored the new field of the tumor biology therapy, which currently was used as the fourth medols and was great attentions from all over the world.

BRM have regulate the body's immune function, recovering the immune function which were inhibited. These medicine function mechanism are multiple, however no matter what mechanisum theirs, they are function through the activing the body immune systems.

BRM, mainly from the microorganism and plants, before called as immune strengthenor, immune stimulator, immune exciting factors or immune regulation, now called as BRM/

The medicine which the author selected on the tumor animal models and had excellent anticancer rat XZ-C can improve immune function, protection of the central immune organs such as thymus and, improving the cell-mediated immune functions, protecting the thymus function, protect the bone morrow function, increase the red blood cells and white blood cells number, active the immune factors, improve the immune surveilence in the blood ect. XZ-C the main anticancer pharmacology function si anticancer and increase of the immune function. After four years of the animal experiments of the selection of the medicine, 48 medicine were selected as the signle medicine for the high anticancer medicine., then after the immune and cell factors levele tests, got 26 medicine separately have phargocyte functions, immune cells function, or increase the antibody- liquid immune system, increased the thymus weight, and promote the bone marrow proliferatin, and improvement of the T cells, and increase the activities of the LAK cells, increasing the IFN activities levels, TNS activity level, strengthening the CSF factors, inhibition of the platelet anticoagulation to inhibiting the cancer thromobosis, antimetastasis, or clearing the free bases etc. The aboving XZ-C has the following function as :

1.) activing the host immune system to promote the host immune function to reach the immune respond to the tumors.

2.) Activing the host immune factors of the anticancer systems to strengthen the host immune function and improve the immunce surviellence of the host immune systems.

3.) protecting the thymus and bone marrow,improve the immune system, and stimulate the bone marrow function to reduce the inhibition of the bone marrow and increase the white blood cell and red blood cells etc.

4.) Reduction of the side effects of the chemotherapy and radioactive therapy to increase the tolerance of the hosts.

5.) The development of the tumors is the imbalance between the biological characteristic of the tumor cells and the the inhibition of the host to tumor XZ-C is the improvement of the immune system and recover the balance of both them.

6.) directly regulate the tumor cell growth and division to have the regulation function of the growth and division.

7.) Increaseing thymus weight and stop the shrinkle of thymus because when the tumor develop thymus goes on shrinkles.

8.) Stimulating the host immune response to the tumors and strengthening the host anticancer abilities and strengthening the sensitivities of the host anticancer mechanism so as to benefits of killing the tumor cells on the ways of the metastasis.

XZ-C can make the body to produce the strong immune reaction to the tumor cells so that it can treat the tumors, which can produce the following immune response: 1). Strengthen the regulation or recover the host immune response to the tumors;2).stimulate the host immune system to active the host immune defense system;3)recover the immune functions.

As the above statement, the basical mechanisu of XZ-C is similar to BRM and the clinical application is similar to those of the BRM.

6. The clinical application principle and the application range of the XZ-C anticancer immune regulation traditional medications

1.) The clinical application of XZ-C: BRM and XZ-C similar to BRM can increase the immune response and strengthen the host immune surveillance function. When the cells start the mutation or the tumors are small, the effects are good. After the surgery or radioactive therapy, the medication therapy can make the tumor reduce to the smallest size which therapy effects are the best.

For the patients who cannot have the operation and are weak and cannot have the chemotherapy and radioactive therapy, the immune therapy has some effects and reduce the symptom and prolong the survival time.

In order to reduce the metastasis and recurrence after the radical surgery, the XZ-C can be used. After the operation removed the big tumors XZ-C can be use to get rid of the remaining cancer cells and the tumor which already spread further away.

If the tumor is not removed, the chemotherapy or the radioactive therapy can be used first, which kill the most of the tumor cells to reduce the number of the tumor cells, then XZ-C can be used to supply.

2.) The clinical observation and application ranges of XZ-C

(1).Antimestasticsid after the operation: recover and improve the immune response after the surgery to improve the life quality and kill the remaining tumor cells after the operatton to prevent the metastasis and inhibit the cell proliferation to prevent the recurrency an d strengthern the longterm curative effects.

The ranges of the application: a. all kind of the middle, and advanced tumor after the surgery. All kind of the tumor after the surgery c. the advanced tumor which can not be removel after the operation investigation d. only can have the intestine recombination or the opening of the colon during the operation.e.can not removal the advanced tumors and lost the indicaton for the surgery. F.the removed tumors plus the tube pump insections.

(2). Improving the life quality, prolonging the survival rate, inhibiting the division of the tumors, control the tumor cell proliferation, improve the body immune response, mainly anti metastasis

Application ranges: a. all kinds of the tumors including the new, further metastasis after the operation;b.all of the cancer with the later metastasis such as the liver, lung, branin or chest cavity, abdominal cavity.

(3).reduce the tumor pain: XZ-C can treat all kind of the pain from the advanced tumors and soft and reduce the tumor size.

(4). Supply with the chemotherapy or the tube pump therapy to protect the liver, kidney and bone marrow and thymus etc immune organs to improve the immune response and change the whole body immune condition, to support and strengthen and increase the period and long time curative effects to prevent the metastasis and spreed and recovery and to improve thelife quality, prolong the life time after the liver cancer patient had the tubes and chemotherapy etc.

(5).Combination with the chemotherapy and radiavivion therapy, can reduce the side effects and increase the curative effects to protect the liver,kindey and bone marrow and other immune organs fucnton to increase the white cell numbers/

(6).the combination of the application of the XZ-C and the traditional xxx: such as the using with xxxx for the liver cancer and theascite or the matatstsis of the abdominal catiy ascite;used th the xxx for the treatment oft liver cancer and jaundice; wused with xxx for the liver tumor with HBSAG POSTIVE AND trf postitvie. Used with ccc for the white cell dectease casuse by the chemotherapy.

3.) The application of XZ-C:

The tumor patietnts mostly have the immune function decreases after the diagnosed, the treatment should be done soon, however the three therapy of the operation, chemotherapy and radicative therapy all can cause the immune function decrase and leasd the decraste the toleratance of the patatient to the surpery or chemotherapy radicative and decrase the immune surveilleance in the host immunce systym. Therefore, it is necessary to start theimmune therapy during the operation or eradicative herpy and chemoterrapy. XZ-C can take by oral as long the thepatiertnte can eart, this is can be taken by oral. After the 1-2 week of the operation, the patient can started to take them. Befre the chmotehrapy and radiative during the peroios beye the radicatcie and chemothery oand after the radicalctive and cheamotherpom the patoeint can comtinuce ot take ZX-C, SO THAT THESE WILL DECRASE OR CONTROL THE RECORURNENVT And metastasis. And decrase the side effect of the radiotherapy and terhotherpay; prevent theimmune system decrease by chemotherapy and imcrease the immn function; promote the bone marrow function, protect eh bone marrow functiinl active the immune cells systems and immune cytokines function to improve the immune surveillance and prevent the recurrenc and metastasis.

16. TYPICAL CASES OF TREATMENT FOR MALIGNANT TUMOR BY XZ-C TRADITIONAL CHINESE ANTICANCER MEDICINE THROUGH IMMUNOLOGICAL REGULATION AND CONTROL

There are a variety of following of typical cases which Z-C anticancer immune regulation, anti-metastatic therapy were applied in our Cancer Research and the National Cooperative Group Hubei

1. Inoperable, nor radiotherapy and chemotherapy, simply taking z-c immunomodulatory anticancer medicine treatment of typical cases

Case 1 Mr. Liu, male, 68year-old, Changzhou, officer, Medical record number:8701735

Diagnosis: the central lung cancer on the right upper of the lung with the metastasis

Disease courses and treatment: in Octocber 1998 he coughed two weeks with the pain in the right shoulder and was treated with inflammation. In Jan 1999 his cough is getting worse and this appetite is decreased and fatigure and getting weak. On CT there is mass on the right upper lung showing the central lung. He had endoscope and biopsy which showed that lung adenocarcinoma in the xxxxxx. He and his family member don't want to have operation. In Feb 1999 after chemotherapy for one course, his reaction to the chemotherapy was strong and stopped to use it. This patient had metastasis in the left lung which showed there are two lesions and he coughed with mucous and blood sputdu and difficult walking. On April 23 2000 he started to take the XZ-C1+XZ-C4+XZ-C7, LMS+MDZ for three months and his general condition is good and he is lively and his appetite is great. In December 2000 his medical condition is stable, and he is lively. His appetite is good and his breath is smooth and his face is red. He walked as the normal person and sometimes he coughs. He persistently takes this medication for more than four years and when he comes back to follow up during the five years, his general condition is great and he walked as the normal healthy person.

Comments: this patient has the central lung cancer in the right upper lung. In April 2000 he started to use XZ-C1+XZ-C4+XZ-C7. XZ-C1 is used to kill the cancer cells only without kill the normal cells; XC-C4 protect the thymus and increase the thymus weight and to protect the bone marrow, XZ-C7 inhibit the lung cancer cells and protect the lung and solve the suptid. After short-term chemotherapy he started to take the XZ-C to strengthen his long-term therapy. XZ-C improve the whole body immune system and he is lively and his appetite is good and his spleen is great and help the patients against the diseases and help the patient's organ functions and the nutrition condition and metabliztion recover so that the patients' healthy condition is recovery.

This patient didn't have the operation. In Feb 1999 he had chemeotherapy, however there is left lung metastasis after chemotherapy. Afterh that,he only took the XZ-C to control the metastasis. He persistently took the medicine for more than four years and his medical condition is great without any complaints. He followed up with us for more than seven years. In May 2005 when he came back to follow up, his general medical condition is great and his appepital is good without other symptoms. His walking and activities and he talks cheerfully and humorously.

Case 2 Mrs. Huang, femal,66 year-old, Wuhan han yan, Medical record number:10102008
Diagnosis: the squamous carcinoma of the low esophagus

Disease courses and treatment: in December 2000 the patients started to vomit and to have progressively swallow difficultly and only swallow the half of xxxx food. EGD showed that there was narrow in the low esophagus, congestion, ulcer and xxx. Pathology showed squamous carcinoma in the lower esophagus. According to his medical condition he should be treated for a surgery, however because he could afford to the medical cost, he started to take XZ-C. After one month, he is energetic and his appetite is getting better and can eat the soft food, noodle and rice soup. After she continued to take these medicine for six months, he is vagour and his appetite is good and can eat the soft food and noodle and rice soup. Until June 2003 she took the medicine more than two and half years and his health condition is good and can eat the regular rice and felt fine as the normal healthy persons. However she stopped to taking the medicine for more than four and half months. Until Octocber 16 2003 he suddenly had the difficulties to swallow the food and vomit the brown food. She could not eat for more than three days. After adding her some fluids and continued to take XZ-C until Octocber 31 2003 she can eat the food again. After that, she never stopped taking the medicine again. Now she is 70 year-old and healthy the same as the normal persons. She is energetic and her appetite is good and can eat regular food. She lived in the seventh floor and everyday she will come down the first floor and sometimes she help others to fill the bicycle wheels.

Comments: This patient had the low grade squamous carcinoma in the low esophagaus which was diagnosed by EGC and pathology. At that time he could only eat the liquid food and half ofXXXX food. She makes her living by filling the bicycle wheels and didn't have money for her surgery so that she started to take XZ-C medicine. After taking the medicine half of year her symptoms turned good. Aftertaking the medicine two andhalf years she recovered as the normal person and didn't have any complain. Because of her incoming condition, she didn't get any other tests and treatment. When she came back to followup, she had taken the medicine more than five years and her condition is good.

To take XZ-C for longterm can improve the patients immune function and the pateitns energy level will increase and the appetites will increase and the sleep will be good. XZ-C4 can protect the bone marrow and thymus to improve the nutrition and the metabolism will turn good and will get rid of the free bases to control and to repair the diseases.

Case 3 Mrs Hang, female, 65year-old, Huangpi in Hubei, Medical record number:10402074

Diagnosis: the middle esophogus carcinoma

Disease courses and treatment condition: In April 2001 the patient had difficulty swallowing and chest and back pain and gradually increased. Until June only can eat the liquid food and vomit the mucous staffs. On June 6 2001 the barium swallow tests in the xxx showed under the aorta branch xxxx 2cm there is a 10cm lenghth narrow and 6cm xxxxxlump in the left wall and the muscous stop. Because of the cost, she didn't have the operation, radioactive and chemotherapy. On June 25 she started to take XZ-C. After three months, her general condition is better and her appetite is getting better and the difficultying swallowing is getting better and can eat the rice soup, noodle. She continued taking the medicine until March 2002 then can take the rice and regular food. In July 2003 she just took XZ-C4+XZ-C2. In April 2005 when she followed up with us, she is energetic and her appetites was great at that time she had been taking XZ-C for more than five year. He condition is stable and can eat the regular food and can do light house work.

Comments: This patient had esophageal cancer which she only took XZ-C to control her condition without the operation, radiactiv therapy and chemotherapy. For more than four years, there was no metastasis and her condition had been controlled and can eat the regular food and rice. She is as healthy as other old persons and can do some choresevery day.

She kept taking her medicine regularly.

Case 4 Ms. Liu, female, 65 year-old, Jianxian in Hubei, officer. Medical record number: 110201
Diagnosis: primary huge liver carcinoma

Disease course and treatment: Because of discomfort in upper abdomen, the patient had CT in XieHe hospital which found that a 6.7 cm x 7.1 cm x 9 cm nodule in right liver, then diagnosed as primary liver carcinoma. She refused to take operation and chemotherapy. In July 11, 1995 she started to take the XZ-C1+XZ-C5. After 2 months, her emotion and appetite get better and her weight increased. In September 20, 1995 on follow-up ultrasound, the nodule was reduced. In November 1995 she had a chemoembolization and didn't have any other therapy. She continues to take the XZ-C for more than 6 years and continues to follow-up more than 10 years. This patient's condition is good. In May 2005 this patient is as healthy as a normal person.

Comments: On July 4, 1995 this patient was diagnosed with primary liver carcinoma by CT and then took XZ-C after 1 week. After 2 month, the CT scan showed that the nodule become smaller. On November 21 the chemotherapy procedure was conducted, and then she continued to take XZ-C regularly and persistently for 10 years. Now this patient is as healthy as a normal individual.

Implication: The chemotherapy+XZ-C have good results on liver carcinoma treatment. The chemotherapy can stop the blood supply to the cancer nodule and chemotherapy can kill some of the cancer cells. There are living cancer cells inside and under the tumor nodule membrane after chemotherapy; the tumor cells didn't die completely and then grew fast after circulation built up. XZ-C can protect thymus and improve the immune ability, protect the bone morrow function and improve the body immune function. In addition, 85% hepatic cancer occurred in the cirrhosis patients so chemotherapy will damage the liver function. XZ-C will protect the liver. The combination of chemotherapy+XZ-C will inhibit the tumor and protect the host to improve the long-term treatment. This is called "take out the bad and keep the good" in Chinese.

Case 5. Mr. Huang, male, 53 year-old, Wuhan. Medical record number: number: 11202225 Diagnosis: primary huge liver cancer, liver cirrhosis after hepatitis, the later stage of Japanese blood fluke, Portal hypertension.

Disease course and treatment: Patient's appetite decreased and he felt uncomfortable in his abdomen. In September 2000 CT showed a 13.6cm x 11.8cm lesion in the right liver lobe. In September 7, 2000 MRI showed a huge 13.1cm x 11.4cm x 12.5cm lesion in right lobe, diagnosed as huge liver cancer in right lobe. The patient had hepatic arterial chemoembolization (HACE) and embolization (HAE) and the chemoembolization medicine were xxxx 25mg+xxx1000g: xxxx10ml+xxxx10mg. Currently his general condition is good. The change of his liver lesions are the following which are stable and getting small: CT showed a 11.1cm x 11.8cm lesion in the right liver lobe on October 12, 2000, a 10.8cm x 9.8cm lesion in the right liver lobe on December 14, 2000, a 10.5cm x 9.5cm lesion on Feb 2001 and a 9.8cm x 8.9cm lesion on September 3, 2001 in the right liver lobe. This patient started to take XZ-C1+XZ-C4+XZ-C5 on January 9, 2002 and his general condition is good, just as his emotion, appetite and sleep are very good. He comes back for check-up every month and takes his medicine regularly. On October 21, 2002 during his follow-up, his general condition is good, emotion is stable, and appetite is good and bowel movement is good and his routine is regular and he exercises regularly. He reports not having had a cold during the last four years. He lived as a normal healthy person.

Comments: This case is primary huge liver carcinoma which had five times embolization and the lesion was getting smaller and had very good response. Last embolization is on November 12, 2001 and the lesion is 9.8cm x 8.9cm. He started to take XZ-C1+XZ-C4+XZ-C5 on Jan 9, 2002. The XZ-C1 can kill the cancer cells and not kill the normal cells; XZ-C4 protects thymus and inhibits thymus shrinkage; XZ-C5 protects liver function. This patient continues to take this medicine for more than 3 years, however when he came back for follow-up in the fourth year, his health condition is general, disease is stable and there is no metastasis and no further development. His emotion is stable, his appetite is good, and he walks as a normal healthy person. The experience from this case is for primary huge liver cancer, first embolization treatment are given to make this lesion smaller and stable, later use XZ-C to support the long-term therapy and to protect the liver function and to improve the immune system and to control the metastasis.

Case 6. Mr. Pu, male, 51 year-old, Yin Zheng, officer. Medical record number: number: 500989 Diagnosis: primary liver cancer

Disease course and treatment: There is a 4.6cm x 3.6cm nodule in left liver and a 1.6cm x 1.6cm nodule in right liver after the patient had CT on October 30, 1997. Diagnosis was liver carcinoma. There is a 5.9cm x 4.0cm x 5.4cm nodule in the left liver lobe and a 2.1cm x 1.8cm lesion in the right liver lobe when the patient had Ultrasound in the XieHe hospital. Liver angiography showed that the patient had liver cancer. HBsAg(+), AFP(-). Because this patient's liver function was poor, he couldn't stand the operation and put on the tube for chemotherapy. This patient is alcohol drinker for 40 years (250ml/per meal average). In 1996 he had Hepatitis B. In 1966 he had blood fluke. On November 25 the patient starts to take XZ-C1+XZ-C4+XZ-C5. In 1998 and 1999 the patient continued to take the medicine. The patient's condition is good, and his face is red and smiles. On November 2, 1999 he came to follow-up and the ultrasound showed the lesion was reduced. He can do light work and feels very well. For more than 2 years, he continues to take XZ-C1+XZ-C4+XZ-C5. After these medicines the patient's energy level is improving and appetite is improving. In June 2002 he went to Beijing for treatment (before he went to Beijing, he was good and walking as the normal person). During the operation there is a 5cm x 6cm nodule in the liver which is the same as 5 years ago and there are cancer cells in the common duct and now metastasis, and no fluid in the abdominal cavity. There is no metastasis in the liver, however because the nodule is close to the hepatic artery entrance, it is very difficult to remove the cancer nodule and then place the drainage tube. After surgery, this patient didn't have urine and had acute renal failure. He passed away on day 6.

Comments: On October 30, 1997 CT showed a 4.6cm x 3.6cm nodule in left liver and in November 1997 there is a 1.6cm x 1.6cm nodule in right liver. Because the liver function was poor, the patient didn't have operation and tube placement and other treatment. On November 25 he started to take XZ-C1+XZ-C4+XZ-C5 and continued for 5 years. His health condition was fine.

Implication: XZ-C can improve the host immune system ability (including the cell and antibody immune function) to protect the central and peripheral immune organs, to protect the liver and kidney, and to produce anticancer factors an dprevent cancer cells metastasis and spread. XZ-C is a medication with no side effects which helps the patient in "fight with bad and help the right". In addition the patient's disease condition was under very good control without metastasis so that therapeutic effect was very good. This patient took XZ-C for 5 years, during which time his condition was stable and the liver cancer lesion was not increasing and there were no metastasis. His general condition was good and not uncomfortable and the patient walked as a normal person. He went to Beijing and was diagnosed as liver cells carcinoma which was in the entrance of the liver and couldn't be removed because of the cancer cells in the common duct. The patient underwent surgery for the placement of the T-tube for chemotherapy. After the operation, this patient didn't have urine and died of acute renal failure. If he had not had the operation which destroyed the liver and kidney function, he might have survived to the present day.

2. Surgical exploration cannot remove tumor, nor do radiotherapy and chemotherapy

Case 1 Mr.Cheng, male, 64 year-old Hubei Xin Zhou, officer, Medical record number::7301454 Diagnosis: the tumor of the mesentaic membranexxxx.

Disease courses and treatment condition:On January 6 1999 the patient suddenly had the uncomfortable in chest and pain and vomit. The emergency diagnosis was "actual GI infection", the surgeons thought of that he had the pancreatitis. On March 3 EGD showed the obstractle of the duodenum. On March 6 1999 during the survey of the abdomen, the tumor which was behind the abdominal membrane including big vessals which during the operation a 6cmx9cm lump in the roots of the small intestine membreance xxxx of hard, stable, fixed and unsmooth on the surface, connected to aorta and the xxxx arterial and pressed the duodenum which it was difficult to remove so that the connection of the duodenus and colon was done because the tumor can not be removed and the patients was told to be treated by the combination of the western and Chinese therapy. On April 1999 she started to take XZ-C1Z+C4. From May 15 1999 to February 2002 she continued to take the medicine and refill her medicine. She is stable and her medical condition is good.

Comments: On March 6 1999 the tumor from the abdomen membrane was foundby the survey of the operation. Because it is connected to the small intestine membrance including the big artery, this tumor can not be removed. But the surface of the tumor was firm and stable, which implied malignant. After taking Z-C years, the patients is stable and no development and no metastasis and healthy.

Case 2. Mr. Fong, male, 50 year-old, Hubei Lou Tang, peasant. Medical record number: 330651
Diagnosis: Pancreas cancer

Disease course and treatment: Because of discomfort in upper abdomen for more than three months, he had jaundice and had opening abdomen surgery showing: No stones in the bile system and enlargement of the pancreas. The tumor couldn't be removed and Pathology showed pancreatic cancer. CT showed enlargement of pancreas head and dilation of the bile duct in liver. After the operation the jaundice extended persistently. On December 11, 1996 he started to take the XZ-C and after one month his medical condition got better and his appetite increased, however he still had little jaundice and weakness and sweating. After taking XZ-C and soup two months the jaundice and pain reduced and got better. After four months, the jaundice was gone completely and his appetite and energy level were good. His pain in abdomen was mild. In July 1998 he returned to work and did mild labor work and his face looks red. He continues to take his medicine for many years. On April 6, 2004 his family introduced a new patient to us and told us that this patient is fine and his activities are as a normal person's and he does his chores very well.

Comments: This patient has pancreas head cancer and jaundice. On November 28 1996 during the operation, this tumor cannot be removed and the Pathology is pancreas cancer with the dilation of the bile duct system in the livers. On December 11, 1996 this patient took ZX-C and soup. After seven months his jaundice is reduced and he continues to take medicine to improve his immune system. Until July 1998 his condition is completely normal. He continues to take his medicine for more than four years and later changed to taking the medicine periodically to support his healthy condition. This patient has followed up for more than nine years and his condition is very good

Case 3. Mr. Lee, male, 53 year-old, Wuhan, farmer. Medical record number: 9901979
Diagnosis: primary huge liver carcinoma, late stage Japanese blood fluke hepatic cirrhosis.

Disease course and treatment: On January 22, 2001 the patient felt pain in the right back. In Feb 26, 2001 ultrasound showed a nodule in the liver. On January 31, 2001 CT showed a 14cm x 1cm lesion in the right liver lobe diagnosed as primary huge liver cancer in the right liver. On March 1, 2001 the open abdomen surgery was done in Tongjin Hospital and the pump implantation in the portal vein because the lesion was huge and couldn't be removed. After the surgery the patient received chemotherapy once. This patient had 30 years Japanese blood fluke. On March 9, 2001 this patient started to take XZ-C medicine. He used XZ-C1+XZ-C4+XZ-C5, LMS, MDZ, and XZ-C3 placed on a fist-size lump in the right rib edge area. After one month of taking this medicine, the patient's condition is getting better and his emotion is stable and happy. His appetite is increasing. The lump in the right rib edge area is getting smaller and softer than before. After he continued to take this medicine for three months, his general condition is good and his appetite and sleep are good. His energy level is recovering and he is walking as a normal person. On October 22, 2001 Ultrasound showed a 6cm x 7.8cm lesion in the right lobe liver and he continues taking XZ-C1+XZ-C4+XZ-C5 and using XZ-C3 on the lump. On November 19, 2003 during his follow-up, ultrasound showed this lesion size the same as before, kidney function is normal and CXR didn't show abnormality, there is no positive lymph node and the lump on the right rib edge is soft and getting smaller and the boundry is clear and not painful. This patient continued to use XZ-C1+XZ-C4+XZ-C5.

Comments: This case is diagnosed as primary huge liver cancer and the lesion can not be removed so that the portal vein pump was placed for chemotherapy once. In March 2001, he started to use the XZ-C1+XZ-C4+XZ-C5 and topical XZ-C3 for 4 years. His general condition is stable and didn't develop further and didn't metastasize.

Case 4. Mr. Kei, male, 54 year-old, Yanxi in Hubei, officer. Medical record number: number: 6301244.
Diagnosis: primary liver carcinoma

Disease course and treatment: The patient had pain on the upper right abdomen for half of a month and his appetites decreased. CT in Yanxia showed nodules in the right front and back lobe and left lobe. The patient was diagnosed with primary liver carcinoma. On August 20, 1998 the patient had opening surgery which revealed that the main tumors were in the entrance of the common duct and there were metastasis in both of left and right liver, which could not be removed. Therefor a tube for the chemotherapy was placed through the hepatic artery. After the operation, the chemotherapy was used once. In October 1998 the second chemotherapy was used. Because the tube was blocked, the patient stopped using the tube. On September 8, 1998 he started taking XZ-C1+XZ-C4+XZ-C5. After taking this medicine one month, the patient's emotion and appetite were good and his body weight increased and his face was glowing with health. On his physical exam the abdomen was soft and flat and the spleen and liver could not be felt; his general condition was good. He could support himself very well and picked up his medication by himself. On June 4, 2002 when he came back for his follow-up, his healthy condition was good; his face was glowing with health, his walking, acting and smiling were like a normal, healthy person. On the physical exam there was no abnormality found.

Comments: On August 20, 1998 liver carcinoma was found in the right and left liver and could not be removed, and a chemotherapy tube was placed, through which the chemotherapy was twice given after CT scan showed many lesions in the left lobe, right front and right back lobe. On September

8 the patient started to take XZ-C1+XZ-C4+XZ-C5. Until 2002 this patient's condition was good and didn't have metastasis.

Implication: When liver cancer could not be removed, the liver artery tube could be placed, then XZ-C1+XZ-C4+XZ-C5 was used to protect Thymus, bone morrow, liver to improve the host immune system function and induce the host to produce more anticancer factors to control the tumors and to control the development of the cancers

3. Typical cases for recurrence after radical surgery, with Z-C immunomodulatory anticancer medication treatment

Case 1 Mr. Mao, male, 48 year-old, Taimen, officer. Medical record number: 100014
Diagnosis: Primary liver carcinoma

Disease course and treatment: On August 1, 1994 because the patient felt fatigued, he had ultrasound in the local hospital and found a 4.1cm x 4.5cm nodule in the left lobe of the liver. On August 26, 1994 the left lobe of the liver was removed in the Xian Ha hospital. Pathological slides showed: liver cell carcinoma without any treatment. After operation, the patient was treated with anticancer immunological traditional medicine **XZ-C1+XZ-C4+XZ-C5** in our outpatient center. After taking these medicines, the patient's appetite increased, energy level increased and he was happy. He takes medicines regularly and comes to our office every month for follow up and refilling of the medicines. He feels very well and goes back to his work. On December 14, 1996 there was another 1.3cm x 1.8cm nodule which was found by B ultrasound in the edge of the left liver. On December 30, 1996 he had that nodule removed. After the operation, he continued to take the medicine. After that, the patient took his medicine persistently and regularly. In May 2010 when he came to follow-up, his general condition was good and his face was glowing with health, his body was as strong as a healthy person's and the patient returned to work for more than 11 years. His appetite is great and his emotion is very good. He eats 600g food per day and his ultrasound is normal.

Comments: On August 26, 1994 this patient had a 4.1cm x 4.5cm nodule removal of left liver. After the operation, the patient received XZ-C for treatment. On December 30, 1996 another 1.3cm x 1.8cm nodule was found and removed. After that, this patient continued to take XZ-C. When he came back for 16-year follow-up, his health condition is good and he can do labor work for many years. This patient is still alive and very well at the time of writing this book.

Case 2 Mr. Chan, male, 65 year-old, Wuhan, retired officer. Medical record number: 280555
Diagnosis: Adenocarcinoma in the pyloric area of the stomach and recurrence after surgery in the remaining stomach

Disease course and treatment: This patient had pain in the upper abdomen for more than one year and in June 1993 he was diagnosed as stomach cancer and had removal of the great curvature in the stomach. After the operation, he had FM chemotherapy once which caused anemia and weakness and wbc is 1900. 8 months after operation, the patient had abdomen pain with vomiting and had left upper abdominal pain for half year. On March 25, 1994 the Barium showed: there was no filled on the upper area of the stomach and part damage of the membranes and the narrow change in the cutting parts. A barium swallow showed recurrence of the stomach cancer. On May 3, 1996 ultrasound showed that there is no lesion inside the liver. Because this patient couldn't eat rice and just eats noodles and liquid food so that he had fatigue and no energy, he didn't want to have operation. In June 1996 he started to take XZ-C. After that he is fine and his appetite is increased and he takes this medicine regularly for more than four years. On May 6, 2000 when he came back to follow-up, his general condition is great and his face looks red and healthy. Walking and activities are normal as the others and he eats rice soup and banana often as his meal.

Comments: In June 1993 the patient had stomach removal. In March 1994 the cancer recurred and the junction part turned narrow. After taking XZ-C+XZ-C4 only, for more than six years his health condition is great.

Implication: For the recurrence of the stomach cancers, the junction of the surgery was not closed completely and the patient could still eat food. After taking the medicines to improve thymus function to control the tumor growth and prevent the tumor growth and metastasis XXXX. The patient's medical condition is stable and he is still alive.

Case 3: Mr. Cheng, male, 62year-old, Wuhan, engineer, Medical record number:s: 210412
Diagnosis: Renal pelvis carcinoma in the right kidney and the recurrence after the bladder carcinoma operation.

Diseases courses and treatment: the patient had cytoscopy which showed the bladder carcinoma in November 4 1995 afterthe bloody urine for two years. On November 21 1995 CT showed that rght renal pelvis tumor. On December 6 1995 the right kidney and urother were removed and his bladder was removed by the xxx and after the operation the local xxxx chemotherapy was used for seven times. On March 8 1996 the cystoscopy showed there was the hard lump in the left wall of the bladder in order to prevent the reccurrence of the tumor, he started to take XZ-C1+XZ-C4+XZ-C6. After taking this medicine he is well and his appetite is getting better. On June 24 1996 the cytoscopy showed that the bladder walls are smooth and the surface is smooth and the new things were gone. He continued to take XZ-C medicine to prevent the recerence and metastasis. Until June 11 1997 the cystoscopy showed the bladder is normal. On December 28 1998 the cystoscopy is normal. On June 26 1999 when he came back to follow up, his condition is stable and he continues to take the XZ-C1+XZ-C4+XZ-C6 for more than ten years to prevent the recurrence and metastasis. On May 6 2005 when he follow-up, he is stable and his condition is good and is the same as the normal individuals.

Comments: this case is the recurrence of the bladder cancinoma after the operation. After taking this medicine more than ten years to prevent the recurrence and metastasis, his medical condition is good and after many cystoscopy, the bladder is normal.

Suggestion: XZ-C can improve the patients immune function and prevent the tumor recurrence and metastasis and control the primary lesions. He is healthy and is in the good condition.

Case 4. Mr. Lin, male, 68year-old, Wuhan, Professor, Medical record number:: 7701534
Diagnosis: the recurrence of the bladder cancer operation.

Disease courses and treatment conditions: After the removal of the bladder cancer was done in April 1994 in the hospital, Pathology showed: transitional cell carcinoma. After the operation the bladder was poured with chemotherapy. Because of the decrease of the white blood cells the chemotherapy stopped. In 1996 he came back to check up and found the cancer recurrence so that the second operation was done by the removal of eight tumors. After the surgery the patient's bladder was poured with XXX+XXXX twice every month for three months. After three months, repeat these medicine for another three months. Twice per month until 1997. In May 1998 the cystoscopy in the XXX hospital showed the xxx in the bladder. In December the ultrasound showed the bladder infection. In April 1999 because of the bloody urine, the cystoscopy showed that there were a four cm2 of the tumor and CT biopsy showed that bladder cancer. In May 1999 the arterial chemotherapy was poured. In June the second time of the poured the XXXX+XXXX+XXX was done. After that the white blood cells decreased into 2x109/l. In September the third time of the poured medicine with xxx+xxxx+xxx, the white blood cells decreased into 1.2x109/L, then inject the XXX to increase the white blood cells. His medical history: stroke in 1992, Hypertension(160/90mmHg), Diabete. In 1984 he had hepatitis and in 1998 had cirrhosis. Family history : two brothers had hepatitis B and then liver cancer, another brother had rectal cancer.

In July 1999 because of the white blood cells decrease after the chemotherapy, he started to take xxxx to protect the bone marrow and take XZ-C1+XZ-C4+XZ-C6. After taking them more than six months, the whole blood count come back again. His energy level is increased and his appetite is getting better and continue taking the medicine. In July 2000 the cystoscopy showed that the bladder was filled well and a 1.3cmx0.6cm xxxxx in the xxxx ranges, considering as the recurrence of the tumors and continued to take the medicine until June 2001, because of the prostate enlargement which caused the frequency and urgency of the urine. CT showed that this lesion was getting bigger than before(in February in 1999), then had arterialy poured once. He continued to take XZ-C1+XZ-C4+XZ-C6 untill July 2002 CT showed that the lesion in CT shrinkled. After taking the medicine, his general medical condition is better and his appetites is good without the bloody urine. He kept coming back to followup and take his medicine for more than six years. His lesion in his bladder is stable without metastasis and enlargement.

Comments: This case is transitional cell carcinoma. After the removal of the cancer, the long- time chemotherapy didn't stop the recurrence. Because of many years of the poured bladder and many times of the cystoscopy with the enlargement of the prostate and the narrowness of the urother, the cystescopy is difficult to be done. After taking XZ-C such as XZ-C1+XZ-C4+XZ-C6, the neoplasm in the bladder didn't develop and didn't metastes. Since he had this disease, it has been 11 years. His general medical condition is well and his appetite is getting better. When he walked more, sometimes the bloody urine occurred.

Case 5 Mrs. Pu, female, 67year-old,Shiyiazhoung, worker, Medical record number::7601511.

Diagnosis: The recurrence after the surgery of the abdominal cavity serous tumors

Disease courses and treatment conditions:because of the belly was getting bigger and ascites, in May 1999 he was hosptilized in Tongjing and ascite(++) and his belly was like to frog and the tumor can be touched. On April 9 the surgery found that there were very many different sizes of the tumor, which were gel-like lump full of the abdominal cavity. One by one were removed, the total weight are 2.5g. During the operations, the chemotherapy tube was put with XXX 500mg. After the operation of four days xxx500MG once/per day and continued to use five days and xxx 100mg once/per day and continuing three days. On June 16 1999 he started to take XZ-C1+XZ-C4 andd after two months she is vigour and her appetite is good and her weight increases. PE: there were no lymph nodes in the superclavial, the abdomen is soft and flat, the ascite(-) and continue to take the XZ-C and refilled her medicine every month until November 26 2000, PE: there was a lump of the fit=size, hard, many nodual on the surface and deep and the clear edges which showed the tumor recurrence. The patient refused to the operation again and to chemotherapy, however he continued to take the XZ-C medicine: XZ-C1+XZ-C4+LMS+MDZ and the anticancer gel on the skin patched. Until Febrauay 24 2002 PE: there was on abnormal and her abdomen was soft and there was a lump which was hard, deep and clear edge and the size is smaller than before and her medical condition is stable. Until December 15 2004 her medical condition is good and her appetite is good and her abdomen is little enlarge and her ascite(++) and there is a fit-size lump with unsmooth surface and many nodule and deep and fix without the metastasis further. After her operation until now she has been following up with us more than six years and her medical condition is stable and the tumor is not metasatasis further.

Comments: This case is the serous tumor in the abdominal cavity. After the removal, the tumor recurrence. After the chemotherapy one week, the reaction is great so that in June 1999 she started to take XZ-C1+XZ-C3+XZ-C4 and she continued to take this medicine for more than six years and her medical condition is stable without the far metastasis and the tumors didn't grow big. She lives well with the tumors.

4. The typical cases of extensive bone metastasis with Z-C immunomodulatory anticancer medication treatment

Case 1 Mrs Pan, female,68year-old, Shengyang

Diagnosis: multiple bone metastasis after the removal of the breast cancer.

Disease courses and treatment: in 1984 the patient had the removal of the right breast cancer I stage, the pathology showed that simple breast cancer without lymph node metastasis. After the xxx +xxxx chemotherapy for two years, she started to use some immune enhancing drug. In January 2001 she felt the right shoulder pain and ECT showed that multiple bone metastasis and the supericlavical lymph nodes enlargement. Since March 27 she had 25 times radicacto therapy on the sites of the right superocliviceal lymph nodes and the whole blood counts decreases and the white cell counts decrease into 2.9x109/L. After the radiactherapy, her condition stable.

On June 15 2001 he started to take XZ-C such XZ-C1+XZ-C2+XZ-C4+LMS+MDZ+VS for two months and her symptom significantly increased. After six months ECT was normal and she is stable. On September 2 2002 on the phone she told us that she is stable and takes her medicine regularly for more than four years. In April 2005 She called us that she is energetic and her appetites is great and walking as the normal healthy persons. On her physical examination, Ultrasound of her liver and gallbladder,Chest X-ray, ECT etc she is normal.

Comments:this patient had right breast cancer after the operation for more than 17 years with bone metastasis and right shoulder pain. After the radiactiv therapy her medical condition is getting better. After taking XZ-C for a long period to protect thymus and bone marrow function, her metastasis was controlled well.

Case 2 Mr. Zhong, male, 66 year-old, Wuxiu, officer, Medical record number:: 11602315
Diagnosis: right kidney clear cell tumors with the bone marrow metastasis and superclavaical lymph node metastasis.

Disease courses and treatment condition: Because of the pain in the right should, the diagnosis was "the inflamtion of the sourround shoulder", which there was a lump as big as XXX behind the right clavical and stern bone, the biopsy showed adenocarcinoma. After CT of abdomen and chest Ultrasound, there was no lesion found. On March 2002 he started to take the XZ-C such as taking XZ-C1+XZ-C4 and plastic XZ-C3. After the plastic gels, the lump was getting soft and shrinkle into small. On March 24 2002 Ultrasound showed a lump of 3.1cmx4.3cm in the right kidney. CT showed : L2,L4 had bone damage and still took the XZ-C and GEM+XXX chemotherapy once. On May 16 2002 the right renal was removed which there was a lump of the size of table tennis. Pathology showed clear cells. Because he was on the immune function medicine, his medical condition was stable and his appetite is good. Although he had the metastasis of his whole body, he still walked as the normal persons. In 2002,2003 and 2004 he came back every month to refill his medicine and his medical condition is stable. Until July 2004 he suddenly lost the ability of speech and headache. CT showed that the bleeding of the brain. After three weeks of the hospitalization,his medical condition was stable and CT showed that the brain bleeding was absorbed and he continues to take XZ-C1+XZ-C2+XZ-C6+LMS+XXX+XXX+xxxx etc. His medical condition is good and he is vigour and his appetite is good.

Comments: this case is the right metastasis lump of the clavic bone with L2 and L4 bone metastasis, the biopsy showed the metastasis adenocarcinoma. After the whole examination the right kidney tumor was found. On May 16 2002 he was diagnosed as right kidney clear cell cancer and the kidney was removed. On March 16 2002 he started to use the XZ-C by taking and plastic. After three years his medical condition is stable and his appetite is good and he is vigour.

5. The cases of simply using Z-C anti-cancer traditional Chinese medications for 5 to 11 years after radical surgery without chemotherapy and radiotherapy

Case 1 Ms Liu, female, 49 year-old, Changsha in Hunan, teacher, Medical record number::260003372
Diangosis: breast infiltrating ductal cancer.

Disease courses and treatment condition: in February 2005 a left breast lump was found which is 2cmx1.5cm, biopsy showed that high degree mutation. On March 8 2005 she had CAF. On May 30 2005 the breast cancer was removed partially, pathology showed the breast cancer so that the breast cancer radiact removal was performed Pathologyshowed that left breast cancer infiltrated ductal cancer. LN0/20 with the C-erB2(++), P53(+), PR(-),ER(-),nm23(+). After the surgery the chemotherapy was used for six cycles. On Octocber 22 2005 she started to take XZ-C to strengthen the curative effects and to prevent the recurrence and metastasis.

Comments:in this case before the operation the lymph nodes under armpit were palpatited. Chemotherapy for six cycle was used before the operation and after the operations to strengthen the long time curative effect. She persistently takes these medicine more than six years and her healthy condition is stable.

Case 2 Mr. Yan, female, 71 year-old, Wuhan, teacher, Medical record number:s:100188
Diagnosis: ascending colon carcinoma

Disease courses and treatment: Because of abdomen pain and bloody stool, the patient was diagnosed as colon cancer by colonoscopy with biopsy. On December 19 1994 he had half of the right colon removal. Pathology showed the medium grade of colon adenocarcinoma involved in serosa. After the operation, he didn't accept other therapy. On July 4 1995 he started to take XZ-C1+XZ-C4 as assistant therapy to prevent the recurrence and metastasis. He only takes XZ-C more than ten years and his healthy condition is very good. In April 2005 when he was 81 years old and came back to follow up with us, he was healthy and played the card every day in the afternoon.

Comments: this case is that after the removal of the ascending colon, the patient just takes XZ-C medicine as the assistant therapy to protect recurrence more than 10 years and his condition is stable.

Case3 Mr. Zhou, male, 49year-old, Wuhan, officer, Medical record number:s: 410804
Diagnosis: lung cancer in the right low labor

Disease courses and treatment: In 1996 the patient started to have cough and chest tightness and low fever and difficult breath and was treated as the Cold. In April 1997 he suddenly started to cough blood and X-ray and CT showed the right lung cancer in low lobe. And at the same month he had right low lobe lung removal and Pathology showed that lung low grade adenocarcinoma. After the operation, his condition is stable and didn't have chemotherapy and radioactive therapy. On May 15 1997 he started to take XZ-C:1,4,7,vitamin C,B6 E,A. After he took these medicine his energy level is increase and appetite was great and his face is red and there were no recuurence and metastasis and no complaints. In June 2004, the patient came back to follow up with us he continues to take these medicine more than three years. Everything is stable. So far his condition is stable as the normal healthy person after he took his medication more than eight years.

Comments: this patient has right low lobe low grade adenocarcinoma. After the operation, he didn't have radioactive and chemotherapy treatment and he only takes the XZ-C medication XZ-C1+C4+C7. After taking these medicine more than eight years, his energy level is high and appetite is good and his healthy condition is great.

Case 4 Mr. Zheng, male, 52 year-old, Wuhan, driver, Medical record number::11302254
Diagnosis: right lung low grade adenocarcinoma with lymph node metastasis

Disease courses and treatment: because of bloody cough he had the CTscan which showed that right low lung tumor and the bronchoscopy didn't show abnormal. On December 12 2001 he had the removal of the right middle and lower lobe and one lymph node between lobe and two lymph node in the entrance were found. Pathology showed that low grade adenocarcinoma with lymph node mestastasis. After the operation he has once chemotherapy. In 2002 he started to take XZ-C to prevent the tumor recurrence and metastasis. He continues to take the XZ-C1+C4+C7+LMS+MDZ for more than three year and his condition is stable and he is energetic and his appetite is great.

Comments: this patient has the right low lobe adenocarcinoma with lymph node metastasis. After the chemotherapy once, then using the XZ-C1+C4+C7 as the supplement treatment. XZ-C1 kills the cancer cells without killing the normal cells. XZ-C4 protects the thymus and bone marrow; XZ-C7 to protect the lung function. He continues to take his medication for more than three years and there was not metatastasis. When he came back to follow up for his fourth year treatment, his condition is stable and his appetite is great and walked as the normal healthy person.

Case 5 Mr. Yin, female, 60 yr, Huangpu, Medical record number::8301655
Diagnosis: sigmoid colon cancer and the removal of half of the left colon.

Disease courses and treatment: In August 1998 the patient had bloody stool and was treated as hemorrhoid. In Octocber 1999 when he had the colonoscopy in Xiehu hospital which there is narrow in the 32cm from the anus. On December 3 1999 he had the removal of half of the left-colon. Pathology showed:sigmoid xxxx adenocarcinoma involved in the whole layers of the colon and the metastasis of the nearby lymph nodules(6/8). On Jan 12 2000 he started to take XZ-C: XZ-C1+XZ-C4+LMS+MDA+VT to protect recurrence and metastasis. After he continues to take the XZ-C more than three years and eight months, his son came to refill the medicine on August 4 2003 and told us that his medical condition was good and did the chores every day and planted a lot of different kinds of flowers and vegatables watering them with ten buckles of water. The patient has been in the good condition and happy and has good energy. After his operation, he continues to take the XZ-C medicines only everyday without other chemotherapy. When he followed up with us, he already took the medicine more than five and half years.

Comments: the case is that sigmoid colon carcinoma with metastasis of the nearby lymph nodes. After the removal of the operation the patient didn't have chemotherapy because of the decrease of the white blood cells so that he took the XZ-C as the assistant therapy to protect the bone morrow and thymus to improve the body immune system to protect the reccurrence and the metastasis. After five and half years, his condition was good.

Case 6 Ms. Yun, female, 63year-old, Jiling, officer, Medical record number::8601705
Diagnosis: the rectal adenocarcinoma

Disease courses and treatment: in Octocbor 1999 the patient has the bloody stool and the the rectaoscopy showed there is a flower-like tumor in the 10cm distance from the ana and Pathology showed the rectal cancer. On November 22 1999 the rectal radioactive surgery was done in the affliatite hospital with Dixon ways. After the operation the patient's condition is stable. On December 2 the chemotherapy was done(urine xxxx 1.0g/day, for five days, xxx 100mg/day for three days). On December 9 the white blood cell counts decrease into 0.09x109/L, on December 10 the white blood cells decrease into 0.06x109/L, injection of the medicine of increasing the white blood cells for five days, the white blood cells into1.1x109/l and had the pneumonia and fever with 40C. On January 2 xxxx after treatment with xxxx+xxxx, the patient still has fever and had the throat infection with three bacteria and can not eat and drink anything. After using XXX for five days, the temperature dropped into 38C. Because this patient had hypertension, diabetes and lung diseases, her medical condition is weak and severe and had twice warrancy from the hospitals. After two months of the treatment, she is stable. On March 20 2000 she started to take XZ-C for half of the years and her medical condition is stable and can do a little chores and can support her daily life by her own. On September 2000 she recurred very well and can shop in the nearby market and do little chores. She has been taken the medicine for more than five years consistently. In May 2005 her daughter come to refill the medicine and told us that she is totally fine and still do some house chores as healthy as other normal healthy individuals.

Comments: this case is the radial rectal cancer removal and the chemotherapy. After these her immune function and bone morrow function were inhibited so that she had throat and both the lung infections, which later are two fungus infections. After the treatment her condition started to get better and started to take the XZ-C which XZ-C1 only inhibited the tumor cells without affecting the normal cells and improve the immune fucntions, XZ-C4 to protect thymus and bone marrow to improve the immune function. The chemotherapy can inhibit the bone marrow so as to lead the bone marrow inhibition to some degrees which can affect the patients for more than 2 to 3 years so that XZ-C which have protect thymus and bone marrow function need to be taken for several years to benefit the bone marrow and immune functions

Case 7 Ms Pen, female, 39 year-old, Shichuang Luchang, officer, Medical record number::7801545
Diagnosis: Thyroid cancer

Disease course and treatment: On April 27 1999 after the removal of the right neck lump, diagnosed as lymphocyte thyroid cancer. On May 6 1999 he had the radical total removal of the thyroid, then he had hourse voice and didn't have chemotherapy. On July 24 he started to take XZ-C:XZ-C1+XZ-C4, LMS,VS and follow-up with us every month and continue to use more than half years. Until Jan 2000 his voice gets better and after continue to take XZ-C another three months his voice come back to the normal. His general conditions get better and his emotion is stable and appetite is good and his energy level came back and he can go back his work. He persistently takes XZ-C1+XZ-C4 to improve his immune function and followed with us more six years and in May 2005 when he came back to us, his general condition is very good.

Comments: this patient has capillary thyroid cancer. After operation his voice was housral and didn't have radiology and chemoactive therapy. He only took the XZ-C to improve his immune function and to prevent recurrence and metastasis.

Case 8 Mrs. Pu, female, 67year-old,Shiyiazhoung, worker, Medical record number::7601511.
Diagnosis: The recurrence after the surgery of the abdominal cavity serous tumors

Disease courses and treatment conditions:because of the belly was getting bigger and ascites, in May 1999 he was hosptilizated in Tongjing and ascite(++) and his belly was like to frog and the tumor can be touched. On April 9 the surgery found that there were very many different sizes of the tumor, which were gel-like lump full of the abdominal cavity. One by one were removed, the total weight are 2.5g. During the operations, the chemotherapy tube was put with XXX 500mg. After the operation of four days xxx500MG once/per day and continued to use five days and xxx 100mg once/per day and continuing three days. On June 16 1999 he started to take XZ-C1+XZ-C4 andd after two months she is vigour and her appetite is good and her weight increases. PE: there were no lymph nodes in the superclavial, the abdomen is soft and flat, the ascite(-) and continue to take the XZ-C and refilled her medicine every month until November 26 2000, PE: there was a lump of the fit=size, hard, many nodual on the surface and deep and the clear edges which showed the tumor recurrence. The patient refused to the operation again and to chemotherapy, however he continued to take the XZ-C medicine: XZ-C1+XZ-C4+LMS+MDZ and the anticancer gel on the skin patched. Until Febrauay 24 2002 PE: there was on abnormal and her abdomen was soft and there was a lump which was hard, deep and clear edge and the size is smaller than before and her medical condition is stable. Until December 15 2004 her medical condition is good and her appetite is good and her abdomen is little enlarge and her ascite(++) and there is a fit-size lump with unsmooth surface and many nodule and deep and fix without the metastasis further. After her operation until now she has been following up with us more than six years and her medical condition is stable and the tumor is not metasatasis further.

Comments: This case is the serous tumor in the abdominal cavity. After the removal, the tumor recurrence. After the chemotherapy one week, the reaction is great so that in June 1999 she started to take XZ-C1+XZ-C3+XZ-C4 and she continued to take this medicine for more than six years and her medical condition is stable without the far metastasis and the tumors didn't grow big. She lives well with the tumors.

Case 9. Mr. He, male, 76year-old, Henan, officer, Medical record number:;9201839
Diagnosis: left renal clear cell cancer.

Disease courses and treatment condition:in 1996 there is a kidney cyst, in 2000 on PE there is a 7.5cmx6.5cm cysts in the left renal. CT and MRI showed that left kidney tumor. On August 31 2000 the removal of the left kidney was done in Tongjing hospital. Pathology showed that middle degree of kidney clear cells carcinoma. After the surgery he started to take the xxxx without chemotherapy and radiactvie therapy. On September 28 2000 she started to take XZ-C1+XZ-C4+XZ-C6 to protect thymus ad bone marrow. After taking the medicine one month, he is vigour and his appetite is still low and contine taking the medicine for three months, his general condition is good and his energy level is high and his sleeping is good. After taking the medicine for one year, Ultrasound of the abdomen, Chest X-ray, and others regular tests are normal and he continues to take XZ-C1+XZ-C4+XZ-C6 to prevent the metastasis and recurrence. After five years of taking these medicine, his healthy condition is stable. On April 10 2005 when he follow-up with us, he is healthy and his face is glowing of the health and his voice is xxxx, and he is energetic and had the hear decrease due to his age. His medical condition is100 by CCCCCC.

Comments: this case is left kidney clear cells. He was 76 year-old when he had his surgery. Because of his age, he didn't have the chemotherapy and radioactive therapy and only take the XZ-C immune therapy as the supplement therapy to protect his thymus and bone marrow to improve the immune functions and protect the recurrence and metastasits. He has been taking the medicine for more than five years and when he came back to followup he was 80 years old. His general medical condition is good and his appetite is good and his face is glowing of the health and his energy level is high and his voice is xxx as the normal healthy person.

Case 10 Mr. Zhen, female, 44 year-old, Wuhan, Medical record number:s: 700121
Diagnosis: Breast adenocarcinoma

Disease courses and treatment: right breast lump was found for three months which the needle biopsy showed breast cancer. On February 20 1995 she had the removal of the breast cancer and once radioactive therapy after the operation. Because of the weakness, she couldn't tolerate it. On May 11 1995 she started to take XZ-C1+XZ-C4 and continued to take them for more than three years. After she took the medicine, her energy level was improving and her appetite was increasing and her weight is increasing. Following up with us every month and her medical condition is stable.

Comments: this patient had the removal of the breast on Feb 20 1995 and once radioactive therapy after the operation. Because of the weakness the radiative therapy was stopped. In May 1995 she started to take the XZ-C1+XZ-C4. After three years her condition is stable. When she came back for her five year follow-up, she is healthy.

Case 11 Ms. Lee, female,33 year-old, Changda in Hunan, worker, Medical record number::3400667
Diagnosis: Left simple breast cancer.

Disease courses and treatment: On November 29 1996 she had the removal of the breast cancer in Changda which showed the right armpit lymph node metastasis(3/5). After one month, CMF was done which she used once/week, for more than four weeks.

On December 25 1996 she started to use XZ-C to protect her bone marrow. After taking the medicine, her whole blood went back to the normal level. From April 2 1997 to May 14 1997 she had radioactive 15 times in right breast inner line, 15 times under the armpit right and 25 times in the right breast outside lines. XZ-C were taken as the supplement therapy without the side effects. The patients is stable and reaction small and even no side effects when she took XZ-C with radiactherapy and chemotherapy. In June 2004 she only took XZ-C. Every three months she came to Wuhan to refill her medicines. Her condition is stable. In Dec 2004 when she came back to follow up with us, she is energetic and appetite is good and her face is glowing of the health. Acting is as the normal healthy persons. She came to refill her medicine from XXXX to WuHAN.

Comments: the curative experience of the treatment:1). During the radiacti and chemotherapy the XZ-C4 can reduce the reaction, during the interval time between the radiac and chemotherapy and after them XZ-C can strengthen longterm curative effects to protect the recurrency.2)after the surgery about six months the radia+chemotherapy +XZ-C can kill the remaining tumor cells or the small tumor lesions, meanwhile to protect the host immune organs. After taking the medicine for six months, the patient's general condition is good so that XZ-C can get rid of the wrong and strengthen the long-time curative effects. After 9 years of the operation, XZ-C can strengthen the long-term therapy.

Case 12 Ms Liu, female, 49 year-old, Changsha in Hunan, teacher, Medical record number::260003372 Diangosis: breast infiltrating ductal cancer.

Disease courses and treatment condition: in February 2005 a left breast lump was found which is 2cmx1.5cm, biopsy showed that high degree mutation. On March 8 2005 she had CAF. On May 30 2005 the breast cancer was removed partially, pathology showed the breast cancer so that the breast cancer radiact removal was performed Pathologyshowed that left breast cancer infiltrated ductal cancer. LN0/20 with the C-erB2(++), P53(+), PR(-),ER(-),nm23(+). After the surgery the chemotherapy was used for six cycles. On Octocber 22 2005 she started to take XZ-C to strengthen the curative effects and to prevent the recurrence and metastasis.

Comments:in this case before the operation the lymph nodes under armpit were palpatited. Chemotherapy for six cycle was used before the operation and after the operations to strengthen the long time curative effect. She persistently takes these medicine more than six years and her healthy condition is stable.

Case 13. Mr. Qian, male, 66year-old, Wuhan, accounting, Medical record number::5401066 Diangosis:rectal carcinoma

Disease courses and treatment conditions:occasionally diarria and constipation with bloody stool for two years. The rectal examination showed that there was a 3cmx3cm lump at the 6 clock point in the xxxx position. On January 20 1998 the colonoscopy showed the polypoid mutation of the rectal colon. On January 24 1998 Dixon which the 40cm of the colon were cut off was done in the xiehae hospital, Pathology showed that rectal cancer with middle division and invade into the muscular layer without lymph nodes metastasis and the margin clear. After thesurgery, on March 3 1998 he started to use the XZ-C and took this medicine persistenly for more than eight years and he come back to work for more than five years He is stable and still continued to use these medicine.

Comments: this case is rectal adenocarcinoma. In January 1998 Dixon was done and Pathology showed that rectal adenocarcinoma, middle-degree. After the operation he only took the XZ-C1+XZ-C4 for more tha eight years. His medical condition is stable.

Suggestions: After the rectal Dixon without the chemotherapy, he only took the immune regulation medicine XZ-C to protect his thymus and bone marrow to improve his immune functions to improve the life quality and prevent the recurrence and metasatasis. He was stable.

Case 14 Ms Year-oldng, female, 32year-old, Zhaoyang, accounting, Medical record number::500993 Diagnosis: rectal villious adenocarcinoma

Disease courses and treatment condition: the patient had bleedy stool. In September 1997 the Colonoscopy and biopsy showed the rectal cancer. On September 17 1997 she had the rectal radial operation which showed that the lump was 1.0cmx1.0cm on the bases and was 4cm distance from the ana. Pathology reported the rectal villious adenocarcinoma and invaded into the all of the wall of the intestines with the menstema lymph node metastasis. After the operation she had chemotherapy once. Because of the decrease of the white blood cells she stop chemotherapy and started to use XZ-C1+XZ-C4. Her medical condition is well and stable. She continued to take the medicine for more than eight years only without chemotherapy and other therapy. She did her chores as the normal persons.

Comments:this case is the rectal radial removal on September 17 1997, during the operation, the metastasis were found in the mestaen membrane lymph nodes and invades the whole wall of the intestines. After the operation she had the chemotherapy once which had been stopped because the side effects were severe. Since December 3 1997 she started to take XZ-C only for more than eight years to prevent the reccurrence and metastasis after the surgery. Her medical condition is well.

Case 15 Mr. Yu, Male, 69year-old, Heilunjing, officer, Medical record number::6001181. Diangosis: the bladder transitional cell cancer

Diseases courses and treatment condition: The bloody urine on Februay 27 in 1998. On March 2 the cystoscopy and ultrasound showed that there was the round lump in the front wall, which is 1.6cmx1.4cm and growed toward to the cavity of the bladder and is the neoplasum of the front wall of the bladder. On March 10 in 1998 the surgery removed the tumor tissues in the bladder and Pathology showed that the bladder transitional cell tumors. He was told that this tumor is the recurrence of the tumors. After the surgery, he had once chemotherapy(on May 26 1998). His reaction to chemotherapy is severe such as the vomiting, nausea, and the whole body is uncomfortable. The left testicule enlarges so that he stop chemotherapy. On June 18 1998 he started to take the XZ-C. He follow up with us very month and his condition is good and his urine is normal and he doesn't have any other symptoms. He follow up with us for more than six years and he is healthy.

Comments: in this case on March 10 1998 the surgery removed three tumors in the bladder and Pathology showed that bladder transitional cell carcinoma. After the operation once chemotherapy was done which the patient had severe reaction to this chemotherapy. On June 18 1998 he started to take the medicine XZ-C1+XZ-C4+XZ-C6. He continued to take this medicine for more than seven years and his healthy condition is good without other therapy and without the recurrence and metasatasis.

Comments:

Case 20 Ms. Zhang, female,39 year-old, Wuhan, account, Medical record number::1700321
Diagnosis: the stomach cancer from the stomach ulcer, low differential adenocarcinoma

Disease courses and treatment: in March 1994 because of the uncomfortable in the upper abdomen for one month and getting worse for one week so that the endoscopy showed the stomach ulceration. On April 20 1994 the major stomach was removed and had chemotherapy for six courses of the treatment after the operation with xxxxx+xxxxx to protect the livers. Pathology showed the low differential stomach canciroma and had lymph nodes metastasis. On November 22 1995 he started to take XZ-C1+XZ-C4+XZ-C8 only to protect the bone marrow and follow up with us for more than ten years. He doesn't have metastasis and recurrence and his condition is great.

Comments: this patient had low degree adenocarcinoma in the stomach and lymph node metastasis. On April 20 1994 he had the removal of his major stomach, then he had six courses of the chemotherapy. On November 22 1995 he took the medicine only and followed up with us for more than ten years. His medical condition is great.

Suggustions: After the operation the combination of the chemotherapy and XZ-C medicine can improve the long-term treatment. XZ-C can prevent the cancer recurrence and metastasis.

Case 17 Mrs Hang, female, 65year-old, Huangpi in Hubei, Medical record number::10402074
Diagnosis: the middle esophogus carcinoma

Disease courses and treatment condition: In April 2001 the patient had difficulty swallowing and chest and back pain and gradually increased. Until June only can eat the liquid food and vomit the mucous staffs. On June 6 2001 the barium swallow tests in the xxx showed under the aorta branch xxxx 2cm there is a 10cm lenghth narrow and 6cm xxxxxlump in the left wall and the muscous stop. Because of the cost, she didn't have the operation, radioactive and chemotherapy. On June 25 she started to take XZ-C. After three months, her general condition is better and her appetite is getting better and the difficultying swallowing is getting better and can eat the rice soup, noodle. She continued taking the medicine until March 2002 then can take the rice and regular food. In July 2003 she just took XZ-C4+XZ-C2. In April 2005 when she followed up with us, she is energetic and her appetites was great at that time she had been taking XZ-C for more than five year. He condition is stable and can eat the regular food and can do light house work.

Comments: This patient had esophageal cancer which she only took XZ-C to control her condition without the operation, radiactiv therapy and chemotherapy. For more than four years, there was no metastasis and her condition had been controlled and can eat the regular food and rice. She is as healthy as other old persons and can do some choresevery day.

She kept taking her medicine regularly.

Case 18 Mr.Huang male, 66year-old, Huanpi, officer, Medical record number::300584
Diagnosis: the middle and low esophagous carcinoma

Disease courses and treatment:in March, he had the difficulty to swallow and the barium swallow test showed that the middle and low esophagum cancer. In May 1996 he had the removal of his cancer without other therapy. On June 19 1996 he started to use the XZ-C as the supplemental therapy to prevent the reccurrence and metastasis. He only takes XZ-C to protect his thymus and bone marrow for more than three years, then he changed into periodly taking the medicine. He is energetic and his appetite is good and walking and other activities are the same as the normal persons. In April 2005 when he came back to follow up with us, his condition is stable.

Comments: after the operation of his esophague, this patient only took XZ-C to assisting his therapymore than nine years, his condition is stable.

6. The typical cases of acute lymphoblastic leukemia with the treatment of Chemotherapy plus Z-C Chinese medications

Case Mr. Zhao, female, 34 year-old, Wuhan, officer, Medical record number:: 9801953
Diagnosis: Acute leukemia

Disease course and treatment: On Novermber 29 the patient was diagnosed as acute leukemia in Beijing hospital and was treated by chemotherapy for seven months. In August 2000 he was treated by bone morrow transplantation, however the results were not good after that because WBC, RBC and platelets are low. Such as wbc0.5x109/l, platelets were 5x100/l, HB46g/l. He depended on the blood transfusion, which were performed once per 8-9 days for 250ml. During his inpatient in Beijing, He had 10 times blood transfusion and 14 times platelets (once per 10 days).In Feb 2001 he came to Wuhan and on Feb 2, 2001 he started to use XZ-C1+XZ-C2+XZ-C8 to protect his thymus and his bone morrow. In April 2001 his WBC and RBC and Pletelets increase and stop to get transfusion. He takes XZ-C1+XZ-C2+XZ-C4 for more than one year and seven months and feel fine and he looked good and healthy and appetites increases and walking and runnig as the normal individual. In September 4 2003 he traveled to America and took his medicine XZ-C1+XZ-C2+XZ-C4 with him and he takes his medicine persistently.

In 2004 he immigrate into Canada and took his medicine XZ-C1+XZ-C2+XZ-C8 regularly and increase blood soups which will be filled once per 3 months. In April 2005 He called me and told us that he was healthy and his medical condition was controlled very well and appetite and sleep very well and started to work on business and energy level is perfectly well.

Comments: This patient has ALL and after seven months chemotherapy in August 2000, he had bono marrow transplantation. However the treatment results were not good because his blood counts were still low which he depended on the blood transfusion. On Feb 2 2001 he started to take

XZ-C1+XZ-C2+XZ-C4. And increase blood soups etc. and after four months his blood counting went back the normal. After one year and seven months his blood counting keeps normal and he is healthy and has taken these medicine for more than 4 years and work in the business field and energy level is normal.

Suggustion: All can be treated satisfiedly by chemotherapy and XZ-C to protect the bone marrow and improve the immune system function. Now he has been followed up more than seven years and his healthy condition is very well.

17. THE IMMUNE FUNCTION OF CHINESE HERBAL MEDICATION FOR ADVANCED CANCER PATIENTS

1. The medication which should be used and can improve immune function in advanced cancer

a. The discovery from the tumor experimental research

Advanced cancer are immunocompromised mice and thymus atrophy.

(1) In 1986 in our laboratory to manufacture tumor-bearing animal models removal of the thymus (THC) can be produced tumor-bearing animal models and injection of immunosuppressive agents can also contribute to the establishment of tumor-bearing animal models. Results of the study show that the incidence and development of cancer and immune function of the host and immune function of organs and tissues is certainly a significant relationship. No removal of the thymus is difficult to manufacture cancer animal models. Repeating several experiments, results were confirmed.

(2) Whether the prior immunocompromised then easy to get cancer, or cancer happens then lead immune function to decrease. The results of our experiments are: first, unocompromised and then tend to have a carcinoma; in the absence of immune function decline, the inoculation of cancer is not successful. The results of this study tips: to improve and maintain good immune function and to protect the immune organs Thymus (TH) can prevent cancer.

(3) The animal model of liver metastasis were divided into A, B groups, A with immunosuppressive agents, group B without our laboratory studies of cancer metastasis and immune relationship. Results: A group was significantly more than the number of liver metastases group B. The results suggest that: the transfer of immunization-related immune dysfunction or immunosuppressive agents, may promote tumor metastasis.

(4) In our laboratory of tumor impacting on the immune organs it was found that with the progress of cancer, TH namely cell proliferation was progressively blocked, volume was significantly reduced. These results suggest that: the tumor can inhibit TH, resulting in atrophy of immune organs.

The above experimental results prove: cancer occurrence, development, metastasis and host immune function decline have significantly affirmative relationship, mice with advanced cancer are immunocompromised and Thymus atrophy. Thus, in advanced cancer treatment should be used Increasing immune function drugs, but cannot be used to reduce or suppress the immune immune drugs.

b. Natural herbal medications: from experimental study to find elevated tumor immune suppression drugs

Our results demonstrate that, with the progress of the tumor, the host has thymus atrophy so that we can use some ways to prevent a host Thymus atrophy.

In order to stop atrophy of immune organs when tumor is progressing, we investigated the ways of making recovery of TH function and the immune reconstruction method and searched to look for anti-cancer drugs increased immune from natural herbal medications. Our laboratory over a long period, a batch of 200 kinds of traditional considered to be "anti-cancer medicine," the herbal flavor carried by tumor-bearing animals in vivo anti-tumor screening experiments. It was found that 152 kinds of invalid, only 48 kinds do have some even better inhibit the proliferation of cancer cells, while increasing the role of immunity, including 26 kinds of Chinese herbal medicine (HM) with enhanced macrophage function or stimulate the animals thymus weight increase, or elevated white blood cell; or promote spleen lymphocyte proliferation, enhance lymphocyte transformation rate of T cell immune function enhancement of NK cell activity enhancement of the role of interferon induced pro, the optimal combination, and then liver cancer, stomach cancer, S180. And other tumor-bearing animal models in vivo anti-tumor experiments, further screening, out of no stabilizing effect of further screening and formed a c z suppressor immune regulation medicine, may protect the chest rise Free, nursing marrow and blood, improve immune function. In animal experiments, based on the success of screening, clinical practice, clinically proven in 10 years a large number of cases, zc immune regulation medicine, can improve the quality of life in advanced cancer patients, increased immunity, enhance physical fitness, improve appetite, prolong survival period, more significant effect.

2. The Experimental research of the medication inhibitory on S180 mice and enhancing the immune effects righting training

1. Objective

40 years of Integrative cancer prevention research and practice, found that many traditional Chinese medicine for the treatment of cancer does have a certain effect; in particular, studies of the efficacy of traditional Chinese medicine righting training for the treatment of malignant tumors showed righting The multi-class medicine can enhance health and improve immune function, improve quality of life and prolong survival. But Chinese medicine treatment of tumors were observed in clinical experience, without experimental research. In order to explore Chinese medicine righting training the spleen, and kidney medicine whether BNI can inhibit tumor growth, and therefore, the following experiment.

2. Method

   (1) Experimental animal: Kunming mice 160, 5-6 weeks old, weighing 27 persons 2. 0g, male and female.

   (2) Tumor-bearing animal models: S180 ascites tumor lines, press 1X1O7X0.2ml tumor cells were seeded in each of the mice was the right forelimb armpit skin.

   (3) Experimental groups. The experimental animals were randomly divided into, A Group: Yiqi treatment group ((n = 20); Group B: blood double up treatment group ((n = 20); Group C: nourishing yin treatment group ((n = 20); D Group: Warming kidney treatment group ((n = 20); E Group: ATCA mixture treatment group ((n = 20); F Group: Xiaochaihutang treatment group ((n = 20); Group G: Compound Capsule treatment group ((n = 20); H Group: tumor-bearing control group ((n = 20) of each group in the first two days after inoculation, respectively, herbal oral 0. 4ml / (only · d),. tumor-bearing control group with normal saline control treatment.

   (4) Preparation of the groups of traditional Chinese medicine: the original party in terms of modern dose decoction made from concentrate, crude drug concentration of 200%. And oral doses of the drug concentration above the normal human dose based on dose into mice come. In this study, the righting training the deficiency of qi and blood make up, nourishing yin, warming yang, supplementation and attack ATCA agent, Xiaochaihutang and compound capsules and other medicine to treat mice bearing S180.

   (5) Observation: systematic observation of the mice in each group had time to tumor, tumor survival time measured their serum protein content, the weight of peripheral blood T lymphocyte counts and immune organs.

3. Results righting training and to righting training is a major component of ATCA agent can significantly delay tumor inoculation mice appeared time, inhibition of tumor growth (A, B, C, D, E group inhibition rate was 40 percent, respectively, 45 %, 44.5%, 31% and 36%), to extend the survival time of tumor-bearing mice, (A, B, extend the lifetime of the CDE groups were 27.6%, 45% .38 5%, 25% and 26.5%). Quxie based Xiaochaihutang, compound capsules not significantly inhibited tumor growth and prolonged survival (compared to E group, P> 0. 05) increase 0 A, serum protein B, C, D, E group content, A / G ratio increase, peripheral T lymphocyte counts increased (and G group P <0. 05, B, C groups P <0. 01), thymic atrophy was significantly inhibited.

4. Conclusion This study shows that the righting training or righting training based medicine treatment can inhibit tumor and enhance immunity, can improve varying degrees of peripheral blood T lymphocytes, are more effective treatment than with Quxie.

5. **Discussion**

   (1) The traditional Chinese medicine righting training inhibitory and prolong survival role. Many cancer patients clinically shown "imaginary" symptoms, such as qi deficiency, blood deficiency, yin, yang and the like. Righting training should be adopted on the treatment of

traditional Chinese medicine. This study investigated the inhibitory effect of all phenomena and righting training supplementation and attack, and the results showed that: deficiency of qi and blood make up, nourishing yin yang, etc. Warming righting training in Chinese medicine and traditional Chinese medicine righting training ATCA-based agent can significantly delay the appearance of tumors in mice inoculated with time, inhibition of tumor growth and prolong survival time of tumor-bearing mice. From each group inhibition rate analysis: blood double up in the experimental group, the inhibition rate was 45 percent; in nourishing yin experimental group, the inhibition rate of 44.5%, followed by deficiency of the inhibition action is also up 40 percent, the effect is also good: Once again, ATCA agent inhibitory rate of 36%: but poor Warming kidney treatment group, the inhibition rate of 31%; opinion should be adopted in terms of inhibition of tumor blood double complement and treatment of nourishing yin. From a prolonged survival rate analysis: supplement qi and blood group of 45%, in order to extend the lifetime of the longest group; followed by nourishing yin group, up 38.5 percent, the effect is also good, as deficiency of warming yang and supplementation and attack the ATCA mixture treatment group, but also to prolong survival, but less nourishing yin qi and blood complement and treatment groups. Quxie based Xiaochaihutang, compound capsule treatment group, shown in this set of experiments not significantly inhibit tumor, we can not prolong survival of tumor-bearing mice, the effect of the worst. Therefore, from the extension of terms of survival to double up and nourishing yin blood treatment is preferred, followed by the deficiency of warming yang and supplementation and attack. From both inhibition of tumor and prolong survival analysis of both qi and blood complement the optimal places, followed by nourishing yin, then followed Buzhongyiqi and ATCA mixture, Warming kidney treatment ineffective. As for Quxie of Xiaochaihutang and compound capsules, from the present experimental results, no significant effect.

In short, each righting training and righting training to varying degrees based treatment inhibited tumor growth and prolong survival role, and to Quxie based treatment had no significant anti-tumor and prolong survival role.

This experiment showed that: righting training to righting training medicine or medicine-based treatment of smaller tumors very significant inhibitory effect, and can significantly prolong survival and improve quality of life, so much as a clinical and postoperative radiotherapy One of adjuvant therapy of chemotherapy. Many reported in the literature using the clinical treatment of malignant tumors righting training have achieved good results, the present results further confirmed that supplement qi and blood, nourishing yin, deficiency of other treatment can suppress tumors and prolong survival, as in Integrative clinical treatment of malignant tumors provide an experimental basis.

(2) Chinese medicine righting training to enhance the immune effect. This experiment showed that the righting training in Chinese medicine and Chinese medicine righting training based treatment could improve in varying degrees of peripheral blood T lymphocytes, such as when the first four weeks, T lymphocyte levels were as follows: 41.5% Buzhong group, blood group, double up 44.8 percent, 38.6 percent nourishing yin group, warming yang group 37.5%, ATCA mixture group 35.6%; suppression thymus atrophy, as the first

two weeks, the deficiency of blood double up, nourishing yin, yang Warming and AT-CA mixture treated thymus index were significant differences with the tumor-bearing control group. Tip righting training anti-tumor effect may enhance immune function. Some people think that a lot of plant polysaccharides have immunomodulatory agents (immunenoclulator) performance, called anti-tumor polysaccharides, these polysaccharides can not directly kill cancer cells, but it can activate the immune system to release cytokines have anti-tumor effects or enhanced LAK cells killing effect on cancer cells. Righting training this drug is rich in plant polysaccharides, such as Zhao Kesheng reported: Huang contempt polysaccharide extract, wherein the molecular weight was found 20 000' -2500. The components of normal and cancer patients peripheral blood mononuclear cells (PBMC) in vitro secretion of tumor necrosis factor (TNF) has significant role in promoting. Chen Kai reported: traditional Chinese medicine Fuzheng anti-tumor was transplanted tumor S18. Natural killer cell activity in mice and interleukin-2 (IL-2) activity can promote, and promote T lymphocyte activation, and promote peritoneal macrophage phagocytosis, increased spleen and thymus weight. In short, the role of righting training the human immune system is very complex, pending further observation and research.

(3) Chinese medicine righting training can enhance the body resistance to disease, improve blood cells and build up their strength. This experiment showed that: righting training this drug can increase serum protein in tumor-bearing mice, raising clearing / globulin ratio. Our clinical observations cancer specialist clinics showed that: liver cancer, esophageal cancer, stomach cancer, colorectal cancer applications to righting training based zc, immune regulation of tumor suppressor liter free medicine. Red blood cells, hemoglobin were higher, leukopenia was also suppressed. Description righting instinct enhance blood cells and proteins, increase strength, improve resistance to disease.

One rule is righting training as a combination therapy of tumors has been widely used clinically. The results showed that: righting training drug treatment can delay the vaccinated mice tumor occurrence time, inhibit tumor growth, prolong survival time of tumor-bearing, enhance immune function and disease resistance, improve quality of life. It can provide experimental evidence for clinical anti-cancer medicine.

3. The immune function of Chinese herbal medicine for advanced cancer patients

Patients with advanced cancer is mostly deficiency, a common immune dysfunction. Tonic righting medicine can enhance immune function, prevention and treatment of the patient's tumor immune dysfunction has important significance.

1. Enhance non-specific immune function

(1) Can stimulate animal immune organs thymus, spleen to gain weight: Ginseng can increased thymus weight 2.2-fold as the control group of young mice.

(2) Enhance macrophage phagocytosis: such as ginseng, Codonopsis, Astragalus (Astragalus), angelica, medlar (Wolfberry), etc. can promote macrophage phagocytosis, especially the role of qi drug is obvious.

(3) Increased peripheral leukocytes count: for example, ginseng, astragalus (Astragalus), Codonopsis, Rehmannia and Millettia etc can significantly increase white blood cell count.

2. Enhancing immune function

(1) to promote lymphocyte proliferation: such as ginseng, can increase the number of lymphocytes, yams, mistletoe, etc. can increase the proportion of peripheral blood T cells.

(2) increasing the lymphocyte transformation rate: such as ginseng, astragalus (Astragalus), Angelica, white fungus and other tonics, lymphocyte transformation rate were increased role.

(3) to enhance red blood cell immune function: such as astragalus (Astragalus), medlar (Wolfberry) can significantly increase the red blood cell C36 mice receptor (RBC-C36) a rosette rate and RBC immune complexes (RBC-IC) rosette formation rate

3. Enhanced humoral immunity

(1) the promotion of antibody production: such as ginseng, Huang Jing, Cynomorium, Curculigo, cinnamon, Dodder, meat from Chengdu, which are to promote the role of antibody production, to varying degrees, increased serum IgG, IgA, IgM and other antibody levels.

(2) increasing the number of antibody-forming cells in the spleen: Longspur bud polysaccharide injection can increase more than double spleen cell culture antibody production and yam polysaccharides can significantly increase forming cells in mouse spleen, hemolytic plaque. However, some tonic medications have double-acting of the function of immune: enhancement and inhibition.

4. The Enhancing role of the immune function in tumor-bearing body with Chinese herbs medications

In medicine, tumor formation and development are inadequate due to the machine off the upright, and that positive qi deficiency associated with tumor occurrence, development, treatment and prognosis of the whole process. Righting training is a basic rule in the prevention and treatment of cancer medicine, and the most prominent is the body's immune function, particularly in the regulation of cellular immune function.

Modern studies have shown that pain occurrence, development and prognosis of tumor-bearing machine is closely related to cellular immune status, patients' immune function is suppressed and the body is in immunosuppression. This immune suppression is extremely significant in terminally ill patients or long after chemotherapy or radiotherapy. Surgery, radiotherapy, chemotherapy or disorders can cause a decline in immune function. Therefore, by Chinese medicine righting training to enhance immune function can enhance the body cancer-fighting ability, improve the effectiveness of surgery, radiotherapy, chemotherapy, improve patient quality of life and prolong survival of patients.

1. The effect of Chinese herbal medication on immune organs

The experiments of protecting immune organs and increasing the weight of immune organs were found:

(1) Daily respectively extract 15 g / kg, 30 g / kg with full Angelica and 12.5mg / kg, 25mg / kg ferulic suspensionto fed mice continuous 7 days could significantly increase mouse spleen and thymus weight.

(2) Gavage mice with Polygonum 6g (kg • d) decoction, continuous 7d can significantly increase thymus weight and also antagonize prednisolone-induced immune organ weight decreases.

(3]) Littoralis polysaccharide 32mg / (kg • d), medication 7d, can significantly increase the weight of thymus gland by intraperitoneal injection in mice.

(4) Cistanche deserticola decoction can significantly increase the weight of spleen and thymus of mice.

It must be noted that some herbs can reduce the weight of your immune organs, prompting the immune organ atrophy, such as Hook, cicada, Puhuang, Sarcandrae, rhubarb, etc., to normal mice fed 0.5g / d rhubarb decoction continuous 8d, allows the mouse thymus atrophy, thymus cortical thinning, decreased cell, spleen weight was significantly reduced, splenic artery sheath surrounding the central lymphocytes (mostly T lymphocytes) decrease, and 10mg / kg per day to mice perfusion continuous medication 10d, no significant effect on the immune organs of mice. Generally small dose had no effect, while large doses decreased.

2. Chinese herbal medicine on mononuclear phagocyte system function

Enhancement medicine polysaccharide, ridge type and a variety of other ingredients to enhance the mononuclear phagocyte system, particularly macrophage activity, enhance its function Free recover from illness. Anti-tumor effect of macrophages are activated by tumor antigen-specific T cells release macrophages, activation of macrophages specifically kill tumor cells: macrophages by cytotoxicity mediated cell killing of tumor cells, such as by activating the macrophages secrete tumor necrosis factor (TNF), a proteolytic drunk, interferon (IFN) and other direct killing or inhibiting the growth of tumor cells.

(1) Wolfberry polysaccharides (LBP): Wang Lingdeng (1995) in the "Shanghai Journal of Immunology" summarizes the research before the second phase of immunomodulatory effects of LBP: LBP 0.125g / (kg • d) mice intragastric 5d, can enhance macrophage phagocytosis that LBP has a certain immune function. Zhang and other studies like LBP on mouse peritoneal macrophages in tumor cell proliferation inhibition activity.

(2) Velvet polysaccharide (PAPS): can significantly improve hydrocortisone immunocompromised mice induced macrophage phagocytosis in 0.01ug / ml concentration that is promoted, and a clear dose-effect relationship. PAPS concentration for use in the strongest when 1ug / ml.

(3)Gypenosides: Gypenosies with 300mg / (kg • d) continuous 7d, can significantly enhance the ability of peritoneal macrophage cells. Shou Zhi Juan (1990) in the "Wenzhou Medical College," Volume 20, reported that daily mice were fed a grain-share blue-infusion 50mg (containing 1.21% total soap celecoxib), once daily for one month under the loose connective tissue and abdominal anti-alveolar macrophages volume increases and enhance phagocytic digestion.

(4) ABPS: can induce the synthesis of IL-1 and tumor necrosis factor a. (TNF-α) in macrophages. ABPS 25mg / kg or 50mg / kg, intraperitoneal injection, can improve the LPS-induced IL-1 production. 100mg / kg, intraperitoneal injection, can promote the formation of TNF-α. Its role of considerable strength was the same as BCG.

(5) Psoralen: with lung cancer caused by carcinogens photo Punta acid ethyl cool, intraperitoneally injection of psoralen 1mg / 20g weight, continuous 10d, can significantly enhance lung cancer mouse peritoneal macrophage phagocytosis.

3. Chinese medication enhancing the role of T cells immune function T cells are very important in the body's immune cells, not only will lead to specific cellular immunity, and is involved in immune regulation, and other functions. Tumor cells are often accompanied by changes in cell surface antigens, because of the immune surveillance of T cells, tumor antigen sensitized T cells directly or indirectly kill tumor cells by directly or indirectly cytotoxicity and released cytokines.

(1) Epimedium polysaccharide (EPS): with EPS 100mg / Kg /d continuous 5d, subcutaneous injection, significantly increased peripheral WBC and T lymph cells.

(2) Alfalfa polysaccharide (MPS): in vitro can enhance PHA, CONA, LPS and pokeweed (PWM) induced lymphocyte proliferation. MPS 125mg / (kg · d) and 250 mg / (kg · d), intraperitoneal injection, spleen lymphocyte index and significantly increased the number of lymphocytes. MPS also partially antagonized by intraperitoneal injection of cyclophosphamide murine lymphocytes amine reducing effect.

(3) Medlar polysaccharide (Wolfberry) (LBP): external mouse can significantly increase the percentage of peripheral T lymphocytes. LBP Smg / (kgx d) abdominal plastic injection continuous 7d, peripheral blood lymphocyte count rises, the control group was 65.4%, 81.6% for the treatment group, but increasing the dose does not continue to improve this effect. In the T lymphocyte mitogen CONA inducing conditions, a small dose of LBP (5-10mg / kg) can also cause lymph proliferative response, that the ratio of P to T cells significantly promote proliferation.

(4) **Paeonia**: 12. 5 / kg and 25g / kg dose orally can significantly improve the mice's T lymph cell transformation, TPG; 25g / kg dose orally, can significantly improve the IL Mice 2 activity. Wulingzhi: dose 12.5g / kg and 25 g / kg push the stomach, not only can significantly improve the T lymphocyte function in mice, and 25g / kg dose of IL-2 also significantly increased the activity of mice.

It must be noted, herbs also have to inhibit T cell immune function, such as Sophora, turmeric, Hook, Millettia, rhubarb, etc., which reduce T cell immune function of medicine must be used with caution.

4. The role of traditional Chinese medicine on LAK cells

(1) Wind polysaccharide in a certain concentration range can be significantly increased workers L-2-induced LAK cell killing activity.

(2) The sea buckthorn with blood circulation. In tumor-bearing mice sea buckthorn juice (3g / kg) can significantly improve their spleen NK cells and LAK activity by injected intraperitoneally.

(3) Cao wenguang etc found that three kinds of Chinese herbs medications of APS, PAS and LBP to 5- 30mg / kg intraperitoneal injection were C57BL / 6 mice and found that three kinds of traditional Chinese medicine and more refined could significantly promote the proliferation of mouse spleen cells. The spleen cells were 2X105 / ml with 125-1 000U / ml of rIL-2 induced 4d, APS group found that injections of spleen cells LAK activity of the group increased by 70% compared with normal saline (NS) - 120%: injection PAS group increased by 20 % -90%; injection LBP group by 26% -80%.

(4) Cao wenguang etc from February 1992 to February 1993 with traditional Chinese medicine LBP 111 joint LAK, IL-2medicine LBP 111 joint LAK, IL-2 treatf7ed 79 cases of radiotherapy, chemotherapy ineffective; LBP oral dose 1. 7mg / kg, LAK total application 1. 2-32X 10^{10}, IL-2 applications total 3. 4- 4. 8X107U / person, specific programs in the conventional therapy is stopped after a month, give LBP, 3 weeks after injection riL-2, giving LBP 4 weeks After a large number of patients with autologous PBL isolated LAK cells in vitro, reinfusion after various inspection, and then continue to give LBP and work L-2, 1 weeks. Results 75 cases of evaluable patients, LAK / IL-2 combined with the efficacy of LBP group (36.36%) than single with LAK / IL-2 effect group (18%), the former joint LBP group before and after treatment and NK activity of PBL 500U / ml IL-2 induced the LAK activity increased level significantly higher than the latter alone LAK / IL-2 group. Show LBP could significantly promote NK and LAK cells antitumor activity.

The medications with Increasing Spleen, warming the positive, increasing kidney, YiQi, protecting Yin etc can increase LAK activity in vivo.

(5) **Free remorse functional regulation of traditional Chinese medicine on RBC**
In 1981 American scholar Siegel and others put forward to the concept of "red cell immunity", based on the immune adhesive phenomena of red blood cells and red blood cell surface type I complement variant (CR1) according with immune complexes (IC), illustrates not only the respiratory function of red blood cells, and is involved in a variety of immune and immune regulate the body's: such as the removal of circulating immune complexes, and promote phagocytosis, immune regulation of lymphocyte. RBC is involved in IFN-7, IL2 antibodies and natural killer cells (NK cells), lymphokine-activated killer cells (LAK cells) and phagocytic immune cells regulation and so on.

(1) It was found that Astragalus (Astragalus polysaccharide (APS) enables cancer patients in vitro activity of erythrocyte C3bR shame attached to the tumor cells and immune function enables cancer patients to enhance.APS erythrocyte immune function in cancer patients after human red cell significant mention prop.

(2) In the group of Trichosanthes root (TCS) compared with the untreated group in the Ehrlich ascites carcinoma in mice, it was found that the untreated group RBD-C3 bR rosette rate was significantly lower than the normal group, the treatment group RBC-C3bR rosette rate significantly higher than the untreated group and slightly higher than the normal group, said Ming He mice RBC-C3bR activity was significantly decreased, while xxx including floor allows RBC-C3bR root activity increased significantly. Trichosanthes root influence on mice erythrocyte SOD activity: After the mice inoculated with cancer cells to 11d, the treatment group erythrocyte SOD activity was significantly higher than the untreated group and the normal group. Late tumor-bearing mice decreased erythrocyte SOD, this experiment shows Chinese medicine TCS (Trichobitacin root) to restore and enhance the activity of SOD.

Trichosanthes root influence on red cell immune cat attached the ability of tumor cells: with Ehrlich ascites tumor cells as target cells, to determine the effect on the mice including the F root red blood cell immunity breast tumor cell attachment capability, found after tumor cell inoculation 11d, treatment mice tumor erythrocyte rosette rate (11.90 Soil 5.00)%, significantly lower than the normal mice (22.13 Soil 6.28)%; while tumors treated mice erythrocyte rosette rate (26. 54 persons 7.27)%, slightly higher than the normal group was significantly higher than the untreated group.

Trichosanthes root erythrocyte immune to cancer patients: its cancer patients hemadsorption ability of tumor cells is also a significant enhancement. Tests found that cancer patients directly enhance rosette rate of RBC-C3bR effect, there is a significant difference with normal saline (NS) group, and promote the role and dose-dependent manner.

5. The types of traditional Chinese medications and its component response regulator (BRMS) action

Chinese medicine has a very important characteristic is biological therapy has the role of two-way adjustment, can make the machine off the normal direction to restore immune function.

In 1983 Jingjianping found that Astragalus can "spleen" 1L-2 model mice was significantly improved, but had no effect on normal mice.

In 1991 Xungxiaolin and others studies the effects of Millettia, Fruit of Purple flower Holly, Psoralen medicine on IL-2 in mouse spleen cells and found that these drugs immunocompromised, hyperthyroidism, normal three groups were showed increased inhibition and no influence, reflecting double-acting medicine. Besides these the effects of traditional Chinese medications in the body are closely related to the amountof anti-tumor substance such as Medlar at low concentrations can promote IL 3-secretion, but high concentrations inhibit IL-3 levels. Total glucosides of peony can work to produce IL-2 in a dose-dependent increase when it is in low concentrations; after the concentration exceeds 12. 5mg it inhibits IL 2-secretion.

Chinese medicine has been used in our country for thousands of years and there are lots of BRMS which can be chosen and the research of anti-cancer immune agents in this area can have a bright future. Chinese medicine have mild adverse reactions by oral intake compared with genetic engineering ERMS and exogenous IL-2, IFN TNF. The advantages of Chinese herbs medications of an anticancer role in the body immune system similar to BRMS can be repeatedly administered, non-toxic side effects, and is available for the tumor and chemotherapy, radiotherapy-induced immune dysfunction, boost the immune cell activation, release of endogenous cytokines, causing inhibition of tumor growth.

In modern cancer treatment learn lift, the medicine can at least play a role in three areas: ① enhance the role of anti-cancer effect inherent institutional members of the body, enhance the body's anti-cancer cell system (NK cells, TK cells, LAK cell factor]; ② Some traditional Chinese medicine has a direct anti-cancer effect; ③ some medicine ingredients can reduce side effects of radiation therapy, chemotherapy, reduce the inhabition to the white cells and help to recover recover and even increase radiotherapy and chemotherapy anti-cancer effect.

18. ANTI-CANCER FUNCTION OF CELL IMMUNE SYSTEM

As we all know, the occurrence and prognosis of cancer development and treatment are decided by two contrast factors: the biological characteristics of cancer cells and the host restrictive ability to cancer cells. If these two are balance, the cancer is controlled; if they are imbalance, cancer will develop.

What are the biological characteristics and the biological behavior of the cancer cells? The previous chapters in this book have been outlined respectively. Under normal circumstances, the host itself against cancer cells has certain constraints defense capability, but in cancer the defense capabilities of these constraints are suppressed and damaged in different degrees so as to lead the loss of the immune surveillance of cancer cells and cancer has immune escape, making cancer metastasis.

1. The human body anticancer mechanism and its influencing factors

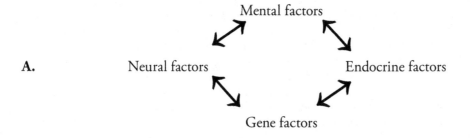

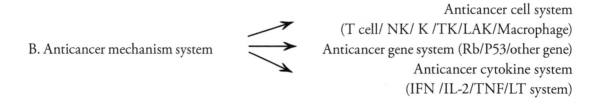

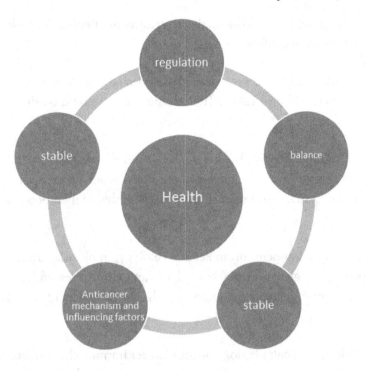

C.

Figure 1 Anticancer mechanism and its influencing factors schematic diagram

The human body has a complete anti-cancer immune system: the anti-cancer immune cells series; anticancer cytokine family; humoral immune series; a series of anti-cancer gene.

Anti-tumor immunological mechanism of the body can be divided ①Cell-mediated immune: including T lymphocytes; NK natural killer cells; K cells; LAK cells; monocyte-macrophages. ②Humoral immune : contains B cells; anti-tumor antibodies. ③ cytokines: interleukin-cell lines have; IFN; TNF; CSF and the like.

These human inherent anti-cancer system and immune substances are their own material in vivo. How biological response modifiers mobilize, activate and enhance the anti-tumor effect occupies an extremely important role in the anti-cancer and anti-metastatic therapy and will have vast work prospects.

Therefore, we have to study which are anti-cancer cells, which are anti-cancer cytokines, which humoral immune can be activated to enhance the anti-cancer metastasis in the human body.

Here, we first review several biological therapies at the history of the 20th century in the treatment of cancer which have impressive results.

In the 1930s, Willam Coley and their successors Coley Nauts treat the advanced cancer with "Coley toxins". More than 200 cases of various types of cancer patients can be analyzed, which more than 30 cases were cured, and life more than 30 years. In the early 1980s Guesada and others treated hairy cell leukemia with IFN-a, which actually made the treatment effective (complete remission /CR + PR/ partial remission) reach over 90%.

In the mid-1980s Rosenberg and others treated patients with advanced metastatic cancer who cannot be treated with other methods with LAK / IL-2. Some patients could be PR(42/228 patients) and CR (9 / 228 cases).

"Biological Therapy" (biotherapy) is also known as "biological regulation therapy" (bioregulator therapy). "Anti-cancer system" is quite complex in our body. From a structural and functional point it is a fairly large network system and under this system a number of members constitutes a "network learning system."

Because of the rapid development of molecular biology, molecular immunology, molecular immunology pharmacology, genetic engineering, basic and clinical research at the molecular level, "cancer establishment" continues to expand and depth, the prospects of its anti-cancer metastasis extremely lure people.

Currently, the research of molecular biology on anti-cancer immunotherapy, are mainly focusing on the "four sub-systems" : "anti-cancer cell therapy," "anti-cancer cytokine therapy", "anti-cancer gene therapy" and "anti-cancer antibody therapy."

The basic characteristics of these molecular biology and molecular immunotherapy are: all of formulations of molecular biology and immunotherapy used are "their selves" in vivo. The fundamental difference from chemotherapy is: it not only did not carry out the role of the damage for the normal body tissue cells, especially the function of cells of the hematopoietic system and the structure and function of the immune system, but mainly there are the regulation and it enhances the role of the immune response; as we all know, radiotherapy and chemotherapy are completely different. Chemotherapy is a kind of non-selective "treatment injury", both kill cancer cells also kill normal cells, which damage the body's normal tissue cells, bone marrow and immune system structure and function suffered serious damage and leads to serious consequences.

Biological therapy is through the regulation of biological response mechanism to make life stable and balance. American scholar Oldam (1984) proposed biological regulation (BRM) theory, which later on this basis, proposed the concept of biological therapy of cancer.

Immune regulation mechanism of life is very important. Immune structure and function are extremely complex and its essence is to identify themselves by tolerance to their own body and removing others to maintain a stable internal environment. Immune defense, immune surveillance and immune homeostasis are three basic types of functions that bodies identify themselves, intolerance to foreign. From the basic point of biological function, immune regulation is one of the basic biological therapies.

On development of cancer there has always been two different views: one view, the tumor occurrence and development are a basic defense mechanism against any restriction body "independent process" so that the treatment for the tumor focused on itself emphatically, few pays attention to the regulation of the immune system; another view is that the tumor occurrence and development are controlled by a variety of factors in vivo, particularly by the regulation of immune factors "involuntary procedure" or "controlled process", are subject to immune surveillance. The cancer cells escape the immune surveillance so that cancer was able to develop. Based on these two different views there are two completely different proposition. The former believe that cancer is a largely unaffected by the body's defense mechanism for any restriction "independent process", which targets the treatment with simply killing cancer cells (regardless of the immune status) which the methods of treatment are radiation therapy and chemotherapy.

Cao guangwen and Du ping presented an important concept which it is about as cancer biotherapy core foundation - the concept of "cancer establishment". And in vivo "cancer establishment" is a fairly large network system, the current basic and clinical research on the anti-cancer organization is expanding and depth, work of anti-cancer treatment has an extremely important role and broad prospects.

About network functionality issues concerning anti-cancer mechanism, currently more study is cytokine network structure and function, the other sides also studied less. This is called as "cytokine network", simply said, various cytokines in structure and function have certain correlations.

2. Anti-tumor effect of various immune functions

The cause of the tumor is very complicated, there are environmental factors, but also the organism internal factors, particularly with the gene mutation, oncogene expression and the decreased immune function.

Modern immunology proposed that immune system has three major functions: the immune defense, immune stable and immune surveillance. There is great significance in the anti-tumor. Immune defenses can resist bacteria, viruses, parasites and other pathogens infection. Immune surveillance function can eliminate mutant cells and prevent tumor occurrence, if the immune dysfunction or loss of immune surveillance monitor can lead to cancer.

After the body normal cells have cancer, cancerous cells on the membrane surface express tumor antigen and the host can recognize such antigens and produces immune response to attack and to exclude tumor cells. Anti-tumor immune response has many ways: both acquired immune response and natural immune response; both cellular immune response and humoral immune response ; both immune cells and immune molecules.

(A) anti-tumor effect of cell-mediated immune

What anticancer human immune cells may be activated, enhanced to do the anti-cancer cell metastasis? Immune cells of participating in vivo anticancer effects are the following:

1. Anti-cancer effect of cytotoxic lymphocytes

Cytotoxic lymphocytes(CTL) play a major role in the anti-tumor immune and have specific cytotoxicity to the same kind of autologous tumor cells and is one kind of anti-tumor lymphocytes subject to MHCI class and (or) class II antigen restrictions. Human CTL cells are CD_4 and CD_8. CTL cells in peripheral blood and spleen have high amounts; thoracic duct, thymus and bone marrow contain a certain amount. The ability of proliferation and accumulation in tumors localized is stronger and the body is more sensitive to radiation and chemotherapy drugs such as cyclophosphamide. CTL is an important effector cell in situ treatment of cancer.

Under certain conditions CTL can produce IL-2, IL-4, IFN, etc., to activate other immune cells, such as anti-cancer killer macrophages, NK cells and anti-B-cell joint anti-tumor effect. Such CTL has a potentially important role in anti-cancer and anti-metastasis.

2. Anti-tumor effect of natural killer cells(NK cells)

NK cells are a group of broad-spectrum anti-NK cell tumor cells, killing activity does not require prior sensitization antigen, do not rely on antibodies, does not depend on the thymus, but also no MHC restricted. The main role is to monitor and to remove cancerous cells. Clinical observations: if NK cell activity is deficient, the incidence of malignant tumors is significantly increased. NK cells are important parts of early anti-cancer immune surveillance.

NK cells bind with tumor cells through tumor cell surface receptor to release perforin protein (Perform, PF) or cytolysin piercing on the tumor cell membrane so that cancer cells die within a fluid outflow. NK cells can release natural killer cell factor (natural killer cell factor, NKCF), this factor can lyse tumor cells. NK cells have a small number, only about 3% of lymphocytes so that it have smaller force for later and larger tumors.

In addition, NK cells produce IL-2, TFN-y and TNF-a, enhance the anti-tumor effects of other cellular and humoral factors.

Distribution of NK cells in organs and tissues is the highest concentrations in peripheral blood and spleen, followed by lymph nodes and peritoneal cells. NK cells is also in the lamina propria alveoli, sinusoidal, intestinal epithelium, skin and bronchial wall, interstitial, esophagus, reproductive tract lymphoid tissue. Low NK cell activity is in bone marrow, thymus undetectable NK activity. NK cells accounted for 5% to 7% of the total number of peripheral blood lymphocytes. NK activity among individual patients is quite different and the level of NK activity in vitro and in vivo is often associated with anti-cancer effect. Therefore, NK activity is often used as a strength and prognosis of cancer immunology indicators and assessment body's anti-cancer therapy response. NK activity was reduced or deficiency often occurs in cancer metastasis. NK activity is often associated with improvement or deterioration of the condition in parallel.

Given the important role of NK cells in anti-tumor immunity, so look for a strong enhancement of biological therapy anti-tumor activity of NK preparation is important. Some micro-organisms or their products, such as BCG (BCG), Corynebacterium parvum (Corynebacteri-urn Parvwm, CP) and certain cytokines such as IL-2, IFN, immune adjuvant interferon inducer can significantly enhance

NK activity. IL-2 and IFN-y combination of NK cell activity enhancement are stronger than a single factor activation. Multiple cytokines enhance the role of NK activity and eliminate residual cancer cells, reducing metastasis and relapse rates. In addition, we developed medicine XZ-C immune regulation agents which can activate NK, IFN-Y.

3. K cells

K cells are in human peripheral blood, spleen and peritoneal cavity, but not much in the thoracic duct and lymph nodes. Advanced cancer patient's serum contains large amounts of free tumor antigen which antigen binds tumor antibody so that K cells can not bind to the tumor cells, and therefore can not play a role in killing tumor. Remove the free tumor antigen, the addition of anti-tumor antibody, or with a non-specific immune stimulants, can enhance K cell activity.

Anti-tumor effect K cells without prior sensitization, do not need to complement participation, but requires the presence of anti-tumor antibodies, so K cells is one of the main anti-tumor antibody effector cells biological therapies.

4. LAK cells LAK cell is the most important modern biotechnology anti-cancer cell. In 1980 Rosenberg and his colleagues found T cell growth factor (TCGF) can short-term induce mouse spleen cells which can give a strong anti-tumor activity. Human peripheral mononuclear cells (PBMNC) can significantly kill a variety of human tumor cell under IL-2 induced. In 1982 Grimn called this kind of IL-2-activated cells which can kill tumor cells that NK cell cannot kill as Lyrnphokine-activa-ted Killer(LAK) cells. LAK cell is a group mainly consisting of mixed lymphocyte with LGL body which is activated by IL-2 cytokines into anticancer cell ; it not only kills the same kind of passaged tumor cells, more importantly, can kill itself.

LAK cells can kill broader spectrum of tumor than NK cells, which LAK cells can kill tumor cells that NK cells cannot kill.

In fact LAK cells are IL-2-activated NK cells and T cells which have similar activity to IL-2-activated NK cells.

From a clinical and practical points all of cells, which are activated into anti-tumor cells by IL-2 cytokines, can be called LAK cells.

5. Macrophages Macrophage plays an important role in tumor immunity. It itself is a kind of effector cells capable of dissolving the tumor cells. If there is significant macrophage infiltration around tumors, the tumor spreads in the lower metastasis rate, the prognosis is better. Conversely, when macrophage infiltration around tumors is small, the rate of tumor metastasis will be higher. Prostaglandin E can inhibit the secretion of TNF gene transcription from macrophages, which antagonist was indomethacin and may counteract this effect.

6. Anti-tumor effect of monocyte-macrophage Its anti-tumor immunity, unless involved in recognizing an antigen and presented the antigen information to T cells and B cells, as

well as participatory role in killing tumor cells antigen. Pathological biopsy tip: there are a lot of tumor monocyte-macrophage infiltration around the tissues, especially in primary and metastatic tumors. If the incidence of patients with a high degree of infiltration, tumor spread and metastasis is low, the prognosis is good; on the contrary, if there is no obvious monocyte-macrophage infiltration surrounding tumor tissue, metastasis rate of tumor spread is high, prognosis is poor.

Monocyte-macrophage tumor cell killing pathways are nonspecific:

(1) An activated macrophage can contact with the tumor cell directly and play a direct killing effect.
(2) The release of TNF and IL-i and other cytokines.
(3) The generation of reactive oxygen species, such as H_2O_2.
(4) The release of lysosomal enzymes and proteolytic enzymes play killing effect.
(5) The release of arginase. L-arginine is an amino acid essential growth of tumor cells. Mononuclear cells stimulates macrophages to release massive arginase and to decompose arginine so as to inhibit tumor growth.

7. Anti-tumor effect of neutrophils

Massive neutrophil can be observed as aggregation and infiltration around the tumor tissue. After activation neutrophil releases: ① reactive oxygen species; ② fat derivatives; ③ cytokines such as IFN, TNF and IL-i, these substances have tumoricidal activity.

Anti-cancer effects of neutrophils: one inhibiting tumor growth, the second is to play a role in killing. Killing time is several hours similar to macrophages, but longer than the time required lymphocytes and NK cells. Although neutrophils life is short, but are huge amounts so that anti-tumor effect must be paid attention. Neutrophils are non-specific anti-tumor effectors and have effects on a variety of tumors.

(B) Anti-tumor effect of humoral immune

In cancer patients serum, anti-tumor antibody can be found, but cannot be detected in all cancer patients. Serum antibody is negative in the majority of progressive or metastasis patients; after surgery or radiation therapy, some patients may turn negative into positive.

Anti-tumor antibodies are divided into protective and closed two: the former is beneficial; the latter is harmful.

1. Protective antibodies

The existing of protective anti-tumor antibodies is closely related to tumor growth and decline. A month or one week before metastasis, serum anti-tumor antibody titer tends to fall, or from positive to negative. There are three kinds of protective antibodies: cytotoxic antibodies, lymphocyte-dependent antibody and cytophilic antibody.

(1) Cytotoxic antibodies: These antibodies need complement participation to kill tumor cells, they are mostly IgM or IgG class.

(2) Lymphocyte-dependent antibody (LDA): such antibodies are mostly IgG, after binding to tumor antigens, which Fc fragment binds lymphocyte surface Fc receptor, the lymphocytes and tumor target cells attach to play a killer role. Such lymphocytes are antibody-dependent killer cells, i.e., K cells.

(3) Cytophilic antibody: It is IgG class antibodies and is macrophages specifically kill tumor way. Unlike activated monocyte-macrophage non-specific cytotoxicity, when addicted to cell antibodies present in body fluids, monocyte-macrophage cells surround the tumor to form a large rosette.

2. Closed factor

Animals and cancer patients have serum blocking factors, it may be proved by experiments. Closed factor is closely related to the presence of tumor ; after tumor is resected, closed factor disappears. If the tumor is blocking factor, the tumor appears relapse. Closed factor has specificity and blocks the same type of autologous or allogeneicfor tumor tissues, however, doesn't block different classes of tumor tissue.

3. The unblocking factor

After tumor resection, not only blocking factor disappears from the serum, and the serum also appeared closed factor antagonist, called deblocking factor (unbiocking factor), deblocking factors also have tumor specificity.

(C) Anti-tumor effect of human cytokine

Which anti-cancer cytokines can be activated, enhanced with anti-metastatic cancer cells in vivo? Cytokines against viruses, parasites, bacteria and cancer immune response in cells plays an important role in the body. It is in clinical trials for cancer treatment and other aspects of bone marrow regeneration. Therefore, cytokine research has a significant increase and there are lots of papers related to the structure and function of cytokine published in the last 10 years. Here is a brief elaboration for interleukins, colony stimulating factor, tumor necrosis factor, interferon and cytokine growth factor 5 categories.

1. Interferon (IFN)

In the 1930s it was discovered that virus-infected cells can protect surrounding cells from virus infection. In 1957 Isaacs and Lindenmann discovered a protein produced by the cells while the body cells are damaged by a virus or stimulation is an interferon. A few years later people realized that the interferon can resist cell differentiation and have immune regulation. Interferon belongs to the cytokine with a variety of biological functions, now known interferon which is divided into three categories: α, β and γ. IFN-α mainly from leukocytes; IFN-β mainly from fibroblasts; IFN-Υ mainly from T lymphocytes.

IFN has anti-proliferative effect on some tumor cells. Its anti-cancer effects may be related to immunoregulatory activity. It increases the activity of NK cells and macrophages.

The main formulations of interferon are: ① a drug name Interferon-alfa-2a, trade names Roferon R -A; ② drug name Interferon-alfa-2b, trade names Intron R -A

Clinical application of interferon: IFN-a is mainly used for ① blood system tumors and lymphomas: for hairy cell leukemia (HCL), chronic myelogenous leukemia, essential thrombocythemia, multiple myeloma, non-Hodgkin's lymphoma. ② solid tumors: Kaposi's sarcoma, renal cell carcinoma, metastatic melanoma. IFN for hematologic malignancies and solid tumors have the effect of slowing its progress; however only part of the role and transient effects.

2. Interleukin (IL)

Interleukin is human immune system natural ingredients, which are a class of cellular kinase, a chemical ingredient is protein, and is a group of molecule family. It mainly works on signal transduction of the immune system and the main function is immune regulation and immune modification. The originally definition of Interleukin is immune system signal transduction between cells. IL is secreted by white blood cells. When they bind to the receptor on the cell membrane, the target cells are activated.

Complex balance between cell activity and immune regulation is kept by the coordination of secretion of IL and immune system cells.

To date, only IL-2 and IL-11 for clinics, their therapeutic effects of cancer treatment and stimulation of hematopoietic cells are under clinical observation.

(1) Interleukin-2 (IL-2):

This lymphocyte line first is described in 1976. It is a T cell growth factor, mainly is produced by activated T helper cells and has a strong regulation immune function.

Biological activity of IL-2: IL-2 is an important material in the body to produce an immune response, which promotes proliferation of all T cel subsets, increases the activity of the cytotoxic T cell lymphocyte, NK cell and monocyte. Lymphocyte in the blood after activated is called LAK.IL-2 can help B cell growth, also promote the release of IFN-a, GM- CSF, TNF.

From 1984 it started to try recombinant IL-2 to treat various malignancies. There are multiple cases reports that IL-2 alone or combined with LAK cells were used to treat renal cell carcinoma and malignant melanoma. In May 1992 FDA approved that IL-2 is used to treat adults with metastatic renal cell carcinoma.

Recombinant IL-2 has been used as a single agent, or in combination with LAK cells, TIL cells, other biological regulatory factors, and other combined chemotherapy for cancer therapy.

(2) IL-4 : IL-4 is produced mainly by activated T cells. ① The effect on B cells: it can stimulate the growth and differentiation of resting B cells, stimulate B cells to replicate DNA, become a B cell growth factor. ②The effect on T cells: it can stimulate T cell growth, increase the production of IL-2, promote the proliferation of cytotoxic T cells and activate LAK cells. IL-4 promote Til growth, increase the cytotoxic effect on melanoma cells.

The clinical application of IL-4: IL-4 clinical trial has entered Phase II renal cell carcinoma, mainly, melanoma and chronic lymphocytic leukemia, Hodgkin's disease and the like.

(3) Interleukin -12 (IL-12): IL-12 has immunomodulatory and anti-tumor effect. Monocytes is mainly source for IL- 12. Its main role is to: stimulate the activity of T cells and NK cell proliferation; to induce T lymphocytes and NK cells to release IFN-y.

The clinical application of IL-12: the stage I, II clinical trials have been finished on the treatment of metastatic renal cell carcinoma and melanoma.

3. Tumor necrosis factor (TNF)

In 1975 Old etc isolated a material produced by activated phagocyte cell, monocytes and lymphocytes in the contact to toxin, called tumor necrosis factor (TNF). In 1984 TNF gene was cloned so that people can get a lot of recombinant TNF.

The biological effects of TNF: In vitro tests showed that TNF effect on cells is cytotoxicity, and can affect tumor microvasculature, resulting in the center of the tumor necrosis. In particular, TNF can induce the expression of tissue factor vascular endothelial cells and promote the formation of fibrin deposition and thrombosis.

In the anti-tumor effect of TNF, T lymphocytes play important role. Many observers prove that TNF and IFN-Y have a synergistic anti-tumor effect.

TNF has been tested in the treatment of melanoma, colon cancer, non-small cell lung cancer, ovarian cancer, but unfortunately none of them showed a clear reduction or therapeutic effect.

TNF and IFN-y work together, IFN-Y can increase the expression of cell surface TNF receptors, thus increasing the effect of TNF on cells. TNF and IL-2 together can treat all types of cancers, its strategy is IL-2 can stimulate cytotoxic lymphocyte activity and TNF can expand the effectiveness of anti-tumor. The side effects of the two drugs have emerged and only one case of breast cancer and one case of renal cell cancer in combination therapy have improved after exacerbations.

4. Hematopoietic growth factors (HGF)

HGF is also known as colony stimulating factor in the past because in vitro it can induce specific cell clones formation.

HGF effects on normal hematopoiesis: blood cells are made from pluripotent stem cell (PPSC). PPSC has small number within the bone marrow and can differentiate into any blood cell. In the bone marrow, each one PPSC split into two sub-cells, one will go to differentiation pathway; another return to the cell bank to maintain a static state. PPSC grows and develops in the sinus-like gap around stroma in the bone marrow.

(1) Neutrophils: a granule cells, total white blood cell count of 50% -70%, its maturation process has six steps, namely bone marrow blasts, before bone marrow cells, bone marrow cells, these three steps need 4-5d, then no mitosis, but continued to mature about 6d, and then released into the peripheral blood. Half of cells are free circulation; half of cells attached to the vessel wall. Cells circulating in the blood will remove into the tissue after 6- 8h, where it can survive 2-3d. Generally the number of circulating cells is three times of the number of cells in the bone marrow so there is always reservation of neutrophils in vivo. Once serious injury, a lifetime of neutrophils is reduced to a few hours.

(2) Platelets: its ancestor cells are megakaryocyte colony forming units. In the bone marrow it is the megakaryocytic mother cell, and then differentiates into megakaryocytes which can release platelets. Platelets can form clots in injured blood vessel walls, while activation of the clotting factor. Platelets in the blood can survive 7-8d.

(3) Lymphocytes: lymphoid stem cells differentiate into pre-T or B lymphocytes. Pre-T lymphocytes mature in the thymus before becoming thymocytes, lymphoblastoid cells and T lymphocytes. They can mediate cellular immunity. They can freely circulate in the blood and peripheral tissues. When it is stimulated by antigen, T cell produces a variety of cytokines, which control specific immune response.

Pre-B lymphocytes mature after moving to the spleen and lymph nodes. When the antigen-antibody appear its response on the cell membrane, B lymphocytes has become mature, and eventually become plasma cells. Plasma cells secrete specific immunoglobulins, namely antibodies, responsible for humoral immunity. B lymphocytes accounted for 20%- 25% of total lymphocytes.

Blood cell growth factors control blood cell development by stimulating cell differentiation and maturation.

Particles colony stimulating factor (G-CSF) have been made to pre-clinical animal studies, such as G-CSF was administrated to accelerate neutrophil recovery after using 5-FU and total body radiation.

Further research in monkeys show: intravenous injection of GM-CSF (granulosa cells of macrophage colony stimulating factor increased white blood cells after 24-72h.

In 1986 clinical trials started and FDA approved the use of G-CSF which can reduce the risk of incidence of infection in bone marrow cancer in patients receiving myelosuppressive chemotherapy in 1991.

The experimental research on Thymus

A. Thymus atrophy in cancer-bearing mouse

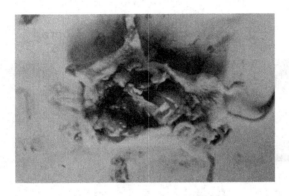

B. The animal model of the experimental research on anti-cancer metastasis and recurrence

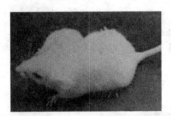

C. Cancer-bearing animal model with the cancerous block is exfoliative as a whole.

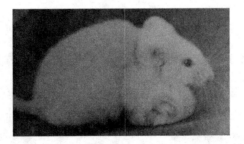

D. The treatment of tumor-bearing group on S180 Sarcoma with Anticancer Z-C medications

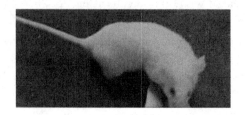

E. The experimental research on Protecting Thymus and increasing immune function as well as protecting bone marrow and hematopoiesis by Z-C medications

Z- C5 Treatment   **Control**

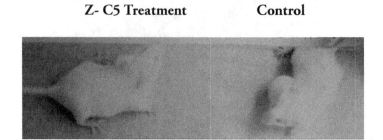

Tumor   Thymus   Spleen   Kindey   Liver

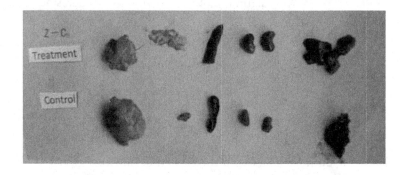

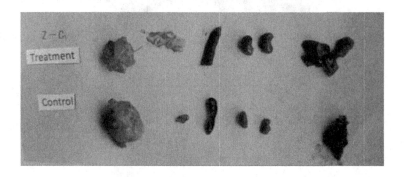

VOLUME IX

The List of Cancer Cases and Some Typical Cases of Cancer treatment with XZ-C immunoregulation and control anticancer medications

CONTENTS VOLUME IX

Preface

一. Immunomodulatory Drug Looks Promising

No matter how complex the mechanism behind cancer is, immune suppression is a key cancer progression. The removal of immunosuppressive factors and restoration of recognition system cells to cancer cells can effectively resist cancer. More and more evidence shows that by regulating the body's immune system it is possible to achieve the purpose of controlling cancer. Many researchers in the field are currently excited by activating the body's anti-tumor immune system to treat cancer. The next major breakthrough in cancer is likely to come from this.

In order to investigate cancer etiology, pathogenesis, pathophysiology, we conducted a series of animal studies. From the analysis of the experimental results the new discoveries and new revelation were found that : thymus atrophy and immune dysfunction are one of cancer etiology and pathogenesis mechanism; therefore at the international conferences Professor Xu Ze proposed that one of the causes mechanisms of cancer may be thymus atrophy, central immune organ dysfunction, immune dysfunction, decreasing immune surveillance and immune escape.

As the results of the experimental studies in the real laboratory it was found: in cancer-bearing mice it showed progressive thymus atrophy and the central immune organ dysfunction and the decreased immune function and the decreasing immune supervision ; therefore, its treatment principle must be to prevent atrophy of the thymus, to promote thymic hyperplasia, to protect bone marrow Hematopoietic function, to improve immune surveillance, which provides the theoretical basis and the experimental evidence for cancer immune regulation and control treatment.

Based on the above revelation about cancer etiology and pathogenesis of the experimental results, it was put forward the new concept and new method of XZ immunomodulatory therapy. After 30 years of clinical validation in the oncology clinics in more than 12,000 cases of cancer patients in the middle and advanced stages, it was confirmed that the treatment principle of protecting thymus and increasing immune function is reasonable and the efficacy is satisfactory. The application of immune regulation medications has achieved good results and improved the quality of life and significantly prolonged the survival time.

XZ-C(XU ZE-China) immune regulation and control theories were the first time put forward by Professor Xu Ze in 2006 in his monograph <<The new concept and new way of cancer metastasis treatment >> which it was believed that under normal circumstances it is the dynamic equilibrium between body's defenses and cancer; cancer is caused by losing the dynamic balance. If the imbalance state has adjusted to the normal level, it can control cancer growth and make it subside.

As we all know, the incidence of cancer development and prognosis is depending on the comparison of two factors, namely, the biological characteristics of cancer cells and the host body's own cancer defense and constraint ability. If these two parts are balance, cancer can be controlled; if these two are imbalance, cancer will develop.

Under normal circumstances, the host organism itself has a certain constraint capacity to cancer, but in cancer patients these constraints are subject to defense suppression and damage in the different levels, leading to the loss of the immune surveillance of cancer cells, to have the immune escape and to have the further development of cancer cells and metastasis.

Through more than four years of basic experimental study investigating the recurrence and metastasis mechanism and after three years of the experiment in vivo anti-tumor cancer-bearing mice screening from the natural herbal medication test, a group of traditional Chinese medications which has better inhibition rate are selected which XZ-C1-10 anti-cancer immune regulation medications are composed of.

二. In medical research why should the accumulation of raw data be paid great attention to?

The purpose of the medical research is to study the disease and to understand the disease and to seek the new methods and the new technologies and the new theories to improve the level of medicine and to prevent and treat the diseases for the people's health services. However, the prominent feature of medical research is that its research object is the human body itself, and its research results are applied to the human body. So its results must be strict scientific, accurate and reliable, harmless to the human body. However, the scientific feature and the reliability of a result, and whether the argument is correct and analysis argument is logical or not, are based on the statistical data processing, analysis, synthesis, induction or generalization from the original data. If you ignore the complete, accurate raw or original data, it is difficult to analyze, sum up the argument, more difficult to draw the correct conclusion. People are the most valuable, many experiments and observations do not allow the researchers to be directly tested on the human body, need to take a simulation method, the establishment of animal models, do the experimental research. After the full grasp of being fully harmless to the human body, and then it can be applied to the human body, thus increasing the experimental procedures to extend the work cycle, especially the national research topics, mostly for the pathogenesis of the underlying theoretical research, especially the national research topics, mostly for the pathogenesis of the basic theory of disease research, these subjects to be completed a few years, technical complexity, difficulty, Involving more disciplines, more staff; If you do not attach importance to the accumulation of raw data, not centralize the management and too scattered; if the time is long, it cannot be statistics and analysis and synthesis and induction and stage summary or summary. Therefore, each medical research and each medical research project leader must attach great importance to and strictly require scientific research of the original data accumulation and management.

三, we must take a serious attitude towards the accumulation of medical research original data

The original information on medical research must be strictly required. Whether it can be obtained the objective information according to scientific research requirements, it is related to the ability to obtain scientific research achievements. The quality and level of the results depends on the level of design and the quality of the original data. If the scientific design is a strategic measure, to collect the original data as tactical measures is the key to success.

On the original data records it must pay attention to being scientific, advanced, innovative (as far as possible not to repeat the low level) and to seeking the truth from facts and it is one on one and the second is the second; the success needs to be recorded as the truth; the failure should be truthfully recorded; the lessons should be recorded as the truth; it should be faithful to the objective information.

For the accumulation of raw materials, it should have a rigorous style, strict requirements. To be realistic, respect for the original information, loyal to the original data (if the method is reliable). It should have a hard work style. The project leader should personally participate in practice and can not have the slightest empiricalism and preconceived. Successful experience is important and the lessons of failure are equally important. It should respect for every objective observation of the material, regardless of what you thought was important or not all at all. And whether you believe that the success or failure of the information is also a record. Sometimes the subject matter is not successful, but it can unexpectedly obtain other results or discoveries. Some new theories, new technologies, new discoveries, and so on in the world were produced as these ways and there are many typical cases. Therefore, we must pay attention to the first hand of the original information, these are valuable wealth. Our laboratory on the scientific research of all the original plan, draft, work contact paper, etc., are one by one to save and complete the end of the project summary of the archive. These raw materials sometimes may trigger our new ideas; the scientific research is not based on unfounded borers think of the inspiration, but it can be repeated in the practice of thinking on the basis of a sudden shock to open a crux.

The academic attitude and the academic style and the way of learning the subject of the scholarship leader are the essential importance. It must have the rigorous style and the serious attitude to seek the truth from facts and the meticulous and hard work spirit. The group members should conscientiously implement and earnestly implement the plan, meticulously.

The Assistant should be structured, categorized according to the order of the subject and be the well-organized collection and the accumulation and the original data storage and comply with the corresponding level. It should at any time provide the necessary information to the project leader in order to organize, summarize, analyze, summarize or summarize the paper.

四How to Summarize, Sort and Express the Clinical Scientific Research Data

It is useful to expound scientific research data or articles by forms. This way is not only concise and clear, but also comprehensive and detailed, which can be understood easily. A large amount of scientific research material and experimental data that was gained from hard and delicate clinical research in several decades can be summarized, sorted and collected by forms concisely, clearly and orderly so that readers can understand the core contents within about ten minutes.

China is a large country with populations of 1.3 billion, so it is a great source of tumor cases. In China, there are a large amount of cancer cases that can be used in clinical observation and analysis. If a clinician observes and analyzes the state of diseases, and positively researches on it, he can find out some new and step further continuously through the accumulation of practical medical experience in long period. As medical research is to improve clinical diagnosis and treatment, as well as medical quality and level, clinical scientific research is an important part of clinic medical work.

1. Preserve clinic case history to keep the information of diagnosis, treatment, recovery and follow-up survey. So it is necessary to fill in form-typed clinic case history in detail completely to gain complete material of clinical verification, which is easy to analyze and do statistics. Without preservation of clinic case history, scientific research on the analysis, statistics and follow-up survey of curative effects can not be developed. Preserving case history is to observe the curative effects. Moreover, restoration and preservation of material are in favor of scientific research on clinic and improving medical quality.

2. Build a schedule to display the treatment of cancer for outpatients, which should be complete and in detail. Those who have return visit after more than three months should fill in the schedule. Filling the schedule with registration in long term is easy to classify, to collect, to sort and count a large amount of material.

3. How to summarize, sorting, analyze and express the clinical scientific research data and experimental scientific research data.

This book is the production of author's practical experience of clinical treatment over sixty years combined with the collection, sorting and classification of research data and experimental data of cancer research in laboratory over thirty years. All the clinical and experimental data come from real work. Actually, it is the collection of articles or material of serial scientific payoffs.

Through experimental research and practical clinic experience combined and many cases of clinical verification over the past fifty years, the author reviews and analyzes the traditional treatment in clinic cases, evaluates and reflects them. He also concludes his own experience of clinical practice from both positive and negative aspects and puts forward new findings, new concept and methods of treatment.

How to put a lot of clinical and experimental research data, so many of the hundreds of research papers, a series of theoretical innovation and new development, collection, collation, classification summary? The author uses the table forms for the production of scientific research materials or research papers and they are easy to read and easy to understand and are easy to guide.

To strive to take our characteristics of anti – cancer metastasis innovation path; to take the modernization of traditional Chinese medicine approach.

To promote the China-Western medicine combination on the molecular level, and to converge with international medicine modernization.

<u>Anti - cancer, anti - cancer metastasis research, scientific and technological innovation, scientific research series</u>

1. LIST OF CASES OF CANCER TREATMENT WITH XZ-C IMMUNE REGULATOR AND CONTROL CHINESE MEDICATIONS

1.) List of partial typical cases of **Liver cancer** treatment with XZ-C immune regulator Chinese medications(case 1 to case 189)

2.) List of partial typical cases of **Pancreas cancer** treatment with XZ-C immune regulator Chinese medications(case 190- case218)

3.) List of partial typical cases of **Stomach** cancer treatment with XZ-C immune regulator Chinese medications(case219-case288)

4.) List of partial typical cases of **Lung** cancer treatment with XZ-C immune regulator Chinese medications(case289-case358)

5.) List of partial typical cases of **Esophagus cancer** treatment with XZ-C immune regulator Chinese medications(case359-case446)

6.) List of partial typical cases of **Breast cancer** treatment with XZ-C immune regulator Chinese medications(case447-case481)

7.) List of partial typical cases of **Colon, Rectal cancer** treatment with XZ-C immune regulator Chinese medications(case482-case649)

8.) List of partial typical cases of **Bile duct cancer** treatment with XZ-C immune regulator Chinese medications(case650-case679)

In our medical record for the patients we made a detail medical record for each patient and the samples are as the following. The following parts are just the examples for several diseases. (We keep all of our patients' epidemiologic information and life habits and clinical information in detail in order to understand the cancers)

1), Some cases of liver cancer were treated by XZ-C immunomodulatory anticancer medications

Liver cancer A

Number	Name	Medical record	Gender	Age	Native place	Occupation	Address	Diagnosis	in accordance with	Unit	Society habit			
											Smoking year	Amount of Smoking	Drinking years	Alcohol consumption
1	Shixx	x	M	57	Zhaoyan	Farmer	Zaoyang	Liver cancer	(CT, MRI) 98/6/22	Zaoyang City Hospital	30	1-2 packages a day	30	3-4 oz/ per
2	Lan xx	x	M	35	Dawu	Teacher	Dawu	massive liver in liver right lobe	CT (98/08)	Dawu County Concord hospital			10	
3	Lunxx	x	M	38	Danyang	Land management cadre	Dangyang	After right liver cancer surgery	U/S, CT (98/07)	Concord hospital	6-7	little		
4	Liu xx	x	M	30	Gongan	engineer	Gongen	massive liver cancer	U/S,CT (98/0707)	County Hospital Ezhou City Hospital	More than 10	One package/ day	10	2-3 oz/ meal
5	Zhen Xx	x	M	50	Zhongyan	Farmers	Zhongxiang	primary liver cancer	CT (98/08)	Zhongxiang City People's Hospital				
6	Ke xx	x	M	54	Hongshi	Agricultural Bank staff	Yellowstone	liver cancer	CT (98/08)	Yellowstone Hospital Concord Medical hospital	More than 30	1-2 package/ day	More than 10	8oz/ meal
7	Shong Xx	x	M	37	Yinchen	headmaster	Ying city	massive liver cancer	U/S, CT, MRI (98/07/01)	Ying City People 's Hospital Concord Hospital				
8	Yanxx	x	M	51	Eizhong	Attending physician	Ezhou	After liver cancer surgery	U/S, CT (98/09)	Ezhou City Hospital Concord hospital				
9	Jiangxx	x	M	57	Henan	Radio station welder	Xiaogan	massive liver cancer	U/S (98/02/10)	Sanjiang spaceflight Red Star Hospital Association	20	One package	More than 10	One pound/ meal

No.	Name		Sex	Age	Origin	Occupation	Location	Diagnosis	Method	Hospital				
10	Zhangxx	x	F	64	Shanhai	Accountant	Wuhan	hepatobiliary and pancreatic cancer with metastasis lung	U/S, CT (98/0/25)	Railway Hospital				
11	Lixx	x	M	36	Huangpi	Farmer	Huangpi	left liver cancer with gallbladder invasion	U/S (98/07)	Union Hospital	10	2-3 package		
12	Wangxx	x	M	47	Wuhan	Cement factory worker	Wuhan	left liver cancer after surgery with lung	U/S (98/04)	Tongji Hospital	10	2 Package/day	10	often
13	Yangxx	x	M	46	Tongchen	Security Section	Wuhan	primary liver cells cancer	U/S, CT (98/09/13)	Wuhan Second Hospital Concord hospital	20	12 cigrettes/day	10	
14	Yan xx	x	F	56	Tiangmen	Farmer	Tanmen	primary liver metastases	U/S, CT,MRI (98/05)	Concord Hospital				
28	Liu ixx	x	M	40	Zhaoyan	Cadre	ZaoyangZaoyang City Xiangyang Road Hongqi Village	Primary liver cancer	CT	Zaoyang City Hospital and concord hospital	20	40 cigarettes/per day	20	8 oz
29	Zheng xx	x	M	61	Henan	Selfemployed	Henan Huaiyang Beimen Township Jia camp aluminum factory	multiple liver cancer	CT	Henan Zhoukou Hospital	Decades	40 cigarettes/per day	several decades	8 oz
30	Wang xx	x	M	40	Shandong	Teacher	Wuhan Electric Power School	Liver cancer	U/S, CT	Concord hospital		5-6 cigarettes/day		
31	Xie xx	x	M	57	Gangxi	Professor	Wuhan xx	Metastasis liver cancer	U/S,CT	Concord hospital				
32	Zhen Xx	x	M	60	Zhanggan	Cadre	Huaxing	primary liver cancer	CT	Concord hospital	More than 20	20 cigarettes/day		
33	Cheng xx	x	M	49	Zhanggang	Cadre	xxx	The liver lumps in right lobe of Liver cancer and ascites	CT, U/S	Concord hospital			20-30 years	16oz
34	Liu Xx	x	F	65	Yinchen	headmaster	Ying city	Primary massive liver cancer	CT	Concord hospital	5-6years	10 cigarettes/day		
35	Zhangxx	x	M	66	Eizhong	Attending physician	Ezhou	Primary liver cancer	U/S, CT	Air force Hospital	40 year	20 cigarettes/day		

36	Hongxx	x	F	54	XX	Worker	xxxx	Liver cancer with bile duct bleeding	Pathology slides	Concord hospital				
37	Qing xx	x	M	58	Hongen	Cadre	Wuhan	Primary diffuse Liver cancer	U/S, CT	People Hospital	20	20 cigarettes/ day		
38	Songxx	x	M	62	Enhui	Cadre	xxx	Multiple liver cancer	U/S,CT	Concord Hospital	10	2-3 package		
39	Huang xx	x	M	59	Hanchun	Peasant	xxx	Multiple diffuse liver cancer	U/S, X-ray and CT	Tongji Hospital	20-30	20 cigarettes/ day		
40	Zheng xx	x	M	32	Hebei	Cadre	xxx	primary diffuse liver cells cancer	U/S, CT	Tongji Hospital	10	20 cigarettes/ day	10	4oz
41	Wuxx	x	M	55	Shanghai	Cadre	XX	primary liver left lobe cancer	U/S, path slide	City three Hospital				

Hepatocellular Carcinoma Patients B

Number	Whether to eat often											Whether to drink often			The method of drinking water	Whether to eat often			Jobs		Characters		Whether to love sports
	Water pickles	Salt pickles	Smoked meat	Dried salted fish	Dry pickle	sausage	Fried food	chili	garlic	onion	fresh vegatable vvegetables	fruit	Fried food	Green tea	Strong tea	Other	meat	Ribs soup	Vegetarian food	General	Tension overcharged	Cheerful	Dull and irritable	
1		√		√							√			√			well water	√ fatty meat						
2	√	√			√			√			√			√			Unsolicited water					√		√
3								√	√		√			√			Unsolicited water						√	No
4								√	√√		√			√			Unsolicited water					√		

468

5	√	√		√	√		√		√		√			Pool water					√	√		
6				√	√		√		√					Well water	√					√		
7							√				√			Unsolicited water	√				√	√	√	No
8							√		√					Well water							√	
9				√	√					√				Unsolicited water	√fatry meat	√	√		√	√		No
10		√		√			√	√						Unsolicited water			√		√		√	
11							√							Unsolicited water	√	√			√	√		√
12										√				Unsolicited water					√		√	No
13		√			√	√	√		√	Eatingmoldyrice	Unsolicited water	√	√		√	√	√		√		√	No
14	√						√							Well water				√	√	√	√	No

Number	Water pickles	Salt pickles	Smoked meat	Dried salted fish	Dry pickle	sausage	Fried food	chili	garlic	onion	fresh vegatable vvegetables	fruit	Fried food	Moldy food	green tea	Strong tea	other	Drinking Water	meat	Ribs soup	Vegetarian food	General	Tension overcharged	Cheerful	Dull and irritable	Whether to love sports
28																					√		√			
29					√					√		√											√	√		
30								√																	√	No
31								√	√√	√	√	√			√			Unsolicited water							√	
32	√	√		√	√						√							Sugar water					√	√		
33								√	√		√			√				Well water	√					√		
34											√							Unsolicited water	√				√	√	√	No
35											√			√				Well water							√	
36													√	√		√		Unsolicited water	√ fatty meat		√		√	√		No

37							√						Unsolicited water		√		√	
38							√					√ √	Unsolicited water		√	√		√
39						√							Unsolicited water		√		√	No
40		√			√	√	√		√	√	Eating mold y rice	√ √	Unsolicited water	√ √	√	√	√	No
41	√						√					√	Well water		√	√	√	No

Hepatocellular Carcinoma Patients C

Number	Chronic disease History	Family three generation of cancer history	Application of pain medication situation			Mass reduction and disappear situation after medications	
			Disappear	Reduction	effective	Tumor location and size	Lump shrinkage after medication
1	In 1991 suffering from pleurisy and removing out the yellow liquid	No		√		In 98/06/22 Check 2 placeholder 1-3cm range in liver	
2	In junior high school suffering from jaundice hepatitis, Liver function is normal, in 1998 acute jaundice hepatitis	Father died because of esophageal cancer				98 /08/18 right palpable 12 x 10 cm²	Reducing to 11 × 8 cm² in 98/08/30 on Physical exam

3	In 1983 had hepatitis B, in 1991,1996 and 1997 hepatitis B +	No					
4	Hepatitis B positive with nosebleeds history	No				On 1998/07/10 CT showed 2.5× 2.5 × 3cm³ in liver side leaves and 10 x 5 x 9 cm³ in right lobe of liver	
5	In 1989 found a large number of ascites and recurrent schistosomiasis in follow-up check health, had checked Hb-SAg (+), and sometimes negative	The third brother had liver cancer without removing; and extensive metastasis and Intubation did not work, 3 months after surgery, this brother died in 1983				In 1998/08 the right lobe of the liver was 8X 10 cm²	
6	check for schistosomiasis; in 1970 Tuberculosis cured	no					
7	In 1983 treatment with hepatitis B half Year and had been delayed intermittent service medicine	no				In 1998/07/01 liver right lobe 8.7 ×7.1cm² size	
8	2 months ago checked hepatitis B	the father had cardia cancer, in 1997 death				98/09 liver mass 4. 3 ×4.4cm2 size	
9	In 1967 had hepatitis B in Sanyang hospitalization For three months and treatment did not turn negative; Tuberculosis has calcified; gastric ulcer	No				98/02/10 U/S showed 15 × 4 × 12cm² lesion in hepatic right lobe	

10	Diabetic	No				98/09/29 Ultrasonographic liver right lobe 2.5×2.4 cm^2 ;pancreatic head 3×3.1 cm^2	
11	Had a history of schistosomiasis for seven years with three positive in small lobe and not treated	No				98/08/03 CT showed in left liver 4.3×9.9cm^2	
12	In 1983 had acute jaundice liver Inflammation and had hospitalization for one month, sometimes liver area had pain, cholecystitis	Father died because of liver cancer					
13	In 1984 acute jaundice liver Inflammation, hospitalization for one month; after one month relapse	No					
14	In 1960s and 1970s has three hospitalization for histosomiasis late stage; endoscopy showed anemia gastric mucosa like	No					

Number	Chronic disease History	Family three generation of cancer history	Application of pain medication situation			Mass reduction and disappear situation after medications	
			Disappear	Reduction	effective	Tumor location and size	Lump shrinkage after medication
28	In 1991 suffering from pleurisy and removing out the yellow liquid	No		√		In 98/06/22 Check 2 placeholder 1-3cm range in liver	

29	In junior high school suffering from jaundice hepatitis, Liver function is normal, in 1998 acute jaundice hepatitis	Father died because of esophageal cancer				98 /08/18 right palpable 12 x 10 cm²	Reducing to 11 × 8 cm² in 98/08/30 on Physical exam
30	In 1983 had hepatitis B, in 1991,1996 and 1997 hepatitis B +	No					
31	Hepatitis B positive with nosebleeds history	No				On 1998/07/10 CT showed 2.5× 2.5 × 3cm³ in liver side leaves and 10 x 5 x 9 cm³ in right lobe of liver	.
32	In 1989 found a large number of ascites and recurrent schistosomiasis in follow-up check health, had checked Hb-SAg (+), and sometimes negative	The third brother had liver cancer without removing; and extensive metastasis and Intubation did not work, 3 months after surgery, this brother died in 1983				In 1998/08 the right lobe of the liver was 8X 10 cm²	
33	check for schistosomiasis; in 1970 Tuberculosis cured	no					
34	In 1983 treatment with hepatitis B half Year and had been delayed intermittent service medicine	no				In 1998/07/01 liver right lobe 8.7 ×7.1cm² size	
35	2 months ago checked hepatitis B	the father had cardia cancer, in 1997 death				98/09 liver mass 4. 3 ×4.4cm2 size	
36	In 1967 had hepatitis B in Sanyang hospitalization For three months and treatment did not turn negative; Tuberculosis has calcified; gastric ulcer	No				98/02/10 U/S showed 15 × 4 × 12cm² lesion in hepatic right lobe	

37	Diabetic	No				98/09/29 Ultrasonographic liver right lobe 2 .5x2.4 cm^2 ;pancreatic head 3× 3.1 cm^2	
38	Had a history of schistosomiasis for seven years with three positive in small lobe and not treated	No				98/08/03 CT showed in left liver 4.3× 9.9cm^2	
39	In 1983 had acute jaundice liver Inflammation and had hospitalization for one month, sometimes liver area had pain, cholecystitis	Father died because of liver cancer					
40	In 1984 acute jaundice liver Inflammation, hospitalization for one month; after one month relapse	No					
41	In 1960s and 1970s has three hospitalization for histosomiasis late stage; endoscopy showed anemia gastric mucosa like	No					

Hepatocellular Carcinoma Patients D

Number	What kind of treatment done				Medication time, type and efficacy	Remarks
	Surgical approach	intervention	Chemotherapy	When the recurrence and metastasis and site size		

1	Not appropriate	For two liver intervention from 98/8/5 to 9/15			From 98/7/14 to 98/09/22 Night pain can not sleep, pain for the stinging 10AM-2PM; Taking XZ-C1, 4,5,2; XZ-C3 topical, after taking the medications, the appetite good; liver pain reduction, obvious medication significantly reduced pain after intervention; no any adverse reactions, hepatomegaly, lump reduced from 3 . 2 x 3. 9 cm2 to 2 . 2x 2 .4 cm2 size	
2		From 98/08 to 98/11 For two liver intervention f			Taking $XZ_{-C1, 4,5}$; $XZ-C_3$ topical medication ; having good appetite, eating a pound, walking activities such as ordinary people, the right upper quadrant mass much softer than before and reduced size, reduced from $12 \times 10cm^2$ to $11 \times 8cm^2$ size	Interventional of vascular occlusion abnormalities and vascular malformations; can not get up after the second intervention and can not eat right upper quadrant pain increased low back pain
3	**On 98/08/05 had half of Liver resection**				From 98 /08/19 to 98/11/15 taking $XZ_{-C1, 4, 5}$, ; after the medication, the spirit is good medicine, appetite is good, the complexion is rosy as ordinary people	
4	Not appropriate	98 /07/21 home pump hemotherapy four times			98 /0 8/ 20-9/24 taking $XZ_{-C1, 4, 5}$, $XZ-C_3$ topical medication; after taking the medications, the appetite is good	Chemotherapy Mitoniyan5Fu heparin with right pulmonary tuberculosis induration
5					From 98 /09/07 -98/11/28 after taking $XZ_{-C1, 4, 5,}$ medication, the mental and appetite are improved than the previous, can get up and take a mile road, morning exercise, liver area is painful, sometimes tingling, mild ascites sign	Fourth younger brother of liver cancer for resection, two years after the death of ascites, mother cirrhosis ascites in patients with ascites blood hospital four times, treatment of schistosomiasis pirimicron three days therapy

6	98/08/20 laparotomy failed to resection	98 /08/30 for the pump in the hepatic artery secondary carboplatin doxorubicin		98/08/20 intraoperative intrahepatic metastasis	98/09/08 so far taking XZ-$C_{1,4,5}$, after taking the medications, the spirit of improvement and the the appetite increased and the weight gain 8 pounds, walking activities as usual, self-care	
7	98 /07/02 surgical exploration failed to remove	98/07/27 and 98/08/27 for these two hepatic artery pump chemotherapy		98/10/08 chest right lower lung metastasis of two 1. 2 cm diameter lesions	98/0 9/20-98/10/18 taking XZ-$C_{1,4,5}$, after taking the drug the generally good, good appetite; 98/07/27 the first pump chemotherapy with adriamycin cisplatin 5-FU digestive tract response, WBC ↓ 2300 ; 8/27 second chemotherapy response large WBC ↓ 1500 lesions have narrowed; 9/19 U/S 5.0 × 5.0cm ^{2}	98 /07/01 sudden lower abdominal pain; 07/02 liver rupture bleeding emergency surgery; the exploration of liver cancer rupture tofu and failure to resection, ligation of liver A
8	98/09/15 for liver resection of the square leaf cholecystectomy				98/09/25- 11/30 taking XZ-C1, 4, 5, after taking the medications, the spirit and appetite is good, physical recovery gradually, AFP and CEA were normal while reviewing	
9	Not appropriate	98/02/18 to 98/11/ for six interventional response		98/09/15 CT considered possible intracystic metastases	98/09/27-98/11/18 after taking XZ-C_4; consciously good, pain symptoms disappeared in the original liver area; before the patient had pain; cough does not hurt; if no moving, the patient is not painful;, cramp-like pain every day.	After the fourth intervention the patient can not speak, right shoulder can not move because of being painful
10	Not appropriate				From 98/09/30 on chest radiographs see lung metastasis	98/09/30-98/10/11 after taking XZ-$C_{1,4,5}$ and Jieshui Xiaotang, the spirit is better, the original muscle aches, and now pain, bloating and lower extremity swelling

11	Not appropriate	On 98/08/07 and 98/09/21 twice Intervention, liver pain after surgery			98/10/03-98/10/18 After taking the $XZ\text{-}C_{1,4,5}$, the patient is generally good, good spiritual and appetite, walking activities such as complexion is rosy; in 98 after embolization and following up check up, there is the liver mass, $8 \times 6.8cm^2$ slightly smaller	
12	On 98 /04/30 had the left liver resection	From 98/06/23 to 98/09/04 had three times Intravenous drug injection		Right liver metastases after secondary chemotherapy; on 98/ 10/19 in Chest X-ray lung metastasis	From 98/10/10- 98/11/22 Taking $XZ\text{-}C_{1,4,5,2}$, application of $XZ\text{-}C_3$ in decoction and decoction of decoction; after the drug the patient is generally good, good appetite, all of the symptoms such as right shoulder pain, bloating, vomiting and spit cough, dyspnea oliguria, a large number of ascites topical, were getting better.	
13	On 98/09/29 had the right liver leaf resection	On 98/11/09 had intervention, MMC + 5FU		On 98/11/13 liver ultrasound reviewed the left lobe and found that 1. $5 \times 7.3cm^2$ occupying from the postoperative complex	On 98/10/11- 98/11/29 after taking the $XZ\text{-}C_{1,4,5}$, the patient was in stable condition, generally good, good spiritual and appetite, walking activities as usual	
14	Not appropriate		98/10/06- 98/10/31 had 5Fu+ CF +HCPT	98/05 liver cancer with peritoneum, pancreatic turnover shift	On 98/10/31- 98/12/07 After taking $XZ\text{-}C_{1,4,5}$, $XZ\text{-}C_3$ external application; the complexin is rosy and there was painful and had intermittent vomiting	

		What kind of treatment done				Medication time, type and efficacy	Remarks
		Surgical approach	intervention	Chemotherapy	When the recurrence and metastasis and site size		
28		Not appropriate	For two liver intervention from 98/8/5 to 9/15			From 98/7/14 to 98/09/22 Night pain can not sleep, pain for the stinging 10AM-2PM; Taking XZ-C1, 4,5,2; XZ-C3 topical, after taking the medications, the appetite good; liver pain reduction, obvious medication significantly reduced pain after intervention; no any adverse reactions, hepatomegaly, lump reduced from 3 . 2 x 3. 9 cm2 to 2 . 2x 2 .4 cm2 size	
29			From 98/08 to 98/11 For two liver intervention f			Taking XZ-$_{C1, 4,5}$; XZ-C_3 topical medication ; having good appetite, eating a pound, walking activities such as ordinary people, the right upper quadrant mass much softer than before and reduced size, reduced from 12 × 10cm² to 11 × 8cm² size	Interventional of vascular occlusion abnormalities and vascular malformations; can not get up after the second intervention and can not eat right upper quadrant pain increased low back pain
30		**On 98/08/05 had half of Liver resection**				From 98 /08/19 to 98/11/15 taking XZ-$_{C1, 4, 5}$, ; after the medication, the spirit is good medicine, appetite is good, the complexion is rosy as ordinary people	
31		Not appropriate	98 /07/21 home pump hemotherapy four times			98 /0 8/ 20-9/24 taking XZ-$_{C1, 4, 5}$, XZ-C_3 topical medication; after taking the medications, the appetite is good	Chemotherapy Mitoniyan5Fu heparin with right pulmonary tuberculosis induration

32				From 98 /09/07 -98/11/28 after taking XZ-$_{C1, 4, 5,}$ medication, the mental and appetite are improved than the previous, can get up and take a mile road, morning exercise, liver area is painful, sometimes tingling, mild ascites sign	Fourth younger brother of liver cancer for resection, two years after the death of ascites, mother cirrhosis ascites in patients with ascites blood hospital four times, treatment of schistosomiasis pirimicron three days therapy
33	98/08/20 laparotomy failed to resection	98 /08/30 for the pump in the hepatic artery secondary carboplatin doxorubicin		98/08/20 intraoperative intrahepatic metastasis	98/09/08 so far taking XZ-$_{C1, 4, 5,}$ after taking the medications, the spirit of improvement and the the appetite increased and the weight gain 8 pounds, walking activities as usual, self-care	
34	98 /07/02 surgical exploration failed to remove	98/07/27 and 98/08/27 for these two hepatic artery pump chemotherapy		98/10/08 chest right lower lung metastasis of two 1. 2 cm diameter lesions	98/0 9/20-98/10/18 taking XZ-C$_{1, 4, 5,}$ after taking the drug the generally good, good appetite; 98/07/27 the first pump chemotherapy with adriamycin cisplatin 5-FU digestive tract response, WBC $\downarrow$ 2300 ; 8/27 second chemotherapy response large WBC $\downarrow$ 1500 lesions have narrowed; 9/19 U/S 5.0 × 5.0cm^2	98 /07/01 sudden lower abdominal pain; 07/02 liver rupture bleeding emergency surgery; the exploration of liver cancer rupture tofu and failure to resection, ligation of liver A
35	98/09/15 for liver resection of the square leaf cholecystectomy				98/09/25- 11/30 taking XZ-C1, 4, 5, after taking the medications, the spirit and appetite is good, physical recovery gradually, AFP and CEA were normal while reviewing	
36	Not appropriate	98/02/18 to 98/11/ for six interventional response		98/09/15 CT considered possible intracystic metastases	98/09/27-98/11/18 after taking XZ-C$_4$; consciously good, pain symptoms disappeared in the original liver area; before the patient had pain; cough does not hurt; if no moving, the patient is not painful;, cramp-like pain every day.	After the fourth intervention the patient can not speak, right shoulder can not move because of being painful
37	Not appropriate				From 98/09/30 on chest radiographs see lung metastasis	98/09/30-98/10/11 after taking XZ-C$_{1, 4, 5,}$ and Jieshui Xiaotang, the spirit is better, the original muscle aches, and now pain, bloating and lower extremity swelling

38	Not appropriate	On 98/08/07 and 98/09/21 twice Intervention, liver pain after surgery			98/10/03-98/10/18 After taking the XZ-$C_{1,4,5}$, the patient is generally good, good spiritual and appetite, walking activities such as complexion is rosy; in 98 after embolization and following up check up, there is the liver mass, 8 × 6.8cm² slightly smaller	
39	On 98 /04/30 had the left liver resection	From 98/06/23 to 98/09/04 had three times Intravenous drug injection		Right liver metastases after secondary chemotherapy; on 98/ 10/19 in Chest X-ray lung metastasis	From 98/10/10- 98/11/22 Taking XZ-$C_{1,4,5,2}$, application of XZ-C_3 in decoction and decoction of decoction; after the drug the patient is generally good, good appetite, all of the symptoms such as right shoulder pain, bloating, vomiting and spit cough, dyspnea oliguria, a large number of ascites topical, were getting better.	
40	On 98/09/29 had the right liver leaf resection	On 98/11/09 had intervention, MMC + 5FU		On 98/11/13 liver ultrasound reviewed the left lobe and found that 1. 5 × 7.3cm² occupying from the postoperative complex	On 98/10/11- 98/11/29 after taking the XZ-$C_{1,4,5}$, the patient was in stable condition, generally good, good spiritual and appetite, walking activities as usual	
41	Not appropriate		98/10/06-98/10/31 had 5Fu+ CF +HCPT	98/05 liver cancer with peritoneum, pancreatic turnover shift	On 98/10/31- 98/12/07 After taking XZ-$C_{1,4,5}$, XZ-C_3 external application; the complexin is rosy and there was painful and had intermittent vomiting	

2) Some Cases of Pancreatic cancer were treated by ZX-C immune regulation and control medications

The Statistics and Treatment of Pancreatic cancer Patients A

Number	Name	Medical record	Gender	Age	Native place	Occupation	Address	Diagnosis	in accordance with	Unit	Society habit				
											Smoking year	Amount of Smoking	Drinking years	Alcohol consumption
190	Chenxx	x	F	60	Wuhan	Union chairman	Wuhan	pancreatic cancer	U/S, CT(94/11)					

191	Zhang xx	x	M	39	Hangpi	Assistant engineer in Electric Power company	Wuhan	duodenum low differentiation of adenocarcinoma with pancreas gland metastasis	Nuclear magnetic resonance (95/03)		20	1 package/ day		
192	Cai xx	x	M	76	Wuhan	Tools Factory worker	Wuhan	Pancreatic tail cancer	GIB U/S, CT and Color Doppler ultrasound (95/06)	Concord hospital	Decades years	1 package/ day	Decades	2oz/ meal
193	Gan xx	x	M	50	Wuhan	Peasant	Wuhan	The head of the pancreas cancer with Periampullary carcinoma	U/S,CT (98/0707)	Chinese medicine hospital	15	little		
194	Yang Xx	x	M	71	Wuhan	Worker	Wuhan	Postoperative head cancer exploration	B ultrasound, exploration (96/03)	Concord hospital				
195	Li xx	x	M	55	Jingshung	Two grading actor	Yellow stone	Pancreatic Gland metastasis after gastric cancer surgery	Gastroscopy (95/11/01)	Yellowstone Hospital Concord Medical hospital	More than 30	1-2 package/ day	5	4 oz/ meal
196	Fang Xx	x	M	43	Luotiang	Village secretary	Lutian	Postoperative head cancer exploration	CT (96/11)	Concord hospital	10	One package/ day	10	2-3oz
197	Cheng xx	x	F	58	Wuhan	Examer	Wuhan	pancreatic cancer with liver right lobe metastasis	U/S, CT (96/12)	The third city Hospital				
198	Du xx	x	F	44	Wuhan	driver conductor	Wuhan	Pancreatic tail cancer with liver metastasis	CT,U/S (97/01/02)	The third city Hospital				
199	Jiangxx	x	F	65	Ezhong	Peasant	Echeng	pancreatic cancer with invasion bile duct	Laparotomy (97/02/18)					
200	Peng xx	x	M	33	Eanlu	Peasant	Luan	Pancreatic head cancer	CT,U/S (96/12)	Union Hospital			1-2 year	8oz
201	Pan xx	x	F	36	Lutiang	Peasant	Luotiang	Pancreatic head cancer	CT(97/07)					
202	Ye xx	x	F	50	Chaixuing	Pharmacy mananger	Chaixuing	Pancreatic tail cancer with liver metastasis	CT(97/08)	Concord Hospital				

Pancreatic cancer B-1

Number	Water pickles	Salt pickles	Smoked meat	Dried salted fish	Dry pickle	sausage	Fried food	chili	garlic	onion	fresh vegatable vvegetables	fruit	Fried food	Green tea	Strong tea	Other	The method of drinking water	meat	Ribs soup	Vegetarian food	General	Tension overcharged	Cheerful	Dull and irritable	Whether to love sports
190											√											√			√
191								√							√							√	√		
192	√	√													√							√	√		
193		√	√	√			√	√	√	√	√						Well water	√ fatty meat	√	√		√	√		
194											√			√			Unsolicited Wter				√		√		
195			√	√			√	√	√		√			√			Unsolicited water	√						√	
196		√	√					√			√		rice	√			Well Water				√			√	
197	√	√	√	√	√			√	√		√						Milk / Well water			√	√		√		

483

198	√	√	√	√	√		√			√			√			Unsolicited water	√ fatty meat			√		√	
199	√	√			√			√			√	√				Unsolicited water				√		√	
200		√		√		√	√	√	√							Unsolicited water	√√ fatty	√	√			√	
201		√		√	√					√						Unsolicited water	√			√		√	
202									√	√						Unsolicited water				√	√	√	√

Pancreatic cancer B-2

Number	Chronic disease History	Family three generation of cancer history	Application of pain medication situation			Mass reduction and disappear situation after medications	
			Disappear	Reduction	effective	Tumor location and size	Lump shrinkage after medication
190				√			
191							
192	10 year ago branch cough Have high blood pressure					In 1995/06 CT showed pancreatic body 6.88 x6.69 cm² mass, pancreas; Tail 1.25 ×1.72 cm² mass	Cervical lymph nodes turn soft but no significant change in size
193							

194		lover one year ago Gingival cancer				In 96/03/15 Intraoperative pancreatic head cancer 3 ×4cm²	
195							
196	check for schistosomiasis; in 1970 Tuberculosis cured	no					
197	In 1983 treatment with hepatitis B half Year and had been delayed intermittent service medicine	no				In 1998/07/01 liver right lobe 8.7 ×7.1cm² size	
198	2 months ago checked hepatitis B	the father had cardia cancer, in 1997 death				98/09 liver mass 4. 3 ×4.4cm2 size	
199	have a history of gastritis	brother died of gastric cancer					
200							
201							
202	In 1930s had Schistosomiasis History, used Antimony agent of schistosomiasis 864, had blood Fluke liver cirrhosis and ulcer of ball collapse						

Pancreatic cancer C

Number	What kind of treatment done				Medication time, type and efficacy	Remarks
	Surgical approach	intervention	Chemotherapy	When the recurrence and metastasis and site size		

190	In 1994/11/22 had hand surgical exploration + drainage				In 1995/01/16-05/16 took XZ-C1, 4, XZ-C3; after taking topical medication the appetite and spirit are improved; after the local topical 3 the situation markedly improved	
191	In 1990/07/06 had radical surgery of intestinal cancer	In 1995/03/28 had posterior catheter chemotherapy for three courses		In 1990/07 had pancreatic metastasis (found in the operation) ; In 1995/03 magnetic resonance had bowel swelling tumors, small bowel transverse colon tumors	In 1995/09/06-present taking XZ-C1, 4, after taking medicine the mental and appetite are good; the physical recovery, walking and life as usual, life is not stable and still smoking	
192	In 1995/06 had abdominal exploration and the tumor can be removed due to cancer huge arterial adhesion			In 1995/06 found right neck lymph nodes metastasis	In 1995/10/26- 1996/03/12 after taking XZ-C1, 4, XZ-C3 topical medication the appetite in improvement; in 1995/12 at the end of ascites drainage improved, with after topical lymphatic softening neck	In 1995/06 the color Doppler ultrasound before the aorta 6.1 x 5.4 cm²
193						In 1996/04/19-04/22 After taking XZ-C1, 4,5, the situation is still good and the jaundice is getting better than before
194	In 1996/03/15 had laparotomy exploration and anastomosis duodenal with total bile duct				In 1996/04/11-1997/11/23 after taking XZ-C1 medication the body weight have improved and the appetite is improved significantly, the mental and sleep is also good ; the jaundice decreased significantly, even to subside	
195	In 1995/11/27 had most of the stomach resections		After five courses of Chemotherapy to 1996/05	In 1996/06/04 CT review found that the pancreas was metastasis	In 1996/06/24-07/27 After taking XZ-C1, 4 the pain disappeared and the mass also disappeared, generally good. Before the patients had recurrent for paroxysmal pain, abdominal lump.	

196	In 1996/11/28 had abdominal exploration failed to remove				In 1996/12/11-1997/04/27 after taking XZ-C1, 4 medication, the patient's appetite was improving, the weight gain; there was no fever and no sweating while high fever when discharge; in the past eating a little food the patient had abdominal pain, drinking water is also pain, currently pain relief by medication obviously, jaundice has been subside	Another patient Tian Yang who is the friend husband was told that appealed full of red and can participate in manual labor and has normal work
197	In 1996/12/25 had abdominal exploration and found that the colon adhesion into blocks, failed resection		Postoperative two course chemotherapy	In 1996/12/25 intraoperative see the right lobe 3 ×3cm² metastatic disease lesions were squamous cell carcinoma	In 1997/01/03-03/17 after taking XZ-C1, 4,5, the situation was improved significantly, the appetite were improved (due to Debiatics the food intake is limited); the hair turned black, physical also increased; On 02/10 had the second course of chemotherapy with strong.Before chemotherapy U/S showed liver metastases disappeared, pancreatic mass significantly reduced	
198	In 1997/01/20 had laparotomy exploration, due to liver metastases pancreatic tail drainage was done with Czech Republic diameter anastomosis	Postoperative intervention twice		In 1997/01/20 intraoperative showed liver metastasis	In 1997/01/27-10/19 after taking XZ-C1, 4,5 and water consumption, then had a course of chemotherapy, ten days after treatment did not eat, vomit and Spit for supportive therapy, abdominal pain, back pain and Continued paroxysmal worsening; in 1997/05 U/S showed the pancreatic tail 6.3x 5.1cm² mass ;In 1997/07 had upper digestive tract Bleeding, the condition is very heavy, after treatment hemostasis in 1997/09 the condition improved significantly	Bleeding has been stopped, can play and out of the bed activities, appetite well, the medical staff recognized as is a miracle, waist to lower extremity with calf above swelling edema with dissipated and, such as ordinary people
199	In 1997/02/18 had Laparoscopic exploration with the anastomosis between gallbladder and jejunum				In 1997/03/09-12/28 after taking the drug XZGC1, 4 the appetite was improved, physical recovery, jaundice subsided, the original swelling and fatigue had been subsided and can live on their own, for light degree of household ; In 1997/12 the patients vomiting spit mucus with Brown color and with duodenum compression, or adhesion caused Pancreatic head swelling uplift, there are umbilical pain	98/09/30-98/10/11 after taking XZ-C1, 4, 5, and Jieshui Xiaotang, the spirit is better, the original muscle aches, and now pain, bloating and lower extremity swelling

200	In 1997/02/27 had laparotomy Exploration of bile and intestinal anastomosis .			In 1997/07/14 U/S re-examination showed pancreatic head Lesions considered from the ampullary occupying disease	In 1997/03- 07/14 showed after taking XZ-C1, 4 the spirit and appetite were improved, weight gain, the body is better than before, Jaundice subsided, ruddy complexion, to restore part of the work, Pick 40-50 lb
201	In 1997/07/12 had laparotomy Exploration and the tumor can not be removed				In 1997/07/30- 10/04 after taking XZ-C1, 4 the appetite has improved
202	In 1997/08/19 had laparotomy Exploration and the tumor can not be removed	After operation, once Treatment with 5GFU, MMC	In 1997/08/19 intraoperative saw pancreatic cancer invasion of the posterior wall of the stomach with liver metastases, pelvic Peritoneal metastasis	In 1997/08/24-11/22 after taking XZ-C1, 4, and Topical medication the spirit is good, appetite is still good, low back Increased pain, burning pain because of gastric ulcer can not take Medication, after taking topical medication the pain was getting better ; after chemotherapy the patient had poor appetite	In 1997/12 had sudden Upper gastrointestinal out Blood, portal hypertension,Esophageal variceal rupture and Bleeding, no time to grab and Save, later the death

3.) Some Cases of gastric cancer were treated by XZ-C immune regulation and control medications

Stomach cancer A

Number	Name	Medical record	Gender	Age	Native place	Occupation	Address	Diagnosis	in accordance with	Unit	Society habit			
											Smoking year	Amount of Smoking	Drinking years	Alcohol consumption
219	Zhou xx	x	F	64	Gongen	Women's Director	Gongen	Gastric Cancer	Gastroscopy	Gongen Hospital				
220	Dang xx	x	F	38	Jingshan	Cadre	Jingshan	gastric cancer and pelvic uterine fallopian tube cancer	Endoscopy B ultrasound (In 1994 and in 1996)					
221	Liu xx	x	M	66	Wuhan	Food worker	Caiyue	stomach cancer, bladder cancer	Gastroscopy, barium meal	Concord hospital	40	1 package/day	40	3oz
222	Shu xx	x	M	58	Henan Xinyang	Driver	Xinyang	The postoperative gastric cancer	gastroscopy, CT (In 1996/09)	Concord hospital, Xinyang City hospital				
223	Cai Xx	x	M	55	Suizhou	Public Security Bureau	Suizhou	gastric cardia cancer	Endoscopy and biopsy (in 1996/11/06)	Concord hospital	30	1 package/day	30	1-2oz/day
224	Xiao xx	x	F	18	Zhejiang	Student	Wuhan	antrum, gastric body cancer right ovarian metastasis	Endoscopic biopsy barium meal (96/10/25)	Concord Medical hospital				
225	Lu Xx	x	M	53	Hefeng County	deputy secretary	Enshi	gastric cancer lymph node metastasis		Concord hospital	20-30	One package/day	20-30	Often
226	Yu xx	x	M	30	Dawu	Cadre	Dawu	postoperative	gastroscope (96/04/20)	Concord Hospital				
227	Wang Xx	x	F	37	Chongyang	deputy director of the Inland Revenue Department	Chong yang	antrum cancer, liver diffuse metastasis	Barium meal (97/01/0 1)	Concord Hospital			Often	16oz
228	Zhao xx	x	M	65	Shanxi	Teacher	Echeng	gastric cancer postoperative	barium meal	Finance and Trade Hospital				

229	Ding Xx	x	F	47	Hubei	administrative cadres	Echen	Postoperative gastroscopy,	biopsy, GI biopsy (97/01)	Concord Hospital				
230	Fong Xx	x	M	65	Huangpi 10 years 1 6 2	special note	Wuhan	gastric cancer with systemic metastasis of large amounts of cancer ascites	endoscopy	Tongji Hospital			10	6oz/day
231	Li xx	x	M	67	Hannan Xingcounty	Cadre	Xingxian	stomach gastric cardia, esophageal cancer liver metastases, a small amount of ascites, pleural effusion	endoscopy (97/03/20) of	Xinyang City Hospital Concord Hospital	40	a package		

Stomach cancer Table B-1

Number	Whether to eat often													Whether to drink often			The method of drinking water	Whether to eat often			Jobs		Characters		Whether to love sports
	Water pickles	Salt pickles	Smoked meat	Dried salted fish	Dry pickle	sausage	Fried food	chili	garlic	onion	fresh vegatable vvegetables	fruit	Fried food	Green tea	Strong tea	Other		meat	Ribs soup	Vegetarian food	General	Tension overcharged	Cheerful	Dull and irritable	
219											√											√			√
220								√							√							√		√	
221	√	√													√							√		√	
222		√	√	√		√	√	√	√		√						Well water	√ fatty meat	√	√	√			√	
223											√			√			Unsolicited Wter				√			√	

224		√	√		√	√	√		√			√			Unsolicited water	√				√	
225	√		√			√			√	rice	√				Well Water				√		√
226	√	√	√	√	√		√	√		√				Milk	Well water		√	√		√	
227	√	√	√	√	√	√			√		√				Unsolicited water	√ fatry meat			√	√	
228	√	√			√		√			√	√				Unsolicited water				√	√	
229	√	√	√	√	√		√	√		√					Unsolicited water	√√ fatry	√	√		√	
230	√	√	Mol dy tofu	√								√	Jamic flower		Unsolicited water	√			√		No
231	√	√	√	√	√	√	√	√	√	√	√	√	√	√	Un solicited water			√	√		

Stomach cancer B-2

Number	Chronic disease History	Family three generation of cancer history	Application of pain medication situation			Mass reduction and disappear situation after medications	
			Disappear	Reduction	effective	Tumor location and size	Lump shrinkage after medication

219			√			
220						
221	Tuberculosis has been calcified	Wife uterine cancer death (93 years)				
222						
223						
224	Gastric ulcer	Grandmother died of gastric cancer; grandmother death of pancreatic cancer				
225	30-year-old history of hepatitis	no				
226						
227		In 1983 the Mother died of cervical cancer ; In 1976 father-in-law had esophageal cancer death				
228	History of hepatitis B dysentery	Grandfather liver cancer ascites				
229	Mother 83 years of cervical cancer death, father-in-law 76 years of esophageal cancer death					
230						
231	Stomach history					

Stomach cancer C

Number	What kind of treatment done					Medication time, type and efficacy	Remarks
	Surgical approach	Postoperative pathological examination	intervention	Chemotherapy	When the recurrence and metastasis and site size		

219	In 1996/09 had gastric cancer surgery	There are 10 lymph nodes metastasis to peripancreatic lymph nodes				In 1996/10/03-97/03/01 taking XZGC1; in 04 after medication the general good, normal meals and sleep, can get up for the light housework	
220	In 1994 Surgical resection of gastric cancer(most) (and in 1996 pairs ofOvarian Cancer Resection) .	In 1996 see the uterus wide adhesion (intraoperative) and Can not be removed		In 1994 had the postoperative chemotherapy of the sixth course of chemotherapy with the strong reaction		In 1996/10/19-1997/05/13 After Taking XZ-C1, 4 medication the general good, good appetite; after eating 3-9 Weitai the Bell pain, abdominal pain went away	
221	In 1991 had bladder cancer resection					In 1996/11/14-12/20 taking XZ-C1,4 with XXX, the spirit and the appetite are good, can eat the general food	
222	In 1996/09/17 for stomach Total removalIn		1996/9/9 Lymphatic metastatic with External invasion of lymph nodes and completely removed		In 1996/11/14 chemotherapy	In 1997/03 in the supraclavicular fossa and cervical root two peanuts large lymph nodes can touch, no significant tenderness	In 1996/11/14-1997/03/08 after Take XZ-C1,4, XZ-C3 topical medication the general is good, can eat and had the spirit, Sleep well
223	In 1996/11/27 had Gastric cancer Radical surgery and left chest Under the arch anastomosis	Gastric mucus adenocarcinoma, stomach Wall full-layer and esophageal one Segment with small curvature of the lymph metastasis			In 1997/01/21 CT saw a small amount of abdominal ascites, retroperitoneal lymph nodes, in Ascites the cancer cells can be checked and lymphatic node is 2.5 × 2.5cm²	In 1996/12/23-97/02/28 after taking XZ-C1, 4 and xxx, the situation improved, the appetite is good, there was reduction of ascites	

224			In 1996/11/18 had magnetic therapy guiding treatment with four times interventions	In 1998/11/13 oral Adriamycin	In 1996/12 U/S showed a small amount of ascites and Pleural effusion, ovarian lesions were found with $1.5 \times 1.7 cm^2$ (right side)	In 1996/12/29-1997/01/05 after taking XZ-C1, 4, XZ-C3 topical and Xiaoshuitang decontamination for ascites, the symptoms were significantly reduced and increased urine output	
225	In 1996/12/23 had stomach Radical surgery	Had Gastric poorly differentiated denocarcinoma, Invasion of stomach full-thickness, Gastric pylorus and common hepatic artery and Portal vein posterior lymph metastasis				In 1997/01/12-03/16 after taking XZ-C1,4 medication, the spirit and appetite got better	
226	In 1996/0 5/01 for gastric cancer Resection			In 1996/06, 07 and 10 three chemotherapy, WBC down to 3200 should not be made		In 1997/01/17-1998/04/18 after taking XZ-C1, 4, the spirit and appetite was good, the weight increased	
227	In 1997/01/14 for gastric cancer Radical surgery	Clean the lymphatic liver within the multiple metastases	In 1997/06/0 8 for Chemotherapy with response seriously, and had palpitation Significantly		In 199702/16 Chemotherapy 5-FU carboplatin, reaction strongly with unfinished that is suspended, in 1997/10 for a treatment Of chemotherapy, reaction with Unfinished suspension	In 1997/01/22-1998/10/30 after taking C1, 4, 5, the general condition is good and the spiritual and appetite were good, walking activities as usual; in 1997/02 One week after chemotherapy, hair all lost, WBC down to 1600; after taking our medication the WBC up to 3600, In 1997/06/06 CT showed liver metastases were multiple.	

228	In 1996/11/27 for the partial excision of the stomach and the small intestine and Sweep lymph nodes There were lymph nodes in	Gastric antrum, pylorus, cardia and small intestine, Stomach abdominal cancer, invasion of muscle Full-thickness, small gonad Lymphatic metastasis		Postoperative mitomycin + 5GFU chemotherapy After a total of four courses		In 1997/01/26-09/30 after taking XZ-C1, 4, the spirit and the appetite were good, poor eating, Can get out of bed activities lower extremity edema	
229	In 1997/01/23 for the stomach Cancer laparotomy	Poorly differentiated adenocarcinoma, large and Small mesentery and gastric fundus cardia cancer		Generally poor and could have Chemotherapy		In 1997/01/14- 04/06 after taking XZ-C1,4, the spirit and the appetite were improved, before had eating Obstruction, difficulty swallowing, after the medication take the patient the semi-flow noodles, abdominal distension, low back pain Limb swelling subsided and black stool got ;the next Abdominal touch than a large mass of fist	
230					In 1997/01 under the left subclavian palpable lymph nodes, right in the lower abdomen Palpable and large mass, U/S had ascites	In 1997/02/04-04/13 after taking XZ-C1, 4 and Water soup the spirit and appetite got better; the original had A large number of ascites and after taking 10 Xiaoshu all of these symptoms subsided. In additional in abdominal mass had significantly prominent with the ball was large, fixed soft, the original completely can not Eating, tea could not enter, after taking medications the patient could eat.	The original bedridden, is now available For getting up to go, the original doctor said no hope, preparation of funeral, now Stable condition improved
231					In 1997 /03/20 CT showed there were liver two metastatic foci with a small amount of ascites and pleural effusion	In 1997/03/25-04/04 after taking XZ-C1, 4, the spirit and appetite were improved	

4) Some cases of the lung cancer were treated by XZ-C immune regulation and control medications

Lung cancer A

Number	Name	Medical record	Gender	Age	Native place	Occupation	Address	Diagnosis	in accordance with	Unit	Society habit			
											Smoking year	Amount of Smoking	Drinking years	Alcohol consumption
305	Dain xx	x	M	68	Hubai		Liupinguang	Upper right lung Cancer	Chest x-ray, CT (99/01)	Concord hospital	30	1 package/ day	No	
306	Cheng xx	x	M	70	Wuhan	Worker	Hangyang	Right lung cancer with obstruction pneumonia and bone metastasis	Chest x-ray, CT	Tongji hospital	40	1 package/ day	40	
307	Pen xx	x	F	53	Xiangfan	Housewife	Xiangfan	Right lung cancer with huge fluid in chest	CT, U/S (99/01)	Xiangfan railroad hospital	No		no	
308	Shu xx	x	M	18	Henan	Student	Xingxian	The lung metastasis from liver cancer	CT (99/02)	Concord hospital	NO		NO	
309	Dengxx	X	M	37	Zhijiang	Technician	Zhijiang	Right lung cancer with diagraph and lung and pleural metastasis	Chest x-ray, CT (99/02)	Zhijiang hospital	20	1 package/ day	occass ionally	
310	Fang Xx	x	F	41	Tianmen	Worker	Tianmen	Left upper lung cancer postoperation	CT (98/10/09)	Province people's hospital	No		No	
311	Zhou xx	x	M	70	Gualin	Driver	Wuhan	Left lower lung cancer	CT (99/01)	Tongjin	50	1 package/ day	50	1 bottle/ day
312	Wang Xx	x	M	73	Wuhan	secretary	Hankou	Lung cancer with decending aorta aneurysm	Chest x-ray (99/04)	The fourth wuhan hospital	20	One package/ day	40	3oz/ day

313	Zhao xx	x	M	44	Hannan	Police office	Xiaogan	Lung cancer with high pressure in portal vein and splenomegly and high function of spleen	U/S, color Doppler ultrasound, CT, AFP	Concord Hospital				
314	Liu Xx	x	M	30	Hubei	Worker	Jinmen	Righ upper lung cancer	Chest x-ray, Pathology slides(98/08)	Concord Hospital	Occas sionally		no	

Lung cancer B-1

Number	Whether to eat often													Whether to drink often			The method of drinking water	Whether to eat often			Jobs		Characters		Whether to love sports
	Water pickles	Salt pickles	Smoked meat	Dried salted fish	Dry pickle	sausage	Fried food	chili	garlic	onion	fresh vegatable vvegetables	fruit	Fried food	Green tea	Strong tea	Other		meat	Ribs soup	Vegetarian food	General	Tension overcharged	Cheerful	Dull and irritable	
305											√	√	√	√			Unsolicited Wter					√	√		
306			√							√	√		√		√		Well water	√				√		√	
307	√	√													√							√		√	
308		√	√	√			√	√	√	√	√						Well water	√ fatty meat	√	√		√		√	
309											√			√			Unsolicited Wter					√		√	

Number																
310		√	√		√		√	√		√			√		Unsolicited water	√
311	√		√			√			√		rice	√		Well Water		√	√
312	√	√	√	√	√			√	√			√		Well water / Milk	√
313	√	√	√	√	√		√			√			√		Unsolicited water / √ fatry meat	√ √
314	√	√			√			√			√	√			Unsolicited water	√ √

Lung cancer B-2

Number	Chronic disease History	Family three generation of cancer history	Application of pain medication situation			Mass reduction and disappear situation after medications	
			Disappear	Reduction	effective	Tumor location and size	Lump shrinkage after medication
305	Chronic bronchus Inflammation with emphysema, Stomach bleeding, enteritis	Father suffering from esophagus Cancer died		√			
306	59 years suffering from blood Worm disease, after treatment of alcohol liver hard						
307		Dad died of stomach cancer					
308							
309							
310		Uncle died of nose and throat cancer					
311	Haptitis and arthritis						
312							

313	In 1995 years of schistosomiasis Cirrhosis, in 1989 hepatitis B (small three positive)	Father died of lung cancer					
314							

Lung cancer C

Number	What kind of treatment done					Medication time, type and efficacy	Remarks
	Surgical approach	Postoperative pathological examination	intervention	Chemotherapy	When the recurrence and metastasis and site size		
305	Not appropriate	Not appropriate		Not appropriate	1999/01/07 CT howed: right upper lung cancer with mediastinal lymph nodes	In 1999/01/21-99/08/09 After taking XZGC1 +4 +7 medications, the patient was in stable condition, the spirit and the appetite were good, every day 3-4 meal, each meal 1-2 two; do not breathe, withdrawal to panting, in cold days or hot days the symptoms increase and hemoptysis, Mostly white sputum, no fever	Exam: lung type III tuberculosis, chronic bronchitis and emphysema, chronic schistosomiasis, cirrhosis, bilateral pleural adhesions
306	Not appropriate		Not appropriate	In 1999/01/14 Chemotherapy : DDP + VPG16 (3 days) HCPT (1 day) DDP + VPG16 (3 days) HCPT (1 day)	In 1999/01 X-ray review: left lung and lower lobe lung cancer, T8-9 vertebral metastatic carcinoma, ECT: L5 bone metastasis	In 1999/01/31- 2000/07/31 After taking XZ-C1 +4 +7 MDI medications, the general condition was good, good appetite, illness was stable effect and could work, X-ray results: lung swelling and Tumor had disappeared, in 2000/07/31 at 11:30 pm had bleeding stroke and died	After Patient had chemotherapy for one course, the review of X-ray showed most of the right lower lung inflammation reduced, right diaphragm had hypertrophic adhesion angle
307	Not appropriate		Not appropriate	Not appropriate	In 1999/01 Thoracic puncture showed bloody pleural effusion and there were cancer cells	In 1999/02/03- 1999/03/03 taking XZ-C1 +4 + 7	Drawing pleural effusion three times for the bloody and there were cancer cells, the current physical weakness with shortness of breath

308	Not appropriate		Not appropriate	Not appropriate	In 1999/02/11 CT showed liver multiple lesions, the largest 11.6 × 7.cm2, in chest there were scattered patchy shadows with Hilar widening, lymphatic metastasis	In 1999/02/11 -1999/04/11 after taking XZGC1 +4 +7 LMS.Indo. and XZ-C3 topical medication, the spirit and the appetite and sleep were good, 2oz/meal, walking activities as usual, laughing as usual, there were secondary liver pain, no other discomfort, the appearance was the same as healthy people	In 1999/03/07 families from Henan New County made a special trip to pick up the medications
309	Not appropriate		Not appropriate	Not appropriate		In 1999/02/27- 1999/03/27 after taking XZ-C1 +4 +7 +2 LMS the spirit and appetite were good;	Patient professional was the painter, car spray Paint for 10 years, nitro paint was harmful; after spraying paint, the gas mist made the patient cough
310	In 1998/11/23 had left low Lung and right lung lobe removed	In 1998/12/30 for X remove	In 1998/12/21-1998/12/30 had Radiation therapy for 10 days, In 1999/01/19-1999/01/26 intra vein Therapy (VPG16, DDP600mp)			In 1999/03/07-1999/04/07 after taking XZGC1 +4 +7 LMS/Indo the spirit and appetite were good	Disease detection: upper left lung squamous cell carcinoma stage II, tongue lobe Lymph nodes (1) and hilar lymph nodes (2) were cancer metastasis
311	In 1967 had Stomach perforation and Subtotal gastrectomy		Not appropriate	Not appropriate		In 1999/04/20-1999/05/22 after taking XZ-C1 +4 +7, XZ-C3 topical, the general situation is still good; in the past had more cough and sputum, however at present Breathing smoothly, up and down the fourth floor and could take care of themselves	The patient has four girls, the old couple often argued, heart muffled every day and liked to eat fermented bean curd and Pickles
312	Not appropriate		Not appropriate	Not appropriate	report: descending aortic aneurysm 3.0 × 1.5cm size with hilar spherical lesion diameter was 5.8cm	In 1999/04/2- In 1999/04/26 after taking XZGC1 +4 +7 medications, the spirit and appetite were good	

| 313 | patients with schistosomiasis Liver cirrhosis + hepatitis B liver cirrhosis+ alcohol liver cirrhosis(Not surgery) | | Due to hypersplenism Progress, Not appropriate | Not appropriate | | | In 1999/04/21-1999/11/29 after taking XZ-C1 +4 + 8+LMS blood soup, Xiaotang Tang medications, the general situation was good, the appetite and sleep were good, three meals a day, a meal 2oz, weight Increase 2 .5 kg; on 10/01 had "cold", a few days later there was abdominal distension, and had abdominal water and urine situation were getting worse | AFP: 355. 7 ng / ml |
| 314 | In 1998/08/25 had top right Lobectomy | | Postoperative chemotherapy III Cycles(had strong gastrointestinal reaction | | There was palpable right cervical lymph | | In 1999/06/10-1999/07/10 after taking XZ-C1 + 4, XZ-C3 External application of medication the patient had a good appetite | Exam: the right upper lung large cell poor differentiation, Adenocarcinoma, 1/5 lymph node had cancer |

5) Some of Cases of Esophageal cancer and cardia cancer were treated by XZ-C immune regulation and control medications

Esophageal cancer and cardia cancer A

Number	Name	Medical record	Gender	Age	Native place	Occupation	Address	Diagnosis	in accordance with	Unit	Society habit			
											Smoking year	Amount of Smoking	Drinking years	Alcohol consumption
394	Cai xx	x	M	55	Shuizhou	Public Security Bureau	Shuizhou	Gastric Cardia Cancer	Endoscopic biopsy (96/11/06)	Concord hospital	30	1 package/ day	30	1-2oz
395	Liang xx	x	M	54	Hunan	power supply bureau	Xiangyang	The lower esophageal cancer	Endoscopic biopsy of esophagus in(96/10)	Concord hospital	30	1 package/ day	30	6-10oz
396	Li xx	x	F	56	Nanzhang	Teacher	Nanzhang	esophageal cancer after surgery with Liver metastasis	Swallow barium	Nanzhang County Hospital				

397	Wang xx	x	F	45	Xiangyang	Peasant	Xingxian	The middle Esophageal surgery with Post-pulmonary metastasis	CT(99/02) Endoscopic biopsy(97/01/10)	Finance and Trade Hospital	NO		5-6	2-3oz
398	Huang xx	X	M	70	Huangpi	Boiler worker	Wuhan	cardia postoperative	CT, endoscopy(97/01)		30	1-2 package/day	20	16oz
399	Li Xx	x	M	61	Xingzhou	Metallurgical Industry Company workers	Xingzhou	Postoperative recovery of cardia cancer	Swallow barium angiography	Fanicail hospital				

Esophageal cancer and cardia cancer B-1

Number	Water pickles	Salt pickles	Smoked meat	Dried salted fish	Dry pickle	sausage	Fried food	chili	garlic	onion	fresh vegatable vvegetables	fruit	Fried food	Green tea	Strong tea	Other	The method of drinking water	meat	Ribs soup	Vegetarian food	General	Tension overcharged	Cheerful	Dull and irritable	Whether to love sports
394													√	√			Unsolicited Wter	√				√	√		
395		√				peanut				√	√	√		√			Well water	√				√		√	
396	√	√												√								√		√	
397			√					√	√	√	√	√					Well water	√ fatty meat	√	√		√		√	
398												√		√			Unsolicited Wter				√			√	

399		√	√		√		√	√		√			√		Unsolicited water	√				√		

Esophageal cancer and cardia cancer B-2

Number	Chronic disease History	Family three generation of cancer history	Application of pain medication situation			Mass reduction and disappear situation after medications	
			Disappear	Reduction	effective	Tumor location and size	Lump shrinkage after medication
394		Father suffering from esophagus Cancer died		√			
395	Renal Diatics	In 1950s Granpa died for esophageal cancer					
396	uterine muscle Tumor surgery	Father because of brain swelling Tumor pain suicide Mother died of uterus cancer					Shrink softening
397	In 1986 had haptitis B with jaundice and three positive						
398	chronic gastritis for years without the system treatment						
399							

Esophageal cancer and cardia cancer C

Number	What kind of treatment done					Medication time, type and efficacy	Remarks
	Surgical approach	Postoperative pathological examination	intervention	Chemotherapy	When the recurrence and metastasis and site size		
394	In 1996/11/27 had gastric cardia cancer cure and left thoracic arch anastomosis				In 1997/11/27 intraoperative found that gastric cardia mucinous adenocarcinoma, invasion of the stomach wall full-thickness and lower esophagus, with the lymph node metastasis of small curvature(10/10); in 1997/01/21 CT showed a small amount of ascites, check the retroperitoneal lymph nodes metastasis 2.5 × 2.5cm	In 1996/12/23-in 1997/02/28 after taking the medication the mental, the appetite and the physical strength had improved; taking XZ-C1,4 Brucea javanica	
395					In 1998/11/07 MRI showed upper left lung 2.2x2.5x 3.2 cm3 metastases	In 1996/12/25 after taking XZ-C1,4, the spirit and appetite, were good, the complexion rosy, could work, and consciously digest well, but could be not supine after eating because of nausea phenomenon	
396	In late 1993 had esophageal cancer by thoracotomy			Had one year of radiotherapy and chemotherapy	In 1995/05 found liver metastasis, barium see 5-6cm² esophageal recurrence	In 1997/01- 04/06 after taking XZ-C1,4,2 ;XZ-C3 topical, had good appetite with the original obstruction, is gradually better; the original had cough seriously withspit, now the cough spit got better, but not much food, malnutrition; the neck Lymph node got shrinkage, softening after application	

397	In 1997/01/25 had esophageal cancer radical surgery,in 1997/06 had left supraclavicular lymphadenectomy				In 1997/06left subclavian lymph node metastasis; in 1998/03 had the left edge of lymph node metastasis; in 1999/01/28 chest x-ray showed lung several metastases	In 1997/02/19 after taking XZ-C1,4, 2 XZ-C3 topical medication, the general was good; from 97/03 to 98/10 the patient stopped medications, then had lymphatic metastasis and took the medications again; in 1997/0 6 had left scapular diffuse Limited swelling, 10 × 2cm2 tenderness, local pain, food can be satisfied, the spirit was poor, can walk	
398	In 1997/01/13 had cardia cancer radical surgery				In 1997/01/13 intraoperative saw lymph node metastasis (4/7) in right supraclavicular lymph nodes with the metastasis	in 1997/02/27- 03/30 after taking XZ-C1,4, 2, XZ-C3 external application for two months, the general is good; in 1997/03 examination found the right neck string of fixed lymph, fusion into a plate, hard, right armpit 3 fingers;The size of the right shoulder lymph nodes can not lift? 97? Yuan? 9CT suspect retroperitoneal lymph nodes and mesenteric lymph node metastasis	
399	In 1997/04/04 had gastric cardia surgery of left thoracic and thoracic esophageal gastric anastomosis		In 1998/03/29- 04/12 had fatigue, nausea and vomiting, dizziness after chemotherapy		In 1998/04/15 barium showed local stenosis;In 1998/06/15 and in 1998/09/21 swallow barium saw esophagus and gastric anastomosis, below the small curvature of the stomach with irregular filling defect recurrence	In 1997/04/29 after taking XZ-C1, 4 the appetite was still good, there is the phenomenon of reflux, eating without obstruction but pain, shoulder pain, and weather-related, for rheumatoid arthritis, left neck tenderness; when eating the hot food, feeling sternal pain	

6) Some cases of Breast cancer were treated by ZX-C immune regulation and control medications

Breast cancer A

Number	Name	Medical record	Gender	Age	Native place	Occupation	Address	Diagnosis	in accordance with	Unit	Society habit			
											Smoking year	Amount of Smoking	Drinking years	Alcohol consumption
447	Jing xx	x	F	75		Teacher	Huangpi	Right side Breast		Concord hospital				1-2oz
448	Peng xx	x	F	47	Wuhan	Worker	Wuhan	Right side breast	Biopsy (95/02/16)	Red community hospital				6-10oz
449	Gui xx	x	F	40	Nanzhang	Teacher	Nanzhang	esophageal cancer after surgery with Liver metastasis	Biopsy and pathology (95/02/28)	Red community hospital				
450	Li xx	x	F	47	Xiangyang	Peasant	Xingxian	The middle Esophageal surgery with Post-pulmonary metastasis	CT, Biopsy (94/11/)	Red community hospital				
451	Cheng xx	X	F	44	Huangpi	Boiler worker	Wuhan	cardia postoperative	Biopsy	Concord hospital				
452	Fang Xx	x	F	45	Hubei	Peasant	Xiaochang	The lymphatic metastasis of the left axillary and the supraclavicular fossa of postoperative breast cancer	Pathology (94/12)	Concord hospital				

Breast cancer B-1

Number	Whether to eat often													Whether to drink often			The method of drinking water	Whether to eat often			Jobs		Characters		Whether to love sports
	Water pickles	Salt pickles	Smoked meat	Dried salted fish	Dry pickle	sausage	Fried food	chili	garlic	onion	fresh vegatable vegetables	fruit	Fried food	Green tea	Strong tea	Other		meat	Ribs soup	Vegetarian food	General	Tension overcharged	Cheerful	Dull and irritable	
447																									
448										√	√	√		√			Well water	√				√		√	
449	√	√												√								√		√	
450							√	√	√	√	√						Well water / fatty meat	√	√	√		√		√	
451		√					√				√			√			Unsolicited Wter				√			√	
452								√																	

Breast cancer B-2

Number	Chronic disease History	Family three generation of cancer history	Application of pain medication situation			Mass reduction and disappear situation after medications	
			Disappear	Reduction	effective	Tumor location and size	Lump shrinkage after medication
447				√			
448	In 1986 had stomach disease						
449							
450	In 1984 had appendectomy						
451							
452							

Breast Cancer 6-C

Number	What kind of treatment done						Medication time, type and efficacy	Remarks
		Surgical approach	Postoperative pathological examination	intervention	Chemotherapy	When the recurrence and metastasis and site size		
447	In 1994 /10 had the right Cancer resection						94/11/14-02/17 after taking XZ-C1,4, he general situation is good	

448	In 1995/03 had Right breast cancer with Radical surgery					In 1995/03/27-04 After taking XZ-C1, 4 for two month, in October the patient came to tell us that the patient was in good condition and because of economic difficulties the patient stopped medication	
449	In 1995/03/29 Left breast cancer Radical surgery					In 1995/0 3/29 – 04/25 after taking XZ-C1, 4 the appetite and sleep were good; In 1995 had little white milk in the right breast	
450	In 1994/11 had the right breast Radical surgery					In 1995/04/14-04/30 after taking XZ-C1, 4, for a month the spirit was good	
451	In 1995/02/20 had the right breast Radical surgery					In 1995/05/11-98/02/26 after taking XZ-C1, 4, the appetite was good; in 1995/11 had no abnormal in chest X-ray, ruddy weight increase of 10 pounds	
452	In 1978 the right breast cancer surgery and in 1990 the left breast Cancer surgery (November)				In 1990/11 had left breast metastasis and in 1993 left armpit Lymph node metastasis; in 1995 underarm (left) 8 × 6 × 6cm3 size, left supraclavicular lymph node metastasis	In 1995/05/08- 08/25 after taking XZ-C1, 4, bruce milk external application, the general was good, the appetite was good; the patient looked good, the wound was significantly reduced, less	

7) Some Cases of the Rectal and Colon cancer were treated by XZ-C immune regulation and control medications

Rectal and colon cancer A

Number	Name	Medical record	Gender	Age	Native place	Occupation	Address	Diagnosis	in accordance with	Unit	Smoking year	Amount of Smoking	Drinking years	Alcohol consumption
											Society habit			
482	Li xx	x	M	67	Wuhan	Worker	Wuhan	Recurrence of rectal cancer and had surgery twice	Rectoscopy (95/10)	Concord hospital	30	A package/ day	30	occasionally
483	Yao xx	x	M	62	Hubei	CADRE	Wuhan	Rectal cancer	Pathology (96/12)	Concord hospital	20	A or two package/ day		occasionally
484	Gui xx	x	M	68	Heilongjiang	Cadre	Wuhan	Rectal cancer	Pathology (96/11/13)	Concord hospital				
485	Li xx	x	F	42	Xiangyang	Cadre	Xingxian	sigmoid colon cancer	U/S	Concord hospital				
486	Cheng xx	X	F	39	Huangpi	Peasant	Wuhan	Colon cancer	U/S (97/03/15)	Concord hospital				
487	Fang Xx	x	M	51	Wuhan	Procuratorate cadre	Wuhan	Colon cancer with liver metastasis	(96/03)	Concord hospital				

Colon and rectal cancer B-1

Number	Whether to eat often													Whether to drink often				The method of drinking water	Whether to eat often			Jobs		Characters		Whether to love sports
	Water pickles	Salt pickles	Smoked meat	Dried salted fish	Dry pickle	sausage	Fried food	chili	garlic	onion	fresh vegatable vvegetables	fruit	Fried food	Strong tea	Green tea	Other			meat	Ribs soup	Vegetarian food	General	Tension overcharged	Cheerful	Dull and irritable		
482			√				√										Unsolicited Wter		√				√			no

483	√	√	√	√	√	√		√	√	√		√		√			√	River water	√				√		√	
484	√	√										√											√		√	
485					√	√	√	√		√					√ fatty meat	Well water	√	√		√		√	
486	√			√			√			√				√		Unsolicited Wter			√		√	
487					√																		

Colon and rectal cancer B-2

Number	Chronic disease History	Family three generation of cancer history	Application of pain medication situation			Mass reduction and disappear situation after medications	
			Disappear	Reduction	effective	Tumor location and size	Lump shrinkage after medication
482	Calcification of tuberculosis with gastritis history of gastritis			√			
483	years of coronary heart disease old myocardial infarction						
484	On 199205\18 stroke, left hypothalamic hemorrhage, right hemiplegia						
485	a history of chronic gastritis						

486	History of chronic headache constipation						
487	In 1982 hepatitis, chronic gastritis history, colitis ; in 1994 barium enema, sigmoid colon mucosal disorder	Father esophageal and cardia Ca; in 1974 passed away					the lump got smaller than before

Colon and rectal cancer C

Number	What kind of treatment done					Medication time, type and efficacy	Remarks
	Surgical approach	Postoperative pathological examination	intervention	Chemotherapy	When the recurrence and metastasis and site size		
482	In 1995/10/17 had rectal resection and anastomosis; in 1996/12/20 had sigmoid fistula		In 1996/09 intubation pump, injection only once	Postoperative chemotherapy 4 times, each time 10 days	On 1996\12\20 during fistula surgery the rectum Ca was found with invasive of the sacrum	On 1997\01\14-02\14 XZ-C1,4, XZ-C3 for external application, after taking the drug the patient had significantly changed, could not get out of bed, there were still red and white frozen; after removing these bloody things, the patient was improved on bloating difficulties and hematuria	Drinking pond water has high incidence of cancer and, the Yangtze River water has the pool sediment
483	On 1997\01\20 for rectal ca radical surgery					On 1997\02-1997\03\16 after taking XZ-C1,4 medication the patient had a good appetite, physical strength had been restored so that the patient could go up and down the stairs, now their own downstairs, on the garden	
484	On 1996\12\09 had rectal caDixon operation					On 1997\02\23-04\22 after taking XZ-C1,4 medications the patient had a good appetite, physical recovery, such as preoperative, blood pressure is not high, good memory, right hemiplegia	
485	On 1997\02\23 had sigmoid colon ca radical surgery		A course of chemotherapy after surgery			On 1997\03\22-04\27 After Taking XZ-C1,4 the spirit of appetite was good, face as usual	

| 486 | On 1997\04 had laparotomy, left colon resection | | | | On 1998\10\28 had laparotomy and abdominal wall and small intestine tumors, invasion and full-thickness abdominal wall and omentum nodular metastasis | On 1997\04\26-06\13 and on 1998\11\0 5 after taking XZ-C1,4 medications the patient was generally good; on 1998\08 found left abdominal mass ; On 1998\10\28 had laparotomy and found invasion of abdominal wall tumor and full-thickness abdominal wall and omentum Nodule metastasis so that the patient had intestinal tumor resection and anastomosis | |
| | | | | | | In 1997/06/03-06/29 After taking the XZ-C1, 4,5, XZ-C3 topical, the patient had good spirit and appetite, looking good; after topical the lump was reduced compared with before; after the drug WBC was up from 6. 4×10^9 /l to WBC7. 0×10^9 /l; on 97 \06\15 physical examination mass was $12 \times 9 cm^2$, on 97\06\ 29 tumor mass was significantly reduced to $7 \times 17 cm^2$ | |

8) Some Cases of Cholangiocarcinoma were treated by XZ-C immune regulation and control medications

Cholangiocarcinoma A

Number	Name	Medical record	Gender	Age	Native place	Occupation	Address	Diagnosis	in accordance with	Unit	Society habit			
											Smoking year	Amount of Smoking	Drinking years	Alcohol consumption
650	Zhang xx	x	F	31	Wuhan	Street Office Director r	Wuhan	common bile duct papilloma malignant transformation of liver metastases	Color Doppler ultrasound, CT (94 /0 4)	Concord hospital	1-2	10 cigerattee/ day		
651	He xx	x	M	51	Xishui	CADRE	Wuhan	Liver hilar cholangiocarcinoma	Pathology (95/04)	Concord hospital	20	10 cigerattee/ day	15	2-3oz
652	Jiang xx	x	M	76	Wuhan		Wuhan	hilar region bile duct cancer surrounding the ampulla	Exploration surgery (95/02))	Concord hospital				
653	Zheng xx	x	F	61	Huanghu	Peasant	Huanghu	gallbladder cancer	U/S (1995/10/08)	Tongji Hospital				
654	Zhang xx	X	F	58	Wuhan	Agricultural Bank cadre	Wuhan	hilar cholangiocarcinoma	U/S,CT (95/11)	Concord hospital				

| 655 | Yang Xx | x | M | 28 | Guizhou | Painter worker | Wuhan | hilar cholangiocarcinoma | (color Doppler ultrasound, CT(95/12)) | Concord hospital | 7-8 | A package/day | | |

Cholangiocarcinoma B-1

Number	Whether to eat often													Whether to drink often			The method of drinking water	Whether to eat often			Jobs		Characters		Whether to love sports
	Water pickles	Salt pickles	Smoked meat	Dried salted fish	Dry pickle	sausage	Fried food	chili	garlic	onion	fresh vegatable vvegetables	fruit	Fried food	Green tea	Strong tea	Other		meat	Ribs soup	Vegetarian food	General	Tension overcharged	Cheerful	Dull and irritable	
650								√			√						Unsolicited Wter	√				√			
651	√	√	√	√	√	√		√	√	√	√	√			√		River water	√ fatty meat				√		√	no
652															√										
653																									
654		√	√				√				√			√			Unsolicited Wter				√			√	
655								√									River water	√ fatty meat							

Cholangiocarcinoma B-2

Number	Chronic disease History	Family three generation of cancer history	Application of pain medication situation			Mass reduction and disappear situation after medications	
			Disappear	Reduction	effective	Tumor location and size	Lump shrinkage after medication
650	In 1989 Found T.B and recovery after 2 months treatment			√			
651	Often cough						
652							
653	There was Schistosoma with Abdominal pain Recurrence more than 20 years	Spouse had brain tumor and died in 1979				In 1995/10/08 U/S showed there was 6. 5x4.5 cm2 mass	
654							
655	history of gastritis, had gastroscopy which showed gallbladder and biliary Stone and Biliary colic in 1993						

Cholangiocarcinoma C

Number	What kind of treatment done					Medication time, type and efficacy	Remarks
	Surgical approach	Postoperative pathological examination	intervention	Chemotherapy	When the recurrence and metastasis and site size		

650	In 1994/08/24 had tumors Resection with anastomosis of bile duct and jejunum				In 1994/04 found bile duct tumor with liver metastasis	In 1995/03/15-03/25 after taking XG-C1, 4; in 01 XZ-C3 outside application, local topical analgesic effect is still good, but less urine, ascites	
651						In 1995/04/23-07/29 after taking XZ-C1, 4 the Appetite was good, abdominal fullness after meals; otherwise, no discomfort; in 1994 gain weight 148 pounds, and now was 114 pounds	
652	In 1995/03/17 had surgery of Exploration due to duodenum and hilar adhesions				In 1995/03/17 found Tumor occupying in hilar and biliary duct, cystic duct, gallbladder ampulla	In 1995/03/22-12/17 after taking XZ-C1, 4 the spirit was good, yellow Jaundice subsided, physical recovery, but poor appetite due to bile completely external drainage	In 1995/02/0 2 had jaundice, yellow urine, one week ago had fever and found obstructive and jaundice Hilar cholangiocarcinoma
653	No application				In 1995/10/08 U/ S showed right hepatic lobular gallbladder Squamous cell lesions of gallbladder invasion	In 1995/10/16-11/15 after taking XZ-C1, 4, the appetite and the spirit had improved, weight gain of 3 pounds	

654	In 1995/12/29 Abdominal exploration of bile enteric anastomosis with Internal drainage					In 1996/01/31-03/29 after taking XZ-C1, 4, the appetite was improved; 39 ℃ fever for three days due to cold; after the temperature went down, the patient had still jaundice.	
655	In 1995/12 had exploration Surgery; due to adhesion the pieces were unable to cut					In 1996/02/11-02/25 after taking XZ-C1, 4, 5, the general situation was well; the wound flew yellow water which every day 3-4 gauzes were used; the whole body was yellow without change, the body depth of yellow, urine dark yellow as tea	

Anti - cancer, anti - cancer metastasis research, scientific and technological innovation, scientific research series

2. THE PARTIAL TYPICAL CASES OF MALIGNANT CANCER WERE TREATED WITH XZ-C IMMUNORUGLATION AND CONTROL OF ANTI-CANCER CHINESE MEDICATIONS

1). Some typical cases of liver cancer treatment

Case 1. Mr. Mao, male, 48 year-old, Taimen, officer. Medical record number: number: 100014 Diagnosis: primary liver carcinoma

Disease course and treatment: On August 1, 1994 because the patient felt fatigued, he had ultrasound in the local hospital and found a 4.1cm x 4.5cm nodule in the left lobe of the liver. On August 26, 1994 the left lobe of the liver was removed in the Xian Ha hospital. Pathological slides showed: liver cell carcinoma without any treatment. After operation, the patient was treated with anticancer immunological traditional medicine **XZ-C1+XZ-C4+XZ-C5** in our outpatient center. After taking these medicines, the patient's appetite increased, energy level increased and he was happy. He takes medicines regularly and comes to our office every month for follow up and refilling of the medicines. He feels very well and goes back to his work. On December 14, 1996 there was another 1.3cm x 1.8cm nodule which was found by B ultrasound in the edge of the left liver. On December 30, 1996 he had that nodule removed. After the operation, he continued to take the medicine. After that, the patient took his medicine persistently and regularly. In May 2010 when he came to follow-up, his general condition was good and his face was glowing with health, his body was as strong as a healthy person's and the patient returned to work for more than 11 years. His appetite is great and his emotion is very good. He eats 600g food per day and his ultrasound is normal.

Comments: On August 26, 1994 this patient had a 4.1cm x 4.5cm nodule removal of left liver. After the operation, the patient received XZ-C for treatment. On December 30, 1996 another 1.3cm x 1.8cm nodule was found and removed. After that, this patient continued to take XZ-C. When he came back for 16-year follow-up, his health condition is good and he can do labor work for many years. This patient is still alive and very well at the time of writing this book.

Implication: After the removal of the liver carcinoma the patient took XZ-C1+XZ-C4+XZ-C5 persistently, these medicines improve thymus function and protect bone morrow function of producing blood cells, protect liver function and improve the whole body immunology function against disease. The operation and the medicine XZ-C can increase the long-term treatment of the cancer patients.

Case 2. Ms. Liu, female, 65 year-old, Jianxian in Hubei, officer. Medical record number: 110201
Diagnosis: primary huge liver carcinoma

Disease course and treatment: Because of discomfort in upper abdomen, the patient had CT in XieHe hospital which found that a 6.7 cm x 7.1 cm x 9 cm nodule in right liver, then diagnosed as primary liver carcinoma. She refused to take operation and chemotherapy. In July 11, 1995 she started to take the XZ-C1+XZ-C5. After 2 months, her emotion and appetite get better and her weight increased. In September 20, 1995 on follow-up ultrasound, the nodule was reduced. In November 1995 she had a chemoembolization and didn't have any other therapy. She continues to take the XZ-C for more than 6 years and continues to follow-up more than 10 years. This patient's condition is good. In May 2005 this patient is as healthy as a normal person.

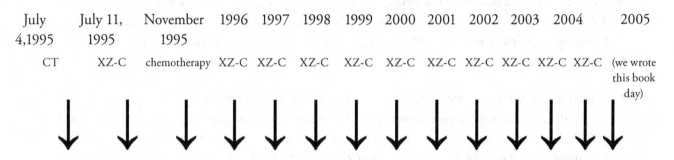

July 4,1995	July 11, 1995	November 1995	1996	1997	1998	1999	2000	2001	2002	2003	2004	2005
CT	XZ-C	chemotherapy	XZ-C	XZ-C	XZ-C	XZ-C	XZ-C	XZ-C	XZ-C	XZ-C	XZ-C	XZ-C (we wrote this book day)

Primary huge   Take XZ-C1+XZ-C4+XZ-C5
liver carcinoma

Comments: On July 4, 1995 this patient was diagnosed with primary liver carcinoma by CT and then took XZ-C after 1 week. After 2 month, the CT scan showed that the nodule become smaller. On November 21 the chemotherapy procedure was conducted, and then she continued to take XZ-C regularly and persistently for 10 years. Now this patient is as healthy as a normal individual.

Implication: The chemotherapy+XZ-C have good results on liver carcinoma treatment. The chemotherapy can stop the blood supply to the cancer nodule and chemotherapy can kill some of the cancer cells. There are living cancer cells inside and under the tumor nodule membrane after chemotherapy; the tumor cells didn't die completely and then grew fast after circulation built up. XZ-C can protect thymus and improve the immune ability, protect the bone morrow function and improve the body immune function. In addition, 85% hepatic cancer occurred in the cirrhosis patients so chemotherapy will damage the liver function. XZ-C will protect the liver. The combination of chemotherapy+XZ-C will inhibit the tumor and protect the host to improve the long-term treatment. This is called "take out the bad and keep the good" in Chinese.

Case 3. Mr. Kei, male, 54 year-old, Yanxi in Hubei, officer. Medical record number: number: 6301244.
Diagnosis: primary liver carcinoma

Disease course and treatment: The patient had pain on the upper right abdomen for half of a month and his appetites decreased. CT in Yanxia showed nodules in the right front and back lobe and left lobe. The patient was diagnosed with primary liver carcinoma. On August 20, 1998 the patient had opening surgery which revealed that the main tumors were in the entrance of the common duct and there were metastasis in both of left and right liver, which could not be removed. Therefor a tube for the chemotherapy was placed through the hepatic artery. After the operation, the chemotherapy was used once. In October 1998 the second chemotherapy was used. Because the tube was blocked, the patient stopped using the tube. On September 8, 1998 he started taking XZ-C1+XZ-C4+XZ-C5. After taking this medicine one month, the patient's emotion and appetite were good and his body weight increased and his face was glowing with health. On his physical exam the abdomen was soft and flat and the spleen and liver could not be felt; his general condition was good. He could support himself very well and picked up his medication by himself. On June 4, 2002 when he came back for his follow-up, his healthy condition was good; his face was glowing with health, his walking, acting and smiling were like a normal, healthy person. On the physical exam there was no abnormality found.

Comments: On August 20, 1998 liver carcinoma was found in the right and left liver and could not be removed, and a chemotherapy tube was placed, through which the chemotherapy was twice given after CT scan showed many lesions in the left lobe, right front and right back lobe. On September 8 the patient started to take XZ-C1+XZ-C4+XZ-C5. Until 2002 this patient's condition was good and didn't have metastasis.

Implication: When liver cancer could not be removed, the liver artery tube could be placed, then XZ-C1+XZ-C4+XZ-C5 was used to protect Thymus, bone morrow, liver to improve the host immune system function and induce the host to produce more anticancer factors to control the tumors and to control the development of the cancers.

Case 4. Mr. Pu, male, 51 year-old, Yin Zheng, officer. Medical record number: number: 500989 Diagnosis: primary liver cancer

Disease course and treatment: There is a 4.6cm x 3.6cm nodule in left liver and a 1.6cm x 1.6cm nodule in right liver after the patient had CT on October 30, 1997. Diagnosis was liver carcinoma. There is a 5.9cm x 4.0cm x 5.4cm nodule in the left liver lobe and a 2.1cm x 1.8cm lesion in the right liver lobe when the patient had Ultrasound in the XieHe hospital. Liver angiography showed that the patient had liver cancer. HBsAg(+), AFP(-). Because this patient's liver function was poor, he couldn't stand the operation and put on the tube for chemotherapy. This patient is alcohol drinker for 40 years (250ml/per meal average). In 1996 he had Hepatitis B. In 1966 he had blood fluke. On November 25 the patient starts to take XZ-C1+XZ-C4+XZ-C5. In 1998 and 1999 the patient continued to take the medicine. The patient's condition is good, and his face is red and smiles. On November 2, 1999 he came to follow-up and the ultrasound showed the lesion was reduced. He can do light work and feels very well. For more than 2 years, he continues to take XZ-C1+XZ-C4+XZ-C5. After these medicines the patient's energy level is improving and appetite is improving. In June 2002 he went to Beijing for treatment (before he went to Beijing, he was good and walking as the normal person). During the operation there is a 5cm x 6cm nodule in the liver which is the same as 5 years ago and there are cancer cells in the common duct and now metastasis, and no fluid in the abdominal cavity. There is no metastasis in the liver, however because the nodule is close to the hepatic artery entrance, it is very difficult to remove the cancer nodule and then place the drainage tube. After surgery, this patient didn't have urine and had acute renal failure. He passed away on day 6.

Comments: On October 30, 1997 CT showed a 4.6cm x 3.6cm nodule in left liver and in November 1997 there is a 1.6cm x 1.6cm nodule in right liver. Because the liver function was poor, the patient didn't have operation and tube placement and other treatment. On November 25 he started to take XZ-C1+XZ-C4+XZ-C5 and continued for 5 years. His health condition was fine.

Implication: XZ-C can improve the host immune system ability (including the cell and antibody immune function) to protect the central and peripheral immune organs, to protect the liver and kidney, and to produce anticancer factors an dprevent cancer cells metastasis and spread. XZ-C is a medication with no side effects which helps the patient in "fight with bad and help the right". In addition the patient's disease condition was under very good control without metastasis so that therapeutic effect was very good. This patient took XZ-C for 5 years, during which time his condition was stable and the liver cancer lesion was not increasing and there were no metastasis. His general condition was good and not uncomfortable and the patient walked as a normal person. He went to Beijing and was diagnosed as liver cells carcinoma which was in the entrance of the liver and couldn't be removed because of the cancer cells in the common duct. The patient underwent surgery for the placement of the T-tube for chemotherapy. After the operation, this patient didn't have urine and died of acute renal failure. If he had not had the operation which destroyed the liver and kidney function, he might have survived to the present day.

Case 5. Mr. Huang, male, 53 year-old, Wuhan. Medical record number: number: 11202225 Diagnosis: primary huge liver cancer, liver cirrhosis after hepatitis, the later stage of Japanese blood fluke, Portal hypertension.

Disease course and treatment: Patient's appetite decreased and he felt uncomfortable in his abdomen. In September 2000 CT showed a 13.6cm x 11.8cm lesion in the right liver lobe. In September 7, 2000 MRI showed a huge 13.1cm x 11.4cm x 12.5cm lesion in right lobe, diagnosed as huge liver cancer in right lobe. The patient had hepatic arterial chemoembolization (HACE) and embolization (HAE) and the chemoembolization medicine were xxxx 25mg+xxx1000g: xxxx10ml+xxxx10mg. Currently his general condition is good. The change of his liver lesions are the following which are stable and getting small: CT showed a 11.1cm x 11.8cm lesion in the right liver lobe on October 12, 2000, a 10.8cm x 9.8cm lesion in the right liver lobe on December 14, 2000, a 10.5cm x 9.5cm lesion on Feb 2001 and a 9.8cm x 8.9cm lesion on September 3, 2001 in the right liver lobe. This patient started to take XZ-C1+XZ-C4+XZ-C5 on January 9, 2002 and his general condition is good, just as his emotion, appetite and sleep are very good. He comes back for check-up every month and takes his medicine regularly. On October 21, 2002 during his follow-up, his general condition is good, emotion is stable, and appetite is good and bowel movement is good and his routine is regular and he exercises regularly. He reports not having had a cold during the last four years. He lived as a normal healthy person.

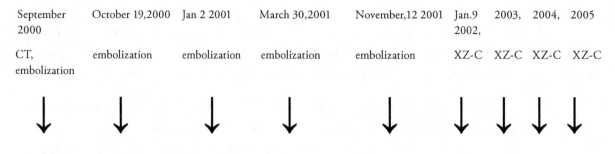

September 2000	October 19,2000	Jan 2 2001	March 30,2001	November,12 2001	Jan.9 2002,	2003,	2004,	2005
CT, embolization	embolization	embolization	embolization	embolization	XZ-C	XZ-C	XZ-C	XZ-C

Lesion in the right liver 13.6cmx11.8cm   embolization

Comments: This case is primary huge liver carcinoma which had five times embolization and the lesion was getting smaller and had very good response. Last embolization is on November 12, 2001 and the lesion is 9.8cm x 8.9cm. He started to take XZ-C1+XZ-C4+XZ-C5 on Jan 9, 2002. The XZ-C1 can kill the cancer cells and not kill the normal cells; XZ-C4 protects thymus and inhibits thymus shrinkage; XZ-C5 protects liver function. This patient continues to take this medicine for more than 3 years, however when he came back for follow-up in the fourth year, his health condition is general, disease is stable and there is no metastasis and no further development. His emotion is stable, his appetite is good, and he walks as a normal healthy person. The experience from this case is for primary huge liver cancer, first embolization treatment are given to make this lesion smaller and stable, later use XZ-C to support the long-term therapy and to protect the liver function and to improve the immune system and to control the metastasis.

Case 6. Mr. Lee, male, 53 year-old, Wuhan, farmer. Medical record number: number: 9901979 Diagnosis: primary huge liver carcinoma, late stage Japanese blood fluke hepatic cirrhosis.

Disease course and treatment: On January 22, 2001 the patient felt pain in the right back. In Feb 26, 2001 ultrasound showed a nodule in the liver. On January 31, 2001 CT showed a 14cm x 1cm lesion in the right liver lobe diagnosed as primary huge liver cancer in the right liver. On March 1, 2001 the open abdomen surgery was done in Tongjin Hospital and the pump implantation in the portal vein because the lesion was huge and couldn't be removed. After the surgery the patient received chemotherapy once. This patient had 30 years Japanese blood fluke. On March 9, 2001 this patient started to take XZ-C medicine. He used XZ-C1+XZ-C4+XZ-C5, LMS, MDZ, and XZ-C3 placed on a fist-size lump in the right rib edge area. After one month of taking this medicine, the patient's condition is getting better and his emotion is stable and happy. His appetite is increasing. The lump in the right rib edge area is getting smaller and softer than before. After he continued to take this medicine for three months, his general condition is good and his appetite and sleep are good. His energy level is recovering and he is walking as a normal person. On October 22, 2001 Ultrasound showed a 6cm x 7.8cm lesion in the right lobe liver and he continues taking XZ-C1+XZ-C4+XZ-C5 and using XZ-C3 on the lump. On November 19, 2003 during his follow-up, ultrasound showed this lesion size the same as before, kidney function is normal and CXR didn't show abnormality, there is no positive lymph node and the lump on the right rib edge is soft and getting smaller and the boundry is clear and not painful. This patient continued to use XZ-C1+XZ-C4+XZ-C5.

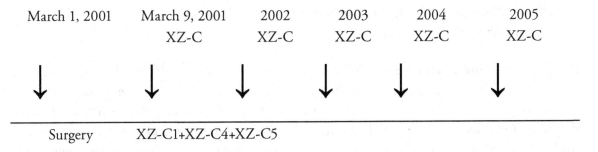

March 1, 2001	March 9, 2001	2002	2003	2004	2005
	XZ-C	XZ-C	XZ-C	XZ-C	XZ-C

Surgery   XZ-C1+XZ-C4+XZ-C5

Comments: This case is diagnosed as primary huge liver cancer and the lesion can not be removed so that the portal vein pump was placed for chemotherapy once. In March 2001, he started to use the XZ-C1+XZ-C4+XZ-C5 and topical XZ-C3 for 4 years. His general condition is stable and didn't develop further and didn't metastasize.

Case 7. Mr. Wang, male, 40 year-old, Shangdou, teacher. Medical record number: 900164 Diagnosis: primary liver cancer

Disease course and treatment: The tumor was removed in the mediastinum on June 28, 1989. The pathology showed the thymoma with lymphocyte type and high malignant tumor and without treatment. In Feb 1995 ultrasound showed a lesion in liver. On Feb 23, 1995 CT showed a 8.2cm x 8.7cm lesion in right posterior lobe and many nodes mixed together. On June 5, 1995 the hepatic artery graph embolization was done. The chemotherapy was injected in the lesion and on November 10, 1995 this right liver lesion was removed and the pathology showed liver cell cancer. On December 21, 1995 ultrasound showed a 3.8cm x 3.2cm lesion in the right liver lobe which was the recurrent lesion after the surgery and there was fluid in the right chest cavity and the right low lung is not distended and CXR showed right low lung metastasis. On December 23, 1995 this patient took the XZ-C1+XZ-C4+XZ-C5 for more than two years and follow-up more than five years. His general condition is good and he continued to teach and work normally without other treatment.

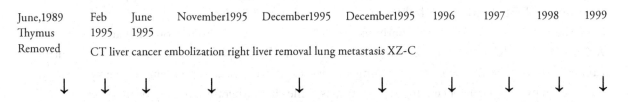

June,1989 Thymus Removed	Feb 1995	June 1995	November1995	December1995	December1995	1996	1997	1998	1999
	CT	liver cancer embolization	right liver removal	lung metastasis	XZ-C				

taking XZ-C1+XZ-C4+XZ-C5

Comments: In May 1995 CT showed a 7.1cm x 6.6cm lesion in the right liver lobe. In 1995 the embolization was done once. On November 10, 1995 this right liver lesion was removed and diagnosed as liver cancer. On December 21, 1995 ultrasound showed a 3.8cm x 3.2cm lesion in the right liver lobe which was the recurrent lesion. On December 23, 1995 this patient took the XZ-C1+XZ-C4+XZ-C5 and his condition is good for more than four years.

Implication: there is very good result for liver cancer while using the combination of embolization +operation removal+XZ-C immune anticancer medicine.

Case 8. Mr. Zhao, 34 year-old, JinZhou, accountant. Medical record number: 380742
Diagnosis: primary huge liver cancer

Disease course and treatment: On Feb 26, 1997 there was a 13cm x 10.4cm lesion between the liver quadrate lobe and left lobe because the patient feel uncomfortable about her stomach and had ultrasound test, then MRI showed a 7.9cm x 11.2 cm x 11.0cm lesion and portal vein had the cancer thrombus. On March 1, the patient had fever of 39°C. On March 2, the patient was transferred to the XieHe hospital because of high fever and there is a 5cm x 6cm hard lump under sternum. On March 10 the embolization was performed and the patient had great reaction to this. This patient had embolization on April 30, on July 9, and on September 18. Then lump decreased significantly. On March 4 the patient started to take XZ-C1+XZ-C4+XZ-C5 to stabilize the lesion and to control the spread and to prevent the metastasis. After taking the medicine, the patient's emotion and appetite are getting better and the general condition is getting better and life quality is getting better. The lump under the sternum couldn't be palpated.

Feb 26,1997	March 3,1997	March 10,1997	April 30,1997	July 9, 1997	Sept 18, 1997,	1998	1999	2000
CT MRK	XZ-C	Embolization	Embolization	Embolization	Embolization	XZ-C	XZ-C	XZ-C

Taking the XZ-C1+XZ-C4+XZ-C5

Comments: For this primary huge liver carcinoma, four times embolization were performed and the patient took XZ-C persistently so that the combination of embolization and XZ-C had good treatment result and life quality increased. The lump under sternum went away. In the past three years the patient's general condition is good.

Implication: The combination of embolization and XZ-C had good results and supported the long-term results. Embolization can kill the parts of cancer cells and decrease lump size, however there are residual alive cancer cells and continued growth so that after embolization the patient took the XZ-C1+XZ-C4+XZ-C5, which can kill 10^5 cancer cells. Taking XZ-C for long-term can control tumors and stablize the lesions, preventing metastasis. An important problem with embolization chemotherapy is that cancer cell division continues while chemotherapy can only be used periodically due to the toxic side effects. The cancer cells can grow back during the intervening period. The embolization can damage most of the cancer cells and XZ-C can support our immune ability to kill the residual cancer cells.

Case 9. Mr. Zheng, male, 48 year-old, Enshi, officer. Medical record number: 500987
Diagnosis: primary liver carcinoma

Disease course and treatment: In January 1996 a thumb-sized lesion was found in the right liver lobe and was treated with protection of liver treatment. In October 1997 a 5.7cm x 5.7cm lesion was found by ultrasound. In October 1997 the patient had open abdominal surgery and the lesion couldn't be removed so a hepatic tube was placed for pump chemotherapy. Pathological diagnosis is liver cells carcinoma.

In December 23, 1997 chemotherapy was given for the second time; however the reaction is great so that the patient didn't have chemotherapy again. In December 25, 1997 the patient started to take the XZ-C. At follow-up, his condition is stable and healthy and he is happy. His appetite is good and energy level is up and he walks and performs other activities as the normal individual. In November 1998 the patient returns to regular work as teacher and his energy level is great.

Jan	Oct	Dec	Dec	April	May	July	Aug	Oct	Dec	Jun
1996	1997	1997	1997	1998	1998	1998	1998	1998	1998	1999

CT CT lesion operation,

Increase XZ-C ---

Taking XZ-C1+XZ-C4+XZ-C5

Comments: In January 1996 a lesion was found in the right liver and in November 7, 1997 the chemotherapy pump was placed during surgery following which chemotherapy was used twice. After the second time in Dec 23, 1997, the patient only received XZ-C1+XZ-C4+XZ-C5 for three years. His condition is good.

Implication: The hepatic arterial chemoembolization and XZ-C1+XZ-C4+XZ-C5 had good result because the chemotherapy can kill most of cancer cells and XZ-C1+XZ-C4+XZ-C5 can kill cancer cells and protect hosts as well as improve the host immune function and get rid of the rest of the cancer cells.

Case 10. Ms. Wei, female, 36 year-old, Chibi in Hubei. Medical record number: 15603095
Diagnosis: Liver cell cancer

Disease course and treatment: The patient had pain in upper abdomen and her appetite decreased and she was tired for more than half month so that she had CT which showed a lesion in left liver and AFP is more than 400ug/L. On June 6, 2004 the left half of the liver was removed and a portal vein chemotherapy pump was placed in Chibi hospital. During the operation, a lesion was found in most of the left liver so that the pump was placed after the removal of the left liver lobe (the end into hepatic portal vein). After operation, the chemotherapy was used twice through the pump and ultrasound showed a 1.7cm x 1.8cm lesion in right liver. Pathology shows: liver cells cancer. On Sept

27, 2004 the patient started to take XZ-C1+XZ-C4+XZ-C5, LMS and MDZ and follow-up every month to fill up the medicine. On April 2008 ultrasound showed no lesion in the liver and AFP is normal. The patient's general condition is good. Her emotion is stable and her appetite is good. Her body weight is increased and her energy lever is good and she works in other city. She continued taking the medicine for more than 7 years and she is healthy.

Comments: After left liver removal and pump chemotherapy which was used twice with right liver lesion, the patient still continued to take XZ-C to protect thymus and bone morrow for more than seven years and her health condition is good. Recently she works in another city and fills up her medicine every month.

Case 11. Mr. Huang, male, 38 year-old, Hubei, worker. Medical record number: 13402661 Diagnosis: primary liver carcinoma

Disease course and treatment: In Feb 16, 2003 during physical exam, the ultrasound found a liver tumor and CT showed a 9.8cm x 5.8cm lesion in positive right lobe for which boundary line is not separate, clear. Diagnosis was liver cell carcinoma. AFP is 91.875ug/l. In March 8, 2003 the right half liver was removed, for which Pathology diagnosis is liver cell carcinoma. The patient only takes XZ-C after operation. He takes XZ-C regularly and persistently for more than 8 years, during which he follows-up every 2 months. His general condition is good. He returns to work for more than four years and energy level is great. On December 10, 2009 he comes back to follow-up and fills his medicine and his general medical control was great and appetite is good and no other complaints. This year he works in another city and he is healthy.

This is the case which after operation the patient survives more than eight years through only taking XZ-C medicine.

March 8,2003	April 2003	2004	2005	2006	2007	2008	2009	2010
Right half liver removal	XZ-C	XZ-C	XZ-C	XZ-C	XZ-C	XZ-C	XZ-C	XZ-C
Liver cell cancers	taking XZ-C1+XZ-C4+XZ-C5							

Comments: This is a case in which, after right half liver removal and the patient only taking XZ-C medicine to improve thymus function and to improve the immune function, the patient survives more than eight years. He comes to work four years now.

Implication: XZ-C medicine can work as an assistant therapy for the surgery to improve the host immune function and to prevent recurrence and metastasis.

Case 12 Mr. Lee, male, 60 year-old, Wuhan, officer. Medical record number: 270003392
Diagnosis: liver cells cancer

Disease course and treatment: In November 2005 during the physical exam B showed a 5.4cm x 4.0cm lesion in right liver lobe. In the same month the patient had right half liver removal. Pathology diagnosed as liver cell carcinoma. After the operation, on November 28, 2005 he started to take XZ-C1+XZ-C4+XZ-C5, LMS and MDZ to protect thymus and bone morrow. He takes the medicine regularly for more than five years and his general condition is good and his appetite is great and he is healthy.

November 2005	November 28 2005	2006	2007	2008	2009	2010
Right half liver removal	XZ-C	XZ-C	XZ-C	XZ-C	XZ-C	XZ-C

Liver cell cancer taking XZ-C1+XZ-C4+XZ-C5, LMS and MDZ

Comments: The patient had a lesion in the right liver, which had right half liver removed. After operation, the patient only takes XZ-C1+XZ-C4+XZ-C5, LMS and MDZ for more than five years and his health condition is good.

2). some typical cases of Pancreatic cancer after adjuvant treatment

Case13. Ms. Yao, female, 73 year-old, Wuhan. Medical record number: 240469
Diagnosis: gallbladder adenocarcinoma

Disease course and treatment: In Dec 1995 the patient felt pain in right upper quadrant getting worse, then admitted to hospital in Feb 1996. On March 26 1996 the patient was diagnosed as gallbladder cancer during operation, then removed of the gallbladder and put T-tube placement to have bile drainage. Pathological diagnosis is papillary adenocarcinoma involved in muscle layers with gallbladder stones. On April 26, 1996 the tube was removed and the patient started to take XZ-C1+XZ-C4. On Jan 23, 1997 the patient had severe pain and was diagnosed as common duct blockage and jaundice by ultrasound. Common duct dilated into 1.5cm. After taking the medicine for 2 months, the jaundice went away, appetite increased, energy level increased. She took the medicine regularly for 15 months. In July 1997 the patient recovered completely, walked normally, activities are the same as a normal individual. She did the chores every day. On December 4, 1999 her son come to office for follow-up: after taking this traditional medicine for one and half years, the patient is doing fine; she is happy and has recovered her energy level and does chores, plays cards and goes to shop. Her activities are the same as other women.

Comments: On March 26, 1996 the patient was diagnosed as gallbladder cancer and the gallbladder was removed. The patient didn't' take any other treatment because of her age and weakness. On April 26, 1996 she start to take XZ-C1+XZ-C4. On Jun 1997 jaundice came after blockage of common duct. She continues to take XZ-C for 2 month and the jaundice went away. She took XZ-C regularly and persistently. Follow-up the patient for four years, she is fine.

Implication: Taking XZ-C1+XZ-C4 for long term treatment can improve quality of life and prevent metastasis and improve the patient's survival rate.

Case 14. Mr. Zhou, male, 53 year-old, XiaoGan, officer. Medical record number: 950004284
Diagnosis: Pancreatic adenocarcinoma

Disease course and treatment: In August 15, 2007 the patient was diagnosed as hepatitis and had CT which showed tumor on the pancreas and blockage of the common duct. The patient had operation for removal of the pancreas and duodenum. Pathology showed malignant pancreas adenocarcinoma and metastasis of the common duct and duodenal wall and the membranes of the pancreas. There are no lymph node metastases around the pancreas. After four weeks chemotherapy the wbc and platelet, and other side effects were significant. On June 16, 2008 the patient started to take XZ-C1+XZ-C4+XZ-C5+LMS+MDZ. This patient's general medication is fine and his appetite is great. He takes his medication regularly and fills his medication regularly for more than four years. In Sept 2010 when he came back to follow up, his medical condition was good and there was no lymph node enlargement and his abdomen is soft and there is no lump palpation. Now the patient is back at work for one year and he is healthy.

August 21, 2007   June 2008 2009 2010
Removal of pancreas and duodenal chemoth chemoth chemo chemo XZ-C

Pancreas cancer   Taking the XZ-C1+XZ-C4+XZ-C5

Comments: This patient had removal of the pancreas and duodenum and after four times chemotherapy, the side effects were significant and then started to take XZ-C for more than four years and now goes back work.

Implication: After the pancreas adenocarcinoma operation, the XZ-C can protect the thymus and protect the bone marrow to control the metastasis and to improve survival rates.

Case 15. Mr. Fong, male, 50 year-old, Hubei Lou Tang, peasant. Medical record number: 330651
Diagnosis: Pancreas cancer

Disease course and treatment: Because of discomfort in upper abdomen for more than three months, he had jaundice and had opening abdomen surgery showing: No stones in the bile system and enlargement of the pancreas. The tumor couldn't be removed and Pathology showed pancreatic cancer. CT showed enlargement of pancreas head and dilation of the bile duct in liver. After the operation the jaundice extended persistently. On December 11, 1996 he started to take the XZ-C and after one month his medical condition got better and his appetite increased, however he still had little jaundice and weakness and sweating. After taking XZ-C and soup two months the jaundice and pain reduced and got better. After four months, the jaundice was gone completely and his appetite and energy level were good. His pain in abdomen was mild. In July 1998 he returned to work and did mild labor work and his face looks red. He continues to take his medicine for many years. On

April 6, 2004 his family introduced a new patient to us and told us that this patient is fine and his activities are as a normal person's and he does his chores very well.

Comments: This patient has pancreas head cancer and jaundice. On November 28 1996 during the operation, this tumor cannot be removed and the Pathology is pancreas cancer with the dilation of the bile duct system in the livers. On December 11, 1996 this patient took ZX-C and soup. After seven months his jaundice is reduced and he continues to take medicine to improve his immune system. Until July 1998 his condition is completely normal. He continues to take his medicine for more than four years and later changed to taking the medicine periodically to support his healthy condition. This patient has followed up for more than nine years and his condition is very good.

3). Some typical cases of gastric cancer after adjuvant treatment

Case 16. Mr. Chan, male, 65 year-old, Wuhan, retired officer. Medical record number: 280555 Diagnosis: Adenocarcinoma in the pyloric area of the stomach and recurrence after surgery in the remaining stomach

Disease course and treatment: This patient had pain in the upper abdomen for more than one year and in June 1993 he was diagnosed as stomach cancer and had removal of the great curvature in the stomach. After the operation, he had FM chemotherapy once which caused anemia and weakness and wbc is 1900. 8 months after operation, the patient had abdomen pain with vomiting and had left upper abdominal pain for half year. On March 25, 1994 the Barium showed: there was no filled on the upper area of the stomach and part damage of the membranes and the narrow change in the cutting parts. A barium swallow showed recurrence of the stomach cancer. On May 3, 1996 ultrasound showed that there is no lesion inside the liver. Because this patient couldn't eat rice and just eats noodles and liquid food so that he had fatigue and no energy, he didn't want to have operation. In June 1996 he started to take XZ-C. After that he is fine and his appetite is increased and he takes this medicine regularly for more than four years. On May 6, 2000 when he came back to follow-up, his general condition is great and his face looks red and healthy. Walking and activities are normal as the others and he eats rice soup and banana often as his meal.

June 1993	March 1994	June 1996	June 1997	June 1998	June 1999	Dec 1999	May 2000
Stomach operation							

taking XZ-C

Comments: In June 1993 the patient had stomach removal. In March 1994 the cancer recurred and the junction part turned narrow. After taking XZ-C+XZ-C4 only, for more than six years his health condition is great.

Implication: For the recurrence of the stomach cancers, the junction of the surgery was not closed completely and the patient could still eat food. After taking the medicines to improve thymus function to control the tumor growth and prevent the tumor growth and metastasis. The patient's medical condition is stable and he is still alive.

Case 17. Mr. Liu, 65 year-old, Wuhan, economist, Medical record number: 2200421
Diagnosis: fundus and cardia stomach carcinoma

Disease course and treatment: In Jan 1995 the patient had stomach pain for six months and had endoscopy which showed stomach pyloric adenocarcinoma and had surgery for primary stomach removal and to connect the esophagus with stomach body. After the operation the patient was weak and thin so he didn't have chemotherapy. On March 16, 1996 he started to take the XZ-C1+XZ-C4 for more than five years persistently, and then changed to periodically taking the medicine.

Jan 1995	March 1996	1997	1998	1999	2000	2001	2002	2003
Operation	XZ-C	XZ-C						

Taking the XZ-C1+XZ-C4

Comments: In Jan 1995 this patient had the removal of the cardia and fundus of the stomach which connected the esophagus with the stomach body. Because of his weakness, he didn't take chemotherapy and takes the XZ-C1+XZ-C4 only for more than ten years and his medical condition is fine.

Implication: After the operation, the medicine XZ-C can control the cancer, preventing recurrence and metastases and has very good curvature results.

Case 18. Mr. Cheng, male, 65year-old, worker. Medical record number: 260518
Diagnosis: Recurrence and metastasis of stomach cancer

Disease course and treatment: On June 1, 1994 the endoscope showed a 3cm x 3cm ulcer in the stomach pyloric area for which the Pathology was adenocarcinoma in the pylorus. In June 1994 the patient had surgery to remove the cancer. Pathology showed cancer cell in the muscular layer and not the lesser curvature and mucous adenocarcinoma. In May 1996 the patient felt pain in the upper abdominal area and decreased appetite and fatigue. On May 14, 1996 he was admitted into the hospital and had fever, pain in the abdomen, low protein and ascites and fluid in the chest. There were many cancer cells in the ascetic fluid. Because of the heavy ascites the patient came to our office and started to take our medicine. After taking this medicine the patient's general medication condition is very well and appetite was great and his ascites is reduced and his energy level is increased. He came back to follow-up regularly. After the surgery six years and recurrence for four years the patient's condition is great and appetite is great and activities are as the normal persons.

Comments: This patient had surgery in June 1994. After that he didn't have any treatment. In May 1996 he had fluid in his chest and his abdominal cavity. Because the ascites is heavy, he started to take the XZ-C and his general medical condition is good and follow-up with us for more than four years.

Implication: One year after surgery this patient had fluid and cancer cells in his chest and abdominal cavity. He takes the medicine persistently and his medical condition was controlled and his life qualities are improved and he survives very well with his cancer.

Case 19. Mr. Wang, male, 53 year-old, Xinzhou, peasant. Medical record number: 800157 Diagnosis: Recurrence of stomach carcinoma

Disease courses and treatment: In February 1994 the patient felt uncomfortable and endoscopy showed stomach carcinoma. In June 1994 he had stomach removal and followed with chemotherapy for two courses of treatment with 5-Fu+MMC. On May 30, 1995 a barium scan showed damage of the junction sides and narrow area for more than five cm and partially obstructed and there is a 5 cm diameter mass in the junction area. On June 2, 1995 he started to take XZ-C1+XZ-C4. After taking his medicine his general medical condition is great and appetite is increased and can eat the rice and bananas. He comes back to follow up regularly for more than two and half years. His health condition is great.

June,1994	July, 1994	August,1994	May 30,1995	June 2,1996	1996	1997
Operation	soph.	Chem.	GI recurrence	XZ-C	XZ-C	XZ-C

Taking the medicine

Comments: The patient had recurrence of stomach cancer after the partial removal of the conjuction of the stomach. In June 1995 he started to take the XZ-C and follow up with us for more than two and half years. His condition is great.

Implications: XZ-C can stable the recurrence of the cancinoma and improve the patient's condition well and had very good results.

Case 20 Ms. Zhang, female,39 year-old, Wuhan, account, Medical record number::1700321 Diagnosis: the stomach cancer from the stomach ulcer, low differential adenocarcinoma

Disease courses and treatment: in March 1994 because of the uncomfortable in the upper abdomen for one month and getting worse for one week so that the endoscopy showed the stomach ulceration. On April 20 1994 the major stomach was removed and had chemotherapy for six courses of the treatment after the operation with xxxxx+xxxxx to protect the livers. Pathology showed the low differential stomach canciroma and had lymph nodes metastasis. On November 22 1995 he started to take XZ-C1+XZ-C4+XZ-C8 only to protect the bone marrow and follow up with us for more than ten years. He doesn't have metastasis and recurrence and his condition is great.

April 20,1994	Chem 6 times	November 22,1995	1996	1997	1998	1999	2000	2005
Operation	XZ-C	XZ-C	XZ-C					

Taking XZ-C1+XZ-C4+XZ-C8

Comments: this patient had low degree adenocarcinoma in the stomach and lymph node metastasis. On April 20 1994 he had the removal of his major stomach, then he had six courses of the chemotherapy. On November 22 1995 he took the medicine only and followed up with us for more than ten years. His medical condition is great.

Suggustions: After the operation the combination of the chemotherapy and XZ-C medicine can improve the long-term treatment. XZ-C can prevent the cancer recurrence and metastasis.

Case 21 MR.Zhou, male, 57 year-old, officer, Medical record number::1900368
Diagnosis: pyloric and greater curvature of the stomach carcinoma from the ulceration

Disease courses and treatment: In September 1995 after the removal of the stomach caner, he had two courses of the chemotherapy and the side effects were significant and his hair lost. Pathology:medium differential adenocarcinoma without the lymph nodes metastasis. On January 5 1996 he started to take the medicine and his medical condition is getting better and his appetite is good. He persistenly takes his medicine for more than four years and his medical condition is stable.

September 1995	1995	1995	Jan 5 1996	1997	1998	1999
The removal of His stomach	Chem(1)	soph.(2)	XZ-C	XZ-C	XZ-C	XZ-C

Comments: the patient had the cancinoma from the stomach ulceration, with medium differential. On September 25 he had the operation and took two period of the chemotherapy after the operation, however the reaction was strong so that he took the XZ-C only since then to prevent the recurrence and metastasis of the cancinoma. He took this medicince for more than four year and his medical condition is great.

Sugguest: After his opearation his immune system function is decreasing so that the chemotherapy was used for short-term and XZ-C1+XZ-C4 for long-term to protect thymus and to prevent the recurrence and metastasis.

Case 22 MR.Yi, male, 58year-old, Shanxing, Medical record number::8801750
Diagnosis: stomach carcinoma

Disease courses and treatment: after the pain in the stomach two years, on April 27,2000 he had the endoscope which showed the stomach cancer which low-grade adenocarcinoma in the body of the stomach so that he had radical removel. After five days of his surgery, he had a chemotherapy. On June 19 2000 he started to use XZ-C1+XZ-C4 to protect his thymus and the patients took the medication persistently. So far he takes this medication for more than eleven years and continues to follow up with us. On Jan eight 2010 when he came back to follow up, his general medical condition was very well.

April 27 2000									
Operation	Chemotherapy once	June 19 2000	2001	2002	2003	2004	2005	2006	2010

Comments:after the radical operation, there is once chemotherapy. Because of the reaction, he kept using the XZ-C to protect his thymus and bone marrow to prevent the immune system and protect the metastasis and recurrence. He kept using the small amount medication to get good health.

Case23 Ms. Zheng, female, 54 year-old, worker Medical record number::12602507
Diagnosis: the stomach adenocarcinoma

Disease courses and treatment: in September 2002 the endoscope showed that stomach cancer. On Octocber 14 2002 he had radical operation. Pathology showed I-II stages and in the deep muscular layer and 2/3 lymph nodes metastasis and once chemotherapy after the operation. WBC decreases and then stop. On Octocber 25 2002 he started to take XZ-C1+XZ-C4. After that he is llively and his appetite is good and his physical strengthen gradually increase and have continues to take this medicine for more than eight year-old. On September 4 2010 when he follow up to us, his healthy condition was great.

Octocber 14, 2002	chemotherapy	Octocber, 25 2002	2003	2005	2006,	2007	2008	2009	2010
Radical	once	XZ-C							

Comments: after this patient had operation and once chemotherapy, his reaction is strong so that he started to take XZ-C to protect his thymus and to prevent his bone marrow to inhibit the recurrence and metastasis. For eight years he takes this medication persistently and his medical condition is healthy.

Case 24 Mr. Liao, male, 60 year-oldu, Wuhanjiongxia, Medical record number::7101403
Diagnosis: the pyloric carcinoma

Disease course and treatment: Because he had pain in the upper back and under stern for more than four months, he had endoscopy and bisopy done which showed the low grade pyloric adenocarcinoma. In December 1998 he had the radical removal of the total stomach the xian hei which the Pathology showed the same results as before and had the metastasis of the lymph nodes in the lesser and greater curvative. He had once chemotherapy and on Jan 31 1999 he started to take XZ-C1+XZ-C4 and he is spirited and his appetite is good and his physical lever is great. He followed up with us for more than twelve years and his general medical condition is great.

December 1998	
Stomach removal	Jan 31 1999
	XZ-C

Comments: this patient had the stomach removal and chemotherapy. After one month later he started to take the XZ-C to protect the thymus and bone marrow. For 12 years his healthy condition is good.

4) Some typical cases lung cancer postoperative adjuvant treatment

Case 25 Mr. Liu, male, 68year-old, Changzhou, officer, Medical record number::8701735
Diagnosis: the central lung cancer on the right upper of the lung with the metastasis

Disease courses and treatment: in Octocber 1998 he coughed two weeks with the pain in the right shoulder and was treated with inflammation. In Jan 1999 his cough is getting worse and this appetite is decreased and fatigure and getting weak. On CT there is mass on the right upper lung showing the central lung. He had endoscope and biopsy which showed that lung adenocarcinoma in the xxxxxx. He and his family member don't want to have operation. In Feb 1999 after chemotherapy for one course, his reaction to the chemotherapy was strong and stopped to use it. This patient had metastasis in the left lung which showed there are two lesions and he coughed with mucous and blood sputdu and difficult walking. On April 23 2000 he started to take the XZ-C1+XZ-C4+XZ-C7, LMS+MDZ for three months and his general condition is good and he is lively and his appetite is great. In December 2000 his medical condition is stable, and he is lively. His appetite is good and his breath is smooth and his face is red. He walked as the normal person and sometimes he coughs. He persistently takes this medication for more than four years and when he comes back to follow up during the five years, his general condition is great and he walked as the normal healthy person.

Comments: this patient has the central lung cancer in the right upper lung. In April 2000 he started to use XZ-C1+XZ-C4+XZ-C7. XZ-C1 is used to kill the cancer cells only without kill the normal cells; XC-C4 protect the thymus and increase the thymus weight and to protect the bone marrow, XZ-C7 inhibit the lung cancer cells and protect the lung and solve the suptid. After short-term chemotherapy he started to take the XZ-C to strengthen his long-term therapy. XZ-C improve the whole body immune system and he is lively and his appetite is good and his spleen is great and help the patients against the diseases and help the patient's organ functions and the nutrition condition and metabliztion recover so that the patients' healthy condition is recovery.

This patient didn't have the operation. In Feb 1999 he had chemeotherapy, however there is left lung metastasis after chemotherapy. Afterh that,he only took the XZ-C to control the metastasis. He persistently took the medicine for more than four years and his medical condition is great without any complaints. He followed up with us for more than seven years. In May 2005 when he came back to follow up, his general medical condition is great and his appepital is good without other symptoms. His walking and activities and he talks cheerfully and humorously.

Case26 Mr. Zhou, male, 49year-old, Wuhan, officer, Medical record number:s: 410804
Diagnosis: lung cancer in the right low labor

Disease courses and treatment: In 1996 the patient started to have cough and chest tightness and low fever and difficult breath and was treated as the Cold. In April 1997 he suddenly started to cough blood and X-ray and CT showed the right lung cancer in low lobe. And at the same month he had right low lobe lung removal and Pathology showed that lung low grade adenocarcinoma. After the operation, his condition is stable and didn't have chemotherapy and radioactive therapy. On May 15 1997 he started to take XZ-C:1,4,7,vitamin C,B6 E,A. After he took these medicine his energy level is increase and appetite was great and his face is red and there were no recuurence and metastasis and no complaints. In June 2004, the patient came back to follow up with us he continues to take these medicine more than three years. Everything is stable. So far his condition is stable as the normal healthy person after he took his medication more than eight years.

Comments: this patient has right low lobe low grade adenocarcinoma. After the operation, he didn't have radioactive and chemotherapy treatment and he only takes the XZ-C medication XZ-C1+C4+C7. After taking these medicine more than eight years, his energy level is high and appetite is good and his healthy condition is great.

Case 27 Mr. Zheng, male, 52 year-old, Wuhan, driver, Medical record number::11302254
Diagnosis: right lung low grade adenocarcinoma with lymph node metastasis

Disease courses and treatment: because of bloody cough he had the CTscan which showed that right low lung tumor and the bronchoscopy didn't show abnormal. On December 12 2001 he had the removal of the right middle and lower lobe and one lymph node between lobe and two lymph node in the entrance were found. Pathology showed that low grade adenocarcinoma with lymph node mestastasis. After the operation he has once chemotherapy. In 2002 he started to take XZ-C to prevent the tumor recurrence and metastasis. He continues to take the XZ-C1+C4+C7+LMS+MDZ for more than three year and his condition is stable and he is energetic and his appetite is great.

Comments: this patient has the right low lobe adenocarcinoma with lymph node metastasis. After the chemotherapy once, then using the XZ-C1+C4+C7 as the supplement treatment. XZ-C1 kills the cancer cells without killing the normal cells. XZ-C4 protects the thymus and bone marrow; XZ-C7 to protect the lung function. He continues to take his medication for more than three years and there was not metatastasis. When he came back to follow up for his fourth year treatment, his condition is stable and his appetite is great and walked as the normal healthy person.

Case 28 Mr. Long, male, 60 year-old, Huangguang, officer, Medical record number: 521028
Diagnosis: Right lung middle and low lobe adenocarcinoma with diaphragm lymph node metastasis

Disease courses and treatment: In January 1997 he started to cough and fever and was treated as pneumonia. In December 1997 CT showed right lung cancer. The bronchoscopy showed that right side central low grade adenocarcinoma with diaphragm lymph node metastasis and then he was treated as intervation treatment and XZ-C treatment. He had his first chemotherapy through the brochial artery on Dec 31 1997 and the second chem. On Jan 20 1998, The third chemotherapy in March 1998. On July 8 1998 he received the 35th radioactive therapy. In September 1998 after the radioactive therapy, the twice chemotherapy were given(one months). From February 14 1998 to March 14 1998, May 9 1998 to June 9 1998, July 1 1998 to August 1 1998 the patients took ZX-C1 +XZ-C4+XZ-C7 by oral. After that the cough decreased an general conditions well, the vital energy and appetites are good, the energy level come back, he walked and acted as the normal person, dry cough. On Auguest 9 1998 because of the radioactive esophagitis which cause the swollen, congestion and difficulty swallowing, horse voice, then XXXX the XZ-C2 and inhaling the Chinese herbs, continue to take XZ-C medicine, his vital viguour and appetites are very well and can take the food.

Common: This patient have the right low lobe lung cancer with diaphragm lymph nodes mestatasits which was treated with intervation+XZ-C, after the long-term usage of the XZ-C regulation and control medicine, his general medical condition is good and appetite is good. Follow-up with us more two years and eight month, the condition is stable.

Suggestion: Left lung cancer with diagraph lymph node metastasis cannot be operated so that he was treated with chemotheray+Radiavtive+Chinese medicine, first radi+chem to kill the tumor cells, then continue to use the XZ-C immune medicine to protect thymus and improve th whole body immune level, so that to strength the curative therapy and protect the recurrence which has the effective effects.

Case 29 Mr. Xie, male, 55 year-old, Xiang Fen, Medical record number::340663
Diagnosis: Right upper lung adenocarcinoma

The disease courses and treatment: The activities of the right shoulder and right hands decreased about half of years and two months cough and little XXX without blood. On November 26, 1996 Chest X-ray showed that there is round lump on the right upper lung, which was confirmed by CT. On December 16 1996 he had the removal of the right upper lung and the pathology showed that right upper lung adenocarcinoma. On December 23 1996 he started to take XZ-C to prevent the recurrence, metastasis and he didn't take any other therapy. After taking XZ-C for a long-term, the patient is stable and his appetite is good and the vigour is very well and the energy level recovered and didn't have any other symptoms. His face glow with health so far it has been three and half years and everything is good as the normal healthy persons. He had many times of Chest X-ray which showed the normal. Ultrosound is normal.

Commens: this patient took XZ-C1+XZ-C4+CX-C7 for three years after the operation, so far he still used the XZ-C without other therapy. He is healthy as the normal persons.

Suggestions: After the lung operation, to take XZ-C for a long term can prevent the reccurence and metastasis for longterm. Because XZ-C protect thymus and bone marrow and can improve the immune function, the immune function of the patients can keep the high level without using radioactive and chemotherapy. Only treated by XZ-C for more than three years, he is well and as healthy as the normal persons.

Case 30 Mr. Huang, male, 54year olds, Xiaogan, the officer, Medical record number:: 4600907
Diagnosis: Lung cancer

Diseases courses and treatment conditions: In September 1996 cough blood and recovered with the antiinfection. In Aprle 1997 coughed again the symptoms can not be treated in the local hospital. On August 15 1997 the bronchoscopy and biopsy showed that lung squamous carcinoma. On August 31 1997 he have the left low lung removal and the pathology showed that left low lung squamous carcinoma with the lymph nodes of the lung entrance metastasis(1/3). Since September 1997 he took XZ-C to prevent the recurrence and matastasis. After taking the medicine, he is vagorous and his appetite is good. Every month he came back to get the medicine. In April 1999 when he came back to follow-up, he is healthy and his face is glowing with health, walking and acting and talk cheerfully and humorously, the superclavica, xxx, xxxxl lymph nodes and liver and spleens have no lesions, his body weight is 63kg. Chest X-ray and CT have changed sincere the surgery. After the surgery he started to take the medicince XZ-C1+XZ-C4+XZ-C7 for more than two and half years without other therapy. He is healthy.

Comments: This patient had the removal of the left low lung on Auguest 31 1997 and the pathology showed that left lung squamous carcinoma with the lymph nodes in the lung entrance metastasis(1/3). On September 19 1997 he started to XZ-C1+XZ-C4+XZ-C7 without other therapy for more than three years and he is healthy.

Suggestions: after the lung removal, to take XZ-C can improve the immune function and strengthen the body and maintain the curative therapy which can form the environment of no benefits for the tumor growth to prevent the tumor recurrence.

Case 31 Mr. Wang, male, 61year-old, Machen, officer.
Diagnosis: the central left lung cancer.

Disease courses and the treatment condition: On July 29 2006 the left lung cancer was found during the physical examinatoion. On August 21 2006 the total lungs in Tongjin hospital and cleaned the lymph nodes and part of the heart capsule+left part of artrium+ the xxx nerve removal. After seven days the left chest cavity had pneumothorax and induced by the tube. After the operation the patient was weak without the chemotherapy and radioactive. On October 10 2006 he started to take XZ-C and he is energetic and his appetite is good. He persistently took his medicince for more than five years. On Octocboer 8 2010 he came back to followup and his health condition is good.

Comments:this patient has the left central lung carcinoma which the surgery is very difficult and have the removal of the total parts of the lung in the heart cavity+ lymph nodes in the digraph+parts of the heart capsule+parts of the left antrium+ xxx nervous. After the operation, the tube was used to induce the fluid. Because of the age he didn't receive any therapy. On November 11 2006 he started to take XZ-C and he took them regularly and he is vagour and his appetite is good formore than five years.

Suggestions: Left central lung cancer, the surgery removal is a difficult procedure. After the operation, the immune function decreases and the patient was weak. After taking XZ-C to protect the thymus and bone marrow, the therapy is excellent. This patient medical condition is stable.

Case 32 Mr. Guang, male, 64 year-old, Fushan in Guangdou, business man, Medical record number::220003302
Diagnosis: right lung adenocarcinoma

Disease course and treatment:in May 2005 CT in the southern hospital showed tha the right lung cancer in the peripheral. On May 16 2005 he had the removal of the right upper lobe lung and Pathology showed that peripheral lung adenocarcinoma in the right lung with XXXXX and no lymph node metastasis. After the surgery once chemotherapy. On July 13 2005 he came to our office for

XZ-C1+XZ-C4+XZ-C7+LMS+MDZ, and continued to take them for more than five years without other therapy. His condition is stable

Comments: this patient had the right upper lobe lung cancer with the removal. After the chemotherapy, he had great reaction so that he stoped. In July 2005 he started to take XZ-C which he refilled every three months. He persistently took his medicine for more than five years and his medical condition is good.

Case 33 Mrs Ling, female, 64year-old, Danan, Medical record number::670003868
Diagnosis: after the removal of the right lung cancer, with both of the sizes metastasis and bone metastasis

Disease course and treatment condition: in March 2006 the patient coughed without the reasons. In May 2006 CT showed the right upper lung cancer and In June he had the removal of the right upper lobe + lymph node in the secondary hospital in the Daniang. The pathology showed that small cell lung cancer. In July 2006 after chemotherapy, CE xxx for two weeks the bone marrow were inhibited for the three degree. In September after the operation CT showed that both lung had metastasis nodules. Because of read my book<< the new ways and new concepts of the cancer treatment>>, he started to take XZ-C1+XZ-C4+XZ-C7+LMS+Vit. He took the medicine persistently for more than four years. His healthy condition is fine and he is energetic and his appetite is good and walking as the normal healthy persons.

Comments: this patient had right upper lobe small cancinoma. After the operation, he had twice chemotherapy and the bone marrow were inhibited to three degree so that he started to use XZ-C medicine to protect his thymus and bone marrow as the supplemental therapy to prevent the recurrence and metastasis.

Suggestions: XZ-C can be used as the assistant therapy after the surgery to improve the immunce function and to prevent the recurrence and metastasis.

5. Typical cases of assistant treatment after operation in sophagi carcinoma

Case34 Mr. Ding, male, 63year-old, Wuhan, officer, Medical record number:s: 600106
Diagnosis: the middle esophagus cancinoma

Disease course and treatment:in January 1994 the patient had the xxx difficulty of the swallow and after the barium swallow tests the diagnosis was confirmed. On Feb 3, he had the removal of the cancer with the reconixxxxx of the esophague and stomach. After one month of the radioavitvotherapy, because of the heart problems, he didn't use the chemotherapy, On April 5 1995 he started to take XZ-C and then he is energetic and appetite is good. From 1996 to 1999, he refilled his medicine every month and take the medicine persistently. In July 2005 his hair was gray. Recently one year his hair started to turn black and currently his black hair is full of his head and his facial skin is mor tenderer than before, his face is glowing of the health. He is the same as the normal persons. So far he has taken the medicine more than 16years and will continue to take his medicine.

Comments: The patient had the removal of the esophageus on Feb 3 1994. After 40 days of the operation he had radioactive and immune therapy and continued to take the medicine more than 16 years and his healthy condition is good.

The experience of this treatment: During the fourty days after the surgery, he received the radioactive and immune therapy. After that he took the immune therapy persistently to protect his bone marrow and thymus. XZ-C1 can inhibit the cancer mutation and XZ-C4 can improve the immune functions and induced the anticancer factors to protect the immune organs and stop the rest cells into the proliferation stages. If persistently using, the body will be the high immune function level and to prevent the recurrence and the health will recover.

Case 35 Mrs. Huang, femal,66 year-old, Wuhan han yan, Medical record number::10102008
Diagnosis: the squamous carcinoma of the low esophagus

Disease courses and treatment: in December 2000 the patients started to vomit and to have progressively swallow difficultly and only swallow the half of xxxx food. EGD showed that there was narrow in the low esophagus, congestion, ulcer and xxx. Pathology showed squamous carcinoma in the lower esophagus. According to his medical condition he should be treated for a surgery, however because he could afford to the medical cost, he started to take XZ-C. After one month, he is energetic and his appetite is getting better and can eat the soft food, noodle and rice soup. After she continued to take these medicine for six months, he is vagour and his appetite is good and can eat the soft food and noodle and rice soup. Until June 2003 she took the medicine more than two and half years and his health condition is good and can eat the regular rice and felt fine as the normal healthy persons. However she stopped to taking the medicine for more than four and half months. Until Octocber 16 2003 he suddenly had the difficulties to swallow the food and vomit the brown food. She could not eat for more than three days. After adding her some fluids and continued to take XZ-C until Octocber 31 2003 she can eat the food again. After that, she never stopped taking the medicine again. Now she is 70 year-old and healthy the same as the normal persons. She is energetic and her appetite is good and can eat regular food. She lived in the seventh floor and everyday she will come down the first floor and sometimes she help others to fill the bicycle wheels.

Comments: This patient had the low grade squamous carcinoma in the low esophagaus which was diagnosed by EGC and pathology. At that time he could only eat the liquid food and half of XXXX food. She makes her living by filling the bicycle wheels and didn't have money for her surgery so that she started to take XZ-C medicine. After taking the medicine half of year her symptoms turned good. Aftertaking the medicine two andhalf years she recovered as the normal person and didn't have any complain. Because of her incoming condition, she didn't get any other tests and treatment. When she came back to followup, she had taken the medicine more than five years and her condition is good.

To take XZ-C for longterm can improve the patients immune function and the pateitns energy level will increase and the appetites will increase and the sleep will be good. XZ-C4 can protect the bone marrow and thymus to improve the nutrition and the metabolism will turn good and will get rid of the free bases to control and to repair the diseases.

Case 36 Mrs Hang, female, 65year-old, Huangpi in Hubei, Medical record number::10402074
Diagnosis: the middle esophogus carcinoma

Disease courses and treatment condition: In April 2001 the patient had difficulty swallowing and chest and back pain and gradually increased. Until June only can eat the liquid food and vomit the mucous staffs. On June 6 2001 the barium swallow tests in the xxx showed under the aorta branch xxxx 2cm there is a 10cm lenghth narrow and 6cm xxxxxlump in the left wall and the muscous stop. Because of the cost, she didn't have the operation, radioactive and chemotherapy. On June 25 she started to take XZ-C. After three months, her general condition is better and her appetite is getting better and the difficultying swallowing is getting better and can eat the rice soup, noodle. She continued taking the medicine until March 2002 then can take the rice and regular food. In July 2003 she just took XZ-C4+XZ-C2. In April 2005 when she followed up with us, she is energetic and her appetites was great at that time she had been taking XZ-C for more than five year. He condition is stable and can eat the regular food and can do light house work.

Comments: This patient had esophageal cancer which she only took XZ-C to control her condition without the operation, radiactiv therapy and chemotherapy. For more than four years, there was no metastasis and her condition had been controlled and can eat the regular food and rice. She is as healthy as other old persons and can do some choresevery day.

She kept taking her medicine regularly.

Case 37 Mr.Huang male, 66year-old, Huanpi, officer, Medical record number::300584
Diagnosis: the middle and low esophagous carcinoma

Disease courses and treatment:in March, he had the difficulty to swallow and the barium swallow test showed that the middle and low esophagum cancer. In May 1996 he had the removal of his cancer without other therapy. On June 19 1996 he started to use the XZ-C as the supplemental therapy to prevent the reccurrence and metastasis. He only takes XZ-C to protect his thymus and bone marrow for more than three years, then he changed into periodly taking the medicine. He is energetic and his appetite is good and walking and other activities are the same as the normal persons. In April 2005 when he came back to follow up with us, his condition is stable.

Comments: after the operation of his esophague, this patient only took XZ-C to assisting his therapymore than nine years, his condition is stable.

6). Some typical cases of breast cancer postoperative adjuvant treatment

Case 38 Mr. Zhen, female, 44 year-old, Wuhan, Medical record number:s: 700121
Diagnosis: Breast adenocarcinoma

Disease courses and treatment: right breast lump was found for three months which the needle biopsy showed breast cancer. On February 20 1995 she had the removal of the breast cancer and once radioactive therapy after the operation. Because of the weakness, she couldn't tolerate it. On May 11 1995 she started to take XZ-C1+XZ-C4 and continued to take them for more than three years. After she took the medicine, her energy level was improving and her appetite was increasing and her weight is increasing. Following up with us every month and her medical condition is stable.

Comments: this patient had the removal of the breast on Feb 20 1995 and once radioactive therapy after the operation. Because of the weakness the radiative therapy was stopped. In May 1995 she started to take the XZ-C1+XZ-C4. After three years her condition is stable. When she came back for her five year follow-up, she is healthy.

Case 39 Mrs Pan, female,68year-old, Shengyang
Diagnosis: multiple bone metastasis after the removal of the breast cancer.

Disease courses and treatment: in 1984 the patient had the removal of the right breast cancer I stage, the pathology showed that simple breast cancer without lymph node metastasis. After the xxx +xxxx chemotherapy for two years, she started to use some immune enhancing drug. In January 2001 she felt the right shoulder pain and ECT showed that multiple bone metastasis and the supericlavical lymph nodes enlargement. Since March 27 she had 25 times radicacto therapy on the sites of the right superoclaviceal lymph nodes and the whole blood counts decreases and the white cell counts decrease into 2.9x109/L. After the radiactherapy, her condition stable.

On June 15 2001 he started to take XZ-C such XZ-C1+XZ-C2+XZ-C4+LMS+MDZ+VS for two months and her symptom significantly increased. After six months ECT was normal and she is stable. On September 2 2002 on the phone she told us that she is stable and takes her medicine regularly for more than four years. In April 2005 She called us that she is energetic and her appetites is great and walking as the normal healthy persons. On her physical examination, Ultrasound of her liver and gallbladder,Chest X-ray, ECT etc she is normal.

Comments:this patient had right breast cancer after the operation for more than 17 years with bone metastasis and right shoulder pain. After the radiactiv therapy her medical condition is getting better. After taking XZ-C for a long period to protect thymus and bone marrow function, her metastasis was controlled well.

Case 40 Ms. Liu, female, 49year-old, Wuhan, account, Medical record number:: 4500884
Diagnosis: Left breast ductal adenocarcinoma

Disease courses and treatment: on May 19 1997 left breast had a lump 3cmx3cm. after the removal, the Pathology showed that left ductal infiltrated cancinoma. On June 3 1997 the second operation of the radiactie left breast cancer was done, which showed that there is no lymph node metastasis. Twice chemotherapy by taking XXXX were used after the operation. Because of the strong reaction to the chemotherapy, she started to take the XZ-C on August 24 1997. After that she is energetic and her appetite is increasing. After three months, she can go back to her work. After four months, the 3cmz3cm of the two lumps were found and the adjecxxxx is not clear, which the biopsy is breast proliferatin. After using the XZ-C1+XZ-C4 the lumps went away. For three years, she only takes the XZ-C medicine and her medical condition is stable and worked as the normal persons.

Comments: this patient had the removal of the breast cancer with twice chemotherapy. On August 24 1997 she only takes XZ-C to protect her thymus and bone marrow. For more than eight years, she is stable.

Suggestions: after the surgery she used twice chemotherapy for short time which the reaction is great so that she only used xz-c to induce the production of the anticancer factors to improve the immune function and to protect the host immune functions.

Case 41 Ms. Lee, female,33 year-old, Changda in Hunan, worker, Medical record number::3400667
Diagnosis: Left simple breast cancer.

Disease courses and treatment: On November 29 1996 she had the removal of the breast cancer in Changda which showed the right armpit lymph node metastasis(3/5). After one month, CMF was done which she used once/week, for more than four weeks.

On December 25 1996 she started to use XZ-C to protect her bone marrow. After taking the medicine, her whole blood went back to the normal level. From April 2 1997 to May 14 1997 she had radioactive 15 times in right breast inner line, 15 times under the armpit right and 25 times in the right breast outside lines. XZ-C were taken as the supplement therapy without the side effects. The patients is stable and reaction small and even no side effects when she took XZ-C with radiactherapy and chemotherapy. In June 2004 she only took XZ-C. Every three months she came to Wuhan to refill her medicines. Her condition is stable. In Dec 2004 when she came back to follow up with us, she is energetic and appetite is good and her face is glowing of the health. Acting is as the normal healthy persons. She came to refill her medicine from XXXX to WuHAN.

Comments: the curative experience of the treatment:1). During the radiacti and chemotherapy the XZ-C4 can reduce the reaction, during the interval time between the radiac and chemotherapy and after them XZ-C can strengthen longterm curative effects to protect the recurrency.2)after the surgery about six months the radia+chemotherapy +XZ-C can kill the remaining tumor cells or the small tumor lesions, meanwhile to protect the host immune organs. After taking the medicine for six months, the patient's general condition is good so that XZ-C can get rid of the wrong and strengthen the long-time curative effects. After 9 years of the operation, XZ-C can strengthen the long-term therapy.

Case 42 Ms Zhang, female, 65year-old,officer, Medical record number::13502682
Diagnosis: Breast ductal adenocarcinoma

Disease courses and treatment conditions:in 2002 on PE, a small lump was found in the breast, which is considered as breast cancer. In 2003 she had breast radiacal removal in Wuhan center hospital, which the Pathology showed that breast ductal adenocarcinoma without metastasis. She has the

Diatebite and chronic renal inflammation. On April 2003 she started to take XZ-C1+XZ-C4 and has been taking the medicine for more than eight years. Every month she come back to refill the medicine and her healthy condition is well.

Comments: This case is the removal of the breast cancer, after the operation due to the chronic renal inflammation so that she started to take XZ-C and XXX soup to protect the thymus and bone marrow for more than eight years to prevent the reccurrency and metastasis. In addition, her kidney inflammation was getteing better and never recurrent. She come back to refill her medicine every two weeks. She is healthy and stable.

Case 43 Ms Liu, female, 49 year-old, Changsha in Hunan, teacher, Medical record number::260003372
Diangosis: breast infiltrating ductal cancer.

Disease courses and treatment condition: in February 2005 a left breast lump was found which is 2cmx1.5cm, biopsy showed that high degree mutation. On March 8 2005 she had CAF. On May 30 2005 the breast cancer was removed partially, pathology showed the breast cancer so that the breast cancer radiact removal was performed Pathologyshowed that left breast cancer infiltrated ductal cancer. LN0/20 with the C-erB2(++), P53(+), PR(-),ER(-),nm23(+). After the surgery the chemotherapy was used for six cycles. On Octocber 22 2005 she started to take XZ-C to strengthen the curative effects and to prevent the recurrence and metastasis.

Comments:in this case before the operation the lymph nodes under armpit were palpatited. Chemotherapy for six cycle was used before the operation and after the operations to strengthen the long time curative effect. She persistently takes these medicine more than six years and her healthy condition is stable.

7). Some typical cases of colon and rectal cancer postoperative adjuvant treatment

Case 44 Mr. Yan, female, 71 year-old, Wuhan, teacher, Medical record number:s:100188
Diagnosis: ascending colon carcinoma

Disease courses and treatment: Because of abdomen pain and bloody stool, the patient was diagnosed as colon cancer by colonoscopy with biopsy. On December 19 1994 he had half of the right colon removal. Pathology showed the medium grade of colon adenocarcinoma involved in serosa. After the operation, he didn't accept other therapy. On July 4 1995 he started to take XZ-C1+XZ-C4 as assistant therapy to prevent the recurrence and metastasis. He only takes XZ-C more than ten years and his healthy condition is very good. In April 2005 when he was 81 years old and came back to follow up with us, he was healthy and played the card every day in the afternoon.

Comments: this case is that after the removal of the ascending colon, the patient just takes XZ-C medicine as the assistant therapy to protect recurrence more than 10 years and his condition is stable.

Case 45 Mr. Yin, female, 60 yr, Huangpu, Medical record number::8301655
Diagnosis: sigmoid colon cancer and the removal of half of the left colon.

Disease courses and treatment: In August 1998 the patient had bloody stool and was treated as hemorrhoid. In Octocber 1999 when he had the colonoscopy in Xiehu hospital which there is narrow in the 32cm from the anus. On December 3 1999 he had the removal of half of the left-colon. Pathology showed:sigmoid xxxx adenocarcinoma involved in the whole layers of the colon and the metastasis of the nearby lymph nodules(6/8). On Jan 12 2000 he started to take XZ-C: XZ-C1+XZ-C4+LMS+MDA+VT to protect recurrence and metastasis. After he continues to take the XZ-C more than three years and eight months, his son came to refill the medicine on August 4 2003 and told us that his medical condition was good and did the chores every day and planted a lot of different kinds of flowers and vegatables watering them with ten buckles of water. The patient has been in the good condition and happy and has good energy. After his operation, he continues to take the XZ-C medicines only everyday without other chemotherapy. When he followed up with us, he already took the medicine more than five and half years.

Comments: the case is that sigmoid colon carcinoma with metastasis of the nearby lymph nodes. After the removal of the operation the patient didn't have chemotherapy because of the decrease of the white blood cells so that he took the XZ-C as the assistant therapy to protect the bone morrow and thymus to improve the body immune system to protect the reccurrence and the metastasis. After five and half years, his condition was good.

Case 46 Ms. Yun, female, 63year-old, Jiling, officer, Medical record number::8601705
Diagnosis: the rectal adenocarcinoma

Disease courses and treatment: in Octocbor 1999 the patient has the bloody stool and the the rectaoscopy showed there is a flower-like tumor in the 10cm distance from the ana and Pathology showed the rectal cancer. On November 22 1999 the rectal radioactive surgery was done in the affliatite hospital with Dixon ways. After the operation the patient's condition is stable. On December 2 the chemotherapy was done(urine xxxx 1.0g/day, for five days, xxx 100mg/day for three days). On December 9 the white blood cell counts decrease into 0.09x109/L, on December 10 the white blood cells decrease into 0.06x109/L, injection of the medicine of increasing the white blood cells for five days, the white blood cells into1.1x109/l and had the pneumonia and fever with 40C. On January 2 xxxx after treatment with xxxx+xxxx, the patient still has fever and had the throat infection with three bacteria and can not eat and drink anything. After using XXX for five days, the temperature dropped into 38C. Because this patient had hypertension, diabetes and lung diseases, her medical condition is weak and severe and had twice warranty from the hospitals. After two months of the treatment, she is stable. On March 20 2000 she started to take XZ-C for half of the years and her medical condition is stable and can do a little chores and can support her daily life by her own. On September 2000 she recurred very well and can shop in the nearby market and do little chores. She has been taken the medicine for more than five years consistently. In May 2005 her daughter come to refill the medicine and told us that she is totally fine and still do some house chores as healthy as other normal healthy individuals.

Comments: this case is the radial rectal cancer removal and the chemotherapy. After these her immune function and bone morrow function were inhibited so that she had throat and both the lung infections, which later are two fungus infections. After the treatment her condition started to get better and started to take the XZ-C which XZ-C1 only inhibited the tumor cells without affecting the normal cells and improve the immune fucntions, XZ-C4 to protect thymus and bone marrow to improve the immune function. The chemotherapy can inhibit the bone marrow so as to lead the bone marrow inhibition to some degrees which can affect the patients for more than 2 to 3 years so that XZ-C which have protect thymus and bone marrow function need to be taken for several years to benefit the bone marrow and immune functions

Case 47. Mr. Qian, male, 66year-old, Wuhan, accounting, Medical record number::5401066
Diangosis:rectal carcinoma

Disease courses and treatment conditions:occasionally diarria and constipation with bloody stool for two years. The rectal examination showed that there was a 3cmx3cm lump at the 6 clock point in the xxxx position. On January 20 1998 the colonoscopy showed the polypoid mutation of the rectal colon. On January 24 1998 Dixon which the 40cm of the colon were cut off was done in the xiehae hospital, Pathology showed that rectal cancer with middle division and invade into the muscular layer without lymph nodes metastasis and the margin clear. After thesurgery, on March 3 1998 he started to use the XZ-C and took this medicine persistenly for more than eight years and he come back to work for more than five years He is stable and still continued to use these medicine.

Comments: this case is rectal adenocarcinoma. In January 1998 Dixon was done and Pathology showed that rectal adenocarcinoma, middle-degree. After the operation he only took the XZ-C1+XZ-C4 for more tha eight years. His medical condition is stable.

Suggestions: After the rectal Dixon without the chemotherapy, he only took the immune regulation medicine XZ-C to protect his thymus and bone marrow to improve his immune functions to improve the life quality and prevent the recurrence and metasatasis. He was stable.

Case 48. Ms Year-oldng, female, 32year-old, Zhaoyang, accounting, Medical record number::500993
Diagnosis: rectal villious adenocarcinoma

Disease courses and treatment condition: the patient had bleedy stool. In September 1997 the Colonoscopy and biopsy showed the rectal cancer. On September 17 1997 she had the rectal radial operation which showed that the lump was 1.0cmx1.0cm on the bases and was 4cm distance from the ana. Pathology reported the rectal villious adenocarcinoma and invaded into the all of the wall of the intestines with the menstema lymph node metastasis. After the operation she had chemotherapy once. Because of the decrease of the white blood cells she stop chemotherapy and started to use XZ-C1+XZ-C4. Her medical condition is well and stable. She continued to take the medicine for more than eight years only without chemotherapy and other therapy. She did her chores as the normal persons.

Comments:this case is the rectal radial removal on September 17 1997, during the operation, the metastasis were found in the mestaen membrane lymph nodes and invades the whole wall of the intestines. After the operation she had the chemotherapy once which had been stopped because the side effects were severe. Since December 3 1997 she started to take XZ-C only for more than eight years to prevent the reccurrence and metastasis after the surgery. Her medical condition is well.

Case 49. Ms. Cheng, female,68year-old, physician, Medical record number:: 15403059
Diagnosis: Colon cancer

Disease coursed and treatment condition: Because the treatment for the obstracle didn't improve, the operation was done in XinHua hospital on April 30 2004 and found the colon cancer, then the right half of the colon was removed. Pathology showed : the colon capillary adenocarcinoma and the obstracle. After the operation, she received once chemotherapy which she can not tolerate. She started to take XZ-C. After that she is energetic and her appetite is good. She took the medicine persistently for more than six years and she is healthy.

Comments: this patient have obstracle from the Colon cancer and had surgery to remove the right half of the colon. After once chemotherapy she couldn't tolerate and then she started to take the XZ-C for more than six year. Her medical condition is well and she is healthy.

Case 50. Ms Zhang, female, 38year-old, Hanchuan, Medical record number::400003595
Diangosis: colon cancer

Disease courses and treatment conditions: the patients had occasionally abdominal pain for more than five months and the Colonoscopy showed the colon lump in the descending colon. On Octocber 4 2005 the left half of the colon and right overian were removed and Pathology showed that the low grade adenocarcinoma and the metastasis to mesentery and right overain. After the operation six cycle of the chemotherapy were done. On August 18 2006 she started to take the XZ-C medicine such as XZ-C1+XZ-C4+LMS+MDZ persistently for more than five years. She is healthy and refilled the medicine every month.

Comments:this case is left half of the colon and right overian removal. After the operation, the six cycle of the chemotherapy was used, then take XZ-C to strengthen his immune systems. She is healthy after she takes the medicine persistently for more than five years.

Case 51 Mr.Luong,male,60year-old, Shichuang,professor Medical record number::8801759
Diagnosis: rectal carcinoma

Disease courses and treatment: in November 1999 there was blood in the stool and he was treated as hemorriod. In Febrary 2000 he was diagnosed as rectal cancer by the colonoscopy with biopsy. On March 2 2000 he had radical rectal cancer removal in Tongjing University, which is Mile models, Pathology: medium grade rectal adenocarcinoma. After the surgery, he had 12 radiactive therapy and once chemotherapy. On May 30 2000 he began to take XZ-C1+XZ-C4+LMS+MDZ. After he took this medicine, his appetite is good and persistently takes small amount medicine to protect thymus and to protect the bone morrow and follow-up with us monthly for more than ten years and his healthy condition is good and every test is normal.

Comments: this patient had the Mile surgery. After theoperation, he had 13 radiactive and one chemeotherapy, then only take the XZ-C to protect thymus and bone marrow. He persistently takes his medicine and every month he refilled his medicine. So far he has been taking his medicine more than ten years and his medical condition is stable.

8). Some typical cases of gallbladder cancer after adjuvant treatment

Case 52 Mr. Shong, male, 51 year-old, Tianmen, officer, Medical record number::14302843
Diagnosis: adenocarcinoma in the distant common ducts

Disease courses and treatment: After one week painless jaundice, the CT showed the tumor of ampulla of vater. On September 7 2003 he had pancreas and duodenum removal in Zhanjiang xxxx central hospital and the operation was done very well and the size of the tumor is the same as the thumb. Pathology: high-grade adenocarcinoma involved in the whole lumon layer and the head of the pancreas. After twice chemotherapy he came to our outpatient center to take XZ-C :XZ-C1+XZ-C4+XZ-C5+LMS+MDZ+Vit. He continued to finish Chemotherapy so that he had chemotherapy and immune regulation medicine. After finished six periods and continued to take XZ-C4+XZ-C5 to protect thymus and to protect his bone morrow. After taking the medicine, his general medical condition is good and his appetite is increasing. So far he had taken XZ-C for 7 years and his general medical is good and his healthy condition is good and healthy condition is good. He comes back to work more than three years and he is physical strength and he look a regular heathy person.

Case 53 Ms. Dai, female, 59year-old, Wuhan, Medical record number::790003988
Diagnosis: Gallbladder adenocarcinoma

Disease courses and treatment condition: because of the gallbladder stone found in PE, the gallbladder was removed on March 22 2007 in Zhengshun Hospital. After the operation the sample was grossed as 1.8cm in the base of the gallbladder ranges from 2.5cmx3cm. Pathology showed that high division of the adenocarcinoma and IHC showed CK(++), CEA(+). EGD showed that the chronic ulcerative gastritis with bile gastritis. H.pyloric (+), after the operation she took the xxxx. She started to take XZ-C such as XZ-C1+XZ-C4+XZ-C5+ LMS+MDZ and treatment of H. Pyloric bacteria. After one month of the XZ-C he is stable and his appetite is good. She have been taken the XZ-C for more than four years and her medical condition is stable.

Comments: This case is gallbladder cancer. Before the operation the diagnosis is gallbladder stone. After the gallbladder removal through laparoscopy, the Pathology showed that high division of the adenocarcinoma. He took XXX for two cycles of the chemotherapy and took XZ-C to assisting the therapy. For more than four years he has been taken XZ-C and his appetite is good and his energy level is good.

Case 54 Mr. Guong, male, 57year-old,Wuhan, Medical record number::260003376
Diagnosis: middle degree of adenocarcinoma in the gallbladder.

Disease courses and the treatment condition: Because of the abdominal pain in September 2005, the test was done and showed polyp in the gallbladder. The gallbladder was removed with laparoscopy on October 18 2009 in Wuhan first hospital. Pathology showed that middle degree gallbladder cancer without the liver metastasis. After the operation, he didn't have the chemotherapy and radioactive therapy. On Octocber 31 2005 he came to our outpatient center and started to take XZ-C1+XZ-C4+XZ-C5+LMS+MDZ to assisting his therapy. After he took his medicine for more than five years, his medical condition is stable.

Comments: this case is gallbladder carcinoma was diagnosed as the polyp of the gallbladder and the removal of the gallbladder through the laparoscopy. Pathology showed that gallbladder carcinoma. Because of the early stage of the carcinomam, he didn't receive other therapy. He only takes XZ-C to assisting his surgery for more than five years. He is healthy as the normal persons.

9. Typical cases of assistant treatment after operation in kidney and bladder carcinoma

Case 55: Mr. Cheng, male, 62year-old, Wuhan, engineer, Medical record number:s: 210412
Diagnosis: Renal pelvis carcinoma in the right kidney and the recurrence after the bladder carcinoma operation.

Diseases courses and treatment: the patient had cytoscopy which showed the bladder carcinoma in November 4 1995 afterthe bloody urine for two years. On November 21 1995 CT showed that rght renal pelvis tumor. On December 6 1995 the right kidney and urother were removed and his bladder was removed by the xxx and after the operation the local xxxx chemotherapy was used for seven times. On March 8 1996 the cystoscopy showed there was the hard lump in the left wall of the bladder in order to prevent the reccurrence of the tumor, he started to take XZ-C1+XZ-C4+XZ-C6. After taking this medicine he is well and his appetite is getting better. On June 24 1996 the cytoscopy showed that the bladder walls are smooth and the surface is smooth and the new things were gone. He continued to take XZ-C medicine to prevent the recerence and metastasis. Until June 11 1997 the cystoscopy showed the bladder is normal. On December 28 1998 the cystoscopy is normal. On June 26 1999 when he came back to follow up, his condition is stable and he continues to take the XZ-C1+XZ-C4+XZ-C6 for more than ten years to prevent the recurrence and metastasis. On May 6 2005 when he follow-up, he is stable and his condition is good and is the same as the normal individuals.

Comments: this case is the recurrence of the bladder cancinoma after the operation. After taking this medicine more than ten years to prevent the recurrence and metastasis, his medical condition is good and after many cystoscopy, the bladder is normal.

Suggestion: XZ-C can improve the patients immune function and prevent the tumor recurrence and metastasis and control the primary lesions. He is healthy and is in the good condition.

Case 56. Mr. Lin, male, 68year-old, Wuhan, Professor, Medical record number:7701534
Diagnosis: the recurrence of the bladder cancer operation.

Disease courses and treatment conditions: After the removal of the bladder cancer was done in April 1994 in the hospital, Pathology showed: transitional cell carcinoma. After the operation the bladder was poured with chemotherapy. Because of the decrease of the white blood cells the chemotherapy stopped. In 1996 he came back to check up and found the cancer recurrence so that the second operation was done by the removal of eight tumors. After the surgery the patient's bladder was poured with XXX+XXXX twice every month for three months. After three months, repeat these medicine for another three months. Twice per month until 1997. In May 1998 the cystoscopy in the XXX hospital showed the xxx in the bladder. In December the ultrasound showed the bladder infection. In April 1999 because of the bloody urine, the cystoscopy showed that there were a four cm2 of the tumor and CT biopsy showed that bladder cancer. In May 1999 the arterial chemotherapy was poured. In June the second time of the poured the XXXX+XXXX+XXX was done. After that the white blood cells decreased into 2x109/l. In September the third time of the poured medicine with xxx+xxxx+xxx, the white blood cells decreased into 1.2x109/L, then inject the XXX to increase the white blood cells. His medical history: stroke in 1992, Hypertension(160/90mmHg), Diabete. In 1984 he had hepatitis and in 1998 had cirrhosis. Family history : two brothers had hepatitis B and then liver cancer, another brother had rectal cancer.

In July 1999 because of the white blood cells decrease after the chemotherapy, he started to take xxxx to protect the bone marrow and take XZ-C1+XZ-C4+XZ-C6. After taking them more than six months, the whole blood count come back again. His energy level is increased and his appetite is getting better and continue taking the medicine. In July 2000 the cystoscopy showed that the bladder was filled well and a 1.3cmx0.6cm xxxxx in the xxxx ranges, considering as the recurrence of the tumors and continued to take the medicine until June 2001, because of the prostate enlargement which caused the frequency and urgency of the urine. CT showed that this lesion was getting bigger than before(in February in 1999), then had arterialy poured once. He continued to take XZ-C1+XZ-C4+XZ-C6 untill July 2002 CT showed that the lesion in CT shrinkled. After taking the medicine, his general medical condition is better and his appetites is good without the bloody urine. He kept coming back to followup and take his medicine for more than six years. His lesion in his bladder is stable without metastasis and enlargement.

Comments: This case is transitional cell carcinoma. After the removal of the cancer, the long- time chemotherapy didn't stop the recurrence. Because of many years of the poured bladder and many times of the cystoscopy with the enlargement of the prostate and the narrowness of the urother, the cystescopy is difficult to be done. After taking XZ-C such as XZ-C1+XZ-C4+XZ-C6, the neoplasm in the bladder didn't develop and didn't metastes. Since he had this disease, it has been 11 years. His general medical condition is well and his appetite is getting better. When he walked more, sometimes the bloody urine occurred.

Case 57. Mr. He, male, 76year-old, Henan, officer, Medical record number:9201839
Diagnosis: left renal clear cell cancer.

Disease courses and treatment condition:in 1996 there is a kidney cyst, in 2000 on PE there is a 7.5cmx6.5cm cysts in the left renal. CT and MRI showed that left kidney tumor. On August 31 2000 the removal of the left kidney was done in Tongjing hospital. Pathology showed that middle degree of kidney clear cells carcinoma. After the surgery he started to take the xxxx without chemotherapy and radiactvie therapy. On September 28 2000 she started to take XZ-C1+XZ-C4+XZ-C6 to protect thymus ad bone marrow. After taking the medicine one month, he is vigour and his appetite is still low and contine taking the medicine for three months, his general condition is good and his energy level is high and his sleeping is good. After taking the medicine for one year, Ultrasound of the abdomen, Chest X-ray, and others regular tests are normal and he continues to take XZ-C1+XZ-C4+XZ-C6 to prevent the metastasis and recurrence. After five years of taking these medicine, his healthy condition is stable. On April 10 2005 when he follow-up with us, he is healthy and his face is glowing of the health and his voice is xxxx, and he is energetic and had the hear decrease due to his age. His medical condition is100 by CCCCCC.

Comments: this case is left kidney clear cells. He was 76 year-old when he had his surgery. Because of his age, he didn't have the chemotherapy and radioactive therapy and only take the XZ-C immune therapy as the supplement therapy to protect his thymus and bone marrow to improve the immune functions and protect the recurrence and metastasits. He has been taking the medicine for more than five years and when he came back to followup he was 80 years old. His general medical condition is good and his appetite is good and his face is glowing of the health and his energy level is high and his voice is xxx as the normal healthy person.

Case 58 Mr. Yu, Male, 69year-old, Heilunjing, officer, Medical record number::6001181. Diangosis: the bladder transitional cell cancer

Diseases courses and treatment condition: The bloody urine on Februay 27 in 1998. On March 2 the cystoscopy and ultrasound showed that there was the round lump in the front wall, which is 1.6cmx1.4cm and growed toward to the cavity of the bladder and is the neoplasum of the front wall of the bladder. On March 10 in 1998 the surgery removed the tumor tissues in the bladder and Pathology showed that the bladder transitional cell tumors. He was told that this tumor is the recurrence of the tumors. After the surgery, he had once chemotherapy(on May 26 1998). His reaction to chemotherapy is severe such as the vomiting, nausea, and the whole body is uncomfortable. The left testicule enlarges so that he stop chemotherapy. On June 18 1998 he started to take the XZ-C. He follow up with us very month and his condition is good and his urine is normal and he doesn't have any other symptoms. He follow up with us for more than six years and he is healthy.

Comments: in this case on March 10 1998 the surgery removed three tumors in the bladder and Pathology showed that bladder transitional cell carcinoma. After the operation once chemotherapy was done which the patient had severe reaction to this chemotherapy. On June 18 1998 he started to take the medicine XZ-C1+XZ-C4+XZ-C6. He continued to take this medicine for more than seven years and his healthy condition is good without other therapy and without the recurrence and metasatasis.

Comments:

Case 59. Mr. Zhong, male, 66 year-old, Wuxiu, officer, Medical record number:11602315

Diagnosis: right kidney clear cell tumors with the bone marrow metastasis and superclavaical lymph node metastasis.

Disease courses and treatment condition: Because of the pain in the right should, the diagnosis was "the inflamtion of the sourround shoulder", which there was a lump as big as XXX behind the right clavical and stern bone, the biopsy showed adenocarcinoma. After CT of abdomen and chest Ultrasound, there was no lesion found. On March 2002 he started to take the XZ-C such as taking XZ-C1+XZ-C4 and plastic XZ-C3. After the plastic gels, the lump was getting soft and shrinkle into small. On March 24 2002 Ultrasound showed a lump of 3.1cmx4.3cm in the right kidney. CT showed : L2,L4 had bone damage and still took the XZ-C and GEM+XXX chemotherapy once. On May 16 2002 the right renal was removed which there was a lump of the size of table tennis. Pathology showed clear cells. Because he was on the immune function medicine, his medical condition was stable and his appetite is good. Although he had the metastasis of his whole body, he still walked as the normal persons. In 2002,2003 and 2004 he came back every month to refill his medicine and his medical condition is stable. Until July 2004 he suddenly lost the ability of speech and headache. CT showed that the bleeding of the brain. After three weeks of the hospitalization,his medical condition was stable and CT showed that the brain bleeding was absorbed and he continues to take XZ-C1+XZ-C2+XZ-C6+LMS+XXX+XXX+xxxx etc. His medical condition is good and he is vigour and his appetite is good.

Comments: this case is the right metastasis lump of the clavic bone with L2 and L4 bone metastasis, the biopsy showed the metastasis adenocarcinoma. After the whole examination the right kidney tumor was found. On May 16 2002 he was diagnosed as right kidney clear cell cancer and the kidney was removed. On March 16 2002 he started to use the XZ-C by taking and plastic. After three years his medical condition is stable and his appetite is good and he is vigour.

Case 60. Mr. Shi, female, 61year-old, Hunan, Medical record number::790003989

Diagnosis: left kidney clear cell tumors

Disease courses and treatment condition:on Octocbr 27 2006 on PE the Ultrasound showed the left kidney lump. On November 8 2006 the left kidney was removed and Pathology showed that clear cell tumors with 0/2 lymph node. After the operation, the treatment of INF and IL-2 for three months without the radiactiv and chemotherapy. On May 10 2007 she started to take ZX-Csuch as XZ-C1+C4+C6+LMS+MDZ etc. She came back to refill up her medication every month for more than four years now. Her medical condition is ok and she is healthy now.

Comments: this case is left kidney clear cells tumor. After the operation, she took XZ-C only and persistently for more than four years. Her medical condition is good and after many tests she is healthy.

Sugguestion: XZ-C immune function medication can improve the immune function and to prevent the recurrence and metatastasis.

Case 61. Ms. Shi, female, 61 year-old, Hubei, Medical record number::790003989
Diagnosis: the kidney cell tumor

Disease courses and treatment condition: in October 2006 PE showe the right kidney lump and no other syptom. On October 2006 the right kidney lump was removed(partial) and Pathology showed the renal cell tumor. After theoperation, the chemotherapy was used. In September 2007 she started to take XZ-C such as XZ-C1+XZ-C4+XZ-C6+LMS+Vit and then every three month she came back to fill her medicine for more than four years now. She is healthy.

Comments:this case is the removal of the partial right kidney and Pathology showed that kidney cell tumors. Since September 2007 she started to take XZ-C1+XZ-C4+XZ-C6+LMS for more than four years. Her medical condition is stable.

10). Some typical cases of Thyroid cancer, retroperitoneal tumor and other postoperative adjuvant treatment

Case 62 Ms Pen, female, 39 year-old, Shichuang Luchang, officer, Medical record number::7801545
Diagnosis: Thyroid cancer

Disease course and treatment: On April 27 1999 after the removal of the right neck lump, diagnosed as lymphocyte thyroid cancer. On May 6 1999 he had the radical total removal of the thyroid, then he had hourse voice and didn't have chemotherapy. On July 24 he started to take XZ-C:XZ-C1+XZ-C4, LMS,VS and follow-up with us every month and continue to use more than half years. Until Jan 2000 his voice gets better and after continue to take XZ-C another three months his voice come back to the normal. His general conditions get better and his emotion is stable and appetite is good and his energy level came back and he can go back his work. He persistently takes XZ-C1+XZ-C4 to improve his immune function and followed with us more six years and in May 2005 when he came back to us, his general condition is very good.

1999,5	1999,7	2000	2001	2002	2003	2004	2005
Thyroid operation	XZ-C						Follow-up

Comments: this patient has capillary thyroid cancer. After operation his voice was housral and didn't have radiology and chemoactive therapy. He only took the XZ-C to improve his immune function and to prevent recurrence and metastasis.

Case 63 Mr.Cheng, male, 64 year-old Hubei Xin Zhou, officer, Medical record number::7301454
Diagnosis: the tumor of the mesentaic membranexxxx.

Disease courses and treatment condition:On January 6 1999 the patient suddenly had the uncomfortable in chest and pain and vomit. The emergency diagnosis was "actual GI infection", the surgeons thought of that he had the pancreatitis. On March 3 EGD showed the obstracle of the duodenum. On March 6 1999 during the survey of the abdomen, the tumor which was behind the abdominal membrance including big vessals which during the operation a 6cmx9cm lump in the roots of the small intestine membreance xxxx of hard, stable, fixed and unsmooth on the surface, connected to aorta and the xxxx arterial and pressed the duodenum which it was difficult to remove so that the connection of the duodenus and colon was done because the tumor can not be removed and the patients was told to be treated by the combination of the western and Chinese therapy. On April 1999 she started to take XZ-C1Z+C4. From May 15 1999 to February 2002 she continued to take the medicine and refill her medicine. She is stable and her medical condition is good.

Comments: On March 6 1999 the tumor from the abdomen membrane was foundby the survey of the operation. Because it is connected to the small intestine membrance including the

Case 64. Mrs. Pu, female, 67year-old,Shiyiazhoung, worker, Medical record number::7601511. Diagnosis: The recurrence after the surgery of the abdominal cavity serous tumors

Disease courses and treatment conditions:because of the belly was getting bigger and ascites, in May 1999 he was hosptilizated in Tongjing and ascite(++) and his belly was like to frog and the tumor can be touched. On April 9 the surgery found that there were very many different sizes of the tumor, which were gel-like lump full of the abdominal cavity. One by one were removed, the total weight are 2.5g. During the operations, the chemotherapy tube was put with XXX 500mg. After the operation of four days xxx500MG once/per day and continued to use five days and xxx 100mg once/per day and continuing three days. On June 16 1999 he started to take XZ-C1+XZ-C4 andd after two months she is vigour and her appetite is good and her weight increases. PE: there were no lymph nodes in the superclavial, the abdomen is soft and flat, the ascite(-) and continue to take the XZ-C and refiled her medicine every month until November 26 2000, PE: there was a lump of the fit=size, hard, many nodual on the surface and deep and the clear edges which showed the tumor recurrence. The patient refused to the operation again and to chemotherapy, however he continued to take the XZ-C medicine: XZ-C1+XZ-C4+LMS+MDZ and the anticancer gel on the skin patched. Until Febrauay 24 2002 PE: there was on abnormal and her abdomen was soft and there was a lump which was hard, deep and clear edge and the size is smaller than before and her medical condition is stable. Until December 15 2004 her medical condition is good and her appetite is good and her abdomen is little enlarge and her ascite(++) and there is a fit-size lump with unsmooth surface and many nodule and deep and fix without the metastasis further. After her operation until now she has been following up with us more than six years and her medical condition is stable and the tumor is not metasatasis further.

Comments: This case is the serous tumor in the abdominal cavity. After the removal, the tumor recurrence. After the chemotherapy one week, the reaction is great so that in June 1999 she started to take XZ-C1+XZ-C3+XZ-C4 and she continued to take this medicine for more than six years and her medical condition is stable without the far metastasis and the tumors didn't grow big. She lives well with the tumors.

11). Some typical cases of Non-Hodgkin's lymphoma treatment

Case 65 Ms. Liu, female, 34 year-old, Xinzhou, Medical record number::7701538
Diagnosis: Non-Hodgkin lymphoma in stomach and liver metastasis

Dieasce course and treatment: in Feb 1999 the patient has little difficulty swallowing and didn't pay attention to. In April he have significantly difficulty swallowing and have difficulty to swallow the water and other fluid foods. In May the endoscopy showed that stomach body and stomach pyloric cancer. And had total stomach removal in June 1999. Pathology showed: Stomach non-hodgkin lymphoma and liver metastasis and lymph node metastasis in the spleen and the stomach lesser and greater curvature. Because her condition is week, she didn't have any chemotherapy after her surgery. On August 18 1999 she started to take XZ-X1+XX-C4. After 2 months, her general condition get better and emotion is stable and her appetites get better. After taking this medicine for more than 3 years, there is not abnormal during her Ultrasond. In November 2002 he feel find and appetites get better so that he takes the medicine periodly. On Jan 18 2004 When he came back to follow up, her general condition is good and appetites are great. On her PE, her abdomen is soft and there is no lump. Sometimes she felt weak on her right hand, however her left arm can work very well and do all of the chores. In April 2005 during her following-up, her general condition is well and everything is find, however she takes the medicince periodly to support her longt-term therapy.

Case 66 Ms Mei, female, 42 year-old, Wuhan, worker, Medical record number::400003599
Diagnosis: Non-hodgkin lymphoma

Disease course and treatment: in November 2005 the patient has pain in both of shoulder, fatigue and there is a thumb-size lump in low jaw. Then there are some egg-size lymph in both of inguinal areas. The lumps were not painful and the patient didn't have fever, however she felt fatigue. Pathology showed that non-hodgkin lymphoma, B cell large cells types which the immunohistochemistry showed:CD30(+), ALD(++), EMA(+), CD20(+),CD79(+),CD3(+),CD43(+),CD15(-). On Auguest 16 2006 the patient didn't have radiative and chemotherapy. On August 22 2006 She came to our office and started to XZ-C4+XZ-C2+LMS+MDZ=XX after PE which showed that the patient's general condition is fine and had a cutting scar in low jaw and there were xxx-size lymph nodes in the back of the neck and there were many lump in both of inguinal area. After 3 months she felt good and appetites increased and continued for three months to take XZ-C2+XZ-C4+XXS+DIANSHEN,the patient's energy level improved and continued to take XZ-C2+xz-c4+xx+dianshen+ganchao for three months, her medical condition turn better. She continues to take the medicine regularly and fills her medicine every month for more than 5 years, which she only takes. On September 26 2010 when she came back to follow up, she is fine and working and acting as the normal individual and her emotion is stable and her appetites are fine and is happy and playing card with her friends.

Comments: The patient had egg-sized lumps in both of inguinal area. Biopsy showed that non-hodgkin lymphoma with B large types. She didn't take chemotherapy and radioactive therapy. On August 22 2006 she started to takeXZ-C2+XZ-C4+LMS+Dianshen+qindai for more than five years which she fills up her medicine every month. Her medical condition is fine.

Suggestion: Non-hodgkins diseases can be treated by takeXZ-C2+XZ-C4+LMS. The patient continues to take her medicine only for more than 5 years and her medical condition is fine.

Case 67 Mr. Gao, female, 38 year-old, worker, Medical record number::550003745
Diagnosis: Non-hodgkin lymphoma, marginal zone lymphoma, recurrence after spleen removal and chemotherapy

Disease course and treatment: in June 2000 the 2cmx3cm lymph nodes on the right neck was biopsied and pathology showed that follicule lymphoma. The chemotherapy was given from June 29 2000 to July 10 2000, from September 2000 to March 2002, from June 2002 to May 2004 because of lung metastasis. In 2005 the spleen enlarged and was removed. Pathology showed: xx lymphoma, small cells types. CT showed that the lymph node in left lung and in both armpits and in diaphragm. After chemotherapy for three weeks, the lymph node disappeared. In November 2005 the lymph node in the back of right ears enlarged and chemotherapy was given for two weeks. In April 2006 the lymph nodes were enlarged in the back of right ear and the left neck. Biopsy showed: marginal Zone lymphoma. Ct showed that LN enlarged in the sizes and increased in the numbers in the entrance of the lungs and central veins.

After the spleen removal and many times chemotherapy this disease came back again. On Jan 7 2007the patient started to take XZ-C4+XZ-C2+LMS+MDZ+XX+XXX+Vit. After the patient took this medicine, her general medical condition is getting better and stable, her appetite is good and now she has been only using these medicine for more than four years regularly.

Common: This case is non-hodgkin lymphoma which was treated by chemotherapy. Since Jan 7 2007 She only took these medicine for more than four years. Her medical condition is stable and appetite is improved. She filled up her medicine regularly once per three month.

12). Some typical cases of Chemotherapy XZ-C traditional Chinese medicine treatment of acute lymphoblastic leukemia

Case 68 Mr. Zhao, female, 34 year-old, Wuhan, officer, Medical record number:: 9801953
Diagnosis: Acute leukemia

Disease course and treatment: On Novermber 29 the patient was diagnosed as acute leukemia in Beijing hospital and was treated by chemotherapy for seven months. In August 2000 he was treated by bone morrow transplantation, however the results were not good after that because WBC, RBC and platelets are low. Such as wbc0.5x109/l, platelets were 5x100/l, HB46g/l. He depended on the blood transfusion, which were performed once per 8-9 days for 250ml. During his inpatient in Beijing, He had 10 times blood transfusion and 14 times platelets (once per 10 days).In Feb 2001 he came to Wuhan and on Feb 2, 2001 he started to use XZ-C1+XZ-C2+XZ-C8 to protect his thymus and his bone morrow. In April 2001 his WBC and RBC and Pletelets increase and stop to get transfusion. He takes XZ-C1+XZ-C2+XZ-C4 for more than one year and seven months and feel fine and he looked good and healthy and appetites increases and walking and runnig as the normal individual.

In September 4 2003 he traveled to America and took his medicine XZ-C1+XZ-C2+XZ-C4 with him and he takes his medicine persistently.

In 2004 he immigrate into Canada and took his medicine XZ-C1+XZ-C2+XZ-C8 regularly and increase blood soups which will be filled once per 3 months. In April 2005 He called me and told us that he was healthy and his medical condition was controlled very well and appetite and sleep very well and started to work on business and energy level is perfectly well.

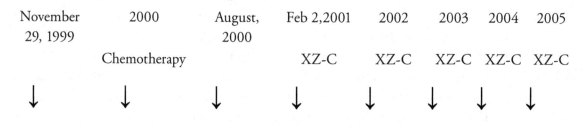

November 29, 1999	2000	August, 2000	Feb 2,2001	2002	2003	2004	2005
	Chemotherapy		XZ-C	XZ-C	XZ-C	XZ-C	XZ-C

ALL bone marrow transplanation

Comments: This patient has ALL and after seven months chemotherapy in August 2000, he had bono marrow transplantation. However the treatment results were not good because his blood counts were still low which he depended on the blood transfusion. On Feb 2 2001 he started to take XZ-C1+XZ-C2+XZ-C4. And increase blood soups etc. and after four months his blood counting went back the normal. After one year and seven months his blood counting keeps normal and he is healthy and has taken these medicine for more than 4 years and work in the business field and energy level is normal.

Suggustion: All can be treated satisfiedly by chemotherapy and XZ-C to protect the bone marrow and improve the immune system function. Now he has been followed up more than seven years and his healthy condition is very well.

Case 69 Ms. Hu, female, 64 year-old, Xisui, account, Medical record number:: 850004087
Diagnosis: Hypothyroidism +multiple bone marrow tumor with toung amyloid change

Disease courses and treatment: In December 2005 the patient's low jaw was sollowed and snored heavily and on Physical exam: her tongue was big and after radiative treatment the enlargement tongue got better, howevery after stop treatment, the large tongue came back again. In December 2007 the soft tissue biopsy in the low jow was done and found that amyloid change of the low jaw amyloid change. Bone marrow biopsy showed that multiple bone marrow tumor. After six weeks chemotherapy, she came to our office. PE: her general condition is find and emotion is stable. Her tongue was enlargement and couldn't speak clearly and her low jaw was firm and bougle. She was in chemotherapy and start to take XZ-C on Octocber 10 2007. This patient had multiple bone marrow tumor and was treated by chemotherapy and had tongue amyloid change and her microcirculation need to improve and her blood need to be active and her swell needs to be treated. After taking XZ-C4,1,6+LMS+MDZ+Radix for three months, her medical condition is stable and after six months her medical condition is significantly improved and her appetites is good and general condition is fine. She fills up her medicine every two months for more than four years.

13). Some typical cases of Ovarian cancer, cervical cancer treatment

Case 70 Peng *, female, 58 years old, Xianning medical records:

Diagnosis: ovarian pulp fluid papillary cystadenocarcinoma

History and treatment: 5 years after menopause (2005) no obvious incentive to vaginal bleeding, the amount of small, untreated. Followed by 2 years (in 2007) in January and no obvious incentive vaginal bleeding, to Xianning Central Hospital B-show: "Pelvic mixed mass". In March, 2007 had the Full uterus ten pairs of accessories + appendectomy. Surgery see: the right side of the attachment area is now a large head of the child, cystic solid, left ovarian atrophy, intestinal and bilateral attachment and pelvic wall adhesions close to the retina package Xiang.

Postoperative pathology: Ovarian pulp papillary cystadenocarcinoma. After surgery due to frail, not for chemotherapy; On June n, 2007 Come to Dawning Tumor specialist outpatient clinic and Taking xz-c immunomodulatory anti-cancer Chinese medicine for postoperative adjuvant therapy.

With XZ a C1 +4 +5 ten LMS + MDZ + Vit adhere to long-term medication for 4 years, monthly outpatient referral and medication, medication after the general situation improved significantly, the spirit of good appetite. July 7, 2010 in the Provincial People's Hospital color Doppler review, liver, spleen, pancreas, kidney no abnormalities, pelvic no abnormal signal, the patient is generally good.

Evaluation: This patient is ovarian cancer, after surgery due to physical weakness, simply to XZ-C immunoregulation anti-cancer traditional Chinese medicine for postoperative adjuvant therapy, The patient has been using these XZ-C medications for a long-term for 4 years. The patient has a comprehensive review recently, good health.

This case suggests: postoperative ovarian cancer can be used xz-c immunoregulation anti-cancer drugs for postoperative adjuvant therapy, the effect is good. Why should xz-c immunomodulatory drugs be used for many years for a long term? because it is consistent with the biological characteristics of cancer cells.

Case 71 Deng **, female, 61 years old, Hunan medical records:

Diagnosis: uterine cancer, rectal cancer

History and treatment: in December 10, 2002 in Henan Province Cancer Hospital examination found cervical squamous cell carcinoma in situ, is the surgical removal of the uterus and ovaries, surgery is not: put, chemotherapy. In February 15, 2006 in the training center hospital found rectal Scm at the differentiation of cancer, on March 6, 2006 in the Chinese Academy of Sciences Cancer Hospital rectal radical calcification, 0i xo :, surgery, postoperative radiotherapy 25 times And oral Xeloda. In July 2005 in Xuchang for intravenous chemotherapy for 4 cycles, later with chest knife too.

Due to easy fatigue, fatigue, anorexia, is the child January 21, 2007 to Wuchang dawn of cancer specialist clinic xz-c immunomodulation anti-cancer Chinese medicine for postoperative adjuvant therapy, serving xz-c1 +4 +5 ten LMS + M DZ + v ft, every 3 months referral and take medicine, long-term adherence to medication has 4 students, health is good recovery.

Evaluation: This patient is uterine cancer, 4 years later the patient has rectal cancer and the postoperative immune function is low, but also for radiotherapy and chemotherapy, so that the patient's immune function further decline, and even easy to be fatigue, and to be anorexia and for a long-term the patient has been using XZ-C immunocompromised anti-cancer Chinese medications for 4 years, and has good health recovery, good spiritual appetite.

Case 72 Xu ", female, 43 years old, farmers disease number:
Diagnosis: uterine squamous cell carcinoma, stage IV

History and treatment: in September 2006 vaginal out of March have been in December 2006 with the crowded hospital examination for the cervix was cauliflower, biopsy for the papillary squamous cell carcinoma, anemia, radiotherapy for 25 times, chemotherapy 4 Cycle, the reaction is large, 2006 grave bladder obscure mirror invasion and bladder. On February 28, 2007 to dawn of the tumor specialist outpatient xz a c immune regulation of anti-cancer Chinese medicine treatment, taking XC1 +4 + ten LMS + MDZ ten lanange root ten cents, long-term adherence to medication, the general situation is good, the spirit of appetite is good, Every three months to clinic outpatient medication, so far nearly 4 years, the health situation is good.

Evaluation: This patient for the uterine squamous cell carcinoma, it was found that has been violated bladder crisp, weak body, is not surgery, the use of radiotherapy 25 and chemotherapy 4 cycles, and then use xz-c immune regulation anti-cancer Chinese medication for the long-term treatment to consolidate the effect. After nearly four years of medication, the patient's health status is good, every three months from the county to Wuhan Haihai medicine, walking, activities, such as ordinary people.

3. THE OBSERVATION OF EXPERIMENTAL AND CLINIC CURATIVE EFFECT ON Z-C MEDICINE TREATING MALIGNANCY

In order to look for the traditional herb medicine with actually curative effect and without toxication and adverse reaction, this surgical tumor research institute has screened 200 kinds of Chinese herbal medicines with so-called anticancer reaction recorded on Chinese herbal medicine books for tumor-inhibition reaction on the solid carcinoma in the tumor-bearing animal models one by one in the past 4 years. Through long-term in-vivo tumor-inhibiting animal experiments, we have screened 48 kinds of Chinese herbal medicines with relatively good tumor-inhibition rate that can prolong the survival time, protect the immune organ and obviously improve the immunologic function. According to the clinical conditions, the anticancer medicines screened are combined into 2 compounds including Z-C_1 and Z-C_4 with better anti-cancer reaction than each single medicine. In the original screening, we carried out the tumor-inhibiting animal experiment for each single medicine and now we further carry out the experimental study on these two groups of compounds for the tumor-inhibiting reaction in the solid tumor of the tumor-bearing rats.

I. Experimental Study on Animal

1. Materials and Method

(1) Experimental animal: 260 Kunming clon white rats, half of male and female respectively, weight:21±2g, 8~10 weeks.

(2) Cell strains and inoculation: hepatic carcinoma H_{22} cell strains, the fresh tumor bodies from the rats with tumor were prepared into the single cell suspended liquid, after dyeing and counting of the cancer cells (1×10^6/ml), 0.2ml normal saline of cancer cell was subject to subcutaneous vaccination at the front axilla at the right side of each rat.

(3) Drugs and experimental group: the traditional herb medicines Z-C_1 and Z-C_4 were entirely developed and prepared by Hubei Branch of China Anti-cancer Research Cooperation of Chinese Traditional Medicine and Western Medicine, the former was a compound and the latter was a medicinal powder. The chemotherapy control medicine used by the chemotherapy group was cyclophosphane (CTX).

Experimental group: the animals with H_{22} cancer cell transplanted were divided into four groups randomly: ① traditional herb medicine Z-C$_1$ group (90 rats). The rats were subject to gastriclavage once every day after 24h of transplantation of cancer cells, 0.8ml per rat every time, equivalent to 1.4mg of the dried medicinal herbs. ②Traditional herb medicine Z-C$_4$ group (90 rats), as to the dose and gastriclavage method, ditto. ③Chemotherapy group (50 rats), from the next day after transplantation of cancer cells, they were subject to gastriclavage with CTX50mg/kg weight every other day. ④Control group (30 rats), they were subject to gastriclavage with normal saline every day from the next day after transplantation of the cancer cells, 0.8ml/rat.

(4) Observation of indexes: measure the weight of the rats every 3d, measure the diameter of the tumor with vernier caliper, measure the immunologic function and blood picture. Half of each group as Group A, subject to tumor-bearing experiment, regular killing of the rats in batches, separation of tumor and weighing of the tumor and then calculation of tumor-inhabiting rate. The tumor was subject to the pathological section and a few of the specimens were subject to the observation of ultra-structural organization. The rest half of each group as Group B. The tumor-bearing experimental rats were drenched for a long time until they met with natural death. Then the tumor was separated and weighed, the long-term inhibition rate and life elongation rate of the tumor was calculated.

2. Experimental result

(1) The tumor-inhibition effect of Z-C Medicine on Rats bearing hepatic carcinoma H$_{22}$: in the second week after administration of Z-C$_1$, the tumor-inhibition rate was 40% and the one in the fourth week was 45% and 58% in the sixth week. The tumor-inhibition rate after administration of Z-C$_4$ was 55%, 68% in the fourth week and 70% in the sixth week. (P<0.01) the tumor-inhibiting rate after administration of CTX was 45% in the second week, 45% in the fourth week and 49% in the sixth week (See Fig. 1 and 2).

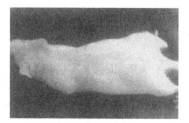

Figure 1 Z-C1, C4 treatment group

30d after inoculation of hepatoma H22

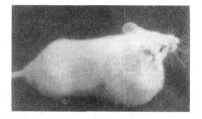

Figure 2 Control group

30d after inoculation of hepatoma H22

(2) The effect of Z-C medicine on the survival time of the rats bearing hepatic carcinoma H$_{22}$: the average survival time of Z-C$_1$, Z-C$_4$ and CTX was longer than the one of the normal saline control group (P<0.01); Z-C medicine played a role in obviously prolonging the survival time. Through comparison with the control group, the life elongation rate of Z-C$_1$ group was 85%, the one of Z-C$_4$ group was 200% and the one of CTX group was 9.8%. The rats

in Z-C$_1$ and CTX in Group B met with death in 75d. 6 rats bearing carcinoma in Z-C$_4$ survived after seven months.

(3) Both Z-C$_1$ and Z-C$_4$ medicine improved the immunologic function and Z-C$_4$ obviously improved the immunologic function, increased the white blood cells and red blood cells, without any effect on the hepatic function and kidney function and without damage to the hepatic and kidney section. CTX decreased the white blood cells and reduced the immunologic function with the renal damage to the kidney section. The thymus in the control group was obviously atrophic (Fig. 1-4) while the one of Z-C$_1$ and Z-C$_2$ therapy group was not atrophic but a little hypertrophic (Fig.1-3).

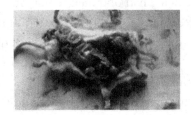

Figure 3 Z-C4 group
30d after inoculation of hepatoma H22
thymus hypertrophy

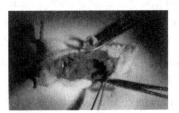

Figure 4 Control
30d after inoculation of liver cancer H22
marked atrophy of thymus

II. Discuss about Z-C Medicine Experiment and Clinic Curative Effect

1. Tumor-inhibition effect of Z-C$_{1-4}$ Medicine on hepatic carcinoma H$_{22}$ rats bearing tumor

It was found that after the medicine was taken to H$_{22}$ tumor-bearing rats for two weeks, four weeks and six weeks, the tumor inhibition rate increased with the prolongation of the administration time, the tumor inhibition rate of Z-C$_4$ in the 6th week reached up to 70%. Through two repeated experiments in succession, the results were stable, which indicated that the tumor-inhibition effect of Chinese herb medicine was slow and it would increase gradually, that is to say, the tumor-inhibition effect was of positive correlation to the accumulated dosage of Chinese herb medicine.

The effect on the survival time of hepatic carcinoma H$_{22}$ tumor-bearing rats from Z-C$_1$ and Z-C$_4$ medicine: it was proven by the experimental results that Z-C$_1$ and Z-C$_4$ medicine could obviously prolong the survival time of the tumor-bearing rats, especially Z-C$_4$, it could prolong the survival time as long as 200%, more than that, Z-C$_4$ could remarkably improve the immunologic function of the organism, protect the immune organ and the bone marrow, alleviate the toxic action and side effect of the radiotherapy and chemotherapy medicines. Furthermore, no toxic action or side effect had been found in the past 12 months after the rats took the medicine. The above-mentioned experimental study offered the beneficial basis to the clinical application.

2. Clinical curative effect

Based on the experimental study, it had been applied to various clinical carcinomas, most of the patients were the ones over Stage III and IV, namely: the ones suffering from the cancer of late stage that could not be removed with exploratory operation; the ones with the exploratory operation without operation indication; the ones meeting with metastasis or reoccurrence in short term or long term after operation of the carcinoma; the ones suffering from hepatic metastasis, lung metastasis or brain metastasis in late stage or the ones accompanied with carcinoma hydrops and hydrops abdominis; the ones suffering from various carcinomas conservative removal operation with the exploratory operation only for the anastomosis of intestines and stomach or colostomy but not for removal and the ones not suitable for the operation, chemotherapy and radiotherapy and so on. Through over 10 years' clinical application and systematic observation, Z-C$_1$ and Z-C$_4$ medicine had obtained remarkable curative effect and no toxic action and side effect had been found after long-term administration. It had been proven by the clinical observation that Z-C$_1$ and Z-C$_4$ medicine could improve the survival quality of the carcinoma patients in medium and late stage in an all-round way, improve the whole immunity, control the hyperplasia of the cancer cells, consolidate and enhance the long-term curative effect. The oral-taken and external-applied Z-C medicine had good curative effect in softening and shrinking body surface metastatic tumor. With the assistance of intervention or treatment with cannula spray pump for medicine, it could protect liver, kidney and bone marrow hemopoietic system and the immune organ and improve the immunity.

3. Good pain alleviation effect of Z-C anti-cancer pain alleviation paste

Pain is the relatively remarkable and painful symptom of the carcinoma patients in late stage, the common pain reliever had no remarkable effect on carcinoma pain, the stupefacient pain reliever had the addiction and dependence, Z-C anti-cancer pain alleviation paste had strong pain alleviation effect with a long maintenance time. It was proven through 298 cases of clinical verification that the effective rate was 78.0%, the total effective rate was 95.3%, after repeated application, there were no toxic action or side effect, without addiction. The paid alleviation effect was stable and it was an effective therapeutic method for the carcinoma patients to get rid of the pain and improve the quality of life.

VOLUME X

Cancer Etiology, Pathogenesis, Pathological Pathology

The Experiment Research

---The experimental study of anticancer recurrence and metastasis

CONTENTS VOLUME X

Preface

Experimental Surgery is extremely important in the development of medical science and is a key to open the close area of medicine. The method of prevention and treatment of many diseases can be applied to clinical after they has achieved stable results and effects in many times of animal studies so as to promote the development of the medical industry.

The experimental research and basic research are important. If it does not have the breakthrough of the experimental research and the basic research, it is difficult to improve the clinical efficacy and is difficult to propose the new understanding and the new concept and the new theoretical insights.

The laboratory is a key to the development of science and the innovation of technology. I deeply experience and appreciate the importance of the lab. I was the first group of university students after the liberation of the college entrance examination. I didn't further degree study, nor went aboard for study, but I made a number of world-class results, The key is that I have a good laboratory. In the 1960s I participated in cardiopulmonary bypass surgery laboratory. In the 80s I built with liver cirrhosis room laboratory. In the 90s I built the Institute of Experimental Surgery in order to conquer cancer as the main direction. In my lab equipment condition is better and there are animals such as mice, rats, guinea pigs, rabbits, dogs, monkeys and other animals, a better operating room sterilization can make various major surgery such as the chest, abdomen operations and postoperative observation successfully, also a variety of designs and conceive of the experimental operation can achieve outcomes or conclusions.

Therefore, laboratory conditions are the key which is to build well-equipped laboratories. If there is no laboratory to perform and to pass the experiment, the design, thinking and imagine cannot be turned into results or become a factual result.

"Oncology" is the most backward subject of the current medical disciplines because the tumor etiology, pathogenesis and pathophysiology are not clear; tumor discipline for scientific research is a virgin land and need to conduct a lot of basic scientific research.

Although countries have invested a lot of money for the treatment of cancer patients, although the traditional three treatment has been nearly a hundred years, but the cancer mortality rate is still the first reason for the death of urban and rural residents in China, the main reasons are the following:

(1) the etiology of cancer is not entirely clear; people is still lack of understanding on the pathogenesis of cancer, cell metastasis mechanism.

(2) the complex biological behavior of cancer and pathophysiology are still lack of sufficient understanding.

To carry out the basic research of cancer, the anti-cancer metastasis and recurrence must be carried out in the basic model of cancer animal models; the nude mice should be used to establish a variety of cancer animal models to study the metastasis of cancer cells and mechanisms (in the author's laboratory used the pure Kunming mice for the cancer animal model about 10,000 many times) because if there is no basic research breakthrough, the clinical efficacy is difficult to improve.

No matter how complex the mechanism behind cancer is, immune suppression is a key cancer progression. Removal of immunosuppressive factors and restoration of recognition system cells to cancer cells can effectively resist cancer. More and more evidence shows that by regulating the body's immune system, it is possible to achieve the purpose of controlling cancer. Many researchers in the field are currently excited by activating the body's anti-tumor immune system to treat cancer. The next major breakthrough in cancer is likely to come from this.

In order to investigate cancer etiology and pathogenesis and pathophysiology, we conducted a series of animal studies. From the analysis of the experimental results the new discoveries and new revelations were found that : thymus atrophy and immune dysfunction are one of cancer etiology and pathogenesis mechanism; therefore at the international conferences Professor Xu Ze proposed that one of the causes mechanisms of cancer may be thymus atrophy, central immune organ dysfunction, immune dysfunction, decreasing immune surveillance and immune escape.

The immune organs have the closest relation to tumor immune system. Thymus is the central immune organ and is the place which T cells get mature and the development and plays the decisive roles to cell immune including the whole immune regulation.

As the results of experimental studies in the real laboratory it was found: in cancer-bearing mice it showed the progressive thymus atrophy, central immune organ dysfunction, decreased immune function, decreasing immune supervision ; therefore, the principle of the cancer must be to prevent atrophy of the thymus, to promote thymic hyperplasia, to protect bone marrow Hematopoietic function, to improve immune surveillance, which provides the theoretical basis and the experimental evidence for cancer immune regulation treatment.

Based on the above revelation about cancer etiology, pathogenesis of experimental results, it was put forward the new concept and new method of XZ immunomodulatory therapy. After 30 years of clinical validation in the oncology clinics in more than 12,000 cases of cancer patients in the middle and advanced stages, it was confirmed that the treatment principle of protecting thymus and increasing immune function is reasonable and the efficacy is satisfactory. The application of immune regulation medications has achieved good results, and improved the quality of life and significantly prolonged the survival time.

XZ-C(XU ZE-China) immune regulation and control rules are is that in 2006 Professor Xu Ze the first time put forward in his monograph <<The new concept and new way of cancer metastasis treatment >> which it was believed that under normal circumstances, it is the dynamic equilibrium between body's defenses and cancer; cancer is caused by losing the dynamic balance. If the imbalance state has adjusted to normal level, it can control cancer growth and make it subside.

As we all know, the incidence of cancer development and prognosis is depending on the comparison of two factors, namely, the biological characteristics of cancer cells and the host body's own cancer defense and constraint ability. If these two parts are balance, cancer can be controlled; if these two are imbalance, cancer will develop.

Under the normal circumstances the host organism itself have a certain constraint capacity to cancer, but in cancer patients these constraints are subject to defense suppression and damage in the different levels, leading to the loss of the immune surveillance of cancer cells, to the immune escape, and to the further development of cancer cells and metastasis.

Through more than four years of basic experimental study investigated the recurrence and metastasis mechanism, and after three years of the experiment in vivo anti-tumor cancer-bearing mice from the natural herbal medication test, a group of traditional Chinese medications which has better inhibition rate are selected and composed of becoming anti-cancer immune regulation medications.

For more than 7 years in more than 6,000 tumor-bearing animal models a series of clinical basic experimental research and basic problems were conducted and explored. The screening of 200 kinds of Chinese herbal medicine for cancer -bearing animal model was carried out by my graduate students. "To explore the spleen on the tumor a long effect and the role of Spleen Yiqi Tang anti-cancer effect of experimental study" was completed by Zhu Siwei Shuo; "the experimental study of Fetal liver and fetal spleen and fetal thymus cells combined with the succession of immunization reconstruction of malignant tumor" by Dr. Zou Shaomin completed;

"the experimental study of the anti-tumor effect of Fuzheng Pei-bao on S180 Mice "was completed by Master Li Zhengxun; the subjects of all of master and doctoral graduate are my total subject s and are closely integrated with the clinical basis of clinical problems, they carried out and completed a large number of hard and meticulous experimental research work, hard work, day and night experimental research work and made a significant contribution to prevent cancer and anti-cancer experimental tumor medical career development.

1. The new discovery of the experimental tumor research of anti-cancer and anti-metastasis and anti-recurrence

Research on Anti-cancer and Anti-metastasis and Anti-recurrence Experimental Tumor ---New Findings

We have done found that in our laboratory from the research on experimental tumor:

1. This lab excised the thymus(Thymus, TH) of the mouse, made the cancer-bearing animal model. The injection of the immunosuppressant was helpful to establish the cancer-bearing animal model. It was proven by the research concludes that the occurrence and development of the cancer had obvious relation to the thymus of the immune organ of the host and its functions.

2. As to the cause and the effect between the inferior immunity and the carcinoma, the experimental results are as follows; the inferior immunity leads to the occurrence and development of the carcinoma; in case of no degeneration of the immunologic function, it is not easy to carry out the successful inoculation. It is suggested by the experimental results: improving and maintaining the good immunologic function is one of the important measures for preventing the occurrence of the carcinoma.

3. When researching the relation between the metastasis of carcinoma and the immunity, we established 60 animal models of hepatic carcinoma metastasis and divided them into two groups including Group A applied with the immunosuppressant and Group B not applied with the Group A was obviously more than the one in Group B. It was suggested by the experimental results that the metastasis was related to the immunity, the inferior immunologic function or the application of the immunosuppressant may promote the tumor metastasis.

4. In the experiment to probe into the influences of the tumor on the immune organ of the organism, we found that the thymus would meet with the progressive atrophia (600 cancer-bearing animal model mice) with the evolution of the cancer and the thymus of the host would meet with the acute progressive atrophia after being inoculated with cancer cells.

5. We found through the experiments: incase that some experimental mice were not successfully inoculated or the tumor was too small, the thymus had no obvious atrophia. In order to understand the relation between the tumor and the thymus atrophia, we ablated the solid tumor of one group of experimental mice after them grew up to the size like a thumb. After one month, it was found that the thymus had mot meet with the progressive atrophia through dissection. As a result, it was inferred by us that the solid tumor might generate one kind of unknown factor to arrest the thymus, which should be further researched by experiment.

6. It was proven by the above-mentioned experimental results: the progress of the tumor could lead to the progressive atrophia of the thymus, then could some measures be taken for preventing the atrophia of the thymus of the host? Therefore, we further did everything to search for the method or drugs to prevent the thymus atrophia of the cancer-bearing mice through the experimental research on the animal. Then, we resumed the experimental research on the functions of the immune organ through transplantation of the cells of the immune organ. Then we probedinto the way to contain the atrophia of the thymus of the immune

organ in the progress of the tumor so as to recruit the functions of the thymus and restore the immunity and made the experimental research on restore the immunologic functions through the transplantation of the thymocyte cells of embryonic liver, spleen and thymus and through the adoptive immunity. It was shown by the results: through the combined transplantation of three groups of cells, namely Group S, T and L (200 experimental mice), CR rate of the tumor in the near term was 40% and the one in the long term was 44.67%, the patient with the completion repercussion of the tumor survived for a long time.

The Research on the roles of searching for and screening the new anti-cancer metastasis medicines from traditional Chinese medicines:

It was found from the results of tumor-inhibiting screening experiment in the tumor-bearing animal bodied applied with 200 kinds of anti-cancer traditional Chinese medicines: among which there were 48 kinds of medicines having the inhibitory action on the cancer cells, through optimization and combination, and then after the tumor-inhibiting experiments on the cancer-bearing animal models such as hepatic carcinoma, carcinoma of lung and gastric carcinoma, we finally produced Z-C$_{1-10}$ anti-cancer traditional Chinese medicine preparation. Z-C1 can obviously inhibit cancer cell without the influence on normal cells, Z-C4 can promote the hyperplasia of thymus and Z-C8 can protect bone marrow to generate blood and thus protects the hematopoetic function of bone marrow. Z-C immune regulating traditional Chinese medicine can improve the living quality of cancer patient in medium and late stages, increase immunity, enhance anti-cancer capacity of the body, strengthen health, improve appetite, and obviously prolong the survival time. We also adopted abdominal muscle transplanted tumor model of mouse(40 pieces of mice for experiment) to observe the inhibitory action on neoformative micrangium of abdominal muscle transplanted tumor of mouse by extract from Chinese herbal medicine XXX and found out the traditional Chinese medicine TC which could inhibit the formation of tumor blood vessel.

On the way to conquer cancer, it must be well worth researching and developing effective cancer preventive and anti-cancer and anti-transferable new types of Chinese herbal medicament. All of the experimental studies should experience clinical verifications, should be observed for 3 to 5 years on large groups of patients or even for 8 to 10 years' of clinical observation. According to evidence-based medicine, there should be long-term follow-up survey and appreciable data to prove that the medicine has favorable curative effect definitely, and the target of curative effect is well living quality and long survival time.

2.The Experimental Research Parts

1. THE EXPERIMENT RESEARCH OF SEARCHING ETIOLOGY OF CANCER FACTOR AND PATHOGENESIS AND PATHOLOGICAL PHYSIOLOGY TO SEEK FOR THE EFFECTIVE CONTROL METHODS

After following up the results, the problems were found-----that recurrence and metastasis after surgery is the key to decide the long-term treatment effects

Therefore, the questions were pointed out---- the clinical surgeons should pay attention to and conduct the research about recurrence and metastasis after surgery.

In 1985 the author visited 3000 of his patients who had general surgical procedures for their different types of cancers. He found that most of the patients had cancer recurrence and metastasis during two or three years after their operation. Some of them recurred and died several months after the operation. Therefore, the author found that even if the operation is successful, the long-term therapy isn't satisfied or is failure. The patients had a big surgery and only were alive for one or two years or three years. Apparently this is not the patient's goals and not our aim. Generally, we only pay attention to five year surviving rate, but five year death rate. For example, the five year survival rate of stomach cancer is 20%; in another side, the five year death rate of stomach cancer is 80% which made the patients' family surprised. After following up many patients we found that the key factors for long-term therapy are recurrence and metastasis. Meanwhile, we found that important questions: to look for the method and ways of preventing cancer from recurrence and metastasis is the key to improve the survival rate after surgery.

Currently there are very high metastasis rate which is related to many factors such as cancer's stage, grade, and differentiation and the host immunology function. Now there are high recurrence rate in outpatient setting. For instance, during one week the author treated forty cancer patients in which the fifteen of the patients were the recurrence after the operations so as to prevent the recurrence and metastasis after the surgery, we must start to do something since the operation time. Because the cancer removal operation can easily leave some remaining cancer cells. The cancer cells will seed and metastasised easily. Once there are remaining, the cancer cells wil recur and metastasis, which cause terrible results. Therefore, Oncology surgery must follow the basic oncology rules. To remove the tumor during the surgery is the same important and strict thing as the sterilized rules during the general surgery, even more strict. There are two goals of performing no-tumor rules: 1. Preventing spread ; 2. Preventing implanation.

The key to the surgical long-term effects and results is recurrence and metastasis. During 20 century the oncology surgery has made extremely success. The task during 21 century is to prevent recurrence and metastasis to improve the long-term surgical results.

If there is no out break on basic research, the clinical efficiency will not be improved. If there questions are resolved, the oncology surgery will have significantly success. Therefore, in 1985 the author built his own experimental research laboratory to conduct the cancer research. First, to make the experiment tumor model, then to start the basic research from the clinical practice.

To look for the tumor pathogenic factors, pathogenesis and metastasis mechanism to search the preventive treating methods through many steps of cancer cells metastasis. Since seven years study, the research projects are all the clinical questions which got explanation from the basic research. After seven years animal research the author finished the following research work by steps and steps.

一.The experimental research of making cancer animal models

Why can human being get cancer? Under what condition can cancer happen? Why can some get cancer, others can not get cancer under the same condition can the same environment? Are there intrinis or extrinis factors or both of them? Therefore, we should make the animal cancer models to study?

The experiment of modeling experiment of cancer metastasis model

In the study of cancer cell transplantation, we conducted dozens of human cancer cells transplanted to mice which thymus was removed in the laboratory in 1985, and a solid cancer transplant model was established. Then we made a cancer metastasis model, simulated lymph node metastasis, we transplanted 10^6 / ml 0.2ml, $H_{22}CC$ in 60 mice paw pad inside the subcutaneous transplantation, after 7-8 days in the foot pad inside the foot it was seen that the tumor with the broad bean size grew and the whole foot ankle was swollen and coved, and 16 days later it was found that the right inguinal lymph nodes were swollen in 8 mice so that a lymphatic metastasis model was established.

After that, we also simulated the blood transfer, injected the H_{22} cell suspension 10^6 / mI 0.4mI into the vein to do intravenous inoculation, gained access to more lung metastasis, causing lung tumor growth, followed by the establishment of experimental liver metastases animal model, 80 Kunming mice were divided into A, B two groups, each group 4. Only group A was injected with cortisone before for 7 days, all injected with 1% paclitaxel 75 mg / kg intraperitoneal anesthesia, and then left a large around 0.5 cm incision, exposure to the spleen, take the living body H_{22} Hepatocarcinoma ascites 10ul thrombolytic injection, local compression 3 - 5 minutes to prevent cancer cells spill out the splenic membrane into the abdominal cavity the injected cancer cells slowly into the lymphatic flow and blood. Animals were fed and raised for 11 days, then broken neck and sacrificed to death, take the metastasis lesion in the liver to count.

The Results:

There were metastasis lesion in A group, B group in the liver, and the number of liver metastases was different, the number of A group was significantly more than B group, mostly 3-5 or more and the size around 1mm; Group B was mostly 1 to 3.

The Experimental results suggest that metastases are associated with immune function ; If immunocompromised, immune dysfunction, or the use of drugs that inhibit immune function, all of these can promote tumor metastasis.

二. The experimental study to explore the relationship between tumor and immune organs to seek immune regulation and control method

Because the laboratory in the exploration of the establishment of experimental animal model of animal research work, found that the removal of thymus or reduce immunity or immune deficiency can be established cancer animal model, then Th and cancer inoculation must have a relationship, thymus for the central immune organs, The spleen is the largest peripheral immune organs, then what is the relationship between the spleen and the tumor? So it is a further study of the immune organs and tumor development and development of the relationship between the next subject of the experimental study.

(一).Experimental study on the effect of spleen on tumor growth

(A).To conduct the experimental study of the tumor and the manufacture of animal models of cancer

At that time, the author was the director of the Department of Clinical Surgery and the director of the Department of Experimental Surgery at the Affiliated Hospital of Hubei Provincial College of Traditional Chinese Medicine, which facilitated the co-ordination of the work of the clinical ward and the animal laboratory. The patients were removed from the on- Blood half an hour that is transplanted in the experimental animals who did more than 100 times (400 animals) were unsuccessful. Then we cut the mouse some thymus (d only c), and then transplant, then successful (210 animals), and some injection of cortisone, reduce the immunity of mice, but also transplant success. Cut 5 days after the thymus transplantation, 5 to 6 days after the growth of large nodules can be soybeans, 10 to 21 days to the thumb big tumor. Transplantation can survive 3 to 4 weeks, but can not pass on.

(1) Through this study found: removal of thymus THC, can produce animal model of injection, injection of cortisone, contribute to the manufacture of animal models.

(2) study concluded that: the occurrence and development of cancer and the host of the body immunity, and immune organs and immune organs and tissues have a very significant relationship.

(3) The results of this study confirm that the immune organ thymus and the immune function have a definite positive relationship with the occurrence and development of cancer, and that the host Th is excised, Resection can not cause the bearing animal model, injection inhibition of immune drugs to reduce the host immune, it helps to produce animal models of cancer, do not inject lower immune drugs, can not produce animal model.

The results suggest that immune organs and immunity are negatively correlated with cancer cell transplantation and grow into solid cancer. Immunodeficiency or immunocompromised transplantation can implant the tumor without being swallowed by the immune cells of the host.

(B) whether it is the first low immunity after cancer or cancer after the immune low

Kunming mice 32. Only divided into group A, group B 'group. Group, each group n = 8. In addition, the thoracic resection (THC) and the transplantation were the same as before, the group A was the first resection of THC, 5 dogs were inoculated with cancer cells 106; 8 groups were injected with cortisone, 7 days after inoculation of cancer cells; Cancer cells, 10 days after resection of THC; D group first inoculated tumor cells, 10 days after injection of cortisone. Results: In group A and 8, all of them were inoculated successfully and grew up. The results of C and D were only 18 days after 14 days. The results showed that the immune function of the host was decreased or the immune organ Thymus is defective to Vix out of the tumor, if the host immune function is good without loss is not easy to grow the tumor, which can be concluded that: the first immune function is low and then the occurrence and development of cancer. If the first decline in immune function is not easy to vaccination success, the study suggests: to improve and protect the immune function, to protect the immune function of good words, is to prevent "dagger cancer occurred important measures.

In view of the spleen is a peripheral immune organs, with important immune function, in the anti-tumor immunity has an important immune as a spleen to explore the peripheral immune organs of the largest tumor growth and the impact of changes in the laboratory conducted the following experiment: Kunming mice were divided into two groups: the spleen group and the spleen group. The spleen group was divided into two groups: the spleen group, the spleen group, the spleen group, the spleen group and the spleen group. In the early stage of tumor on the inhibition of tumor Health, 25% inhibition rate, in the late stage of the tumor, the spleen atrophy, the loss of inhibition, spleen cell transplantation several inhibition of tumor growth, the inhibition rate of 54%

The conclusion of this study is: the effect of spleen on tumor growth, showing biphasic, early have a certain inhibitory effect, late loss of inhibition, splenocyte transplantation can enhance the role of inhibition of tumor growth.

(二) to explore the tumor on the immune organs thymus, spleen of the experimental study

In the previous experimental study, we have explored the effects of central immune organ thymus and peripheral immune organ spleen on the growth of cancerous cell transplanted tumors. The findings and conclusions of the experimental results are as described above.

So, in turn, then think about it, swollen on the immune organs thymus and spleen will find what impact?

The rats were randomly divided into four groups. The cells were sacrificed at the 3rd, 7th and 14th day after inoculation of cancer cells and inoculated with cancer cells. Observation of thymus, spleen weighing and cancer tissue sections.

The results showed that: in the early stage of tumor growth, spleen congestion, enlargement, cell proliferation active, in the late stage of the spleen Sheng was atrophy, cell proliferation blocked. Thymus inoculated cancer cells, immediately showed acute atrophy, cell proliferation by injection volume was significantly reduced, significantly reduced weight, indicating that the immune function is inhibited.

The results of this experiment suggest that the tumor will significantly inhibit the thymus, not only inhibit thymus function, but also cause the immune system atrophy.

(三) to explore the anti-cancer effect of traditional Chinese medicine Jianpi Yiqi Decoction

The above study found that the spleen has a certain effect on tumor growth, spleen cell transplantation can improve the inhibition rate of the tumor. Although the spleen referred to by the traditional Chinese medicine and the two doctors refer to the spleen in theory, the pathogenesis and clinical is completely different. But this two reminds us of the experimental results only Kunming mice, since both are spleen, with the name of different functions, whether the use of spleen Qi method, combined with the above three modern, composition of traditional Chinese medicine spleen and stomach compound, animal (N = 30) and the control group (11 = 10) were inoculated with 01 cancer cells. The experimental group was treated with Jianpi Yiqi Decoction for 14 days (P <0.05). There was no significant difference between the two groups, To observe the tumor growth, tumor-bearing mice quality of life and survival.

Experimental results: Serving Spleen Yiqi Decoction can delay the time of tumor nodule after tumor cell transplantation, inhibit tumor growth, prolong the survival time of tumor-bearing mice, and have certain anti-cancer effect.

三, to explore the tumor progression to prevent thymic atrophy and to find immune reconstruction method of experimental study

When we produced the animal model, we found that THC was able to mold successfully and replicate the same experiment with three batches. The results clearly show that Thymus has a definite relationship with tumorigenesis. In the above study of the relationship between tumor and immune organs in the experimental study, the results also clearly prove that the progress of the tumor can quickly make Thyrnus progressive atrophy, indicating that the tumor significantly inhibited the thymus, not only inhibit its function, but also cause immunity Organ atrophy.

If so, then we can use some way to stop the host's thymus atrophy, so that the thymus to restore function, so that immune reconstruction, therefore, we further design, want to use the immune organ cell transplantation to restore the immune organs, reconstruction of its organ function, It is an experimental study on the immune function of fetal liver, spleen and thymocyte transplantation. A closed group of Kunming mice was used. The experimental group was divided into six experimental groups and two control groups. The spleen cells, fetal thymocytes and fetal liver cells were transplanted respectively. The tumor growth of each group was observed systematically., Regression, survival time, cellular immune index and histopathological examination, compare the efficacy of each group. The results showed that the three groups of cells were transplanted, the rate of complete tumor regression was 40%, the rate of complete regression was 46. 67%, and the tumor was completely depleted. Part of the rate of withdrawal, the recent 26.67%, long-term 13.33%, part of the survival rate of the average extension of 1 month to _, the immune indicators significantly improved immune organ hypertrophy. Immunological tissue sections were shown to show that cell proliferation was active. The results of this experiment show that the system has been reconstructed more than the partial reconstruction, through the whole system of synergies, better play anti-tumor immune function, improve efficacy.

四, from the natural medicine to find drugs to inhibit tumor neovascularization

In 1986, our laboratory cancer cells can only promote the breeding of cancer cells, but can not form a solid tumor mass, the experiment we accidentally found in the test tube cancer cell culture if the drop of 1-'2 drops of chicken soup, which promote cancer cells quickly Breeding into a plexus, if the drop of a drop of aminophylline and then quickly spread,

Since then we have been warned cancer patients do not eat chicken. It is known that cancer cells have several steps, first of all, cancer cells fall off, and then into the blood vessels into the blood flow, microcirculation and then invade the microvascular, to reach the transfer of organs, implantation, first bloodless stage, Through the blood flow to not grow up, followed by the rapid formation of new blood vessels, the tumor increased rapidly.

In this transfer process, if we can block one of the links, we can prevent tumor metastasis. We consider the the tumor neovascularization can be root of the cancer cell metastasis and of growing into cancer nodules and it is one of the key links, so it is Designed to Find Anticancer Angiogenesis from Natural Drugs.

(1) The experimental study on neonatal microvascular observation of transplanted tumor of mouse abdominal muscles

Twenty Kunming mice were injected with EAC cell fluid into the abdominal muscles to make the newborn microvascular model of abdominal tumor. The microvessel formation and microvessel flow rate and flow rate were observed by microcirculation photomicrography.

The results showed that: 1 day after inoculation without neovascularization, the first two days that can be seen from the original host microvessel issued a slender, curved neovascularization into the tumor, the first 3-4 days of neonatal microvascular density increased.

(2) the experimental study of the effect of different doses of TG on immune function in mice

The rats were randomly divided into TG group, TG group, TG3 group and D group G group. The rats were sacrificed on the 13th day, and the rats were sacrificed.

The results showed that different doses of TG rats had different immune organs, low dose of 20 mg / kg when the thymus weight gain, high dose so mg / kg thymus atrophy.

(3) The experimental study of the inhibitory effect of extract of Rhizoma Coptidis on the neovascularization of mouse abdominal muscle transplanted tumor

The mice were sacrificed on the self - made observation platform, and then the mouse observation platform was placed on the microscope stage of the incubator. The mice were sacrificed on the microscope. The morphology and number of neovascularization were observed by HH4 microcirculation detection system. And microscopic photographs were taken to measure the neonatal microvessel density of the tumor and the average diameter and velocity of the veins.

The results showed that TG (20mg / kg) significantly inhibited tumor angiogenesis in the early stage of tumor.

From the experimental results of this group, it can be seen that IG can significantly inhibit the growth of new microvessels in the intratumoral and peritumoral tissues, and reduce the density of new microvessels entering and exiting the tumor.

Current domestic and foreign scholars have focused on trying to inhibit tumor neovascularization in order to control the growth and metastases of tumors. Fotkman reported in June 1998 that his laboratory has developed two drugs that inhibit tumor neovascularization called angiostatin And endostatrn, in the tumor-bearing animal experiments, so that the human body transplanted to the test mouse cancer significantly reduced, he used anti-angiogenesis inhibitors blood vessels, so that the capillary atrophy and cut off the nutritional supply of the tumor, so as to achieve cancer purpose. They reported that they planned to conduct very limited tests on people in 1999. Our laboratory in July 1997 completed the TG experimental study, because TG is already blindly traditional Chinese medicine, which means Chinese medicine in Chinese medicine books have been used for hundreds of years, but also long-term clinical application, but never in the past For the treatment of tumor neovascularization. So from September 1998, we have tried to clinically outpatients, for anti-cancer, anti-metastasis comprehensive treatment of one of the comprehensive treatment, has been in December 1999 has been used in more than 80 cases ll, stage cancer patients, cancer The initial observation of the control, recurrence, and metastatic outcome is good and is currently continuing to be observed in clinical validation.

1. The new discovery of the experimental tumor research of anti-cancer and anti-metastasis and anti-recurrence

Research on Anti-cancer and Anti-metastasis and Anti-recurrence Experimental Tumor ---New Findings

We have done found that in our laboratory from the research on experimental tumor:

1. This lab excised the thymus(Thymus, TH) of the mouse, made the cancer-bearing animal model. The injection of the immunosuppressant was helpful to establish the cancer-bearing animal model. It was proven by the research concludes that the occurrence and development of the cancer had obvious relation to the thymus of the immune organ of the host and its functions.

2. As to the cause and the effect between the inferior immunity and the carcinoma, the experimental results are as follows; the inferior immunity leads to the occurrence and development of the carcinoma; in case of no degeneration of the immunologic function, it is not easy to carry out the successful inoculation. It is suggested by the experimental results: improving and maintaining the good immunologic function is one of the important measures for preventing the occurrence of the carcinoma.

3. When researching the relation between the metastasis of carcinoma and the immunity, we established 60 animal models of hepatic carcinoma metastasis and divided them into two groups including Group A applied with the immunosuppressant and Group B not applied with the Group A was obviously more than the one in Group B. It was suggested by the experimental results that the metastasis was related to the immunity, the inferior immunologic function or the application of the immunosuppressant may promote the tumor metastasis.

4. In the experiment to probe into the influences of the tumor on the immune organ of the organism, we found that the thymus would meet with the progressive atrophia (600 cancer-bearing animal model mice) with the evolution of the cancer and the thymus of the host would meet with the acute progressive atrophia after being inoculated with cancer cells.

5. We found through the experiments: incase that some experimental mice were not successfully inoculated or the tumor was too small, the thymus had no obvious atrophia. In order to understand the relation between the tumor and the thymus atrophia, we ablated the solid tumor of one group of experimental mice after them grew up to the size like a thumb. After one month, it was found that the thymus had mot meet with the progressive atrophia through dissection. As a result, it was inferred by us that the solid tumor might generate one kind of unknown factor to arrest the thymus, which should be further researched by experiment.

6. It was proven by the above-mentioned experimental results: the progress of the tumor could lead to the progressive atrophia of the thymus, then could some measures be taken for preventing the atrophia of the thymus of the host? Therefore, we further did everything to search for the method or drugs to prevent the thymus atrophia of the cancer-bearing mice through the experimental research on the animal. Then, we resumed the experimental research on the functions of the immune organ through transplantation of the cells of the immune organ. Then we probedinto the way to contain the atrophia of the thymus of the immune

organ in the progress of the tumor so as to recruit the functions of the thymus and restore the immunity and made the experimental research on restore the immunologic functions through the transplantation of the thymocyte cells of embryonic liver, spleen and thymus and through the adoptive immunity. It was shown by the results: through the combined transplantation of three groups of cells, namely Group S, T and L (200 experimental mice), CR rate of the tumor in the near term was 40% and the one in the long term was 44.67%, the patient with the completion repercussion of the tumor survived for a long time.

The Research on the roles of searching for and screening the new anti-cancer metastasis medicines from traditional Chinese medicines:

It was found from the results of tumor-inhibiting screening experiment in the tumor-bearing animal bodied applied with 200 kinds of anti-cancer traditional Chinese medicines: among which there were 48 kinds of medicines having the inhibitory action on the cancer cells, through optimization and combination, and then after the tumor-inhibiting experiments on the cancer-bearing animal models such as hepatic carcinoma, carcinoma of lung and gastric carcinoma, we finally produced $Z-C_{1-10}$ anti-cancer traditional Chinese medicine preparation. Z-C1 can obviously inhibit cancer cell without the influence on normal cells, Z-C4 can promote the hyperplasia of thymus and Z-C8 can protect bone marrow to generate blood and thus protects the hematopoetic function of bone marrow. Z-C immune regulating traditional Chinese medicine can improve the living quality of cancer patient in medium and late stages, increase immunity, enhance anti-cancer capacity of the body, strengthen health, improve appetite, and obviously prolong the survival time. We also adopted abdominal muscle transplanted tumor model of mouse(40 pieces of mice for experiment) to observe the inhibitory action on neoformative micrangium of abdominal muscle transplanted tumor of mouse by extract from Chinese herbal medicine XXX and found out the traditional Chinese medicine TC which could inhibit the formation of tumor blood vessel.

On the way to conquer cancer, it must be well worth researching and developing effective cancer preventive and anti-cancer and anti-transferable new types of Chinese herbal medicament. All of the experimental studies should experience clinical verifications, should be observed for 3 to 5 years on large groups of patients or even for 8 to 10 years' of clinical observation. According to evidence-based medicine, there should be long-term follow-up survey and appreciable data to prove that the medicine has favorable curative effect definitely, and the target of curative effect is well living quality and long survival time.

Cancer Etiology, Pathogenesis, Pathological Pathology

The Experiment Research

---The experimental study of anticancer recurrence and metastasis

1. The research team : Academician Qiu Fazu, Honorary President of Tongji Medicine University, medical leading scientist of general surgery in China directed the scientific research design in the experimental surgery lab

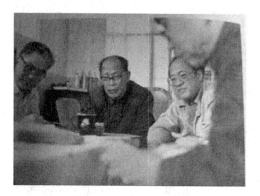

2. The independently invented fruit with independent innovation and independent intellectual property as a series of Products of Z-C medications as the following **examples:**

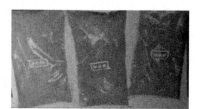 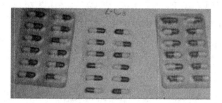

One of The Study on New Concept and Way of Treatment of Carcinoma

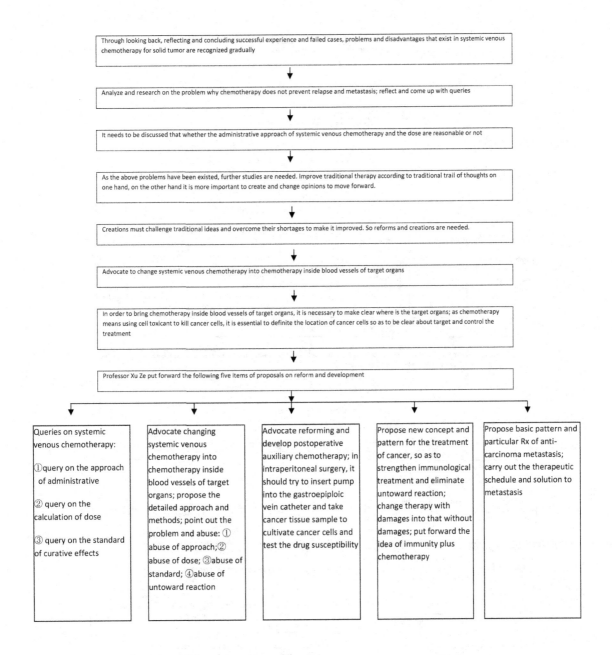

Through looking back, reflecting and concluding successful experience and failed cases, problems and disadvantages that exist in systemic venous chemotherapy for solid tumor are recognized gradually

↓

Analyze and research on the problem why chemotherapy does not prevent relapse and metastasis; reflect and come up with queries

↓

It needs to be discussed that whether the administrative approach of systemic venous chemotherapy and the dose are reasonable or not

↓

As the above problems have been existed, further studies are needed. Improve traditional therapy according to traditional trail of thoughts on one hand, on the other hand it is more important to create and change opinions to move forward.

↓

Creations must challenge traditional ideas and overcome their shortages to make it improved. So reforms and creations are needed.

↓

Advocate to change systemic venous chemotherapy into chemotherapy inside blood vessels of target organs

↓

In order to bring chemotherapy inside blood vessels of target organs, it is necessary to make clear where is the target organs; as chemotherapy means using cell toxicant to kill cancer cells, it is essential to definite the location of cancer cells so as to be clear about target and control the treatment

↓

Professor Xu Ze put forward the following five items of proposals on reform and development

| Queries on systemic venous chemotherapy:

①query on the approach of administrative

② query on the calculation of dose

③ query on the standard of curative effects | Advocate changing systemic venous chemotherapy inside blood vessels of target organs; propose the detailed approach and methods; point out the problem and abuse: ① abuse of approach;② abuse of dose; ③abuse of standard; ④abuse of untoward reaction | Advocate reforming and develop postoperative auxiliary chemotherapy; in intraperitoneal surgery, it should try to insert pump into the gastroepiploic vein catheter and take cancer tissue sample to cultivate cancer cells and test the drug susceptibility | Propose new concept and pattern for the treatment of cancer, so as to strengthen immunological treatment and eliminate untoward reaction; change therapy with damages into that without damages; put forward the idea of immunity plus chemotherapy | Propose basic pattern and particular Rx of anti-carcinoma metastasis; carry out the therapeutic schedule and solution to metastasis |

IV. Study on New Concept and Way of Treatment of Carcinoma (3)

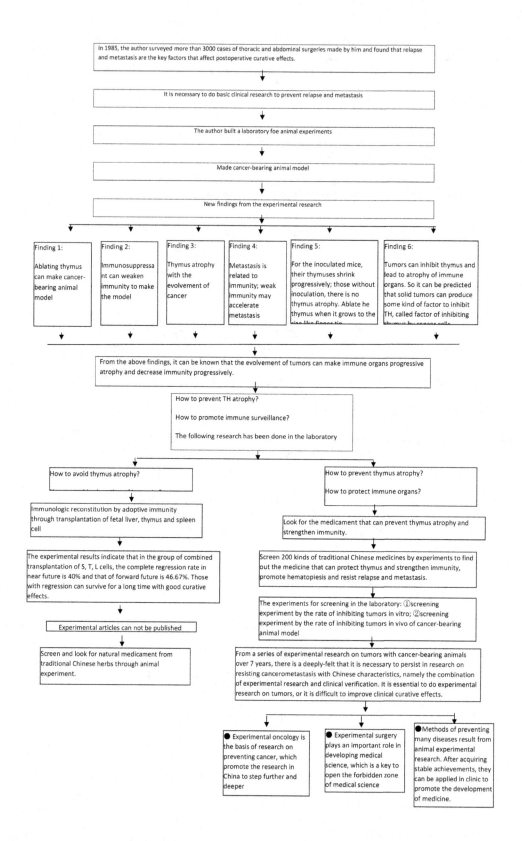

In 1985, the author surveyed more than 3000 cases of thoracic and abdominal surgeries made by him and found that relapse and metastasis are the key factors that affect postoperative curative effects.

It is necessary to do basic clinical research to prevent relapse and metastasis

The author built a laboratory foe animal experiments

Made cancer-bearing animal model

New findings from the experimental research

Finding 1:
Ablating thymus can make cancer-bearing animal model

Finding 2:
Immunosuppressant can weaken immunity to make the model

Finding 3:
Thymus atrophy with the evolvement of cancer

Finding 4:
Metastasis is related to immunity; weak immunity may accelerate metastasis

Finding 5:
For the inoculated mice, their thymuses shrink progressively; those without inoculation, there is no thymus atrophy. Ablate he thymus when it grows to the size like finger tip.

Finding 6:
Tumors can inhibit thymus and lead to atrophy of immune organs. So it can be predicted that solid tumors can produce some kind of factor to inhibit TH, called factor of inhibiting thymus by cancer cells.

From the above findings, it can be known that the evolvement of tumors can make immune organs progressive atrophy and decrease immunity progressively.

How to prevent TH atrophy?

How to promote immune surveillance?

The following research has been done in the laboratory

How to avoid thymus atrophy?

Immunologic reconstitution by adoptive immunity through transplantation of fetal liver, thymus and spleen cell

The experimental results indicate that in the group of combined transplantation of S, T, L cells, the complete regression rate in near future is 40% and that of forward future is 46.67%. Those with regression can survive for a long time with good curative effects.

Experimental articles can not be published

Screen and look for natural medicament from traditional Chinese herbs through animal experiment.

How to prevent thymus atrophy?

How to protect immune organs?

Look for the medicament that can prevent thymus atrophy and strengthen immunity.

Screen 200 kinds of traditional Chinese medicines by experiments to find out the medicine that can protect thymus and strengthen immunity, promote hematopiesis and resist relapse and metastasis.

The experiments for screening in the laboratory: ①screening experiment by the rate of inhibiting tumors in vitro; ②screening experiment by the rate of inhibiting tumors in vivo of cancer-bearing animal model

From a series of experimental research on tumors with cancer-bearing animals over 7 years, there is a deeply-felt that it is necessary to persist in research on resisting cancerometastasis with Chinese characteristics, namely the combination of experimental research and clinical verification. It is essential to do experimental research on tumors, or it is difficult to improve clinical curative effects.

● Experimental oncology is the basis of research on preventing cancer, which promote the research in China to step further and deeper

● Experimental surgery plays an important role in developing medical science, which is a key to open the forbidden zone of medical science

●Methods of preventing many diseases result from animal experimental research. After acquiring stable achievements, they can be applied in clinic to promote the development of medicine.

3. EXPERIMENTAL STUDY ON EFFECTS ON THE GROWTH OF TUMOR FROM SPLEEN

The experimental research of the effects of the spleen on the tumor growth

In recent years, effects of spleen on the anti-tumor immunity are receiving more and more attentions from people. Its anti-tumor effects are extremely complicated. At present there are many differences and doubts. For further investigating effects of spleen on the growth of tumor and understanding the relation between spleen and tumor immunity, the experimental surgical method is adopted to prepare Ehrlich ascites tumor model. Group without spleen should respectively remove spleen before and after the inoculation of cancer cells. Then by contrasting it to the group with spleen, we perform the following experiment to observe whether the splenectomy will affect tumor immune state.

[Material and Method]

1. Experimental Animal Grouping Kunming mice, no gender classification, mice age 50~60d, weight 15~20g, and quantity of 300. According to the group with or without spleen, different sequence of splenectomy and inoculation of cancer cells, they are divided into 5 groups. Then on the basis of various amounts of inoculated cells (1×10^4 ml or 1×10^7 ml) and different inoculated regions (abdominal cavity or subcutaneous), each group is further separated into subgroups A and B. The specific grouping is shown in the following table 1.

Table 1 Summary table of experimental animal grouping

Group Inoculation Method	cancer cells concentration 1×10^4/ml		cancer cells concentration 1×10^7/ml	
	percutaneous	transabdominal	percutaneous	transabdominal
Group I simulating spleen removal	I A$_1$ (15)	I A$_2$ (15)	I B$_1$ (15)	I B$_2$ (15)
Group II (spleen removal before inoculation)	II A$_1$ (15)	II A$_2$ (15)	II B$_1$ (15)	II B$_2$(15)
Group III (inoculation before spleen removal)	III A (30)		III B (30)	
Group IV (spleen removal before inoculation+ splenic cells)	IV A$_1$ (15)	II A$_2$ (15)	IV B$_1$ (15)	IV B$_2$ (15)
Group V (administration of Chinese medicine)	V A (15)		V B (15)	

The Fourth Section Experimental Study

Group I: Control group with spleen. Firstly simulating spleen removal, after 7d transabdominal or percutaneous inoculation of Ehrlich ascites cancer cells 0.1ml, the number of cancer cells is 1×10^4 or 1×10^7 (table 2).

Table 2 Control group of simulating spleen removal (Group I)

Group I	Inoculated Cancer Cell Number	Inoculated Regions	Mice Number
I A$_1$	0.1×10^4	right armpit subcutaneousness	15
I A$_2$	0.1×10^4	abdominal cavity	15
I B$_1$	0.1×10^7	right armpit subcutaneousness	15
I B$_2$	0.1×10^7	abdominal cavity	15

Group II: Group of spleen removal before inoculation. Firstly spleen removal, after 7d percutaneous or transabdominal inoculation of Ehrlich ascites cancer cells 0.1ml, the number of cancer cells is 1×10^4 or 1×10^7 (table 3).

Table 3 Group of spleen removal before inoculation

Group II	Inoculated Cancer Cell Number	Inoculated Regions	Mice Number
II A$_1$	0.1×10^4	right armpit subcutaneousness	15
II A$_2$	0.1×10^4	abdominal cavity	15
II B$_1$	0.1×10^7	right armpit subcutaneousness	15
II B$_2$	0.1×10^7	abdominal cavity	15

Group III: Group without spleen, i.e. group of inoculation before spleen removal. Firstly inoculation of cancer cells, after 7d spleen removal. Both are right armpit subcutaneous inoculations. The number of cancer cells is 1×10^4ml or 1×10^7ml (table 4).

Table 4 Group of inoculation before spleen removal

Group III	Inoculated Cancer Cell Number	Inoculated Regions	Mice Number
III A	0.1×10^4	right armpit subcutaneousness	15
III B	0.1×10^7	right armpit subcutaneousness	15

Group IV: Group of spleen removal before inoculation, and further transabdominal transplantation of splenic cells or clear liquid of splenic tissue. Firstly remove spleen, after 7d inoculate cancer cells. In another 1d, transabdominal injection of living spleen cell suspension or supernatant liquid of splenic tissue (table 5).

Table 5 Group of spleen removal before transplantation of splenic cells or clear liquid of splenic tissue

Group IV	Inoculated Cancer Cell Number	Inoculated Regions	Processing Factor	Mice Number
IV A$_1$	0.1×10^4	trans-sub right armpit	injection of supernatant liquid of splenic tissue	15
IV A$_2$	0.1×10^4	transabdominal	injection of supernatant liquid of splenic tissue	15
IV B$_1$	0.1×10^7	right armpit subcutaneousness	transplantation of splenic cells of newborn mice	15
IV B$_2$	0.1×10^7	abdominal cavity	transplantation of splenic cells of adult mice	15

Group V: Group of taking Traditional Chinese Medicine (TCM) complex prescription with efficacy of strengthening the spleen and replenishing qi (table 6).

Table 6 Group of taking Traditional Chinese Medicine (TCM) complex prescription with efficacy of strengthening the spleen and replenishing qi

Group V	Inoculated Cancer Cell Number	Inoculated Regions	Processing Factor	Mice Number
V A	$10^7 \times 0.1$	right armpit subcutaneousness	firstly take TCM for 10d, after inoculation continue to take medication for 3 weeks	15
V B	$10^7 \times 0.1$	right armpit subcutaneousness	after inoculation take medication for 3 weeks	15

2. Instruments and Materials

(1) An animal sterile operating room and a set of sterile surgical instruments.
(2) Hank liquid, improved Hank liquid, calf serum, PRH, triple-distilled water, 0.9% sodium chloride solution for injection, ketamine, soluble phenobarbital, heparin sodium, trypan blue stain, Giemsa stain, Wright's stain, hydrochloric acid baking soda, L-glutamic acid, sensitization and non- sensitization zymosan.
(3) Centrifugal machine with 400 rounds per minute, glass homogenizer, medicine vibrator, filtering metal gauze (size 1000), funnel, thermostat, baker, low temperature water tank, microscope, relative sterile workbench.
(4) Animal feed are refined pellet feed. The drinking water is tap water. Rearing cage is plastic mouse cage.

3. Tumor Inoculation and Model Preparation Ehrlich ascites tumor cell strain is introduced from Wuhan Biological Research Institute Cell Room. Ascites containing cancer cells are

extracted from ascetic-type tumor animal abdominal cavity of mice Ehrlich ascites tumor. Firstly use improved Hank liquid to clean and centrifugate ascites for 3 times with 800 rounds per minute of centrifugal speed and five minutes. Remove supernatant liquid, and respectively combine deposited cancer cells with Hank liquid to make up the cancer cell suspensions, containing $1×10^4$ ml or $1×10^7$ ml inoculated cells. The trypan blue dead cells exclusion test proves that the living cell rate is above 95%. Then inoculate cancer cells to experimental mice through right armpit subcutaneousness and abdominal cavity. Each mouse is inoculated with cancer cell suspension of 0.1ml, i.e. amounts of containing cancer cells are $1×10^4$ ml or $1×10^7$ ml.

4. Splenectomy Combine ketamine with soluble phenobarbital to execute intraperitoneal anesthesia. Dosages are 0.4mg/10g and 0.2mg/10g. After anesthesia, fix the mouse on surgery board. Shear the belly fur. Use iodine (2.5%) and ethanol (75%) to disinfect the belly. Bespread the sterile cloth on it. An incision is made into each layer of abdominal wall tissue through left lower abdomen. Then enter into abdominal cavity. Expose and dissociate the spleen. Use silk thread of size 0 to ligate the splenic stalk. Excise the spleen. Ensure the strict sterile operation, gentle action and thorough hemostases. During the operation, notice whether there is a splenulus. In case there is, excise it together. For simulating spleen removal of control group, only open the abdominal cavity; pull but do not excise the spleen. Antibiotics are not used in and after the operation. Infection of incisional wound is 1.0%. After operation, continue to feed the mouse with refined pellet feed.

5. Preparations of Splenic Cell Suspension and Supernatant Liquid of Splenic Tissue

(1) Preparation of splenic cell suspension: Execute newborn Kunming mice of 24~48h or adult mice. An incision is made into abdominal wall to take out the spleen. Cut off peripheral envelope and adipose tissue of spleen. Use Hank liquid to irrigate them in sterile glass culture dish for 3 times. Then put spleen into the glass homogenizer. Add in Hank liquid for 5ml. Grind up the splenic tissue. Filter it with stainless silk net of size 100. Centrifugate the filtering medium (1000 rounds per minute, 10 min). Remove supernatant liquid. Use Hank liquid to dilute deposited cells and make up the splenic cell suspensions of $5×10^7$/ml. Suspensions are dyed by trypan blue stain and proved that the living cell rate is above 97%. Then transplant splenic cell suspensions into abdominal cavity of experimental mouse. Each mouse can only accept splenic cell suspensions of 2ml which belong to one receptor.

(2) Preparation of splenic cell homogenate: After excising the spleen, use quick freezing (-20 centi degree) and rapid rewarming to induce the cracking of dead splenic cells proved by trypan blue stain and microscopic examination. Then centrifugate the filtering medium (1000 rounds per minute, 10 min). Reserve supernatant liquid and remove deposits. Inject supernatant liquid through abdomen into the experimental mouse.

6. Observation Item

(1) Observe success ratio of cancer cell inoculation, occurrence time of subcutaneous tumor nodi and speed of tumor enlargement.

(2) Every day use vernier caliper to measure diameter and size of subcutaneous tumor nodi; measure mouse' weight; observe metastasis condition and moving degree.

(3) Observe the quality of life, fur color, vitality, state of nutrition, breath, mental state of tumor-bearing mice and survival time of bearing tumor.

(4) Observe abdominal shape and prohection of ascetic-type tumor-bearing mice. Also according to prohection state, divide ascites content into 5 grades.

Grade 0: the abdomen is not of fullness, without ascites, note as (-).

Grade 1: slight prohection of abdomen, with a little ascites, note as (+).

Grade 2: prohection of abdomen, with medium content of ascites, note as (++).

Grade 3: obvious prohection of abdomen, with more ascites, note as (+++).

Grade 4: shape of frog abdomen, with plentiful ascites, note as (++++).

During necropsy, measure the content of ascites, microscopic examination of cancer cell shape, count living cell rate and content.

(5) Determine immunologic functional condition of red blood cells of tumor-bearing mice: test for measuring C_3b receptor garland with semi quantitative method.

(6) Necropsy and pathological section: dissect each dead experimental mouse. Observe tumor's size and weight, infiltrating and metastatic condition, morphological structure and involvement condition of visceral organs; measure the content of ascites; extract tumor tissue, liver, spleen, thymus gland, lung and other visceral organs to carry out the examination of pathological section.

[Experimental Result]

1. Resulting comparison and analysis on different groups with right armpit subcutaneous inoculation of small dose of 0.1×10^4 ml Ehrlich ascites tumor cells.

(1) Comparison on occurrence time of tumor nodi with different processing method (T test), see table 22-7.

**Table 7 Comparison on occurrence time (d) of tumor nodi
with different processing method (T test)**

Group	Group I A$_1$ (Control group with spleen)	Group II A$_1$ (Group of spleen removal before inoculation)	Group IIIA (Group of inoculation before spleen removal)	Group IVA$_1$ (Spleen removal before inoculation＋supernatant liquid of splenic tissue)
Occurrence time (d)	8	7*	9	9*

Note: ① *. Compared with Group I A$_1$, P<0.05 has remarkable significance; ② In Group I A$_1$ (control group with spleen), one experimental mouse (accounts for 7.6%) suffers no tumor nodi after inoculation of cancer cells. It survives for a long term (i.e. survival time is above 90d). No tumor is found during dissection. Treat it as inoculation failure. Not for statistical treatment; also in Group IVA (group with transabdominal injection of supernatant liquid of splenic tissue), 3 experimental mice (accounts for 25%) fail to be inoculated.

According to table 7, the earliest occurrence time of tumor nodi in above groups belongs to group of spleen removal before inoculation (Group II A$_1$). Control group and group with injection of supernatant liquid of splenic tissue have the later occurrence time.

(2) For different processing methods, maximum diameter comparison of each group's tumor nodi on the seventh, fourteenth and twentieth day, see table 8.

Table 8 Size comparison of each group's tumor nodi on the seventh, fourteenth and twentieth day after subcutaneous inoculation of 0.1×10^4 ml cancer cells (maximum diameter mm)

Group	Group I A$_1$ (Control group with spleen)	Group II A$_1$ (Group of spleen removal before inoculation)	Group III A (Group of inoculation before spleen removal)	Group IVA$_1$ (Spleen removal before inoculation＋supernatant liquid of splenic tissue)	P
seventh	0	3.3±0.48	0	0	<0.01
fourteenth	11.43±5.99	14.4±6.2	11.8±7.45	8±4.33	<0.01
twentieth	18.92±9.98	21.12±8.28	19.7±5.98	13.89±7.63	<0.01

Note: Values *P* in the table are gained through analysis of diameter variance (*F* test).

From above results in the table, the tumor which belongs to group of spleen removal before inoculation (Group II A$_1$) appears first and grows fast. Before the fourteenth day, its tumor volume reaches biggest. On the twentieth day after inoculation, tumors' sizes of control group (Group I A$_1$), group II A$_1$ (group of spleen removal before inoculation), group of inoculation before spleen removal (Group III A) reach unanimity. While tumors which belong to group of injecting supernatant liquid of splenic tissue (Group IV A₁) have the smallest volume. That explains that during early growing stage of tumor (before the seventh day), spleen has tumor inhibitory action. But during medium and advanced stages (experimental group sets: medium stage is from eighth day to fourteenth day since the inoculation; since the fourteenth day, it is tumor advanced stage), the inhibitory action of spleen weakens or disappears. Furthermore, it can be observed that after cancer cells inoculation of spleen removal group, since the fourteenth day, tumor nodi often bear liquefaction, necrosis and ablation, which result in the shrinkage of tumor volume. Even some incisions have healed. Why does such phenomenon appear? That needs to have a further observation.

(3) Comparison of mean survival time (MST) for groups of subcutaneous inoculation with 0.1×10^4 ml cancer cells, see table 9.

Table 9 Comparison of each group's mean survival time (MST)

Group	Group I A₁ (Control group with spleen)	Group II A₁ (Group of spleen removal before inoculation)	Group III A (Group of inoculation before spleen removal)	Group IVA₁ (Spleen removal before inoculation＋supernatant liquid of splenic tissue)	P
MST (d)	41.61±12.24	38.73±19.63	44.8±15.95	50±27.21	<0.05

Note: Values *P* in the table are gained through *F* test.

From table 9, mean survival times of groups I A₁, II A₁, III A are close to each other. T test shows there is no difference among these three groups, $P > 0.05$. While for injection of supernatant liquid of splenic tissue, mean survival time of this group is obviously longer than those of other groups, $P < 0.05$. The significant difference exists.

2. Resulting analysis of each group's transabdominal inoculation with 0.1×10^4 ml cancer cells After inoculation of cancer cells, experimental mice can survive above 90d without any ascite or tumor nodus. Also a dissection of corpse shows no tumor. The above results are treated as inoculation failures. It explains the fact that vaccinal cancer cells are rejected by the organism and no tumor forms.

(1) Comparison of inoculation failure rate for each group's transabdominal inoculation of 0.1×10^4 ml cancer cells without ascites, see table 10.

Table 10 Comparison of each group's inoculation failure rate (T test)

Group	Group I A$_2$ (Control group with spleen)	Group II A$_2$ (Group of spleen removal before inoculation)	Group II A$_2$ (Spleen removal before inoculation+supernatant liquid of splenic tissue)
failure rate	26%	0**	54%*

Note: **. indicates the comparison with control group, T test $P<0.01$, with high degree of significant difference; *. indicates $P<0.05$, with significant difference.

Results of table 10 show that all experimental mice in the group of spleen removal before inoculation form ascites, and failure rate is zero. The inoculation failure rates of control group with spleen and injection group of supernatant liquid of splenic tissue are 26% and 54% respectively. It process that tumor is easy to grow in the mouse without spleen after inoculation of tumor. That is, the removal of spleen promotes the growth of tumor. On the contrary, injection of supernatant liquid of splenic cells will suppress the growth of tumor.

(2) Comparison of survival time for each group's transabdominal inoculation of 0.1×10^4 ml cancer cells, see table 11.

Table 11 Comparison of each group's survival time (F test)

Group	Group I A$_2$ (Control group with spleen)	Group II A$_2$ (Group of spleen removal before inoculation)	Group IVA$_2$ (Spleen removal before inoculation+supernatant liquid of splenic tissue)	P
survival time (d)	51.46±29.35	35.6±18.93	57.6±14.85	<0.05

From table 11, the mean survival time of group with spleen removal before inoculation is 35.6±18.93 days. While mean survival times of control group with spleen and injection group of supernatant liquid of splenic tissue are 51.46±29.35 days and 57.6±14.85 days respectively, and P<0.05. Significant differences exist among these three groups. In three groups, group of spleen removal before inoculation has the shortest survival time. Group with spleen owns long survival time; while group without spleen owns short survival time. That shows the removal of spleen promotes the growth of tumor and shortens survival times of tumor-bearing mice. On the contrary, injection of supernatant liquid of splenic cells will suppress the growth of tumor and prolong survival times of tumor-bearing mice.

3. Results of each group's subcutaneous inoculation with 0.1×10^7 ml cancer cells

(1) Comparison on occurrence time of each group's subcutaneous tumor nodi, see table 12.

Table 12 Comparison on occurrence time of each group's subcutaneous tumor nodi

Group	Group I B$_1$ (Control group with spleen)	Group II B$_1$ (Group of spleen removal before inoculation)	Group III B (Group of inoculation before spleen removal)	Group IV B$_1$ (Spleen removal before inoculation+transplantation of fetal mouse's splenic cells)	P
Occurrence time (d)	5.5	5	7.5	9	<0.05

Mice of group IIIB are removed spleens on the seventh day after inoculations. So after seven days group IIIB and control group with spleen (Group I B$_1$) are in the same condition. The table shows that for the group with spleen removal first, occurrence times of subcutaneous tumor nodi are slightly earlier than these of other groups. While for group IVB$_1$ (transplantation of fetal mouse's splenic cells), occurrence times of tumor nodi are obviously later than these of other groups. It proves that the removal of spleen promotes the growth of tumor. While transplantation of splenic cells intensively suppresses the growth of tumor.

(2) Comparison of maximum diameter average on each group's subcutaneous tumor nodi on the seventh, fourteenth and twentieth day after inoculation, see table13.

Table13 Comparison of maximum diameter on each group's tumor nodi on the seventh, fourteenth and twentieth day (mm)

Group	Group I B$_1$ (Control group with spleen)	Group II B$_1$ (Group of spleen removal before inoculation)	Group III B (Group of inoculation before spleen removal)	Group IV B$_1$ (Spleen removal before inoculation+transplantation of fetal mouse's splenic cells)	P
seventh	5.07±1.847	10.88±5.278	2.83±1.948	3.0±1.56	<0.01
fourteenth	19.85±4.598	21.12±5.3	20.3±6.07	11±5.69	<0.01
twentieth	30.9±7.87	24±7.86	25.25±4.77	16±4.95	<0.01

Note: Values P in the table are gained through F test.

(3) Comparison of each group's mean survival time (MST), see table14.

Table 14 Comparison of each group's mean survival time
(subcutaneous inoculation of 0.1×10^7 ml cancer cells)

Group	Group I B$_1$ (Control group with spleen)	Group II B$_1$ (Group of spleen removal before inoculation)	Group III B	Group IV B$_1$ (Spleen removal before inoculation+transplantation of fetal mouse's splenic cells)	P
MST (d)	33.1±13.15	49.56±24.39	38.7±14.45	50.75±19.30	<0.01

From table 13 and 14, on the seventh day after inoculation, for the three groups-control group with spleen (Group IB$_1$), group of spleen removal before inoculation (Group IIB$_1$) and group of inoculation before spleen removal (Group IIIB), their maximum diameter averages of tumor nodi are $\overline{X}$ (IB$_1$) = (5.07±1.847) mm, $\overline{X}$ (IIB$_1$) = (10.88±5.278) mm, $\overline{X}$ (IIIB) = (2.83±1.948) mm respectively. $P<0.01$. Significant differences exist among these three groups. Tumors which belong to the group of spleen removal before inoculation (IIB$_1$) have the maximum volumes. Now on the seventh day, in fact groups IB$_1$ and IIIB have the spleen, which is in proliferative active phase. While group IIB$_1$ has no spleen. The tumor volume of group with spleen is smaller, and the tumor volume of group without spleen is larger. It indicates that the spleen can suppress tumor during early stage or the removal of spleen can promote the growth of tumor. While on the fourteenth day after inoculation, their average maximum diameters of tumor nodi are $\overline{X}$ (IB$_1$) = (19.85±4.598) mm, $\overline{X}$ (IIB$_1$) = (21.12±5.3) mm, $\overline{X}$ (IIIB) = (20.3±6.07) mm respectively. $P>0.05$. Significant differences disappear among these three groups. On the twentieth day after inoculation, the tumor volume of control group with spleen is larger than that of other groups. The maximum diameter $\overline{X}$ = (30.9±7.87) mm. At this time, the spleen of tumor-bearing mouse has extremely shrank, and lost the tumor inhibitory action. From the experiment, since the fourteenth day after inoculation, most mice tumors of group with spleen removal begin to bear liquefaction and necrosis. Some lumps ulcerate and ablate, whose volumes shrink. The reason that tumors in this period suffer from liquefaction, necrosis and ulceration is not clear at present. That needs to have a further observation.

Therefore, during the early stage of tumor, spleen can suppress the growth of tumor. For the group with spleen, the tumor growth rate is slower. Tumor volume is smaller. While on the advanced stage of tumor, the inhibitory action of spleen weakens or disappears. The tumor size of all groups reaches unanimity.

Furthermore, it can be seen from the stable that tumors of the group (IVB$_1$), which removes spleen before inoculation and transplants splenic cells of fetal mice, have obviously slower growth rate than that of other groups. The tumor volume is smaller. Its survival time is longer that that of other groups. These conditions prove that splenic cells of homogeneous variant fetus have obvious tumor-inhibitory action.

4. Results of each group's transabdominal inoculation with 0.1×10^7 ml cancer cells

(1) Comparison on occurrence time of ascites for each group, see table 15.

Table 15 Comparison on occurrence time of ascites for each group of transabdominal inoculation with 0.1×10^7 ml cancer cells

Group	Group I B_2 (Control group with spleen)	Group II B_2 (Group of spleen removal before inoculation)	Group IV B_2 (Spleen removal before inoculation＋transplantation of splenic cells)
Occurrence time (median, d)	5	3*	4*

Note: **. indicates the comparison with control group, T test $P<0.05$, with significant difference.

(2) Occupying percentages of ascites content greater than (++) for groups on the fifth, seventh and fourteenth day after transabdominal inoculation of 0.1×10^7 ml cancer cells, see table 22-16.

Table 16 Comparison on ascites content of transabdominal inoculation with 0.1×10^7 ml cancer cells

Days after inoculation (d)	Group I B_2 (Control group with spleen)	Group II B_2 (Group of spleen removal before inoculation)	Group IV B_2 (Spleen removal before inoculation＋transplantation of splenic cells)
2	0%	75% **	10% *
7	28%	100% **	70% *
14	100%	100%	100% *

Note: **. indicates the comparison with IB_2 (control group), T test $P<0.01$; *. indicates $P<0.05$; no *. indicates $P>0.05$.

(3) Comparison of survival time (d) for each group's transabdominal inoculation of 0.1×10^7 ml cancer cells, see table17.

Table 17 Comparison of each group's survival time

Group	Group I B_2 (Control group with spleen)	Group II B_2 (Group of spleen removal before inoculation)	Group IV B_2 (Spleen removal before inoculation＋transplantation of splenic cells)
survival time (d)	20.15±4.59	15.56±10.94*	16.67±8.34

Note: *. indicates the comparison with IB$_2$, *P*<0.05, with significant difference; no *. indicates the comparison with IB$_2$, *P*>0.05, without significant difference.

Integrating tables15, 16 and 17, results show that for the group with spleen removal first (IIB$_2$), tumor growth rate is faster. Amounts of ascites are more. Survival time is shorter. Also visceral organs are easier to metastasize. Those explain that removal of spleen can promote the growth of tumor. Transabdominal transplantation of splenic cells of homogeneous variant adult mice can partially suppress the growth of tumor. But its inhibitory action is weaker than that of control group with spleen and group with transplantation of fetal mouse's splenic cells.

5. Results of necropsy and pathological examination Each mouse accepts the postmortem necropsy. Visually observe tumor shape, involved visceral organs and diffusion condition. And extract tissues for pathological section examination. The result shows that Ehrlich ascites tumor cell strain owns features of stable proliferation, strong invasiveness and so on. Subcutaneous inoculation is easy to induce the form of solid tumor. Necropsy proves that after inoculation tumors or ascites are easy to form in some regions, easily infiltrating to surrounding tissues. The metastases of cancer cells rarely happen to mice with subcutaneous inoculation. While for mice with transabdominal inoculation, cancer cells easily metastasize to liver, kidney and lymph node in advanced stage. Only two of two hundred and seventy experimental mice suffer from splenic metastases, proving the weak affinity of spleen to cancer cells. This group of experiments has also found phenomena that for the group of spleen removal before transabdominal inoculation, multiple carcinomatous metastases appear in visceral organs of abdominal cavity. Metastatic ratio is up to 50%. These metastases invade liver, kidney, pancreas and mesenteric lymph nodes, always implicating more than two visceral organs. While for control group with spleen and group with transplantation of homogeneous variant splenic cells, carcinomatous metastases rarely occur. Metastatic ratios are 20% and 25%, which are obviously lower than those of the group without spleen. It shows that spleen can suppress the growth of tumor. While the group without spleens lose the inhibitory action, consequently leading to easy diffusion and metastasis of tumor.

Furthermore, dynamic observation of this group of experimental mice shows that thymus and spleen of tumor-bearing mice present a series of changes with the process of illness, which own certain regularity. About seven days after inoculation, the thymus presents acute and progressive atrophy. Its volume shrinks; the diameter of each normal lobule shortens from 5~8cm to about 1mm; the weight reduces from (70±10) mg to (20±5) mg. While soon after the inoculation of cancer cells, spleen becomes congested and tumid. The volume enlarges; weight increases; texture becomes fragile. Microscopic examination shows the increase of germinal centers and active cell proliferation. On the fourteenth day after inoculation, the spleen also quickly presents progressive atrophy. Its volume shrinks; the weight reduces from (140±15) mg to (50±10) mg. Germinal centers obviously decrease; cell proliferation is suffocated. The spleen also suffers from hyperplasia of fibrous tissues, fibrosis with gray color and rigid texture.

6. Testing results of erythrocytic immune function This group of experiments choose 100 mice to carry out the erythrocytic C$_3$b receptor garland test. The result shows that after the removal of spleen, bonding ratio of C$_3$b receptor garland of tumor-bearing mice is on a progressive declining tendency.

That explains that after the removal of spleen, immunological adhesive competence of red blood cells drops to some extent.

[Discussion]

1. As seen from experimental results, spleen can suppress the growth of tumor. After the removal of spleen, compared with the control group, the growth rate is faster; the occurrence time and volume of subcutaneous tumor nodi is earlier and larger in the same period. For group with transabdominal inoculation of cancer cells and group with the removal of spleen, occurrence time of ascites is earlier; ascites content is greater; cells content is also higher. Survival time is shorter than that of control group. Necropsy finds that cancer metastatic rate of the group with the removal of spleen is 30% above that of control group (metastases to liver, kidney, pancreas and mesenteric lymph nodes). From table 22-13, group IIB$_1$ (spleen removal before inoculation) and group IIIB (inoculation before spleen removal) accept splenectomy in different time. On the seventh day after inoculation, maximum diameter averages of their subcutaneous tumor nodi are $\overline{X}$ (IIB$_1$) = (10.8±5.28) mm and $\overline{X}$ (IIIB) = (2.83±1.948) mm respectively. The former is obviously longer than the latter one. But on the fourteenth day after inoculation, the tumor of group IIIB quickly proliferates after the removal of spleen. The difference between them almost disappears. $\overline{X}$ (IIB$_1$) = (21.2±5.3) mm, $\overline{X}$ (IIIB) = (20.3±6.07), $P>0.05$, without significant difference. It prompts that the removal of spleen promotes the growth of tumor, i.e. spleen can suppress the growth of tumor.

In recent two decades, people find that spleen not only performs a great role in anti-infection, but also has the all-important influence on anti-tumor immunity. The active mechanism may be by producing Natural Killer cell, macrophage (Mϕ), Lympholine-Activated Killer cell, TH/Ti cell, B cell, Ts cell, etc. to realize the cellular immunity; and by secreting lymphokines of Tufisn factor, TNF factor, IL-2, interferon, addiment, antibody, etc. to kill tumor cells. Ge Yigong once used rat Lw56 pulmonary sarcoma model to the effect of removing spleen on tumor growth. Mr Ge holds that success ratio of tumor inoculation after the removal of spleen is higher than that of group with spleen. The metastatic ratio increases. Results are similar to this group of experimental results.

This group of experimental results also prompts that after the removal of spleen, bonding ratio of C$_3$b receptor garland of organism peripheral blood is 40% below that of healthy group with spleen. It explains that erythrocytic immune function of organism reduces after the removal of spleen.

2. Spleen's inhibiting action on tumor growth mainly occurs in the early stage of tumor course. While in the advanced stage of tumor, spleen's inhibiting action on tumor growth weakens and disappears. As seen from tables 22-8 and 22-13, in the early stage of tumor (within 7d), the tumor of group without spleen has a faster tumor growth rate than that of control group with spleen. The volume of subcutaneous tumor nodi is large and ascites content is great. While in the advanced stage (after 14d) of tumor, tumor nodi of control group with spleen and group with the removal of spleen basically have the same volume. No significant comparability. No obvious difference between survival times. Necropsy and pathological examination of three hundred experimental mice find that spleen of tumor-bearing mice present a series of regular changes with the process of illness. In the early stage

of tumor (within 7d after inoculation), due to the cytostimulation, the spleen becomes congested and tumid. The volume enlarges; cell proliferation accelerates; germinal centers increases. While in the advanced stage (since 14d after inoculation) of tumor, the spleen presents progressive atrophy. Its volume shrinks; germinal centers fall sharply. The spleen also suffers from hyperplasia of fibrous tissues. The fibrosis of spleen occurs; therefore, its anticancer immunization weakens or disappears. Even it can pass through the suppressor T cell. Macrophage and immune inhibiting factor can suppress the anticancer immunization of organism and promote the growth of tumor. That explains that spleen's effect on tumor immune state is bidirectional, has obvious time phase and is relevant to stadium. In early stage, the spleen owns the anti-tumor action. In advanced stage, the spleen owns immune inhibiting action. But the basic reason that leads to the immune inhibiting state of organism is the tumor itself. Spleen just plays a certain part in the forming process of this state.

1. Transabdominal injection of supernatant liquid of healthy splenic cells and transplantation of homogeneous variant splenic cells can suppress tumor growth. For group of injection with supernatant liquid of splenic cells or transplantation of splenic cells (Group IV), comparative results with other groups show that the tumor growth rate is slower; the occurrence time of tumor nodi is later; the volume is smaller; ascites content is less. After the inoculation of small dose of 0.1×10^4 ml cancer cells, success ratio of inoculation for tumor-bearing mice is obviously lower than that of other groups. Moreover, after a little ascites or subcutaneous lesser tubercle firstly appearing in several mice, the tumor can disappear naturally. The survival time is above 90d (as long-term survivors). Especially splenic cells of homogeneous variant fetal mouse (group IVB_1) have obvious tumor-inhibitory action. The tumor inhibition rate is 54%. The survival time is 17d longer than that of control group. Pathological examinations of this group of tumor-bearing mice find that after transplantation of homogeneous variant fetal splenic cells, splenic islands grow on the abdominal cavity and (or) mesentery of seven mice (account for 50%). Pathological examination proves it as living splenic tissues. Fetal splenic cells have features of weak antigenicity, deficient quantity and strong cell proliferation, etc. After the transplantation of splenic cells of homogeneous variant mice, there is no sharp rejection. And moreover, it is not subject to blood group ABO. Do not need the cross test of different blood groups. Here in China some people use traumatic splenic cells to prepare LAK cells for treating advanced malignant tumors, which achieves better curative effects on inhibiting tumor growth and prolonging mouse's lifespan.

At present, adoptive immunotherapy of tumors with transplantation of fetal splenic cells has not yet been reported in the literature. This group of experiments needs to have a further observation.

4. Negative correlation between anti-tumor immunological action of the organism and the quantity of cancer cells This group of experiments finds that anti-tumor immunological action of the organism is obviously affected by the quantity of inoculated cancer cells. The less the quantity of cancer cells, the stronger and more significant the anti-tumor effect; on the contrary, the weaker the anti-tumor effect. As for 0.1×10^7 ml inoculated cancer cells, immunological action of the organism is obviously suppressed. The tumor growth rates of group without spleen and group with spleen have bigger difference in the early stage. While after medium stage (after 7d), the difference will quickly disappear. There is also no significant difference in survival time. But for 0.1×10^4 ml inoculated cancer cells,

anti-tumor action of the organism is relatively significant. The inoculated failure rate of group with spleen is obviously higher than that of group without spleen. The growth rate of tumor is slow; the volume of tumor nodi is small; and the survival time is long. Furthermore, after the transplantation of homogeneous variant splenic cells for small dose of inoculated cancer cells group, anti-tumor immunological action goes up remarkably. The growth rate of tumor decreases obviously. Some tumor nodi even can naturally disappear after its formation. Also the survival time is long. These results show the negative correlation between anti-tumor action of the organism and the quantity of inoculated cancer cells. While there is a positive correlation between cancer's immunological inhibiting action on the organism and the quantity of inoculated cancer cells. The spleen participates in tumor immunoregulation, which has double influences on immune state of tumor-bearing mice. In early stage, the spleen shows a certain anti-cancer action. As the development of tumor, the number of tumor cells is increasing. The spleen is shrinking gradually. Then the anti-cancer action is converted into immunological inhibiting action. But the basic reason of immune inhibiting state is the tumor itself. The progress of cancer, an increase in the number of cancer cells and the reinforcement of inhibiting action lead to the atrophia of spleen, thymus gland and other immune organs.

5. Experimental result prompts of this group

(1) The spleen has certain anti-tumor effects. In tumor's early stage, spleen can suppress the growth of tumor. While in advanced stage of the course of disease, the anti-tumor action of spleen weakens or disappears. The spleen even can promote the growth of spleen.

(2) Adoptive immunotherapy of tumors with transplantation of homogeneous variant splenic cells of fetal mice can reinforce anti-tumor immunological action of the organism, and suppress the growth of tumor.

(3) There is a negative correlation between anti-tumor action of the organism and the quantity of inoculated cancer cells. The more the quantity of cancer cells, the more easily the immunological action of the organism is suppressed or damaged. The faster the growth rate of tumor, the worse the prognosis.

4. EXPERIMENTAL STUDY ON TREATMENT OF MALIGNANT TUMOR BY ADOPTIVE IMMUNOLOGIC RECONSTITUTION THROUGH COMBINED TRANSPLANTATION OF FETAL CELLS

I. Experiment on Adoptive Immunologic Reconstitution of Fetal Liver, Spleen and Thymus Cells through Combined Transplantation

In this paper, the author introduces the experiment on the systematic adoptive immunologic reconstitution with the mice bearing Ehrlich ascites cancer (EAC) subcutaneous solid tumor through combined transplantation using the same kind of fetal liver, spleen and thymus cells. In this experiment, set up groups of monomial transplantations of fetal liver, spleen and thymus respectively; the groups of bigeminal transplantation of fetal liver and spleen cells, fetal liver and thymus cells as well as fetal spleen and thymus cells, and then observe the time of the growth, regression and survival, index of cellular immunity as well as all items of pathological examination in each group respectively; compare the curative effects of each groups. The research results show that the curative effect of trigeminal group is better than that of the bigeminal group which is better than the individual groups in turn. For the experimental group of trigeminal cell transplantation, the complete regression rates of the tumor in near and forward future are 40% (n=15) and 46.67% (n=15) respectively, and the partial regression rates (the percentage of the tumor regression is more than 50%) are 26.67% and 13.33% respectively. Those whose tumors regress completely can survive for a long time and the lifetimes of those whose tumors regress partially are prolonged for more than a month on average, and their immune index improves obviously and the immune organs are of hypertrophy. The sections of immune organ tissue reveal the active cell proliferation. Moreover, the pathological sections of tumor tissue show that a large amount of lymphocytes soak around the tumor tissue and in stroma, and then form parcel; flaky concretion, liquefaction necrosis, karyorrhexis and other pathologic phenomena emerge in the central tumor tissue. For the experimental groups of bigeminal cell transplantation, except a few cases of partial regression, there is no complete one. All the improvement of the immune indexes, the prolonged lifetime, and the soakage of lymphocytes in tumor tissue are less obvious than those of the experimental trigeminal group. As to monomial groups of cell transplantation, the results of regression, lifetime and immune indexes as well as the pathological examination results are less apparent than the former two groups, but better than the control group of the tumor-bearing mice. It can be implied that compared with partial reconstitution, systematic adoptive immunologic reconstitution can develop the anti-carcinomatous immunologic function and improve the curative effects though overall systematic synergism.

Thanks to the theory of biological response modifier (BRM), treatment of tumor has been experiencing a profound reform. The fourth generation of the modality of tumor therapy, biological treatment of tumor has become the focus in the field of tumor therapy after surgeons, chemotherapy and radiotherapy. According to a large number of clinical and experimental researches, it can be found that the organismal immune state exhibits progressive inhibition with the evolution of the stadium. Therefore, how to restore and reconstitute the anti-carcinomatous immunologic function is the core of the research of tumor biological treatment. The adoptive immunotherapy developed by Rosenberg who is the representative has got outstanding achievement in this field. Except transferring the active factors amplified in vitro and various kinds of artificial immunologic factors, fetal immune organs and cell transplantation are promising researches. Although the technique of biotherapy is expensive, it possesses several advantages like economy, convenient technique and easy popularization in that the sources of embryo are broad in China, which is worthy of thorough research and exploration. In recent years, many scholars at home have developed the research on transplantation of fetal liver, spleen and thymus from the level of cells to tissue and then to the level of organs for curing advanced malignant tumors and they have achieved some curative effects. The thorough researches can explain the source, proliferation, differentiation and the function of lymphocytes as well as the function and effects of reconstituting immune organs and peripheral immune organs clearly. Currently, in many cases of adoptive immunologic treatment with transplanting fetal immune organs, only single fetal organs is utilized, cell transplantation of fetal liver, spleen and thymus cells as well as tissue transplantation, etc. there is no similar literature or reports on the question that it is possible to carry out adoptive reconstitution systematically and integrally. The combined transplantation of fetal liver, spleen and thymus cells, in which the transplantation of fetal liver cells has analogous function of marrow transplantation and is combined with the transplantation of fetal thymus and spleen cells, can make the adoptive reconstitution approach to the systematical and integral level. But it is worthy of researches and exploration that whether it can bring synergism into play and improve curative effects.

1. 【Material and Methods】

Animals and tumor model

Experimental animals: 200 cross bred Kunming mice in closed flock, 5 to 6 weeks old, 18±2.1g in weight, no gender limitation.

Facilities for model of planting tumors: prepare mice of ascitic type after the anabiosis of the root of Ehrlich ascites tumor; when the ascites are formed, draw out the ascites of the cancer cells and centrifuge washing with Hank for three times(800r/min), five minutes for one time; remove the supernatant liquid, then dilute the liquid with the precipitated cancer cells to the concentration of 10^7/ml; use eosin exclusion teat to verify that the percentage of living cells is above 95%; inoculate the experimental mice under the skin of the right hollow viscera, 1ml for each mouse; after a week, all the mice have tumor nodes with the diameter of 9.5±1.5mm in the point of inoculation to make the subcutaneous solid tumor model bearing Ehrlich Ascites tumor.

Grouping

Group the experimental animals with random into control group bearing tumors (Group B, n=9), observation group for combined transplantation of fetal liver, spleen and thymus cells in forward future (Group CI, n=15), observation group in near future (Group CII, n=15, carry on combined transplantation to this group once a week for successive 5 weeks and then execute the mice), treatment group with transplantation of fetal liver cells (Group F), treatment group with transplantation of fetal spleen cells (Group G), treatment group with transplantation of fetal thymus cells (Group H), treatment group with combined transplantation of fetal liver and spleen cells (Group I), treatment group with combined transplantation of fetal liver and thymus cells (Group K), $n_F=n_G=n_H=n_I=n_J=n_K=$ 12. When the model is prepared, carry out correspondent cell transplantation once a week for each group respectively for five times in a row. As to the control group, use Hank as comparison.

Preparing of the suspension of fetal liver, spleen and thymus

Use the female mice that copulate naturally by stages and have been pregnant for 15 to 18 days; paunch them aseptically to take out the fetal mouse, liver, spleen and thymus; rinse them through the Hank individually under 4℃, then individually mix them with aseptic homogenate to the full; dilute the mixture with Hank under 4℃ and filter them to collect the suspension with adequate cells; Sample the suspension and do bacterial culture and pyrogen experiment; if the experimental results are negative, divide them and package as standby.

The approach and method for cell transplantation

Transplantation of fetal liver cells: use the prepared suspension of fetal liver cells for caudal vein injection, 0.2ml for each mouse at a time.

Transplantation of fetal spleen cells: use the prepared suspension of fetal spleen cells for intraperitoneal injection, 0.2ml for each mouse at a time.

Transplantation of fetal thymus cells: use the prepared suspension of fetal thymus cells for intramuscular injection in the back leg, 0.2ml for each mouse at a time.

The treatments for the experimental mice mentioned above begin after a week from cancer cell inoculation, once a week for successive five weeks. As to the control group, use the same amount of Hank as comparison.

Observation item

General items: after cancer cell inoculation, observe the time when tumor emerges; measure the size of the tumor nude with a vernier caliper every two days (the average vertical diameter, mm), the quality of life, the situation of the tumors and the lifetime (d).

Dynamic observation on T cells in peripheral blood: in this experiment, use Alpha Naphthyl Acetate Esterase (ANAE) staining method to take count of the T cells in peripheral blood. Prepare six pairs of nitrogen magenta solution and 2% ANAE solution respectively, store them in the shade under 4℃; before using the prepared solution, add 89ml, 1/15mol/L, pH=7.6 phosphate buffer into the 6ml nitrogen magenta solution gradually and mix up fully, then add 2.5ml, 2% ANAE solution gradually, then mix up to the full. The final sample is amber with pH being 6.4 as solution for incubation. Put this into the water bath of 37℃ for warm-up. Cut the tip of the mouse's tail, and get the section. After the section has dried by natural wind, soak it into the solution for incubation for 1 to 3 hours, then wash it clear by tap water and air it. Use 1% methyl green to dye for 1 to 3 minutes, wash with tap water. After airing, observe the section under microscope. There are black red granules, namely ANAE positive cells in different size and quantity (the amount generally is 2 to 5). Count 200 lymphocytes and then calculate the percentage of T lymphocytes. Observe the percentage dynamically after a week from having built the model and from treatment respectively and measure it every two weeks.

Dynamic observation on the conversion rate of lymphocytes: Measure the conversion rate with the morphologic method of microdose whole blood culture in vitro. Prepare RPMI 1640 complete medium (1640 is the product of Japanese Juchheim, containing 10.4g dry powder in each bag), which consists of 1ml, 20%, 30.0g/L L- glutamine of killed calf blood serum, 3ml 60.0g/L aseptic $NaHCO_3$, 10000U penicillin and 10000µg streptomycin. Sanitize the tail strictly and cut the tip for 0.2mm; collect blood aseptically for 0.1ml with heparinization microdose sampler; add 1.8ml complete medium and then o,1ml PHA; cultivate the sample in the water-jacket incubator under constant temperature of 37℃ for 72 hours and stir it once a day. After the cultivation, draw most of the supernatant liquid out and add 4ml 8.5g/L NH_4Cl to mix up; place the mixture in the water-bath of 37℃ for 10 minutes, then centrifugalize it in 2500r/min, discard the supernatant liquid; Add 5ml fixation fluid (9 units of methanol and an unit of glacialaceticacid; place the sample under ambient temperature for 10 minutes and centrifugalize it in 1500r/min for 5 minutes, discard the supernatant liquid and reserve the precipitate. Add Hank to the precipitate to the volume of 0.2ml, mix the precipitate and Hank and drop on a clean glass to stretch uniformly. After natural airing, dye it with Giemsa for 5 minutes, then wash with tap water. After drying, observe 200 lymphocytes under the microscope and calculate the percentage of the conversion rate of the metrocyte. As same as T cells, observe the percentage dynamically after a week from having built the model and from treatment respectively and measure it every two weeks.

Measuring the green weights of immune organs: do comprehensive autopsy in detail for each dead or the executed mouse, cut the thymus and spleen and observe their sizes, then weight them with a torsion balance; calculate the ratio of the green weight of the immune organs to the body weight for each mouse.

Pathological examination: do systematic pathological autopsy to each dead and the executed mouse, observe the tumor soakage and tumor metastasis; reserve tumor tissue, thymus, spleen, lung, liver, kidney, etc. for tissue pathological section ant attach importance to observe the lymphocyte soakage in tumor tissue and the pathologic changes in the immune organs.

2.【Experimental Results】

1. Comparison of the average lifetime of the mouse in each group (geometrical average) and the persistence in different ages of tumors

According to Table 1, the lifetimes of all treatment groups are prolonged obviously compared with the control group with P being less than 0.05. Especially, the effect of the treatment group of trigeminal cell transplantation is most obvious, with P being less than 0.01. Other treatment groups have significant difference compared with the trigeminal treatment group with P being less than 0.5. In Group CI, the tumors in 7 cases regress completely, which gain a long-term survival and no tumor relapse. The rate of tumor regression in 2 cases is more than 50%, in which the two mice survive for 2 months and die of tumor relapse. Regarding the persistence in different ages of tumor, in the third week after bearing tumor, all treatment groups have significant differences compared with the control group. With the extent of the stadium and observation period, compared with the control group, Group CI shows notable differential all along, but other treatment groups lose the difference from the control group gradually and show the significant difference from that of Group CI.

Table 1 comparison of the average lifetime of the mouse in each group and the persistence in different ages of tumors

Group	N	Lifetime(d) $\overline{X}$ +S	The persistence in different ages of tumor							
			1week	2week	3week	4week	5week	6week	2weeks	3months
GroupB	9	13.3±1.2	100	55.6	11.1	11.1	0	0	0	0
GroupF	12	22.5±1.6△*	100	83.3	58.3*	50	33.3	33.3	0△	0△
GroupG	12	21.4±1.9△*	100	75	75*	50	33.3	16.7△	0△	0△
GroupH	12	26.2±1.4△*	100	100	100*	58.3*	41.7	33.3	0△	0△
GroupI	12	27.4±1.7△*	100	91.7	91.7*	50	33.3	33.3	8.3△	0△
GroupJ	12	28.3±1.8△*	100	83.3	83.3*	66.7*	41.7	41.7	16.7	0△
GroupK	12	23.5±1.5△*	100	100	100*	58.3*	33.3	25	16.7	0△
Group CI	15	47.2±2.0**	100	93.3	93.3*	73.3*	66.7*	60*	46.7*	46.7*

Note: ①in Table 1, Group B is the control one bearing cancer; Group F is the treatment group with fetal liver cells; Group G is the treatment group with fetal spleen cells; Group H is the treatment group with fetal thymus cells; Group I is the group of combined treatment of fetal liver and spleen cells; Group J is the group of combined treatment of fetal liver and thymus cells; Group K is the group of combined treatment of fetal spleen and thymus cells; Group CI is the group of combined treatment of fetal liver, spleen and thymus cells; ②*means that comparing the each treatment groups with the control group, P <0.05; **means P <0.01; △ means comparing the treatment groups with Group CI, P <0.01.

2. The curative effect and the analysis on the effect

Table 2 the analysis on the curative effect

Group	N	Curative rate	The rate of apparent effect	Effective rate	Rate of inefficiency	Total effective rate
GroupB	9	$0^{\triangle\triangle}$	0	0	100	0
GroupF	12	$0^{\triangle\triangle}$	0	34.4(4)	66.4(8)	$33.4(4)^{\triangle\triangle}$
GroupG	12	$0^{\triangle\triangle}$	0	25(3)	75(9)	$25(3)^{\triangle\triangle}$
GroupH	12	$0^{\triangle\triangle}$	8.3(1)	33.4(4)	58.3(7)	$41.7(5)^{\triangle *}$
GroupI	12	$0^{\triangle\triangle}$	8.3(1)	33.4(4)	58.3(7)	$41.7(5)^{\triangle *}$
GroupJ	12	$0^{\triangle\triangle}$	26.67(2)	41.7(5)	41.7(5)	$58.3(7)^{*}$
GroupK	12	$0^{\triangle\triangle}$	26.67(2)	33.4(4)	50(6)	$50(6)^{*}$
GroupCI	15	46.7^{**}	13.3(2)	20(3)	20(3)	$80(12)^{**}$

Note: *means $P < 0.05$ compared with the control group, ** means $P < 0.01$ compared with the control group; $\triangle$ means $P < 0.05$ compared with Group CI, $\triangle\triangle$ means $P < 0.01$ compared with Group CI

The standards of curative effects:

① Cure: The tumors regress completely, the suffers regain long-term survival without relapse;

② Apparent effects: The tumors regress partially (the regression rate is more than 50%), and the survival time is more than 2 months;

③ Being effective: The lifetime is prolonged for more than one time without obvious tumor regression.

④ Inefficiency: The tumors grow progressively leading to death in short term (3 to 4 weeks).

According to Table 2, the curative effect of Group CI reaches 46.67%, and is obviously different from other groups with $P < 0.01$. There is no obvious difference among each group as to the rates of apparent effect and being effective respectively. The comparison of the total effective rate shows that except the treatment groups of unitary fetal liver or spleen cells, the total effective rate of all other treatment groups have visible distinction from the control group, with their curative effects being in the rank that the trigeminal is better than the bigeminal which is above the monomial. Moreover, in the groups of monomial cell transplantation, the curative effect of TH cells treatment group is the best, and in the groups of bigeminal cell transplantation, the curative effect of the group containing TH cells is better than that of the groups without TH cells, which indicates that thymus cells play an important role in the course of treatment, but sole liver or spleen cell transplantation have little effects. However, if two of liver, spleen or thymus cells are combined, the curative effect can be improved. And the combination of the three can improve the curative effect significantly.

3. Observing and comparing the growth rate of tumors, the regression and prognosis

In this experiment, the mimic clinical method is used to file case history for all the experimental mice in each groups to record their growth rate of tumors, regression and the prognosis. Measure the average vertical diameter every two days. For the cases of death, all the terminal measured values are regarded as effective sample parameter in the following measures within the same group. After a week from the establishment of the model, tumors grow rapidly with the average vertical diameter being 9.5±1.5mm. After a week from beginning the treatment, tumors continue to grow. Until the second week, the results of each group become differential that the mice bearing tumors have progressive exhaustion with the tumors growing rapidly in the control group; within four weeks, all mice are dead. In the group of sole cell transplantation, the life quality of the experimental mice are improved apparently with their tumors growing slowly, but all the mice bearing cancer die within two months. In the groups of bigeminal cell transplantation, the growths of the tumors are inhibited obviously. Five cases have partial regression but all the mice die with three months. In the group of trigeminal cell transplantation, there are nine cases with apparent tumor putrescence, fall off and ulcer, then scab. In other seven cases, the tumors regress completely, and then canker, scab. In two cases, the regression rate of tumors is more than 50%. As to other cases, except the mice in two cases die in the second and the third week respectively, tumors in the residual cases are in dead state until the death from exhaustion. The sufferers whose tumors regress completely regain long-term survival without relapse for more than six months, and they have normal capacities to become pregnant and give birth. From the above observation, it can be found that the sole or bigeminal cell transplantation is able to inhibit the growth of tumors, improve the life quality and prolong the lifetime; the trigeminal cell transplantation can not only inhibit the growth of tumors, but also result in apparent complete or partial regression and prolong the lifetime.

4. Dynamic observation on the number of T lymphocytes in peripheral blood and the conversion rate of lymphocytes

From table 3 and 4, after a week from the establishment of the model, the cellular immune indexes of the experimental groups decline obviously with the average decrease being more than 50% compared with that of the control group (the number of T cells in the normal group X is 62.5±1.7 and that of lymphocyte transformed X is 66.8±4.8), indicating that the development of tumors does inhibit immune function. After a week from beginning treatment, all immune indexes are improved（P＜0.05）and there are no apparent differential among all treatment groups from the comparison between the treatment groups and the control group as well as the comparison of the indexes before and after the treatment. Seen from the growth of tumors, the immune indexes are improves, but the inhibition of tumors is not apparent. The continuous dynamic observation shows in the groups of sole and bigeminal cell transplantation, the inhibition of tumors and the improvement of immune indexes last for a certain period (3 to 4 weeks), after that period the immune indexes tent to decline, so that the state of the mice bearing cancer deteriorates, which is consistent with the reports on the clinical monitor of immunologic functionand the prognosis. In the group of trigeminal cell transplantation, the immune indexes have persistent improvement, especially the tumors regress obviously. For those who regain long-term survival, the above indexes measured two months later are still close to the indexes of normal mouse. By contrast, for those suffering deterioration, the indexes measured before their deaths have declined below the level before treatment. The above indicates that the cellular immune indexes do reflect the curative effects and can be regarded as a good prove for prognosis; at the same time it can indirectly prove that immunocyte transplantation is able to achieve the aim of immunologic reconstitution for cancer-bearing organisms.

Table 3 dynamic observation on the number of T lymphocytes in peripheral blood (ANAE)

Group	N	The number of T lymphocytes ($\overline{X} \pm S$)							
		n	1 week	n	2 weeks	n	4 weeks	n	6 weeks
GroupB	9	9	3.42±4.8	5	29.1±2.9	1	32	0	
GroupF	12	12	31.4±3.6	10	54.6±5.12$^{\triangle *}$	6	48.7±2.2$^{\triangle}$	4	36.7±4.9
GroupG	12	12	35.5±3.9	9	52.5±4.7$^{\triangle *}$	6	46.6±3.3*	2	33.4±5.1
GroupH	12	12	32.6±4.1	12	56.6±4.1$^{\triangle *}$	7	50.9±2.1$^{\triangle}$	4	40.7±3.8$^{\triangle}$
GroupI	12	12	36.2±2.7	11	53.4±3.5$^{\triangle *}$	6	55.3±3.6$^{\triangle}$	4	39.3±4.2$^{\triangle}$
GroupJ	12	12	30.8±4.3	10	55.8±3.8$^{\triangle *}$	8	56.4±1.9$^{\triangle}$	5	42.6±2.7$^{\triangle}$
GroupK	12	12	33.7±3.4	12	57.3±4.4$^{\triangle *}$	7	55.8±2.8$^{\triangle}$	3	41.3±4.5$^{\triangle}$
GroupCI	15	15	31.8±3.1	14	59.6±2.6$^{\triangle *}$	11	62.5±1.7$^{\triangle}$	9	67.8±3.4$^{\triangle}$

Note: * means P<0.05 compared with the control group; $\triangle$ means P<0.05 in the comparison before and after the treatment

**Table 4 the dynamic observation of the conversion rate
of the lymphocytes in peripheral blood**

Group	N	The conversion rate of lymphocytes ($\overline{X} \pm S$)							
		n	1 week	n	2 weeks	n	4 weeks	n	6 weeks
GroupB	9	9	3.25±5.4	5	25.51±3.6	1	28	0	
GroupF	12	12	31.6±3.7	10	51.2±2.7$^{\triangle *}$	6	54.2±6.1$^{\triangle}$	4	36.1±5.4
GroupG	12	12	29.8±4.3	9	48.4±4.6$^{\triangle *}$	6	52.8±1.8*	2	33.5±2.5
GroupH	12	12	34.1±4.1	12	56.5±2.1$^{\triangle *}$	7	52.4±3.7$^{\triangle}$	4	40.7±1.9$^{\triangle}$
GroupI	12	12	28.5±5.1	11	53.4±3.5$^{\triangle *}$	6	50.5±2.9$^{\triangle}$	4	37.3±3.2$^{\triangle}$
GroupJ	12	12	29.4±2.9	10	58.1±3.5$^{\triangle *}$	8	60.6±3.4$^{\triangle}$	5	46.5±4.5$^{\triangle}$
GroupK	12	12	30.7±1.8	12	54.9±5.2$^{\triangle *}$	7	57.5±4.3$^{\triangle}$	3	45.8±3.9$^{\triangle}$
GroupCI	15	15	31.5±3.2	14	55.8±2.8$^{\triangle *}$	11	63.9±3.2$^{\triangle}$	9	66.8±4.8$^{\triangle}$

Note: * means P<0.05 compared with the control group; $\triangle$ means P<0.05 in the comparison before and after the treatment

5. Anatomic observation of immune organ and comparative analysis of immune organ's green weight

The observation results are seen in table 5 and table 6. In this experiment, in order to see the changes in immune organs of cancer-bearing organisms and the relevance to the curative effects, another near-future observation group of trigeminal cell transplantation is set up (Group CII, n=15, the tumors in six cases regress completely and the regression rates in four cases are more than 50%). After building the model, give the treatment to the mice in Group CII for five times and then execute them. At the same time, set a normal group for comparison, using Hank to simulate the model and execute the mice in the sixth week. Anatomize the mice and observe the changes in their immune organs; measure the green weight of the immune organs and calculate the ratio of immune organs to the body weight; compare the values in Group CII with those of the other groups. From the results, it can be found that in all the cases that in all experimental groups, the tumors develop progressively and lead to death, the thymus shrink apparently and the degree of atrophy is relevant positively to the tumor development. The atrophied thymus is dull-colored and of crisp texture. As to spleen, its change is not as obvious as that of the thymus. In most cases, the spleens are congested and swelling. Only in a few cases the spleens are atrophied. However, in Group CII in all the cases that the tumors regress completely and partially, the thymus and spleens are hypertrophied, so as the indexes of thymus and spleen increase. Through statistical disposition, these indexes are not only differential apparently from the death cases in each group (or the cases without tumor regression), but also different from the normal control group.

Table 5 the comparison of the green weight of the immune organs between the death cases and the normal control group.

Group	N	Thymus(mg)/body weight(g) $\overline{X} \pm S$	spleen(mg)/body weight(g) $\overline{X} \pm S$
Normal	10	2.97±0.38	3.80±0.23
Group B	9	1.02±0.32[**]	4.01±1.32
Group F	8	1.21±0.41[**]	4.213±0.87
Group G	10	1.18±0.46[**]	4.45±1.63
Group H	8	1.28±0.25[**]	4.47±1.24
Group I	8	1.34±0.43[**]	4.67±0.48
Group J	7	1.47±0.28[**]	4.56±0.62
Group J	9	1.43±0.35[**]	4.89±1.47
Group CII	5	1.96±0.37[**]	5.12±1.56

Note: * means P<0.05 compared with the control group; ** means P<0.01 compared with the normal control group

Table 6 the comparison of the green weight between the cases of complete or partial tumor regression and the cases without apparent regression in Group CII

Immune organ(mg/g)	Normal group (N=10, $\overline{X}$ ±S)	Group with tumor regression (N=10, $\overline{X}$ ±S)	Group without tumor regression (N=10, $\overline{X}$ ±S)
thymus	2.79±0.38	4.65±2.21△*△*	1.96±0.37
spleen	3.80±0.23	10.15±2.29△*△*	5.12±1.56

Note: ** means P<0.01 compared with the normal control group; △△means P<0.01 in the comparison between the group with tumor regression and the group without tumor regression.

1. The comparison of pathological examination

In this experiment, anatomize the mice in each group and observe the pathologic section. Observe the tumor soakage and metastasis as well as the changes in immune organs like thymus, spleen, etc. Reserve the viscera like tumor tissue, lung, kidney, thymus and spleen as tissue pathological section for observation. The results show that with the course developing, the range of local tumor soakage expends and the tumor becomes hypertrophied without apparent remote organ metastasis. The thymus shrinks obviously, which has positive relevance to the evolution of the tumor. As to the spleen, it is congested and swelling. In the near-future observation group of trigeminal cell transplantation, the thymus, spleen and liver in the cases of complete or apparent partial regression do not become hypertrophied obviously, which exhibits significant differences from the normal group. When the mice in the cases of complete regression are anatomized, no residual cancer cells can be found in the part of tumor inoculation with both naked eyes and microscope. At the 3rd or 4th week when the tumor putrescence is the most apparent, reserve the tumor tissue as pathological section for observation. It can be found that there are large amount of lymphocytes soakage around the tumor tissue and in the stroma which wrap the tumor tissue resulting a wide range of tumor cells are liquefied and solidified to be dead. The sections of immune organs show that the thickness of the thymus cortical area and the denseness of lymphocytes as well as the increase in epithelial reticular cell, phagocytotic phenomenon and thymus corpuscles. In the spleen, the white pulp area enlarges and the lymph nodes increases, also the lymphocytes become dense. In the control group, the sections of tumor tissue show that the tumor cells soak into the deep-layered muscular tissue and there are cancer embolus formed by tumor cell transplantation in the blood vessels but no lymphocytes soakage. As to the thymus, the cortex atrophy and the cells are sparse, the blood vessels are congested. In the spleen, the amount of lymphocytes decreases significantly and the cells are sparse. In other treatment groups, the tumor sections show that the boundary of the tumor are clear with a little lymphocyte soakage and the changes in thymus and spleen is between the group of trigeminal cell transplantation and the control group. Moreover, the arrangement of the cells is dense with light atrophy.

【Discussion】

1. Therapeutic evaluation

It can be found from the results of the above experiment that the adoptive immunological therapy through transplantation of immunocyte with the origin of embryo can inhibit the growth of tumor and improve the life quality in different extend and force the tumor to regress completely or partially, and then improve the immune indexes apparently and prolong the lifetime, which indicates that immunocyte transplantation with the origin of embryo can reconstitute the anti- carcinomatous immunologic functionfor cancer-bearing organisms. The combined reconstitution of central immunity and the peripheral immunity at the same time is the best and better than the partial reconstitution of bigeminal and monomial cell transplantation.

2. Possible mechanism

The possible mechanisms to take effect are mainly the following: ①After the cancer-bearing organisms accept the same kind of xenogenous embryo cell transplantation, the immune system of the organism gets non-specific simulation to produce immune hyperplasia so as to improve the immunologic function to resist tumors. ②Cell transplantation belongs to organ transplantation, which can keep active for a certain period of time in the acceptor. By immunocyte transplantation with the origin of embryo, fetal liver cells can provide stem lymphocytes, which is combined with thymus and spleen cell transplantation so as to achieve the combined reconstitution of central immunity and peripheral immunity and enable the organism to gain adoptive immunity. A large number of researches home and abroad on the proliferation, differentiation and function of fetal immune organs and histiocytes show that when fetal immune organs are in their 16 weeks, they put up obvious proliferation to the original simulation of division, which becomes more intensive in the 24th week. In the 8th week of pregnancy, lymph tissue begins to emerge in the fetal thymus and lymph nodes as well as the cells with secretion in the 20th week. All these researches indicate that fetal immunocytes are able to bring immunoreaction into play. ③Some researches show that both the supernatant liquid from fetal thymus tissue cultivated outside the body and thymus extractive have the ability to promote the formation rate of the acceptor's E- wreath and the transformation of lymphocytes obviously. Therefore, fetal immunocyte transplantation can strengthen the cellular immunity of the cancer-bearing organism for cancer-bearing organism. ④ low immunogen of the fetal organs and the homology between the transplanted fetal organs and the acceptor's immune organs are in favor of forming immunologic tolerance to the transplanted for the acceptor, which can not only avoid rejection or have light rejection, but also simulate each other to achieve synergetic effects so as to reconstitute immunity. Moreover, as the curative effects of the trigeminal cell transplantation group are much better than those of the other groups, it is be believed that the effects result from the relatively complete reconstitution of central immunity and peripheral immunity at the same time which lead to the synergetic effects. In a word, the mechanism is much more complex than the above mentioned. It will be useful to step further to make the mechanism clear if the level of the immune factors that are closely relevant to anti-tumor immunity like IL-2, TNF, INF, etc. and the activity of the immunocytes that relate directly to anti-tumor immunity like NK, LAK, TIL, etc. in peripheral blood can be detected and the transplanted cells can be marked to make clear their distribution and survival inside the acceptor.

1. Problems about the barrier of transplantation

Although fetal organs have low immunogen, it is still impossible to avoid rejection, just in different degree. Therefore, the problem about the barrier of transplantation exists and directly relate to the success of transplantation and that whether the transplant can continue to act inside the acceptor. In this experiment, the animals used belong to the hybrid species in closed flock, which ensures largely that the mice in each experimental group have relatively close genetic background. It is probably the important reason for the success of transplantation with tissue matching except the low immunogen of embryonic tissue. Apart from those, it is possible that the mismatch of histocompatibility leads to the cases with inconspicuous curative effects in Group CI and Group CII. Thus, the key of improving curative effects may lie in studying and solving the barrier of transplantation.

2. The choice of the approach and method of transplantation

The transplantations of fetal immune organs from the level of cells, to tissue, then to the level of entire organ belong to adoptive immunity. In terms of the current repots, for fetal liver and spleen, blood cell transplantation is the best; for thymus, spleen and tissue, omentum embedding is the best. Although the technique of cell transplantation is simple and easy to be successful, it can only last for a short time. Therefore, the best approach of transplantation needs further observation and research.

II. The Progress of Study on Treatment of Tumor by Adoptive Immunity through Transplantation of Immunocyte with the Origin of Embryo

According to a large amount of clinical and experimental researches, the immunity of the tumor-bearing organisms tent to be in progressive inhibition with the course the disease. So how to reconstitute the anti-tumor immunity is the core of the research on immunological therapy. In 1980s, the fourth generation of tumor treatment mode, namely biological treatment of tumor, brought tumor therapeutics into a new era, when the adoptive immunotherapy was the most outstanding achievement. For those whose tumors were in the advanced stage, several kinds of the conventional therapies were of no effects. However, adoptive immunotherapy of LAK, TIL and gene-modified TIL, which is represented by Rosenberg gained prominent curative effects, attracting the attention all over the world. In this technique, it is needed to gain a great amount of artificial synthesized IL-2 with high purity by biotechnology and plentiful immune competent cells through cultivate and proliferation in vitro in a long term to reach the aim, so the cost was very expensive. Currently, this project is still in depth research. As only a few institutes at home have developed the research in this area, there is no doubt that the above mentioned therapy is an extremely prominent research direction in treatment of tumor, however it is some difficult to become popularized in China. Besides, treatment of tumor by adoptive immunity through transplantation of immune cells, tissue and organs with the origin of embryo is another prominent research in the treatment of tumor by adoptive immunity, which is featured by simple technique, low cost and popularity. In recent years, some researchers have used embryonic liver, spleen and thymus to do transplantation from the level of cellular tissue to organs with vessel pedicles, which has been applied in the treatment of advanced malignant tumor gaining some curative effects, and paid much attention gradually.

i. Research status of fetal liver cell transplantation (FLT)

In 1958, Uphoff was the first one to fetal liver cells into the mice who died from ray of fatal dose with the remarkable effects of regaining hematopiesis. From then on, that fetal cell transplantation can be applied in curing the diseases in hemopoietic system and in the therapy of regaining hematopiesis after chemotherapy and radiotherapy for those with malignant tumors is researched extensively. In the following researches it has been found that FLT can not only reconstitute hematopiesis, but also reconstitute immunity. Wu Zuze and other researchers have found that FLT is able to reconstitute T and B lmphyocytes. They have also found that founder cells in fetal liver and spleen nodes are possessed with the basic features of several kinds of hematopoietic stem cells or lymph myeloid stem cells through the comparative research on the proliferation and differentiation between fetal liver cells and myeloid hematopoietic stem cell. Fetal liver cells contain a small amount of macrophages and lymphocytes. After 5 months from being pregnant, the amount of T lymphocytes begins to increase gradually, which is thought to be the substantial foundation of applying FLT to cure hematopoietic disorders immunologic deficiency disease to reconstitute hematopiesis and immunity. These features of fetal liver cells, especially the ability to reconstitute immunity make FLT play an important role in improving immunity. In recent years, there have been more and more researches on applying FLT to treatment of tumor.

ii. Research status of treatment of tumor through fetal spleen cell transplantation

1. Research on the relationship between spleen and the growth of tumor

It has been thirty years since Old and others began to study the influence of spleen to the growth of tumor. During this period, many scholars have done a large number of experiments and clinical researches on the effect of spleen in anti-tumor immunity, but they can not get a consistent conclusion as they hold that spleen has both positive and negative effects on anti-tumor immunity. With more deep researches on splenic surgery and its function, most scholars tent to confirm the anti-tumor immune function. As spleen is the biggest immune organ in bodies, it is the place where Th and Ts cells become mature. The antibodies, Fibronetin, Tufftsinr-1NF and IL-2, etc. immune factors secreted by Th and Ts cells as well as killer cells like LAK and NK, etc. play an crucial role in anti-tumor immunity. Ge Yigong, etc. have found when researching the effect of ablating spleen to the growth of W256 rat's sarcoma that in the group of spleen ablation, the survival rate of the tumor inoculation and the diameter of tumor are higher apparently than those of the control group. Meanwhile, in the former group, the postoperative changes of T cell subgroup in peripheral blood are manifested by the reduction in T and Th cells and slight increase in Ts cells which is on the low level continuously after inoculation and have remarkable differential from the group without tumor and the tumor-bearing control group($P < 0.001$). That is consistent with the research on the effects of spleen to the growth of tumor that was done before. They have also found that after ablating spleen, there was positive correlation between the decline in the ratio of Th/Ts in T cell subgroup and the diffuse and metastasis of tumor. Lersch has reported that lymphocytes inside the spleen of tumor-bearing mice decline progressively with the growth of tumor, which is consistent with the experimental results mentioned above. All these researches can indicate that spleen plays an important role in anti-tumor immunity.

2. Researches on treatment of tumor through fetal spleen cell transplantation

Based on the understanding of the action of spleen in anti-tumor immunity, many scholars have begun to develop the experimental and clinical researches on treatment of tumor through fetal spleen cell or tissue transplantation. Ma Xuxian, etc. report that fetal spleen cell transplantation has been used in nine cases of advanced malignant tumor. All sufferers in these cases feel better after the treatment. The author also has found that fetal spleen cell transplantation can inhibit the growth of tumor apparently when studying the effects of spleen to the growth of tumor. What's more, some scholar has studied the feature and approach of fetal spleen transplantation and found that transplantation through vein is the best, intramuscular injection and celiac injection follow. For tissue transplantation, omentum embedding is the best; both HVGR and GVHR are few. The mechanism of spleen cell transplantation is still in research.

iii. Research status of treatment of tumor through fetal thymus transplantation

Among immune organs, thymus has the closest relation to anti-tumor immunity and the researches on thymus are the most profound. Thymus plays a decisive role in cellular immunity and even the entire immunoregulation as thymus is the central immune organ where T cells develop and grow up.

1. Research on the relationship between thymus and the growth of tumor

The function of thymus has close connection with the occurrence of tumor that can lead to thymus atrophy, low level of thymosin or lack of analogous thymic factor. For those experimental animals, that the thymus are ablated or irradiated by dead dose ray can promote the tumor metastasis. Therefore, fetal thymus transplantation or thymic epithelial cell transplantation as well as injection of thymosin can put off thymus atrophy and reconstitute immune function. The above researches indicate that thymus plays an extremely important role in anti-tumor immunity.

2. The application of fetal thymus transplantation in treatment of tumor

Many scholars have done plentiful researches on treatment of tumor through fetal thymus transplantation. Zhou Shifu, etc. have performed the treatment of tumor through fetal thymus transplantation for 14 tumor cases. After 46 hours, the immune indexes have been improved and the conditions of the sufferers have been remitted and improved. Song Ruze, etc. have used the treatment of advanced malignant tumor through fetal thymus tissue omentum transplantation and gained the same curative effects. Liu Dungui, etc. have used cell transplantation, tissue transplantation and transplantation of thymus with vessel pedicle to treat advanced liver cancer resulting in that tumors in some cases shrunk significantly and the lifetime was prolonged for six months. All these can indicate that fetal thymus transplantation is an effective approach of immunotherapy of tumor.

Moreover, some scholars have studied on the features of the immune organs in different ages with the origin of embryo like the activity and the saving time, etc. They have found that the activity of fetal organs after five months' pregnancy is best. The researches on the approach of transplantation show that fetal liver and spleen cell transplantation through vein is the best, and omentum embedding is best for spleen and thymus tissue transplantation.

All these researches provide precious theoretic and experimental basis for treatment of tumor by adoptive immunity through immune organ transplantation with the origin of embryo and contribute to further studies.

5. TG'S INHIBITION ON ANGIOGENESIS OF TRANSPLANTATION TUMOR OF MICE

Since Folkman presented the concept that the growth of tumor depends on vascularization in 1971, the following researches further confirm that angiogenesis is a key factor for the growth of tumor. Thereafter researchers have brought forth the concept of anti-angiogenic therapy, that is, by preventing neovascularization and (or) spread of new-born rete vasculosum and (or) destroying new-born blood vessels to stop the production or establishment of small solid tumor, and finally to prevent the growth, evolution and metastasis of tumor. At present, foreign experts have done a lot of studies in this respect and made gratifying progress. Therefore anti-angiogenic therapy is expected to be an effective means to cure tumor. But domestic relative studies start fairly late; and very few reports are given to it except some counts about capillary density of tumor tissues.

Along with the deepening research of Common Threewingnut Root, its new pharmacological actions are constantly to be found, such as anti-tumor action and two-way regulating action on immune system. Especially the recently discovered Common Threewingnut Root, which inhibits in vitro the formation of lumen that induced by the migration, proliferation and differentiation of vascular endothelium cells, has a better inhibiting action on neovascularization. In order to further explore the inhibiting action of Common Threewingnut Root on new-born blood vessels of tumor in vivo, the writer adopts transplantation tumor model of mouse's abdominal muscles. Based on the observation of formation characteristics of tumor blood vessel and its relation with tumor, researchers' new findings in recent years and the writer's experimental results both prove that Common Threewingnut Root has the two-way regulating action with dose dependent on immune system. Choose adequate doses of TG with no effect on the body's immune function to carry out the experimental study of TG's inhibiting action on new-born blood vessels of transplantation tumor of mouse's abdominal muscles. The study is to know about TG's inhibiting capability on tumor angiogenesis, which can provide experimental references for further anti-tumor study in terms of blood vessels.

I. Experimental Study on Observation of Angiogenesis of Transplantation Tumor at Mouse's Abdominal Muscle

This experiment depends on the anatomical position and structural features of mouse's abdominal muscle, adopts EAC transplantation tumor model of abdominal muscle, fixes and displays blood vessels with transparent specimen, which are all for finding out the formation characteristics of tumor blood vessel and its relation with tumor.

[Material and Method]

1. Materials

   (1) Animals: 20 Kunming mice, 18~22g, a 50:50 proportion of male and female.
   (2) Cancer-bearing mouse: Kunming mouse with the intraperitoneal inoculation of EAC cells.
   (3) Instrument and apparatus: mouse retaining plate, 1ml injector, test tube and heparin tube, glass slide, ophthalmic scissors, microsurgery scissors and surgical clamps, small cutting needle, 1-0 silk thread, ophthalmic needle holder, glass petri dish, light microscope, Olympus Japanese microscopic observation and photographic system of type BH-2.
   (4) Reagent: Wright stain, 0.2% physiological saline of trypan blue, Hank solution, depilatory, 1% pentobarbitale sodium solution, 10% formaldehyde solution, tertiary butyl alcohol solution of 70%, 80%, 90%, 95% and 100%, methyl salicylate.

2. Method

   (1) Prepare EAC cell suspension (6.0×10^7/ml): Aseptically draw ascites of cancer-bearing mouse with the inoculation for 7~9d; put ascites in a sterile tube; draw another little ascites in a heparin tube for cell count; store tubes in ice blocks. Drop remaining ascites in the empty needle on a glass slide, cover with another slide and stain the specimen with Wright stain, finally use it for differential counting of cells, the proportion of cancer cells $\geqq$ 95% (if insufficient, choose another cancer-bearing mouse). Dilute ascites in the heparin tube with physiological saline to 10 times and 100 times; respectively take 0.95ml blending with 0.1ml trypan blue physiological saline of 0.2%; use the counting method of white blood cells to count the total number of tumor cells and dead tumor cells, calculate the survival rate, which should be $\geqq$ 95% (if insufficient, choose another cancer-bearing mouse). Finally dilute ascites in the tube with sterile pre-cooling Hank solution to 6.0×10^7/ml and use it for the inoculation.
   (2) Inoculation in the area of peritoneum: Use depilatory in advance to clean a mouse's ventral seta two days ago; anaesthetize it injecting with 1% pentobarbitale sodium (0.3mg/10g weight) into the abdominal cavity; lie on its back and fix it on mouse retaining plate; sterilize the abdominal skin; cut open the skin about 1.2cm long from the middlemost place about 1cm below the processus xiphoideus; conduct the blunt separation to one side gently and carefully, then find an area on this side with few blood vessels in the abdominal muscle; inoculate 0.04ml EAC cell suspension with the concentration of 6.0×10^7/ml, then present a full small "swelling" without any collapse, which explains the correct inoculation location without penetrating the peritoneum. Finally stitch the skin and isolate this mouse for protection until it regains consciousness safely.

   Note: During the process of inoculation, always store the test tube with cancer cell suspension in ice blocks so as to ensure the constant survival rate. And also require a fast and stable manipulation.

(3) Group and make transparent specimen: 20 inoculated mice, randomly divide into 10 groups with 2 mice of each group. Since the first day after the inoculation, pull off the cervical vertebra to execute one group each day for making transparent specimen. The specific making procedures are as follows.

Submerge and fix the execute mice in formaldehyde solution with the concentration of 10% for 24h. Take out the mice, cut open their skin, peel off the whole abdominal muscle membrane, rinse it with distilled water for 1 min, and submerge it orderly in the tertiary butyl alcohol with different concentration (70%, 80%, 90%, 95% and 100%) to dehydrate for 6~8h. Finally submerge it directly into the methyl salicylate until the tissue is completely transparent.

(4) Observe and shoot tumor vessels: Use Olympus microscope of type BH-2 to observe the transparent specimen in the small petri dish with methyl salicylate. Note the shape, quantity and distribution of new born capillary around tumor tissues and in the tumor. Then take microscopic photos and use Olympus microcirculation microscopic photographic system to observe the flow rate of new born capillaries.

[Experimental Result]

On the first day after the inoculation, there is no new born vessel in the inoculation area, around which the original host's capillaries slightly exude. On the second day, tumor cell mass swells. It is clear that original host's capillaries put forth slim but crooked new vessels, which invade into the tumor. There is no continued vessel segment. On the third and fourth day, the tumor tissue has a further growth. The density of new vessels outside the tumor increases; the caliber is irregular; vessels array in disorder. In the tumor, incontinuous and imperfect new vessels with maldistribution and various thicknesses are obviously in the direction of muscle fiber. Some vessels are comma-shaped or bud-shaped, and irregular bud-shaped vessels connect each vessel. On the fifth and sixth day, the tumor presents the progressive growth. Capillaries outside the tumor twist or distend or cluster to distribute with various thicknesses; vessels in the tumor start to interlace with each other or show irregular sinusoid dilatation. On the seventh and eighth day, the color in the tumor becomes red. Capillaries outside the tumor distend, twist and come in different shape and size; in the tumor only a few incontinuous and short vessels present an irregular distribution, most vessels have no any figure and fuse in the shape of flake or mass. On the ninth and tenth day, there is only a red mass-shaped zone in the tumor, which is fused by vessels. Brown area of hemorrhage and necrosis appears in the centre of the tumor. Vessels with extreme dilatation and distortional appearance can be made out in some areas.

Transplantation tumor model of mouse's abdominal muscles helps to have a more intuitional observation, from inflammation changes of stimulating the angiogenesis since the first day after inoculation to tumor vessels that gradually appear later. It reflects the formation characteristics of tumor's new-born capillaries and their relations with the tumor. That is, new-born capillaries generally register as the abnormal route, irregular arrangement, irregular diameter, the lack of continuity and integrity, and even comma-shaped or bud-shaped immature differentiation and growth. The relation between capillaries and tumor is the continued proliferation and enlargement of tumor cell cluster along with the formation and growth of new-born capillaries in the inoculation area. Simultaneously, the tumor mass characterized by progressive growth causes the blood vessels in the central part to bear the rise in blood pressure, dilatation, and necrosis, which appear as a red fused mass.

II. Experimental Study on Effects of TG with Different Dosages on Immunologic Function of Mice

In recent years, reports about Common Threewingnut Root having the two-way regulating action with dose dependent on immune system have continued to arise. TG is a refined product that separated and abstracted repeatedly from the crude drug—Common Threewingnut Root. In order to have a better understanding of the two-way regulating action, this experiment chooses three different doses of TG to act on the phagocytic function of mice celiac macrophages ($M\Phi$) and immune organs. Their drug reactions can basically reflect TG's effect on the immune function of mice.

TG's effect on the phagocytic function of mice celiac macrophages ($M\Phi$)

[Material and Method]

1. Materials

  (1) Animals: 40 Kunming mice, 18~22g, a 50:50 proportion of male and female.
  (2) Drugs and reagents: ① TG turbid liquor: Pulverize TG tablets; use 0.5% Carboxythmethyl Cellulose (CMC) to respectively prepare turbid liquors of three different concentrations, TG_1 10mg/10ml, TG_2 10mg/20ml and TG_3 40mg/10ml; ② 0.5% CMC solution; ③ 2% chicken red blood cell (CRBC) suspension: Sterile venous sampling of 2ml under the chicken wing; put the blood sample in a heparin tube; clean it for three times with physiological saline; after centrifugation, abandon the supernatant fluid and white blood cell layer at the interface; when the specific volume of blood cells keeps stable, use physiological saline to prepare 2% (V/V) red cell suspension; ④ Sterile calf serum; ⑤ 1:1 acetone- methanol solution; ⑥ 4% (V/V) Giemsa-phosphate buffer.
  (3) Instrument and apparatus: Gastric lavage needle, thermotank, and for the rest, please sees "Experimental Study on Observation of Angiogenesis of Transplantation Tumor at Mouse's Abdominal Muscle".

2. Method

  (1) Grouping: 40 mice are randomly divided into 4 groups with 10 mice of each group, group TG_1, TG_2, TG_3 and control group.
  (2) Gastric lavage: According to the proportion of 0.2ml/10g (weight), respectively inject TG suspension into the stomach with corresponding concentrations (group TG_1 20mg/kg, TG_2 40mg/kg and TG_3 80mg/kg) and 0.5% CMC solution for 12 days.

(3) Induction and functional examination of celiac MΦ: On the tenth day after gastric lavage, sterile injection of 0.5ml calf serum into each mouse's abdominal cavity. On the thirteenth day, inject 1ml CRBC suspension with the concentration of 2% into each mouse's abdominal cavity. 30min later pull off the cervical vertebra to execute the mouse. Cut open the abdominal wall skin from the middlemost place. Inject 2ml physiological saline into the abdominal cavity and turn the mouse's body. Aspirate 1ml celiac lotion, averagely drop it on two glass slides and put slides into an enamel box with wet paper cloth. 30 min after moving the box into 37°C thermotank for warm cultivation, rinse the two glass slides with celiac lotion in physiological saline, dry by airing, fix in 1:1 acetone- methanol solution, dye them with 4% Giemsa-phosphate buffer, rinse with distilled water and dry by airing. Finally conduct the count of MΦ (200 MΦ on each slide) under the oil immersion lens of microscope. See the following mathematical equation to calculate the phagocytose percentage.

$$\text{Phagocytose Percentage} = \frac{\text{Amounts of } M\Phi \text{ that phagocytizes CRBC}}{200 \ M\Phi} \times 100\%$$

(4) Statistical treatment: The data is represented by average ± standard error ($\overline{X} \pm S$), and analyzed by *t* test.

[Experimental Result]

Determination result about TG's effect on the phagocytic function of mice celiac MΦ can be seen in table 1.

Table1 TG's effect on the phagocytic function of mice celiac MΦ ($\overline{X} \pm S$)

Group	Dosage(mg/kg)	Case load	Amounts of MΦ that phagocytizes CRBC (%)
Control group	-	10	44.83±0.41
TG$_1$	20	10	47.20±0.35*
TG$_2$	40	10	45.72±0.25
TG$_3$	80	10	44.40±0.45*

Note: Compare to the control group, *$P<0.05$

As seen from the table 1, in low doses of 20mg/kg, TG can obviously activate the phagocytic function of MΦ ($P<0.05$); in median doses of 40mg/kg, TG has no obvious effect on the phagocytic function of MΦ ($P>0.05$); in high doses of 80mg/kg, TG will inhibit the phagocytic function of MΦ ($P<0.05$). The above results indicate that TG can affect the phagocytic function of mice celiac MΦ and have the obvious characteristic of dose dependent, that is along with the gradual increase of TG dosage, the phagocytic function of mice celiac MΦ can respectively present three different effects of being activated, no obvious effect and inhibition.

TG's effect on immune organs of young mice

[Material and Method]

1. Materials

   (1) Animals: 40 three-aged Kunming mice, 10~12g, a 50:50 proportion of male and female.
   (2) Drugs and reagents: TG suspension and 0.5% CMC solution: Preparation is same as stated before.
   (3) Instrument and apparatus: Analytical balance and for the rest, please sees "Experimental Study on Observation of Angiogenesis of Transplantation Tumor at Mouse's Abdominal Muscle".

2. Method

   (1) Grouping and gastric lavage: see "Experimental Study on Observation of Angiogenesis of Transplantation Tumor at Mouse's Abdominal Muscle".
   (2) Weighing of thymus gland and spleen: On the thirteenth day after the experiment, pull off the cervical vertebra to execute the young mouse. Cut open its skin, chest cavity and abdominal cavity. Excise the whole thymus gland and spleen. Use filter papers to suck dry the blood and finally weigh thymus gland and spleen on an analytical balance.
   (3) Statistical treatment: The data is represented by average ± standard error (**<IMAGE>**±S), and analyzed by *t* test.

[Experimental Result]

Weighing results of thymus gland and spleen can be seen in table2. As seen from the table 2, TG at different dosages has different effect on immune organs of young mice. In low doses of 20mg/kg, TG can stimulate the weight gain of young mouse's thymus gland ($P<0.05$); in median doses of 40mg/kg, though there is a trend in weight loss, no obvious difference exists when compared with control group ($P>0.05$); in high doses of 80mg/kg, thymus gland appears as obvious atrophia compared with control group ($P<0.01$). Only in high doses, TG can inhibit the growth of young mouse's spleen ($P<0.05$); while in median and low doses, there is no obvious effect ($P>0.05$).

Table2 TG's effect on immune organs of young mice ($\overline{X}$ ±S)

Group	Dosage(mg/kg)	Case load	Thymic weight (mg/10g weight)	Spleen weight (mg/10g weight)
Control group	-	10	26.38±1.22	70.43±0.76
TG$_1$	20	10	30.20±0.74*	72.65±0.83
TG$_2$	40	10	23.48±0.88	69.88±0.56
TG$_3$	80	10	21.12±0.76**	68.44±0.42*

Note: Compare to the control group, *$P<0.05$, ** $P<0.01$

Experiments about TG's effect on the phagocytic function of mice celiac MΦ and weight of young mice's immune organs can basically reflect TG's two-way regulating action with dose dependent on mice's immune function. That is, along with the gradual increase of TG dosage, there are three different immune effects of enhancement, no obvious effect and inhibition. It prompts that the application range of TG can be expanded by different effects of choosing different dosages of TG on immune system.

III. Experimental Study on Inhibition of TG of Different Dosages on Angiogenesis of Transplantation Tumor at Mouse's Abdominal Muscle

i. Observation on new-born capillaries of transplantation tumor at mouse's abdominal muscle

Researches in recent years have found that Common Threewingnut Root has the characteristic of inhibiting migration and proliferation of endothelial cell to suppress angiogenesis. In order to have a further exploration of its inhibiting action on tumor angiogenesis, this experiment bases on the previous experiment and chooses adequate doses of TG (40mg/kg) that have no effect on mice's immune function. Through observation in vivo by microcirculation microscope, experts can carry out an experimental study on angiogenesis of transplantation tumor at mouse's abdominal muscle.

[Material and Method]

1. Materials

   (1) Animals: 40 Kunming mice, 18~22g, a 50:50 proportion of male and female.
   (2) 6.0×10^7/ml EAC cell suspension; see [Experiment 1] for preparation.
   (3) 20mg/10mg TG suspension and 0.5% CMC solution; see [Experiment 2] for preparation.
   (4) HH-1 microcirculation detection system (microcirculation microscope, photomicrography system and display system, video light mark blood flow meter, etc.), other required reagents and instruments are same as those mentioned in the previous experiment.

2. Method

   (1) Inoculation: see this chapter "Experimental Study on Observation of Angiogenesis of Transplantation Tumor at Mouse's Abdominal Muscle".
   (2) Grouping: 40 inoculated tumor-bearing mice are randomly divided into medication administration group and control group with 20 mice of each group. Then each group is also randomly divided into four groups with 5mice of each group, which is the third day, sixth day, ninth day and twelfth day.
   (3) Gastric lavage: Since the first day after inoculation, medication administration group and control group begin to undergo the gastric lavage of 20mg/ml TG suspension and 0.5% CMC solution according as the proportion of 0.2ml/10g (weight).
   (4) Observation of new-born tumor capillaries: Respectively on the third day, sixth day, ninth day and twelfth day, observe new-born capillaries of tumor at mouse's abdominal muscle among

the proper group of medication administration group and control group (groups of the third day, sixth day, ninth day and twelfth day). Specific method and procedure are as follows: ① Carry out the anesthesia with the injection of 1% sodium pentobarbital (0.3mg/10g weight) in abdominal cavity before operation, carefully cut open the skin below the processus xiphoideus to the lower abdomen, conduct blunt separation of skin to the middle axillary line of one side, and then cut open the abdominal muscle along the white line. This operation should be careful and gentle. If there is a little oozing of blood, use small gauze dipped in tepid physiological saline to stanch the bleeding. ② Make the mouse lie on side on the self-made observation platform, overturn the abdominal muscle that is detached from one side of the skin, and fix incision edge on the outer margin of the window of observation platform, which lets the half-side abdominal muscle cover the whole window and makes the tumor mass be located in the middle of the window. ③ Put the observation platform with mouse on the microscope carrier that is in a thermotank (Refer to the preparation of Tian Niu and make an improvement), and drop 37°C Ringer-Locke liquor in the overturned abdominal muscle to moisten it. ④ Start the cold light source and bring into focus for observation.

(5) Observation project: Use HH-1 microcirculation detection system to observe the shape and quantity of new-born capillaries in and around the tumor, and take microscopic photos. Measure the density of new-born capillaries which enter and leave the tumor, as well as the average diameter and flow rate of tumor arterioles and venules. Use a vernier caliper to measure the maximum diameter and transverse diameter of tumor, and calculate its maximum transverse section.

(6) Statistical treatment: The data is represented by average ± standard error (**<IMAGE>**±S), and analyzed by *t* test.

[Experimental Result]

1. Changes in the shape and quantity of new-born capillaries in and around the tumor. See table 3.
2. The density of new-born capillaries which enter and leave the tumor (the number of new-born capillaries around tumor cell cluster/mm^2). See table 4.

The above results indicate that the density of new-born tumor capillaries of group TG is obviously lower than that of control group ($P<0.05$), which shows that TG has an inhibiting action on tumor vascularization. Especially on the third and sixth day, this manifestation is more apparent ($P<0.05$). The angiogenesis speed of control group is faster during the previous six days, but then it gradually slows down. While the angiogenesis speed of group TG during the previous six days is slower than that during the next six days and capillaries are obviously smaller that those of control group, indicating that TG significantly slows down angiogenesis speed during the previous six days and suppresses the angiogenesis. During the next six days, the angiogenesis speed of group TG gradually increases to that of control group on the tenth day to twelfth day. It shows that during the next six days TG's inhibiting action on tumor vascularization begins to remit. But as seen from table 25-4, on the twelfth day the density of new-born tumor capillaries of group TG is still obviously below that of control group, indicating that the comprehensive effect of drugs still appears as the inhibition of tumor vascularization up to now.

Table 3 TG's effect on the shape and quantity of new-born capillaries in and around the tumor

Observation Date	Control Group	Medication Administration Group of TG
The Third Day	Obvious, unbalanced and new-born capillaries in the tumor; unbalanced and crooked capillaries around the tumor; capillaries unevenly enter and leave the tumor. The whole tumor body is light red.	No crooked new-born capillaries enter and leave the tumor; capillaries around the tumor grow straight in the original direction; no obvious, unbalanced and new-born capillaries in the tumor. The whole tumor body is milky white.
The Sixth Day	Abundant capillaries with various thicknesses around the tumor branch from minute blood vessels of the host, twist into the tumor and form a nodular capillary network, which make the whole tumor body become light red.	Slender earthworm-shaped capillaries grow around the tumor; there are new-born capillaries without dilatation and distortion in the tumor. The whole tumor body is light red.
The Ninth Day	Abundant twisty and spreading capillaries grow around the tumor; abundant unbalanced and new-born capillaries appear in the tumor and intertwine with each other to form the shape of fasciculation and twist. There are new-born vascular buds resembling a pointed cone or cyst. The whole tumor is flesh-colored.	A small quantity of new-born circuitous capillaries start to grow around the tumor; capillaries in tumor grow in number and begin the irregular dilatation. The whole tumor body is light red.
The Twelfth Day	Abundant capillaries around the tumor look like a string of beads, or intertwine with each other to cause an irregular arrangement, or penetrate the tumor and form into concentrated clumps; capillaries in the tumor extremely distend and fuse into the shape of mass or anal sinus, which form a vast light-tight area of hemorrhage and necrosis in the centre of the tumor. The whole tumor body is maroon.	New-born slender capillaries around the tumor grow in number without interlaced phenomenon. Capillaries in the tumor distend and fuse, but there is no the area of hemorrhage and necrosis. The whole tumor is flesh-colored.

Table 4 TG's effect on the density (the amount of capillaries/ mm^2) of new-born tumor capillaries ($\overline{X}$ ±S)

Group	Case load	The Third Day	The Sixth Day	The Ninth Day	The Twelfth Day
Control Group	5	3.40±0.14	8.34±1.05	11.26±1.28	13.1±0.90
TG Group	5	1.84±0.12**	3.64±0.64**	6.58±1.20*	9.90±0.92

Note: Compare to the control group, *P<0.05, ** P<0.01

3. The average diameter and flow rate of tumor arterioles and venules

Results can be seen in the table 5, 6, 7 and 8.

Table 5 TG's effect on the diameter (μm) of tumor arterioles ($\overline{X}$ ±S)

Group	Case load	The Third Day	The Sixth Day	The Ninth Day	The Twelfth Day
Control Group	5	15.0±0.71	18.8±1.07	20.8±0.84	21.4±0.75
TG Group	5	14.2±0.97	19.0±1.14	18.0±0.71*	19.2±0.58*

Table 6 TG's effect on the diameter (μm) of tumor venules ($\overline{X}$ ±S)

Group	Case load	The Third Day	The Sixth Day	The Ninth Day	The Twelfth Day
Control Group	5	22.6±0.68	24.0±0.71	25.6±0.51	26.8±0.58
TG Group	5	22.4±0.93	23.2±0.86	23.4±0.75*	19.2±0.68*

Table 7 TG's effect on the flow rate (mm/s) of tumor arterioles ($\overline{X}$ ±S)

Group	Case load	The Third Day	The Sixth Day	The Ninth Day	The Twelfth Day
Control Group	5	0.42±0.014	0.45±0.022	0.39±0.011	0.36±0.015
TG Group	5	0.43±0.018	0.47±0.013	0.42±0.012	0.41±0.013*

Table 8 TG's effect on the flow rate (mm/s) of tumor venules ($\overline{X}$ ±S)

Group	Case load	The Third Day	The Sixth Day	The Ninth Day	The Twelfth Day
Control Group	5	0.35±0.016	0.32±0.014	0.28±0.014	0.23±0.016
TG Group	5	0.34±0.014	0.35±0.013	0.32±0.012	0.29±0.015*

Note: Compare to the control group, *P<0.05

As seen from the above tables, on the ninth and twelfth day, diameters of tumor arterioles and venules of TG group are obviously thinner than those of the control group ($P<0.05$); on the third and sixth day, there is no significant difference between the two groups ($P>0.05$). On the twelfth day, flow rates of tumor arterioles and venules of TG group are faster than those of the control group ($P<0.05$); on the third, sixth and ninth day, there is no significant difference between the two groups ($P>0.05$). It indicates that TG also has an influence on minute blood vessels (feeding the tumor) of the original host. Especially during an advanced stage, narrowing the diameter and quickening the flow rate can affect the amount of tumor blood supply.

4. The maximum cross section of tumor

Results can be seen in the table 9.

Table 9 TG's effect on the tumor size (<IMAGE>±S, mm)

Group	Case load	The Third Day	The Sixth Day	The Ninth Day	The Twelfth Day
Control Group	5	9.46±0.65	21.78±1.90	34.11±1.62	65.99±2.21
TG Group	5	4.91±0.76**	14.01±1.27**	27.09±2.16*	62.64±2.45

Note: Compare to the control group, *$P<0.05$, ** $P<0.01$

The above results indicate that in the previous nine days TG inhibits the growth of tumor ($P<0.05$); especially in the previous six days, this effect is more obvious ($P<0.06$). On the twelfth day, there is no significant difference between the tumor size of TG group and that of control group ($P>0.05$). It prompts that TG can obviously inhibit the growth of tumor in an early stage. While in the middle-late stage, this effect decreases. Finally in the advance stage, there is no significant inhibiting action.

Determination of plasma endothelin (ET) in mice with transplantation tumor at abdominal muscle

ET is a kind of biologically active peptide synthesized by epidermic cells with extensive biological effects. Recently, increasing researches indicate that ET has an intimate relation with the growth and development of tumor, and also can participate in and promote the vascularization. In order to have a further understanding of tumor, ET and TG's effect on ET of tumor mice, experts carry out the following experiments.

[Material and Method]

1. Materials

(1) Animals: 60 Kunming mice, 18~22g, a 50:50 proportion of male and female.
(2) EAC cell suspension of 6.0×10^7/ml, 20mg/10ml TG suspension and 0.5% CMC solution: Preparation is same as stated before.

(3) Endothelin radioimmunoassay kit.

(4) The gamma (γ) radioimmunoassay counter of SN-682.

(5) Other required reagents are same as those mentioned in the previous experiment.

2. Method

(1) Grouping and gastric lavage according to the table 10.

Table 10 Grouping and gastric lavage of experimental mice

Animals (mice)	Grouping	Gastric lavage (0.2ml/10g)
20 uninoculated mice	Normal group ① 10 mice	physiological saline×6d
	Normal group ② 10 mice	physiological saline×12d
40 inoculated mice	Control group ① 10 mice	0.5% CMC×6d
	Control group ② 10 mice	0.5% CMC×12d
	Administration group ① 10 mice	20mg/10ml TG×6d
	Administration group ② 10 mice	20mg/10ml TG×12d

*. The inoculation method refers to "Experimental Study on Observation of Angiogenesis of Transplantation Tumor at Mouse's Abdominal Muscle".

(2) ET determination: Six days after gastric lavage, collect specimens of blood from the eye socket of mice with 2ml of each mouse in normal group ①, administration group ① and control group ①. Put the blood sample in the tube with 10% EDTA · Na 230μl and 40μl aprotinin. Lightly shake the mixture well. Centrifuge for 10min with 3000 revolutions per minute at 4°C. Separate plasma and store it at -20°C for determination. Twelve days after gastric lavage, for the mice of remaining groups to adopt the same method to collect specimens of blood, separate plasma. Use the specific radioimmunoassay and gamma (γ) radioimmunoassay counter of SN-682 to measure both the present and previous plasma. Operating procedures should be seriously carried out according to instructions of radioimmunoassay kit.

(3) Statistical treatment: The data is represented by average ± standard error ($\overline{X}$ ±S), and adopt analysis of variance — F test to carry out the comparison among groups.

[Experimental Result]

Determination results of plasma endothelin (ET) in mice can be seen in the table 25-11.

Table 25-11 TG's effect on the plasma endothelin (ET) in mice with transplantation tumor at abdominal muscle ($\overline{X}$ ±S, pg/ml)

Group	Case load	The Sixth Day	The Twelfth Day
Normal group	10	93.6±4.72	93.4±4.83
Control group	10	126.4±3.87**	132.8±4.02**

| Administration group | 10 | 106.4±4.49*△△ | 114.6±5.41*△ |

Note: Compare to the normal group, *P<0.05, ** P<0.01; while compare to the control group, △ P<0.05, △△ P<0.01

The above results indicate that ET of administration group and control group is obviously higher than that of normal group (P<0.05), which shows that the tumor can increase the plasma endothelin (ET) of mice. While ET of administration group is apparently lower than that of control group, and this phenomenon is significant during the previous six days (P<0.01), which shows that TG can reduce the increase of plasma endothelin (ET) caused by the tumor and effects in the early stage are stronger.

Results of observation on new-born capillaries of transplantation tumor at mouse's abdominal muscle with microcirculation detection system indicate that TG can inhibit the growth of new-born capillaries in and around the tumor, reduce the density of new-born capillaries which enter and leave the tumor and suppress the growth of tumor. Furthermore, those effects of TG are significant in the early stage, and TG can change the diameter and flow rate of tumor arterioles and venules in the advanced stage to narrow the diameter and quicken the flow rate. Determination results of plasma endothelin (ET) show that the tumor can increase the plasma endothelin (ET) of mice. But TG can reduce the increase of plasma endothelin (ET) caused by the tumor with stronger effects in the early stage.

[Discussion]

1. Analysis and evaluation on the observation method of new-born capillaries by building the transplantation tumor model of mouse's abdominal muscles

At present, the methodology of tumor capillaries research is still in the process of constant exploration and improvement. Generally choose the rabbit cornea, chorioallantoic membrane (CAM) and yolk sac of chick embryo, and hamster cheek pouch for in vivo techniques; and also insert manual apparatus into rabbit ear chamber and subcutaneous air pouch of rat's back, which are called "sandwich" observation room, as the location of transplantation tumor for viviperception. In recent years, corrosion casting and immunohistochemistry are also used to display and identify vascular composition. Each of the above methods has its merits and drawbacks. At present, experts are still exploring to find a kind of simple, economical model and method with high quantitative feature and repeatability for the angiogenesis research. Therefore, combining concrete conditions of this laboratory, the writer has studied and designed the transplantation tumor model of mouse's abdominal muscles, applying improved microcirculation observation techniques to observe new-born capillaries of tumor. This method is easy, convenient and intuitional, and finally becomes a new approach for the tumor capillaries research on the methodology.

(1) Model evaluation: The approach of transplanting tumor at mouse's abdominal muscles is adopted to study and observe the relation between tumor and capillaries, as well as the drug effect on tumor capillaries, which has the reliable theoretical and practical basis.

The abdominal muscle layer of mouse is thinner. A thin layer of aponeurosis lies between the exterior of abdominal muscle layer and skin. The interior of abdominal muscle layer links closely with the abdominal membrane. The Hunter's line divides the abdominal muscle layer along the centre position into right and left halves, which are provided blood circulation by inferior epigastric arteries and veins. The right and left halves diverge one more into tiny branches (arterioles and venules) and capillary branches, which form rich anastomoses around the abdominal muscle of each side. The center position has fewer vascular branches and ramus anastomoticus and becomes an area with rare vessels, where is convenient for the observation of new-born capillaries.

When EAC cell suspension is injected into the abdominal muscle layer, tumor cells will quickly begin the infiltrative growth and expand along the flat surface of abdominal muscle without any adhesion of skin and organs in the abdomen. When the tumor grows up to a certain extent, it will gradually break through the abdominal muscle layer, penetrate inward through the abdominal membrane, move into organs in the abdominal cavity through implantation metastasis and finally produce ascites.

Consequently, the better choice is to inoculate in the area with rare vessels and observe tumor capillaries during the period of the tumor not yet penetrating through the abdominal membrane, which can both make a clearer observation of the emergence and change of new-born capillaries and avoid many factors' combined effects on new-born capillaries, such as ascites and tumor diffusion caused by the tumor's penetration through the abdominal membrane.

Combined with this experiment content, in order to have a better reflection and observation of the transplanted tumor in abdominal muscle and the whole growing and developing process of new-born capillaries, the writer has carried out repeated trials and finally chosen EAC cell suspension with the concentration of 6.0×10^7/ml for inoculation. According to the growth status of tumor, the writer arranges 10 days' observation and 12 days' treatment. Divide four time spans of the third day, sixth day, ninth day and twelfth day to reflect the tumor's reaction to drugs in the early, intermediate and advanced stages.

The transplantation tumor model of mouse's abdominal muscles can intuitively and clearly reflect the formation and change of new-born tumor capillaries, and it also provides new idea and method for studying new-born tumor capillaries' selection of transplantable parts and preparation of animal model. There are a few points that should be remembered when preparing the model: ① Inoculation site should be chosen in the abdominal muscle with rare vessels, not penetrating the peritoneum. The mark is a full small "swelling" without any collapse on the inoculation site. ② The experimental operation should be gentle and careful. Try to keep away from the tiny venous tributary (generally only 1~2 vessels) that links skin and abdominal muscle, so that no local hemorrhage is caused. Then the inoculation effect and the growth of new-born tumor capillaries after inoculation will be unaffected. ③ Appropriately increase the number of experimental mice to reduce errors of different location of rare vessels of abdominal muscle caused by individual difference.

(2) Evaluation of observation method

① Observation of transparent specimen: The tissue of abdominal muscle membrane is thinner. After transparent treatment, other sites are all transparent except vessels are red. Naked eyes can clearly see vessels' routes. Microscope observation can show the shape, distribution and interrelation of capillaries. The transparent specimen is not only convenient and intuitive but also preserves the natural form of vessels and associative perception. When preparing the transparent specimen, do not inject with Chinese ink or other pigments, but directly display vessels through natural color of blood, which prevent particle size, dispersion degree and viscosity of perfusate from affecting the specimen quality and changing the shape of vessels due to improper injection pressure. The transparent specimen must completely reflect the condition in vivo so as to make displayed vessels be closer to the reality.

The transparent specimen of abdominal muscle- membrane can clearly display various vessels in the abdominal muscle, involving the route, shape and distribution of capillaries around and in the tumor as well as localized congestion, oozing of blood and bleeding, which make it more convenient for observing new-born capillaries inside and outside of the tumor. The transparent specimen can only show the change of capillary form after animals have died, but it cannot reflect their blood flow state. Therefore, combined with the dynamic state of vital blood flow and functional parameters to have observation, it will be more favorable to have a complete understanding of new-born tumor capillaries' features.

② In vivo observation with microcirculation microscope: The mouse's abdominal muscle membrane is thinner with the shape of film and is easy to transmit light, whose vascular form and fluid state can be clearly seen through the microcirculation microscope. Inoculated tumor cells begin the infiltrative spreading growth in the abdominal muscle. In the early stage, the abdominal muscle membrane still can transmit light and display the vascular form in tumor tissue due to unobvious increase in thickness. In the advanced stage, the tumor tissue grows and thickens; the pressure of central part increases; necrosis and hemorrhage arise, which appear as a light-tight solid mass; vessels in this part cannot be seen, but the form of vessels in other transparent parts of tumor can be seen at present. The microcirculation microscope is used to observe new-born capillaries inside and outside of transplantation tumor at abdominal muscle and those which enter and leave the tumor as well as tumor arterioles and venules, which can completely reflect the relation between tumor and vessels as well as drugs' effect on new-born tumor capillaries in the respect of vascular form and fluid state.

The above two observation methods can complement each other with joint application. Observation of transparent specimen can cover the shortage of not observing vessels in a light-tight part of tumor in vivo; while in vivo observation makes up for the observation of dynamic state of blood flow. The above methods can only make one-off observation and cannot have a continuing dynamic monitoring in a long term, so they also remain inadequate. In order to have a more accurate and deeper research, the methodology needs the further improvement and completeness.

2. Evaluation of experimental drugs Common Threewingnut Root generally refers to the plant belonging to Tripterygium of Celastraceae. There are three varieties in China, which are Common Threewingnut Root, Tripterygium Hypoglaucum and Common Threewingnut Root of North-East

(Tripterygium regelii Sprague et Take). This kind of drug has an acrid-bitter flavor and medicinal properties of cold and hot. The drug passes through main channels of liver and spleen as well as twelve regular channels, which has efficacies of clearing away heat and toxic material, expelling wind and removing dampness, relaxing the muscles, stimulating the blood circulation and removing obstruction in channels, reducing swelling and alleviating pain, destroying parasites and relieving itching. This drug, which contains about 70 components, is recorded in *Sheng Nong's herbal classic* at the earliest. Since the 1970s, it has been used in treating rheumatoid arthritis, which results in certain curative effect. In recent twenty years, it has been widely used in treating chronic nephritis, hepatitis, purpura haemorrhagica and all kinds of skin diseases. At the same time, the research of pharmacological action also becomes deeper, widely covering adrenal gland, immunity, generation, micturition, central nerve and blood system. Experts all agree that this drug can enhance adrenal cortex function, relieve inflammation and alleviate pain, resist fertility and prevent tumor activity. Only as to its effect on immune system, experts each sticks to their own viewpoint. There were many controversies and inferences. In an early period, experts embarked on the research of its effect on immune system because of its unique effect on treating rheumatoid arthritis. The earliest result indicates that this drug can suppress immunity. As more and more researches are done deeperly, most researchers gradually tend to the viewpoint of "two-way regulation". They hold that Common Threewingnut Root has the two-way regulating action with dose dependent on immune system. For instance, Zheng jiarun, Yan Biyu, Luo Dan, Lei Yi and Fan Yongyi respectively report that Common Threewingnut Root has the two-way regulating action on mouse's thymic weight, human thymocyte hyperplasia, NK activity of mouse's spleen cells, T and B cell function of mouse's spleen and proliferation of T cells in vitro. Through the experiment of the effect of TG with different dosages on $M\Phi$ function of mice abdominal cavity and immune organs by the writer, it reflects that Common Threewingnut Root has the two-way regulating action on immune system. The above results indicate that Common Threewingnut Root does not have the only effect of immunological suppression. Many experiments have proved that a small dosage of Common Threewingnut Root can enhance the immunization to some extent. While within a certain limits, there will be a reversible manifestation between enhancement and inhibition. It can also show nearly no appreciable effect on immunologic function. When further increasing the dosage, this drug will show the complete inhibiting action on immunization. The inhibiting action of Common Threewingnut Root is obviously related to its dosage.

Given the above conclusions, the writer chooses the dosage of TG, which has no appreciable effect on immunologic function, to carry out the experiment. It can avoid drugs' influence on immunologic function, which may complicate the research of TG's inhibiting action on tumor capillaries. At the same time, it can provide experimental considerations and exploring foundations for experiments and clinical researches of TG's anti-tumor action on the premise that Common Threewingnut Root will not damage the body's immunological function.

The drug of this experimental research is a kind of prepared product after repeated separation and abstraction. The amount of active principle is higher and the untoward effect is less. In order to have a further exploration of angiogenesis inhibition of active principle in this drug, various chemical compositions and monomers after the second separation and purification still need further study.

3. Features of tumor angiogenesis Under normal conditions, the angiogenesis only limits in embryonic development, repair in trauma and endometrial regeneration. Furthermore, the host can strictly control its growth with various mechanisms. But in the recent twenty years, experts haven't found any mechanism which can suppress tumor angiogenesis. It indicates that tumor angiogenesis has its own features.

Through the observation on new-born capillaries of transplantation tumor at mouse's abdominal muscle, it is easy to find that as the formation and growth of capillaries in the inoculation area, tumor cell cluster constantly proliferates and its volume continually expands. It starts with the exudation of original host's capillaries, and then slender and crooked new-born capillaries gradually come out with the characteristics of disorganized arrangement, uneven distribution and irregular diameter. Especially these capillaries, which enter into the tumor, have incontinuous routes, lack completeness and present the shape of comma or bud. The above signs indicate that those capillaries are not fully mature and cannot form complete and continuous basilar membrane. Furthermore, they are not blocked and packed by well-differentiated vascular walls with multilayered structure, which make vessels expand irregularly in the shape of nodositas or sinus. Along with the progressive growth of tumor, dust-color area of hemorrhage and necrosis appears in the centre of the tumor. Capillaries in adjacent sites are hard to be seen because of extreme dilatation, which may be due to the constantly rising pressure within tumor caused by the continuous proliferation of tumor cells. The pressure of central part in tumor is relatively highest, and the central part is far away from new-born capillaries that penetrate from the outside of tumor, so the central part is easy to suffer from necrosis because of ischemia, involving the necrosis and hemorrhage of vessels. But there still are different-shaped tumor capillaries with active proliferation at the margin of tumor, which can ensure the required nutrition for the further infiltrative growth. This phenomenon also indicates that the tumor grows indefinitely and cannot be adjusted and controlled.

At present, experts have been adopting various methods to study tumor vessels. The existing achievements have proved that the formation of tumor vessels is different from the angiogenesis in a normal physiological state. It has its own special uniqueness, such as infantile differentiation, incomplete vascular wall and out of the body's control, etc. While the whole process and regulatory mechanism of tumor angiogenesis remains obscure and are still in further exploration. This experiment just superficially reflects the relation between tumor and vessels, as well as some features of tumor vessels. The deeper study also needs the breakthrough of methodology, and the continued clarification of biological characteristics of tumor vessels in terms of the physiology and pathology of angiogenesis, biochemistry and molecular biology.

4. Exploration of TG's inhibiting action on new-born tumor capillaries Since Common Threewingnut Root is explored and applied, domestic and foreign medicine circles have been starting to pay great interest and attention to it and carrying out multi-disciplinary study and exploration one by one for broadening the application range. The recent researches show that Common Threewingnut Root can inhibit the migration and proliferation of vascular endothelial cells (EC). Zhu Jinbo and another two Japanese scholars utilize self-made F-2 and F-2C of EC strain to study the effect of Common Threewingnut Root on the process of angiogenesis. The result shows that Common Threewingnut Root can directly act on EC and inhibit its migration, proliferation, differentiation and

the formation of lumen, which prompts that Common Threewingnut Root has a better inhibiting action on angiogenesis. The experimental study of TG's inhibiting action on new-born capillaries of transplantation tumor at mouse's abdominal muscle finds that TG can suppress tumor angiogenesis with stronger effects in the early stage. Presumably TG's active mechanisms may include the following respects.

(1) Directly act on new-born tumor capillaries: The experimental results indicate that TG can obviously suppress the growth of capillaries in and around the tumor and reduce the density of new-born capillaries which enter and leave the tumor. Thus it can be inferred that TG may directly act on endothelial cells of tumor vessels, suppress the migration and proliferation of cells and reduce the formation, differentiation and growth rate of tumor vessels.

(2) Directly act on tumor cells: TG's direct damaging effect on tumor cells has been proved in an early period. It is generally acknowledged that TG comes into the effect of cell toxicant by directly interfering with DNA replication of tumor cells and suppressing RNA and protein synthesis. During the process of angiogenesis, the tumor cell itself can produce multiple angiogenesis factors, such as fibrocyte growth factor (FGF), angiogenine, transfer growth factor (TGF) and tumor necrosis factor (TNF-2), etc. Furthermore, the tumor cell can release some chemical mediators to induce the angiogenesis of host and tumor. The above substances that are released by tumor cells and can induce angiogenesis are collectively called "tumor angiogenesis factor (TAF)" by Folkman. TG can reduce the production of TAF by directly killing tumor cells, which indirectly inhibits the angiogenesis.

(3) Change of tumor blood flow: Determination result of the average diameter and flow rate of host's tumor arterioles and venules shows that TG can change the blood flow in the tumor and affect the growth and change of tumor and its new-born capillaries by acting on the blood supply of tumor.

(4) Reduction of plasma ET content: The recent researches indicate that ET has the effect of growth factor on promoting cell proliferation, which can stimulate the growth of endothelial cell and the proliferation of vascular smooth muscle cells. ET has an intimate relation with the tumor, which can promote the transcription and expression of proto-oncogene and the growth and differentiation of tumor, increase the blood flow of tumor tissue and stimulate the angiogenesis. The determination result of mouse's plasma ET indicates that ET of inoculated group is obviously higher than that of normal group. It proves that ET has an intimate relation with tumor and the tumor can increase mouse's plasma ET content. While ET of TG group is apparently lower that that of control group, which indicates that TG can obviously lower mouse's plasma ET content and reduce the growth effect on promoting tumor and angiogenesis caused by ET.

Furthermore, TG has a feature in this experiment that its inhibiting action on tumor angiogenesis in the advanced stage is weaker than that in the early stage. In addition to TG's pharmacological characteristic of suppressing angiogenesis, its inhibiting power is also related to drugs' accumulative action. It is conjectured that TG accumulates in vivo and plays an extensive pharmacological effect with prolongation of medication time, and thus affects its inhibiting action on tumor angiogenesis.

This research result indicates that TG can suppress tumor growth by inhibiting tumor angiogenesis with no significant effect on the immune system, and moreover, TG's effect in the early stage is significant. This study provides references for the further multi-field and multi-angle TG researches, and also new ideas for the research of TG anti-tumor mechanisms. Without doubt, this conclusion still needs extensive repeated experiments to be verified. At the same time, drug purification and methodology improvement are necessary for the further deeper study.

Inhibiting the formation of new-born tumor capillaries to suppress the tumor growth is a new idea on oncology that emerges in recent years.

This topic is on the basis study of formation features of new-born capillaries of transplantation tumor at mouse's abdominal muscle as well as capillaries' relation with tumor and TG's two-way regulating action with dose dependent on the immune system of mouse, and thus by choosing the TG dosage (40mg/kg weight) of no obvious effect on mouse's immune function to carry out experiments of TG's effect on the shape and quantity of new-born capillaries of transplantation tumor at mouse's abdominal muscle, the density of new-born capillaries which enter and leave the tumor, the average diameter and flow rate of tumor arterioles and venules, tumor size and plasma ET. The above experiments find that TG can inhibit tumor angiogenesis through various mechanisms of direct action on new-born tumor capillaries as well as tumor cells, the change of tumor blood flow and the reduction of plasma ET content, and moreover, TG's effect in the early stage is significant. This research result shows that the anti-tumor study of TG from the angle of vessels has certain significance and needs the further study confirmation and deepening.

IV. The Significance of Inhibition of Angiogenesis in Treatment

Tumorigensis is a complicated process and is affected by many factors, involving the foundation of tumor vascular net. Many researches have proved that tumor growth must depend on angiogenesis. By inhibiting certain steps or the whole process of tumor angiogenesis to control tumor growth is of great importance to tumor therapy and prevention of tumor's distant metastasis.

i. The relation between tumor angiogenesis and the generation and growth of tumor

At present, the question about tumor generation mainly focuses on the study of oncogene; nevertheless, malignant change of tissues, tumor formation and tumor gene activity are just necessary conditions instead of the whole. Folkman Judah and other scholars in Children's Hospital of Harvard Medical School do a series of studies about the generation of pancreatic islet B cell tumor of mutant mice. The study result finds that tumor gene activity is related to the proliferation of B cells, and moreover, angiogenesis plays an important role during the generation of B cell tumor. The generation of tumor is caused by getting angiogenic ability of hyperplastic tissue. The research proves that one of evident characteristics of most precancerous lesions is the lack of obvious neovascularization. Compared with the tumor with abundant new-born vessels, the transition from precancerous condition and lesion to blood vessel phase may be the "switch" for tumor generation. It indicates that the induction of angiogenesis and the consequent neovascularization are both ahead of the tumor generation. Once the tumor is found, its further growth must depend on the continuous generation of vessels. This concept has been put forward by Folkman in 1971. He holds that tumor cells and vessels combine into a highly integrated ecological system. If there is no angiogenesis, the tumor will not swell. Many experimental research evidences in recent years further support the above views.

The growing period of solid tumor cells can be divided into invading prophase without vessels and invading growth phase of vascularization. During the invading prophase, the growth of tumor cells mainly depends on diffusion to gain nutrition. When the diameter of solid tumor exceeds 1~3cm and cell number is up to about 10^7, tumor's central part and its continued growth must be provided with oxygen and nutrient substance by vessels. ① Observe the black tumor cell cluster of mouse that is cultured in agar. When the cluster grows to 1mm³, the proliferation of its peripheral cells and the necrosis of central cells are equivalent. When the tumor body continues to swell, the proliferation and necrosis achieve a dynamic equilibrium. If the tumor grows in the organism, then this phase can also be called the blood vessel phase of tumor growth. Breaking this state needs the growth of new and functional capillaries so as to provide adequate oxygen and nutrient substance. ② Observe the growth rate of transplantable tumor in the subcutaneous transparent cavity of mouse. The tumor shows a slow linear growth before angiogenesis. While after angiogenesis, the tumor shows a rapid exponential rise. ③ Implant tumor tissue masses into the rabbit cornea. The tumor stands back from the host's vascular bed. The new-born capillaries around the cornea are found to gather toward the tumor. The growth rate averages 0.2mm/d. After new-born capillaries grow into the tumor, the tumor mass begins to grow rapidly and exceeds 1cm³. ④ The tumor grows in the isolated perfused organ of mouse. Because there is no vascular proliferation, the tumor limits in 1mm³. If this tumor is transplanted into the mouse, it will rapidly grow to 1~2cm³ after angiogenesis. ⑤ Suspend tumor cells in the aqueous humor of anterior chamber of rabbit eyes. Because there is no vessel, the tumor size is less than 1mm³. If this tumor is transplanted into iris vessels, it will grow rapidly with 1.6 times of its original volume in two weeks. ⑥ When the human retina blastoma is transplanted into the vitreous body or anterior chamber, the growth of this tumor will be limited due to the lack of vessels. ⑦ Use ³H- thymine to label tumor cells of fixed cancer. The label index of tumor cells reduces with the increase of distance between the nearest open capillaries and tumor cells. The mean value of label index of tumor cells is the function of label index of tumor vascular endothelial cells. ⑧ Transplanted tumor in CAM. During the avascular period (≥72h), the growth of tumor is restricted. A set of experiments show that the tumor diameter is no more than (0.93±0.29) mm. In 24 hours after the vascularization, the tumor starts growing rapidly. On the seventh day, the average diameter of tumor is (8.0±2.5) mm. ⑨ Oophoroma metastasizes to the abdominal membrane. Before the vascularization, this tumor grows slowly and its size seldom exceeds 1mm³. ⑩ If the tumor diameter is less than 1mm, there will be no vascularization in the metastatic cancer of rabbit cornea. All other metastatic cancers, whose diameter is greater than 1mm, have the formation of vessels.

All these above can indirectly or directly prove that tumor growth must depend on vascularization and the vascularization is a key factor for tumor development.

ii. The anti-tumor action of angiogenesis inhibitors

In the early 1970s, along with the presentation and research of the concept that tumor growth depends on vascularization, researchers also bring forth the relevant concept of anti-angiogenic therapy. That is to say, by preventing neovascularization and (or) the expansion of new-born vascular net and (or) destroying new-born vessels to stop the generation or establishment of small solid tumor and also arrest the growth, development and metastasis of tumor. Ways of adopting anti-angiogenic therapy: ① Suppress tumor to release tumor angiogenic factors (TAF); ② Neutralize the tumor angiogenic factors (TAF) that have already been released; ③ Inhibit the reaction of vascular endothelial cells (EC) on angiogenic factors; ④ Disturb the synthesis of basilar membrane; ⑤ Destroy the formed new-born tumor vessels, etc. In conclusion, ideal tumor angiogenesis inhibitors must be able to suppress one or more procedures or the whole process of tumor angiogenesis.

At present, people have done a lot of researches in this respect. Experimental results indicate that angiogenesis inhibitors (AI) can inhibit the growth of tumor. ① According to more domestic reports, the combination of heparin and hydrocortisone is acknowledged as an effective angiogenesis inhibitor. Experiments prove that their combined application can suppress the angiogenesis in CAM, promote tumor regression, prevent metastasis and inhibit the neovascularization of rabbit cornea that caused by tumor. That this kind of inhibitor is used to cure some mice tumors can bring about a striking effect. For instance, after the oral administration of heparin (200U/ml) and subcutaneous injection of hydrocortisone (250mg), 100% reticulum cell sarcoma, 100% Leuis lung cancer and 80% B16 melanoma can have a complete regression. What's more, 80% tumors will not suffer from the relapse after regression. ② Fumagillin is a kind of antibiotic which is naturally secreted by aspergillin. For the in vitro experiment, Fumagillin can inhibit the proliferation of endothelial cells. For the in vivo experiment, Fumagillin can inhibit the angiogenesis caused by tumor and also suppress the tumor growth of mice. For example, 30mg/kg of Fumagillin can inhibit the growth of Lewis lung cancer and B16 melanoma. ③ 1μg/ml TNP-470 (a kind of Fumagillin synthetic analogue) can inhibit the growth of cultural endothelial cells of human umbilical vein. 3~10mg/kg TNP-470 can suppress the growth of nude mice's transplanted tumor of human oophoroma. ④ Platelet factor 4 (PF_4) is a kind of 28kDa protein that is released by the dense body when blood platelets aggregate together. There is a great affinity between PF_4 and heparin. Taylor and other scholars have found that PF_4 can effectively inhibit the growth of CAM vessels. Recently Maione and others have discovered that recombination of human PF_4 ($rHuPF_4$) can suppress the reproduction and migration of human endothelial cells, and also produce an avascular area in chick embryo CAM. Sharpe has carried out the research about mice melanoma and human colon cancer, which proves that human PF_4 ($rHuPF_4$) has an inhibiting action on the growth of solid tumor. ⑤ α-Difluoromethylornithine (DFMO) is a kind of nonreversible ornithine decarboxylase inhibitor. It can inhibit the angiogenesis caused by melanoma in chick embryo CAM, and then inhibit the tumor growth in CAM. ⑥ The latest approved angiogenesis inhibitor - Angio stain is a kind of 38kDa protein, which can inhibit the generation of endothelial cells and angiogenesis in the Lewis mice tumor. When Folkman injects Angio stain into the mouse with transplanted tumor, this new type of inhibitor can keep this transplanted tumor in a state of dormancy, that is to say, the multiplication rate of tumor is equal to the death rate of cells. In addition, Angio stain can suppress the growth of human tumor.

At present, people have realized that the anti-tumor effects of many anti-tumor methods directly or indirectly act on the structure or function of tumor vessels, such as anti-tumor angiogenesis, the change of tumor blood flow and its regulation, etc. That by inhibiting the angiogenesis of malignant tumor to suppress the growth and metastasis of tumor is a new way to fight against cancer, and meanwhile adopting angiogenesis inhibitors to cure tumors will open up a new and promising therapeutic area clinically. For instance, cooperating operation, chemotherapy, radiotherapy and immunological therapy will certainly improve the overall tumor treatment level.

Tumor cells produce multiple tumor angiogenesis factors (TAF), such as basic fibroblast growth factor (bFGF), acid fibroblast growth factor (aFGF), endothelial cell growth factor (ECGF), vascular endothelial cell growth factor (VEGF), platelet derivation endothelial cell growth factor (PDECGF), epidermal cell growth factor (EGF), transforming growth factor (TGFα, TGFβ), tumor necrosis factor (TGF-α), granulocyte colony stimulating factor (G-CSF) and granulocyte macrophage colony stimulating factor (GM-CSF), etc. TAF has the promotional effects on tumor generation, development and metastasis. Exploring the generative mechanism of tumor capillaries and the inhibition of capillaries' formation and growth is one of the effective measures to prevent and cure tumors, and may also become a new promising anti-cancer therapy after the surgical treatment, radiotherapy, chemotherapy and biological therapy.

ANNEX: PATHFINDER AND FOOTPRINT(SCIENTIFIC FOOTPRINTS)

(To overcome cancer, where is the direction of the road?
- where is the road? Where are you going? How to go?)

Pathfinder and Footprint (Research Footprint)

CONTENTS ANNEX

1. THE CAUSES AND REASONS

(1) why do I study cancer?

I am a clinical surgeon, why do you study cancer?

This is due to a result of a group of cancer patients after the results of petition.

In 1985, I carried out the petition (according to the operation room registration list of the letter) for my own patients which were more than 3000 cases of chest, general cancer after radical surgery operations were done by me.

The results showed that most of the patients were postoperative 2-3 years recurrence and metastasis. This makes me realize that although the operation is successful, but the long-term efficacy is not satisfactory, postoperative recurrence and metastasis are the key factors affecting the long-term efficacy of surgery. Also it prompted us to prevent postoperative recurrence and metastasis is the key to extend the survival term.Therefore, we must carry out clinical basic research, if there is no basic research breakthrough, the clinical efficacy is difficult to improve, so we established the Institute of Experimental Surgery, conducted a series of experimental research and clinical verification work.

(2) from the results of follow-up it was found that :

① the postoperative recurrence and metastasis are the keys to long-term effect of surgery;

② it was suggesting that clinicians must pay attention to and must study the prevention and control methods of the postoperative recurrence and metastasis to improve the long-term efficacy of surgery

2. PATHFINDER

(1) Why to pathfinder? How to find this way? To overcome cancer, where is the direction of the road?

- where is the road? Where are you going? How to go?

Over the past 100 years, many people with lofty ideals and research elites are looking for.

(2) how to find path?

Our research is carried out by following the following scientific research routes:

①

1). To find the problem

Through the large number of patients follow-up, it was found that the impact of long-term effect of postoperative key factors are postoperative recurrence, metastasis.

2).Ask the question

It is necessary to study the problem of recurrence and metastasis in order to improve the long-term curative effect, and put forward the goal or "target" of anti-metastasis.

3). To research the problems

Set up a series of projects, experiments, explore the transfer mechanism and find anti-recurrence transfer technology and new drugs, screening 200 kinds of traditional Chinese medicine, to find 48 kinds of anti-cancer, anti-metastasis effect

4). To solve the problems

Clinical validation and clinical research, to explore the pattern of cancer metastasis and to find a new model of anti-metastasis therapy, and rose to independent innovation theory system and the new anti-metastatic treatment model and the new program.

② from the clinical → the experimental → the clinical → the re-experimental → the re-clinical, back to the clinical to solve the problem.

③ the theory and the practice are closely integrated, the topics are from the clinical, to find the focus of clinical problems and clinical breakthrough, after experimental research and clinical validation, and then applied to clinical, to solve clinical problems.

④ from the combination of Chinese and Western medicine → macroscopic combination→ molecular level, with modern cancer cell molecular metastasis mechanism and the latest theory of the "eight steps", "three stages", from 200 kinds of ancient Chinese medications to find and screen anti-metastasis medications which also protect the immune organs, activate the cytokines and immune factors so that the ancient Chinese medications become modernization and merge with international standards and so that modern medication and ancient Chinese herbal medication can combine at the molecular level, BRM level.

⑤ the establishment of experimental surgery Institute conducted a series of cancer animal experimental research and clinical basic research, if no basic research breakthrough, the clinical efficacy is difficult to improve.

⑥ the establishment of the dawn of cancer specialist clinic:

(A) the establishment of outpatient medical records, to retain outpatient medical records, full follow-up, long-term follow-up, the phone at any time at any time to answer, to guide rehabilitation and diet precautions;

(B) the establishment of detailed medical records (including the patient's epidemiological data) in-depth analysis of each case after the successful experience of treatment and failure of the lessons and the particularity of the disease (eg analysis of information);

(C) referral of the case summary analysis of 6 months to 1 year of follow-up, referral that more than 3 years of the cases were excerpted medical records, write medical records, analysis and treatment experience and lessons (example: summary of medical records). Dawn tumor specialist outpatient department has 21 years, outpatient medical records remain no missing.

⑦ through the laboratory of laboratory research laboratory to establish a variety of cancer animal model, it was carried out a series of experimental studies; explored the cause of cancer, pathogenesis and recurrence, metastasis mechanism and carried out the regulation of cancer invasion, recurrence, transfer effective experimental study; through the experimental research, it accessed to a series of new discoveries from the experimental study.

(3) how to find this way? It should be based on clinical problems and experimental studies to search

Foe 20 years the road which we are looking for was to walk on step by step as this :

① It was found by follow-up results: postoperative recurrence and metastasis are the key to long-term efficacy of surgery, and thus the revelation:

A – it must find the road of the study of prevention and treatment of cancer recurrence and metastasis

(Method, medication, technology, basic theory)

② through the animal experimental study results it was found:

With the progress of cancer, thymus was atrophy; in the host after inoculated cancer cells the thymus had acute progressive atrophy, cell proliferation was blocked, the volume was significantly reduced, and thus revelation:

B – it must be looking for the path to prevent thymic atrophy, promote thymic hyperplasia, increase the immune function.

(Method, medication, technology, basic theory)

③ through the animal experimental study results it was found:

Experimental results confirmed that first the immunization is low, and then easy to occur in cancer and to develop, if there is no immune function decline, it is not easy to vaccination success. Experimental results suggest that improving and maintaining good immune function and maintaining a good central immune organ thymus are one of the important measures to prevent cancer from occurring.

Another experimental result in our laboratory suggested that metastases are immune-related, immune dysfunction, or the use of immunosuppressive agents to promote tumor metastasis. The revelation:

C – it must be looking for the way for cancer patients with immune reconstruction

(Method, medication, technology, basic theory)

④the revelation through the understanding of our proposed new concept and the new theory of cancer metastasis therapy:

The key to cancer treatment is anti-metastasis, how to eliminate the cancer cells in the process of being transferred

D – it must find the way to eliminate cancer cells in the way of transfer

(Method, medication, technology, basic theory)

Through the above research results we basically found the way to take the immune regulation, and gradually established the XZ-C immunomodulation therapy for cancer.

For 28 years we have walked out of the new path of a traditional Chinese medications with immune regulation and regulation of immune activity, to prevent thymus atrophy, promote thymic hyperplasia, protect bone marrow hematopoietic function, improve immune surveillance, at the molecular level of combining Chinese medications with Western medication to overcome of cancer.

3. THE FOOTPRINTS (RESEARCH FOOTPRINTS)

1. anti-cancer, anti-cancer metastasis research, scientific research results, scientific and technological innovation series

The following argument in XZ-C (XU ZE - China) series of monographs are all the first time to be put forward to in the international and all are original papers.

①"thymus atrophy and immune dysfunction are one of the cause and the pathogenesis of cancer"

- Putting forward New findings of experimental studies on the etiology and pathogenesis of cancer

- see "new concept and new method of cancer treatment" P.13 in the monograph

② "theoretical basis and experimental basis of protecting Thymus and increasing immune function of XZ-C immunoregulation treatment"

- put forward the theoretical basis and experimental basis of immunoregulation therapy for cancer

- Because of the above experimental study it was found the new revelation, so the treatment principle must be to prevent thymus atrophy, promote thymic hyperplasia, protect bone marrow hematopoietic function, improve immune surveillance, control malignant cells immune escape.

- see the monograph "new concept and new method of cancer treatment" P.17

③ "cancer treatment should change the concept and establish a comprehensive treatment concept"

- put forward the new concept of cancer treatment principles

- The goal or target of cancer treatment must be both for both the tumor and the host, the establishment of a comprehensive treatment view

- should overcome the simple cancer cells in the one - sided treatment view

- see the monograph "new concepts and new approaches to cancer treatment" P.28

④ **"the new model of combination of cancer multidisciplinary comprehensive treatment"**

- Advise on the new concept of cancer treatment portfolio model

--The new model of multidisciplinary comprehensive treatment is:

Long-term treatment mainly: surgery + biotherapy + immunotherapy + Chinese medication, Chinese and Western combination therapy

Short-term treatment, supplemented: radiotherapy and chemotherapy, not long-term, not excessive

- see the monograph "new concept and new method of cancer treatment" P33

⑤ **"The analysis and evaluation and questioning and four comments of solid tumor systemic intravenous chemotherapy"**

--Discussion on the Problems and Disadvantages of Whole Body Venous Chemotherapy

- questioning and commenting on the route, dose calculation and curative effect evaluation of systemic intravenous chemotherapy

- see the monograph "new concept and new method of cancer treatment" P.57

⑥ **"the initiative in abdominal solid tumor systemic intravenous chemotherapy should be the target organ for intravascular chemotherapy and the traditional cancer chemotherapy reform initiative"**

- because in the systemic intravenous chemotherapy cytotoxic from the superior vena cava route can not directly reach the portal vein system; the vena cava system and portal venous system are generally not connected; the drugs administered through the superior vena cava is difficult to reach the portal vein

- In the abdominal solid tumor (stomach, colorectal, liver, gallbladder, pancreas, spleen, abdominal and other malignant tumors) where the cancer cells? It is mainly in the portal vein system and the postoperative adjuvant chemotherapy by the elbow vein → vena cava route of administration is unreasonable, does not meet the anatomy, physiological pathology because it can not directly into the portal vein system

therefore, it should change the route of administration, instead of target organ endovascular treatment.

- see the monograph "new concept and new method of cancer treatment" P.63

⑦ **"in the human body there are three main forms of cancer expression"**

--Advice on the new concept of cancer metastasis therapy

---proposed this third form of expression is the cancer cells in the process of being transferred, the treatment of cancer should be aimed at the above three forms of existence, in particular, it should be aimed at the transit of cancer cells

- see the monograph "new concept and new method of cancer treatment" P.38

⑧ **"the whole process of cancer development," two points and a line"**

--Advice on the theory of cancer metastasis therapy

--- One of the purposes of cancer treatment is to prevent the whole process of metastatic cancer and the metastasis can be summarized as "two points and a line"

- traditional cancer treatment only attaches importance to "two points" while ignoring the "first line"

The new concept that should pay attention to both "two", but also to cut off "line"

- see the monograph "new concept and new method of cancer treatment" P.43

⑨ **"anti-cancer metastasis therapy trilogy"**

Advice on the theory of cancer metastasis therapy

- The "eight steps" of the transfer of cancer cells are grouped into "three stages" and attempts to break each step

- see the monograph "new concept and new method of cancer treatment" P.47

⑩ **"open up the third field of anti-cancer metastasis"**

- put forward the new concept of cancer metastasis therapy theory innovation and it was found and put forward the third field of human anti-cancer metastasis

- Circulation system has a large number of immune surveillance cells. To annihilate the transit of cancer cells in the "main battlefield" is in the blood circulation.

Proposing that to conquer cancer and launch a total attack is unprecedented work

11. In the international for the first time it was proposed: "the XZ-C research program of conquer cancer and launch a total attack"

- The Overall Strategy Reform and Development of Cancer Treatment in China
- to avoid empty talk, focus heavy hard work and start to go; No matter how far away from the cancer, should always start to go
- proposed to attack the cancer and launch a total attack, which is unprecedented work

(12) In international for the first time it was put forward : "the necessity and feasibility report to overcome the cancer attack on"

- In China's cancer treatment the overall strategic reform from to focus on treatment into the prevention and treatment of both

- XZ-C proposed to the general idea and design of capture of cancer

- What is the total attack against cancer? What does the total attack target?

- XU ZE proposed the ideas, strategies, planning, blueprint to overcome cancer, launched the general offensive.

(13) In the international for the first time it was proposed: "to build the hospital of cancer occurrence and development during the whole process"

(Global Demonstration Cancer, Hospital)

- Problems in the Mode of Running Hospital in Current Tumor Hospital
- the path of how to overcome cancer is to study the establishment of hospitals with prevention and treatment of cancer during the whole process of the development and occurrence and the reform of the current focusing on treatment with light defense mode
- XU ZE on the strategic thinking of fighting cancer, planning a map, prevention and treatment of cancer, the development of the whole process

(14) In the international for the first time it proposed: "to build the basic design of the general idea of conquering cancer and science city"

- is equivalent to the design of a Chinese framework for cancer design
- How to set up the basic idea and design of the total attack of cancer
- How to overcome cancer? It must set up a "cancer animal experimental center"; "Innovative Molecular Oncology School of Medicine"; "Cancer and Multidisciplinary Research Institute"

How to overcome cancer? It must be "to build a cancer attack to start the general attack of the medical, teaching, research, science base - Science City"

(2) The published monographs on cancer research

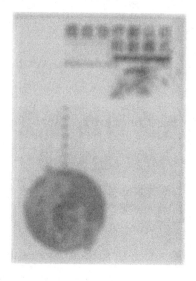

This first book at the
age of 67was published
by Bejing in 2001

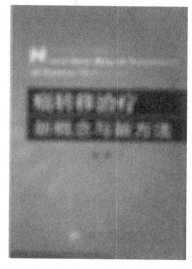

The second book was published
at the age of 73 in 2006

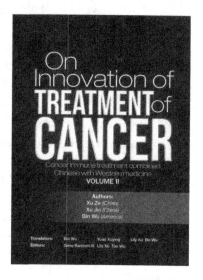

The book was published
in English at 2015

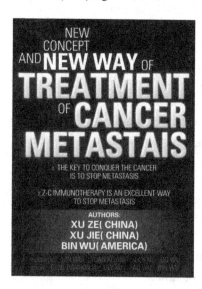

It was published in
August in 2016

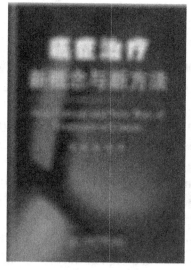

The third book was published
at the age of 78岁
2011年10月北京出版

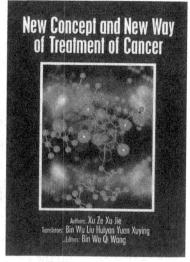

This book was published
at the age of 80 in
English in March 2013

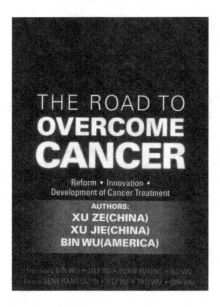

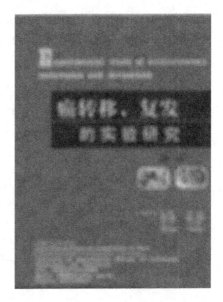

This book was published in December 2016

This is all of our achievement of the research in 2009

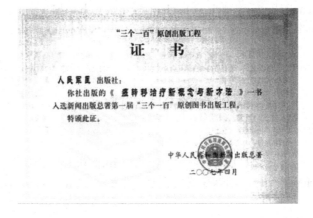

After Professor Xu Ze was retired, he still continues the research. Science journey is non-stop and continues to obtain the following series of scientific research.

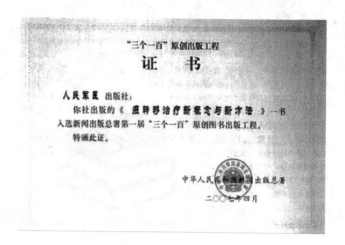

In 1996, I was 63 years old and was retired. After I retired, I hid in a small building for more than 30 years and sola strives and continue to conduct a series of experimental research and clinical validation observation and made the following series of scientific research achievement and did the summary collection, then Published the following monographs.

Three monographs are in Chinese version and distributed in the country.

Four monographs in English version and were published in Washington and were distributed in the international and worldwide.

This seven monographs are the scientific research of our difficult trek and the hard climbing step by step in four different scientific research stages and the mountain results of the four different levels.

1).In 67-year-old sixtieth year it was published the first monograph "new understanding and new model of cancer treatment" by Hubei Science and Technology Press in January 2001

2).In 73 years old seventy years it was published the second monograph "new concepts and new methods of cancer metastasis treatment" by Beijing People's Medical Publishing House in January 2006

In April 2007 the People's Republic of China Publishing House issued a "three hundred" original book certificate.

3).In 78 years old seventy years it was published the third monograph "new concept and new methods of cancer treatment" by Beijing People's Medical Publishing House in October 2011

Followed by American medical doctor Dr. Bin Wu translated into English, the English version on March 26, 2013 published in Washington, the international distribution

4).The New Book and the New Way Of Treatment of Cancer, published in Washington, DC in March 2013, in English, the international distribution of the third edition.

5).In 82-year-old it was published the fifth monograph "On Innovation of Treatment of Cancer" - "cancer treatment innovation" published in full English, worldwide in December 2015 in Washington,

6). At the age of 83 it was published the sixth monograph "New Concept and New Way of Treatment of Cancer Metastais" - "new concept and new method of cancer metastasis therapy" in August 2016 in Washington in the full English version, the global release

7).In 83 years old the seventh monograph "The Road To Overcome Cancer" - to overcome the road of cancer in December 2016 in Washington, published in full English, the global release.

(3) at the International Conference of International Oncology it was reported cancer research papers, scientific papers on the international

(1) received the American Cancer Research Society AACR to Xu Ze's invitation, is in September 2013 at the International Conference on International Oncology in Washington, "XZ-C immunoregulation anti-cancer therapy," aroused widespread attention in the international tumor medical community And highly valued.

(2) Participated in the 12th International Conference on Cancer Research in the American Society of Cancer Research (AACR) in Washington, USA, from 27 to 30 October 2013, which attracted the attention of the medical profession.

(3) On February 14, 2014, Dr. Bin Wu gave a lecture on "Thymus Atrophy, Immune Function is One of the Etiology and Pathogenesis of Cancer" in the Academic Lecture Hall of the Library of the University of Hobbs, Washington. And the theoretical basis and experimental basis of the treatment principle of "treatment of bone marrow" ("protection of thymus to improve immunity"), "protection of bone marrow" (protection of bone marrow stem cells) by the participants were warmly welcomed and highly valued.

(4) United States Stanford University School of Medicine, University of California, San Francisco, Harvard University School of Medicine and other world-class tumor immune scientists fully affirmed Professor Xu Ze's research results, and agreed that through immunization to enhance cancer patients themselves anti-recurrence, It is agreed that it is the most effective anti-cancer route after chemotherapy, radiotherapy and chemotherapy after strengthening the anti-recurrence and metastasis immunity of cancer patients by immunoregulation and can improve the quality of life of patients with advanced cancer.

(4) Visit the Stoutin Cancer Institute in Houston, USA

In order to strengthen the exchange and cooperation of international scientific and technological organizations, on December 10, 2009, we were invited to visit the Stoutin Cancer Institute in the United States. We were warmly welcomed and warmly received by the Institute. Many professors, researchers, nude mice animal model laboratory and anti-cancer drug analysis laboratory responsible person participated in the discussion, exchange, with a slides to report the latest scientific research.

We presented to the United States Stoutin Cancer Institute of my Institute of "cancer metastasis, recurrence of the experimental study" color Atlas, introduced the experimental study of radical surgery in the tumor-free technology and removal of thymus to produce animal model of animal experiments Research, and the exclusive development of the ZC immune regulation of anti-cancer, anti-transfer of traditional Chinese medicine products Z-C1-10 of the situation. And presented my published monograph "cancer metastasis treatment of new concepts and new methods", the Department of the book award of three hundred original books, by the Institute of the warm welcome and appreciation.

(5) The basic Envisage and design of XZ-C's launching the total attack

Xu Ze Professor proposed the following of the general idea of the total attack of conquering cancer and the basic design of science city

Dawn spirit of scientific research

Hard work and struggle ------
: 18 years of cold window, hard work

Review and reflection --------------
: Follow-up, summed up the successful experience of treatment (In the second monograph there are the typical case); reflection failure treatment lessons (in the first monograph there are cases of failing to prevent from recurrence, failed to stop metastasis)

open up Innovation
: 48 kinds of good tumor inhibition rate were screened out of 200 kinds of Chinese herbal medicine in the animal experiments ; 11 years of clinical validation of Z-C immunoregulation of traditional Chinese medicine series; it was realized to rise to theoretical knowledge, new concepts, new models.

Facing future medicine ------
: Recognizing the inadequacies and problems of traditional therapies in the

twentieth century,recognize the
direction of the 21st century

Look forward to look ------------ Suggest:

• Establishment of Innovative Molecular Tumor Hospital

- Cultivating advanced cancer researchers for the country.

• Establishment of innovative molecular tumor hospital (at the molecular level of Western medicine combined)

- benefit more cancer patients and serve more cancer patients.

• Establishment of Innovative Molecular Cancer Institute

- Research cells begin to change

- to the CT can be found between a long time,

To achieve three early goals,

"Target" metastasis, cancerous lesions, precancerous state.

• Build innovative molecular cancer pharmaceuticals

- out of a new way to overcome the cancer with our characteristics

(6) It has been the formation of XZ-C anti-cancer immune regulation theoretical system

The book of "New concepts and new methods of cancer treatment," was published by Professor Xu Ze with 20 years of self-reliance, hard work, completed a series of basic and clinical research an the results were summarized to nearly 100 research papers which were published in the form of this new books.

This book has formed the XZ-C immune regulation of the theoretical system of cancer and provided the theoretical basis and experimental basis of undergoing clinical application observation and verification for the cancer treatment.

The Theoretical System of XZ-C Immunomodulation and Treatment of Cancer

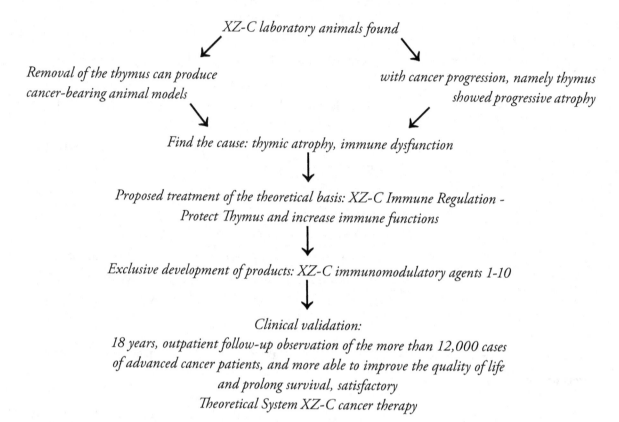

XZ-C laboratory animals found

Removal of the thymus can produce cancer-bearing animal models

with cancer progression, namely thymus showed progressive atrophy

Find the cause: thymic atrophy, immune dysfunction

Proposed treatment of the theoretical basis: XZ-C Immune Regulation - Protect Thymus and increase immune functions

Exclusive development of products: XZ-C immunomodulatory agents 1-10

Clinical validation:
18 years, outpatient follow-up observation of the more than 12,000 cases of advanced cancer patients, and more able to improve the quality of life and prolong survival, satisfactory
Theoretical System XZ-C cancer therapy

Exclusive research and development products: XZ-C immunomodulation anti-cancer traditional Chinese medicine products (Introduction)

Self-developed XZ-C (Xu Ze China) immunoregulatory anti-cancer series of traditional Chinese medicine preparation, from experimental research to clinical validation, in animal experiments on the basis of successful clinical practice, after 30 years more than 12,000 clinical cases of clinical validation, it had the significant effect. Clinical application can improve symptoms, good spirit, good appetite, significantly improve the quality of life, significantly extend the survival period and are the independent innovation and independent intellectual property rights.

The new drug research from the Chinese medication to find and screen anti-cancer and anti-metastasis:

The aim of this study was to screen out the medications XZ-C1-10 with anti-cancer and anti-metastasis and anti-recurrence which had no drug resistance, no toxic and side effects, high selectivity, long-term oral anti-cancer, anti-metastasis and anti-relapse.

(XZ-C immunomodulation series of traditional Chinese medicine product profile, see the first volume, the eighth volume)

(7) In 83 years old ripe old age (April 2016) it was proposed to move with the "new moon plan (Cancer moon shot)" together forward because from 2013 onwards Xu Ze already put forward "to overcome the cancer attack on the necessity and feasibility report" and put forward the "attack the cancer launched a total attack, Cancer science city report" which is planning, design.

"New Moon Plan" (US) and the dawn of the C-type plan (in)

- common progress, toward the scientific temple to overcome cancer

① "Cancer moon shot (Cancer moon shot)" profile

January 12, 2016 US President Barack Obama in the State of the Union issued a national plan to overcome cancer:

Project name: "new moon program"

Goal: to overcome cancer
Nature: A national plan to overcome cancer
Announcer: President Obama
The head of the program: Vice President Biden
Announced on January 12, 2016
The program specific program: unknown
② Shuguang C-type plan profile

a. before January 12, 2016, it was put forward the "capture of cancer launched a total attack on the XZ-C research program" progress
b. before January 12, 2016, it was put forward "to capture the cancer as the research direction has been carried out scientific research, scientific and technological innovation series"
c. The dawn of the C-type plan (in July 2015 to develop)

I "attack the cancer launched a total attack"

II "to build the whole anti-rule hospital"
III "to build to overcome the Cancer Science City"
IV "set up multi-disciplinary research group"
V "Vaccine is human hope"
VI "immunoregulatory drug prospects gratifying"

③ analysis of the situation

a. analyze their respective technological advantages
b. analyze the current status quo
c. analyze the next step in the future
d. "dawn of the C-type plan" to achieve technological innovation outline
e. how to implement this unprecedented human event?
f. Expected results

(8) The anticancer drug use is currently an urgent need

① anti-cancer, anti-cancer metastasis research is the urgent need for the development of the current tumor discipline, "oncology" is the most backward of the current medical disciplines of a discipline, its "name" are not yet unified, it was written as "tumor" Cancer "," cancer "," malignancy "," newborn ".

Because a disease name is defined, it must be clear about its etiology and pathogenesis. As the etiology of tumor, pathogenesis, pathophysiology are not clear, so the tumor discipline for scientific research, or a virgin land, to be a lot of basic scientific research.

② anti-cancer metastasis, recurrence, must be carried out in the study of cancer animal model, the current number of large hospitals have not established a laboratory, can not carry out the basic research of cancer, nude mice should be used to establish a variety of cancerous animal models to study cancer metastasis The law and mechanism (the author of the laboratory with pure mice Kunming mice to do animal animal model about 10,000 times), because if no basic research breakthrough, the clinical efficacy is difficult to improve.

③ anti-cancer, anti-cancer metastasis research focus on the study of unknown knowledge, research workers should look forward to the future of science, science is an endless frontier, scientific research workers must be beyond the development of the old knowledge, Continue to go beyond, continue to develop, keep moving forward.

(9) How to innovate science and technology? How to leave a scientific research footprint?

An old cement road, every day hundreds of thousands of people go, will not leave footprints, only a newly made cement road, every step will leave the eternal footprints, so scientific research must have innovative thinking, must be innovative Results.

30 years (1985 -) our research history, cancer research work, in animal experiments, clinical basic research, clinical validation work has made a series of scientific and technological innovation research results, here only the results of the directory (scientific footprints), each scientific research Belong to the original innovation or independent innovation, are for each eternal scientific research footprint.

(10) 85 years old ripe old age published "agglutination of wisdom, to conquer cancer - for the benefit of mankind" medical monograph, XZ-C proposed: how to overcome cancer? How to prevent cancer I see? how to cure cancer see me?

Professor Xu Ze proposed the planning of the project of how to overcome the cancer?

This medical monograph is practical, applied, research, implementation of how to overcome the outline of cancer. This set of scientific research programs, scientific research design, scientific research planning, blueprint for national, provincial and state reference applications, in order to carry out the cancer against the ambitious, for the benefit of mankind.

The main project of this implementation is:

To overcome the cancer and to launch a total attack and defense + control and treatment at the same level and progress together

To create a multidisciplinary research base related to cancer - Science City

Two wing works are:

A wing - how to prevent cancer? To reduce the incidence of cancer
B wing - how to cure cancer? To improve cancer cure rate

The aims:

A: reduce the incidence of cancer
B: to improve cancer cure rate, extend the survival terms, improve the quality of life

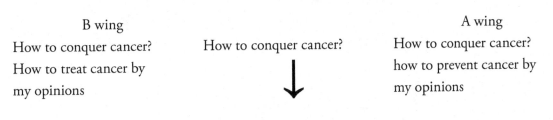

B wing
How to conquer cancer?
How to treat cancer by
my opinions

How to conquer cancer?

A wing
How to conquer cancer?
how to prevent cancer by
my opinions

•conquer cancer and launch the total attack
•build multidiscipline and cancer research scientific city
• prevention+control+ treatment at the same attention

Figure 1 XZ-C presents a schematic diagram

Printed in the United States
By Bookmasters